Level 3

Diploma in Adult Care
SECOND EDITION

Maria Ferreiro Peteiro

The City & Guilds textbook

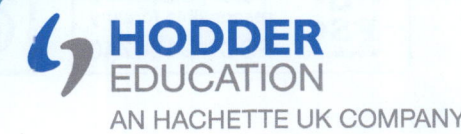

Although every effort has been made to ensure that website addresses are correct at time of going to press, Hodder Education cannot be held responsible for the content of any website mentioned in this book. It is sometimes possible to find a relocated web page by typing in the address of the home page for a website in the URL window of your browser.

Hachette UK's policy is to use papers that are natural, renewable and recyclable products and made from wood grown in well-managed forests and other controlled sources. The logging and manufacturing processes are expected to conform to the environmental regulations of the country of origin.

Orders: please contact Hachette UK Distribution, Hely Hutchinson Centre, Milton Road, Didcot, Oxfordshire, OX11 7HH. Telephone: +44 (0)1235 827827. Email education@hachette.co.uk Lines are open from 9 a.m. to 5 p.m., Monday to Friday. You can also order through our website: www.hoddereducation.co.uk

ISBN: 978 1 3983 7932 9

© Maria Ferreiro Peteiro 2023

First published in 2018.

This edition published in 2023 by

Hodder Education (a trading division of Hodder & Stoughton Limited),

An Hachette UK Company

Carmelite House

50 Victoria Embankment

London EC4Y 0DZ

www.hoddereducation.co.uk

The authorised representative in the EEA is Hachette Ireland, 8 Castlecourt Centre, Dublin 15, D15 XTP3, Ireland (email: info@hbgi.ie)

Impression number   10 9 8 7 6 5 4 3 2

Year   2027 2026 2025

All rights reserved. Apart from any use permitted under UK copyright law, no part of this publication may be reproduced or transmitted in any form or by any means, electronic or mechanical, including photocopying and recording, or held within any information storage and retrieval system, without permission in writing from the publisher or under licence from the Copyright Licensing Agency Limited. Further details of such licences (for reprographic reproduction) may be obtained from the Copyright Licensing Agency Limited, www.cla.co.uk

City & Guilds and the City & Guilds logo are trade marks of The City and Guilds of London Institute and used under licence. The City and Guilds of London Institute accepts no liability for the contents of this book.

City & Guilds Logo © City & Guilds 2022

Cover photo © Monkey Business - stock.adobe.com

Typeset in India.

Printed and bound by CPI Group (UK) Ltd, Croydon, CR0 4YY

A catalogue record for this title is available from the British Library.

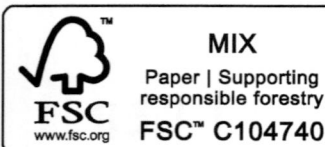
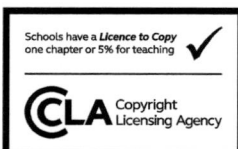

Contents

About the author and Acknowledgements iv

How to use this book v

Introduction vi

300 Responsibilities and ways of working in adult care settings/services 1

301 Safeguarding and protection in adult care settings/services 32

302 Understanding mental capacity and restrictive practice 85

303 Understanding duty of care 107

304 Effective communication in adult care settings/services 132

305 Handling information in adult care settings/services 194

306 Promoting and implementing person-centred practice 233

307 Promoting choice and independence in adult care settings/services 272

308 Supporting individuals with their health and wellbeing 287

309 Promoting equality, diversity, inclusion and human rights in adult care settings/services 316

310 Promoting health and safety in adult care settings/services 354

311 Supporting infection prevention and control in adult care settings/services 389

312 Implementing health and safety in adult care settings/services 407

313 Continuous development when working in an adult care worker role 428

314 Understanding personal wellbeing 469

Glossary 491

Index 497

About the author and Acknowledgements

About the author

Maria commenced her career in Health and Social Care 32 years ago, living and working in a lay community in France alongside individuals with a range of disabilities and health conditions. Her journey continued through a variety of services and settings in the UK, which included working within and leading provision for young and older adults who have learning disabilities, physical disabilities, dementia, mental health needs, challenging needs and sensory impairments. Maria then embarked on delivering a range of Health and Social Care programmes and qualifications in both college and work-based settings. The experience she gained in work and academic settings led Maria to become a qualified assessor, internal and external quality assurer and the chief verifier for vocational-based qualifications in Health and Social Care and Children and Young People's Services. Maria has combined her experience in the social care sector with teaching adults with mental health needs, learning disabilities and additional needs to drive, which is proving to be exciting, enjoyable and very rewarding.

Author's acknowledgements

I wish to thank Ruth Murphy, Rachel Edge and the Hodder team for all their fantastic support and hard work in updating this publication. A very special thank you must also go to my wonderful husband, Chris, whose patience and understanding I couldn't have done without! And, to my dog Simba for his boundless energy that just gave me no choice but to keep going and going…

Picture credits

The publishers would like to thank the following for permission to reproduce copyright material.

Unit 300 © Alexander Raths – Fotolia; **fig. 1.3** © Jules Selmes/Hodder Education; **fig. 1.4** © Denise Hager/Catchlight Visual Services/Alamy Stock Photo; **fig. 1.6** © JackF/stock.adobe.com; **Unit 301** © Diego cervo/stock.adobe.com; **fig. 2.1** © Alexander Raths – Fotolia; **fig. 2.2** © Monkey Business Images/Shutterstock.com; **fig. 2.6** © Olesia Bilkei/stock.adobe.com; **Unit 302** © Satjawat/stock.adobe.com; **fig. 3.1** © Deanm1974 - Fotolia; **fig. 3.2** © Satjawat/stock.adobe.com; **Unit 303** © Dglimages/stock.adobe.com; **fig. 4.1** M.Dörr & M.Frommherz/stock.adobe.com; **fig. 4.2** © Katarzyna Białasiewicz/123RF; **fig. 4.2** © JackF/stock.adobe.com; **fig. 4.4** © JackF/stock.adobe.com; **Unit 304** © Clarissa Leahy/Image Source/Alamy Stock Photo **fig. 5.1** © Amelaxa/stock.adobe.com; **fig. 5.2** © Belahoche/stock.adobe.com; **fig. 5.3** © Monika Wisniewska - Fotolia.com; **fig. 5.5** © Monkey Business Images/Shutterstock.com; **Unit 305** © Syda Productions/stock.adobe.com; **fig. 6.1** © Xixinxing/stock.adobe.com; **fig. 6.2** © Stepan Popov/stock.adobe.com; **fig. 6.3** © Jdwfoto/stock.adobe.com; **fig. 6.4** © M.Dörr & M.Frommherz- Fotolia; **fig. 6.6** © Photographee.eu - Fotolia.com; **fig. 6.8** © B. BOISSONNET/BSIP SA/Alamy Stock Photo; **Unit 306** © Jacob Lund/stock.adobe.com; **fig. 7.4** © Belahoche/stock.adobe.com; **Unit 307** © Nejron Photo/stock.adobe.com; **fig. 8.1** © Monkey Business/stock.adobe.com; **fig. 8.2** © Tatsiana/stock.adobe.com; **Unit 308** © Maksim Shmeljov/stock.adobe.com; **fig. 9.1** © AnnaStills/stock.adobe.com; **fig. 9.3** © Zinkevych/stock.adobe.com; **fig. 9.5** © Rawpixel.com/stock.adobe.com; **Unit 309** © Monkey Business/stock.adobe.com **fig. 10.1** © Rawpixel.com/stock.adobe.com; **fig. 10.2** © Deanm1974 - Fotolia; **fig. 10.3** © Antonioguillem/stock.adobe.com; **Unit 310** © Gina Sanders - Fotolia; **Unit 311** © Maridav/stock.adobe.com; **fig. 12.2** Adapted from World Health Organization Guidelines on Hand Hygiene in Health Care. Contains public sector information licensed under the Open Government Licence v3.0. /http://www.nationalarchives.gov.uk/doc/open-government-licence/version/3/; **Unit 312** © Ake1150/stock.adobe.com; **fig. 13.1** © Schlierner/stock.adobe.com; **fig. 13.2** © Bilderzwerg/stock.adobe.com; **Unit 313** © Jules Selmes/Hodder Education; **fig. 14.1** © Jules Selmes/Hodder Education; **fig. 14.4** © Stockbroker/MBI/Alamy Stock Photo; **fig. 14.5** © Woodapple - Fotolia; **Unit 314** © Inesbazdar/stock.adobe.com; **fig. 15.2** © DC Studio/stock.adobe.com; **fig. 15.3** © Prostock-studio/stock.adobe.com

This book contains public sector information licensed under the Open Government Licence v3.0.

How to use this book

This textbook covers all 15 mandatory units for the City & Guilds Level 3 Diploma in Adult Care.
The book refers to Lead Adult Care Workers, and Lead Personal Assistants – this is meant to include those who are not currently in this role, but are working to become leaders. It is therefore for leaders and potential leaders.

Key features of the book

Learning outcomes

Learn about what you are going to cover in each unit.

LO1 Learning outcomes

AC 1.1 Assessment criteria

Learning outcomes and assessment criteria are clearly stated and fully mapped to the specification.

Getting started

Short activity or discussion to introduce you to the topic.

Key term

Understand important terms and concepts.

Reflect on it

Learn to reflect on your own experiences, skills and practice, and develop the skills necessary to become a reflective practitioner.

Reflective exemplar

Explore examples of reflective accounts tailored to the content of the unit and understand how you can write your own accounts.

Research it

Enhance your understanding of topics with research-led activities encouraging you to explore an area in more detail.

Evidence opportunity

Test your understanding of the assessment criteria, apply your knowledge and generate evidence.

Dos and don'ts

Do	Useful advice and tips for best practice.
Don't	Advice on what to avoid in specific situations.

6Cs

Understand how each of the 6Cs (care, compassion, competence, communication, courage and commitment) can be applied in each unit.

Case study

Learn about real-life scenarios and think about issues you may face in the workplace.

Legislation

Summaries of legislation relevant to the study of each unit. Legislation is frequently updated so it is important to ensure you keep up to date with the most recent version of legislation and regulations by doing your own research as well.

Introduction

The qualification

Becoming a care worker is a choice that people make at different points in their life. Perhaps you decided you wanted to become a care worker when you were at school, or perhaps you have had a role in another profession and made the decision later in life. Whenever you made the decision to enter the care profession, for whatever reason, or whether you decided to work in a residential care home or assist someone to live independently in their own home, it is certain that the profession you are entering is a rewarding one; one where you provide a valuable service to those you care for.

The Level 3 Diploma in Adult Care is for learners who work in adult care settings. The qualification is suitable for those workers who have senior responsibilities for the delivery of care and support and/or for supervising the work of others. For example, you may be working as, or working to become, a Lead Adult Care Worker, Lead Personal Assistant, Key Worker, Domiciliary Care Worker, Senior care Assistant or Support Worker.

This book contains all fifteen mandatory units that you will need to complete for the City & Guilds Level 3 Diploma in Adult Care. The mandatory units cover your responsibilities working in adult care, safeguarding and protection, mental capacity and restrictive practice, the duty of care you have to those you support, communication, how you must handle information, person-centred practice, promoting choice and independence, how to support individuals with their health and wellbeing, equality, diversity, inclusion and human rights, health and safety, infection prevention and control, continuous development and understanding personal wellbeing.

Study skills

To complete the diploma to the best of your ability, you will need to ensure you develop the skills that are essential not only in providing high-quality care in the setting, but also when preparing assignments and documentation for your portfolio and other assessments. Here, we briefly discuss some of the skills that you will need to learn and develop for study as you progress through the diploma.

Spelling, punctuation, grammar

Being able to clearly express what you want to say is essential for good communication and ensuring others understand you. In your role, it is likely that you will write letters, reports and add notes to care or support plans and documents that will be seen by others. Ensuring that the information in these documents can be easily understood is important so that others are able to understand what is written and to ensure efficient practice. It also means that those you work with will view you as someone who is competent with good command of vocabulary, spelling, punctuation and grammar; this will reflect positively on you as a professional. Writing in full sentences, placing words in sentences in the correct order and using the correct punctuation shows that you take pride in your work. You will also need to apply these skills when you provide evidence and assignments for your portfolio so that you are able to demonstrate your knowledge and convey this in a grammatically correct, clear and accessible way.

Skills of reflection

Reflection is one of the key skills you will need to develop as a care worker. It encourages you to think back on your practice and consolidate what you have learned so that you can make changes and improvements. It involves thinking back over a situation or event that happened and understanding what you gained from the experience and the improvements or changes you will make, or have already made. For example, you may have attended a training update on safeguarding and, as a result, gained a greater insight into your role and the responsibilities for safeguarding individuals from abuse. This in turn means that your awareness on how to do this in your day-to-day work activities has been raised.

It is important to remember that reflecting involves thinking about what did not go well but also what did go well. It can be very tempting to just think about the negatives, and what went badly in a situation. This, of course, will help you to improve. However, it is important to think positively, and also focus on what went well so that you are able to repeat your behaviour and skills in other situations and also pass on good practice. In this way, you are always developing in your role and providing the best possible care which is why it is so important that you take time to reflect.

In each of the units, you will find an example of a reflective account. These will guide you with the different steps involved in writing your own reflective accounts, including:

- an introduction that sets the scene
- an account of the occasion, details of what happened
- a reflection of what worked well
- a reflection of what did not go as well
- a reflection of what you could do to improve
- all the assessment criteria it is directly linked to.

Research

Research involves exploring and finding out information about a topic to further develop your knowledge and understanding of it. Depending on the topic, research can be carried out in different ways such as by using the internet, books and/or journals. You are likely to use research skills not only for studying for this qualification but also in your personal life and at work. For example, you may have carried out research in relation to the best restaurant to go to in your local area or you may have been asked to explore different activities that an individual you care for can participate in at work. In health and/or social care, there are many examples of how and why research is used. For example, to find a cure for Alzheimer's, to gain a better understanding of diabetes or to find out how to improve work practices when supporting individuals with care or support needs.

If you think about an occasion when you successfully carried out research, you will have used a range of different skills and have gone through a process to be able to carry it out effectively. You would have begun by thinking about the purpose of carrying out the research, what you wanted to find out and why. You would then have set out a plan for how to do this, including deciding on the methods of collating the information, the sources of information to use and a timescale for doing this. You would then have moved on to collating the information, interpreting the information you collated before finally reviewing your research against the original purpose of your research and presenting your findings. In this way, you are able to develop your knowledge and skills beyond the setting and discover new, up-to-date background information which will help you to keep on top of what is happening in your profession and related stories.

Reading

In your role, you will read various documents; it might be this textbook, news articles as part of research or care plans, for example. You will therefore need to know when you need to read documents in depth, and when you can 'skim' read. Skim reading refers to reading to gain an overview or insight into the context of a topic. For example, you may 'skim' through a unit by reading the introduction or titles of each section to gain an insight into what the unit is about. However, in order to fully understand the unit and content of any document, you will need to carefully read the content in detail and not just the key points like when you skim read. It is important that you understand when you should read documents in detail and when you can skim read.

Time management

Managing your time effectively involves being able to achieve timescales set for the completion of, for example, assignments. This means being able to complete them on time while not compromising on the quality of your work, and allowing yourself enough time. To be able to manage your time effectively you need to be realistic about what you can and cannot do. There is no point in setting yourself an unrealistic target; not only will you not achieve this but not doing so will make you feel negative about yourself. Planning how to best manage your time is key! Perhaps you have children so you plan to study in the evenings or at night when they have gone to bed and you have no distractions, or perhaps you care for a family member and find mornings a better time to study. Make a plan and stick to it by ensuring you review it from time to time to check that you are on track.

Referencing

Referencing the work and ideas of others means that you will not be plagiarising (a topic you will learn more about below). Referencing shows that you have carried out research in detail, and that you have read widely. It also shows that you have thought about and connected the ideas of others such as theorists and authors. It means you can show that you have a valid and credible basis for your work and ideas. Referencing also enables those reading your work to explore in more detail the topic you have referenced and to find out more about it.

Plagiarism

Plagiarism occurs when you do not acknowledge the work or ideas of others and claim that it is your own. This is unethical and illegal and has serious consequences including not being allowed to continue to study for your qualification. Therefore, referencing the work and ideas of others when submitting your work and assignments is a must.

Command words

The knowledge-based command words that you will find across this book and the specification will include 'describe', 'explain' and 'evaluate' for example, and will set out what you are expected to know or understand. The skills-based command words will include 'demonstrate', 'use' and 'work with others', for example, and these will set out what you will be expected to do or show through your work practice. Your assessor will be able to provide more guidance on the definitions of command words.

Assignments and work products

Work products

Work products can include plans and records of what you have produced during your everyday work activities. For example, you may have evidence of a social activity you carried out with an individual in the form of a short video film, or an entry you made in an individual's care plan about a change that has occurred in their needs, such as in relation to the support they require for their mobility.

Work products may also include other records that you and others may contribute to such as your supervision record (you and your manager would discuss this) or an individual's risk assessment (you and your colleagues would contribute to this). Sometimes work products can be included in your portfolio, but you should speak to your assessor who will be able to provide more guidance on this.

You will also need to ensure confidentiality when you include any work products in your portfolio that relate to an individual you care for or others including the individual's family, friends, or those you work with.

Assignments

Assignments are opportunities for you to show how you apply the knowledge and skills you have gained during your studies. An assignment could include a scenario or a brief that sets out the tasks that you are required to complete. For example, you may be given a scenario of an individual with care needs who discloses that they are being abused; you may be tasked with showing your knowledge and understanding of what actions to take when an individual makes a disclosure of abuse and how to report it. Or you may be given a brief that requires you to plan and deliver a recreational activity with an individual. You will also be asked to demonstrate skills as part of other tasks.

Assessment

How will I be assessed?

In order to achieve the Level 3 Diploma in Adult Care, you will need to have a completed a portfolio of evidence covering the assessment criteria for each unit that you study, including the mandatory and optional units required. City & Guilds advise that the majority of assessment for this competence-based qualification will take place in the workplace under real work conditions.

The portfolio will contain evidence of your knowledge, skills and behaviours. The portfolio can be a physical paper-based file or a digital e-portfolio, and can include personal statements, reflective accounts, records of discussions, witness testimonies, assignments and work products, some of which we discuss below.

Observations

These are real-life observations of your practices in the setting where you work and will more often than not be carried out by your assessor.

Your assessor

Your assessor will be the main person who will plan and discuss the observations of your work practices with you and will be responsible for recording your observations. Expert witnesses may also on occasions be used but you will agree this with your assessor; this is discussed in more detail below. Observations of your work practices must reflect your everyday work activities and will therefore be carried out in the adult care setting where you work. You will be responsible for obtaining permission from those in your care setting for your observations to take place. This may, for example, involve seeking permission before the observation takes place and you may need to gain this permission from your employer, the individuals with care or support needs, individuals' families, friends, other professionals and others you work with.

It may not be possible to plan all of your observations as some of them may be 'unexpected events' that occur in your work setting, such as a fire drill or an individual having difficulties communicating. Your assessor will be responsible for collating this unplanned evidence if they deem it suitable to do so.

Witness testimonies

Witness testimonies can be used as evidence of your work practices that have been witnessed. Your manager, for example, will be able to provide witness testimonies of your practice in the setting.

Witness testimonies can be provided orally or in writing and must be recorded. They must include your name, the date, time, venue and details of the work activity observed as well as the details of the witness including their name, designation/role and contact details (for example, telephone number or email address). Again, it will be a good idea to ensure it is okay to include this information.

Expert witnesses

Expert witnesses may be able to observe your working practices if they have current expertise in a specialist area, such as diabetes care or when the observation is of a sensitive area such as end of life care. However, expert witnesses can be used only in specific circumstances and when agreed with your assessor.

Professional discussions

Professional discussions are planned and structured and are carried out between you and your assessor; it is an in-depth discussion that is led by you. It is a good way of presenting evidence through discussion, clearly showing the knowledge you have gained, the skills you have developed and the behaviours you have. It is a way of showing how you have met the requirements of the qualification. Your portfolio can form the basis of the discussion and so can other pieces of evidence that you may have collated, such as work products. Witness testimonies can also be discussed.

Personal statements and reflective accounts

Written accounts detailing knowledge and skills related to the assessment criteria can also be included in your portfolio.

Recognition of prior learning

Relevant prior credited learning that you have undertaken will also be recognised. This can take the form of not only certificated courses but may also include work placements or volunteering opportunities you have undertaken.

End-point assessment

The Level 3 Diploma in Adult Care is linked to the Lead Adult Care Worker Apprenticeship. If you are completing this qualification as part of an apprenticeship, you will need to complete the end-point assessment. You can find out more about this at: www.hoddereducation.co.uk/cityandguilds/adultcareextras

6Cs

The 6Cs are values which underpin Compassion in Practice, the national strategy that was developed for nurses, midwives and care staff, and was launched in December 2012. They are values which should underpin your practice; you are expected not just to know what these are, but also be able to demonstrate them in your practice.

- **Care** is at the heart of the work we do, helping to improve the lives of individuals we support, and something we should always be striving to improve.
- **Communication** is key to forming and maintaining strong successful relationships with those we support and work with.
- **Compassion** and treating those we support with kindness and empathy are essential for upholding bonds and ensuring individuals trust us to care for them with respect and dignity.

- **Courage** allows us to speak up for those we care for especially when we have concerns, and doing the right thing for them in order to ensure that their rights are upheld. It also means having the courage to try and test new practice.
- **Competence** means fulfilling our roles to the best of our ability, understanding the needs of those we provide support for, and having the expertise and knowledge to effectively carry out our roles.
- **Commitment** means to be dedicated to providing high-quality care and helping to improve the lives of those we provide support for.

You can find out more about the Skills for Care definitions of the 6Cs here: www.skillsforcare.org.uk/resources/documents/Developing-your-workforce/Care-Certificate/Care-Certificate-Standards/Standard-5.pdf

The 6Cs are also addressed in each unit in this textbook with clear links to how they are relevant to the content of the unit or assessment criteria.

Knowledge, skills, behaviours

Knowledge: This includes your understanding of the units you study and reasons for why you practise the way you do at work. It will also include understanding of a range of topics and areas such as legislation, different cultures, how to build good relationships, how to communicate and interact with others, and expectations that others, such as your employer, colleagues, others you work with, individuals and individuals' families, have of you. Knowledge will also cover more than just your knowledge and understanding of health and/or social care; it will include wider knowledge of cultures and the people you will work with, for example.

Skills: There are a wide range of skills that you will learn, practise and develop in your role and as you complete this diploma. This will include skills in communicating with your colleagues, safeguarding individuals, reporting and recording and also the skills that make you unique and bring out your qualities such as showing compassion, warmth, kindness and empathy. You will also develop and be required to show the skills you have when studying for this qualification such as your ability to interpret information, describe an event or analyse a task so that you can make improvements.

Behaviours: These include how you put into practice the personal qualities you have. For example, how do you use verbal and non-verbal communication to show your empathy towards a colleague who is finding a task difficult to complete? How can you be supportive and encouraging? How do you convey your happiness when an individual tells you that they have achieved the goal that they have been working towards? Your behaviours reflect the kind of person you are, for example, professional, kind and considerate.

The book refers to Lead Adult Care Workers, and Lead Personal Assistants, this also includes those who are not currently in this role, but are potential leaders.

Online resources

Online at www.hoddereducation.co.uk/cityandguilds/adultcareextras you will find additional resources, including:

- **Suggestions for using the activities.** Summaries of all the activities in the unit that can be used to show your knowledge and skills for the assessment criteria. This also includes other suggestions for using the activities and presenting your knowledge and skills. These are suggestions and your assessor will be able to provide more guidance on how you can evidence your knowledge and skills.
- **Further reading.** This includes references to books, websites and other sources for further reading and research.

You can access more information about this City & Guilds qualification and specification by searching for 'Adult Care' or '3095' on their website: www.cityandguilds.com

300 Responsibilities and ways of working in adult care settings/services

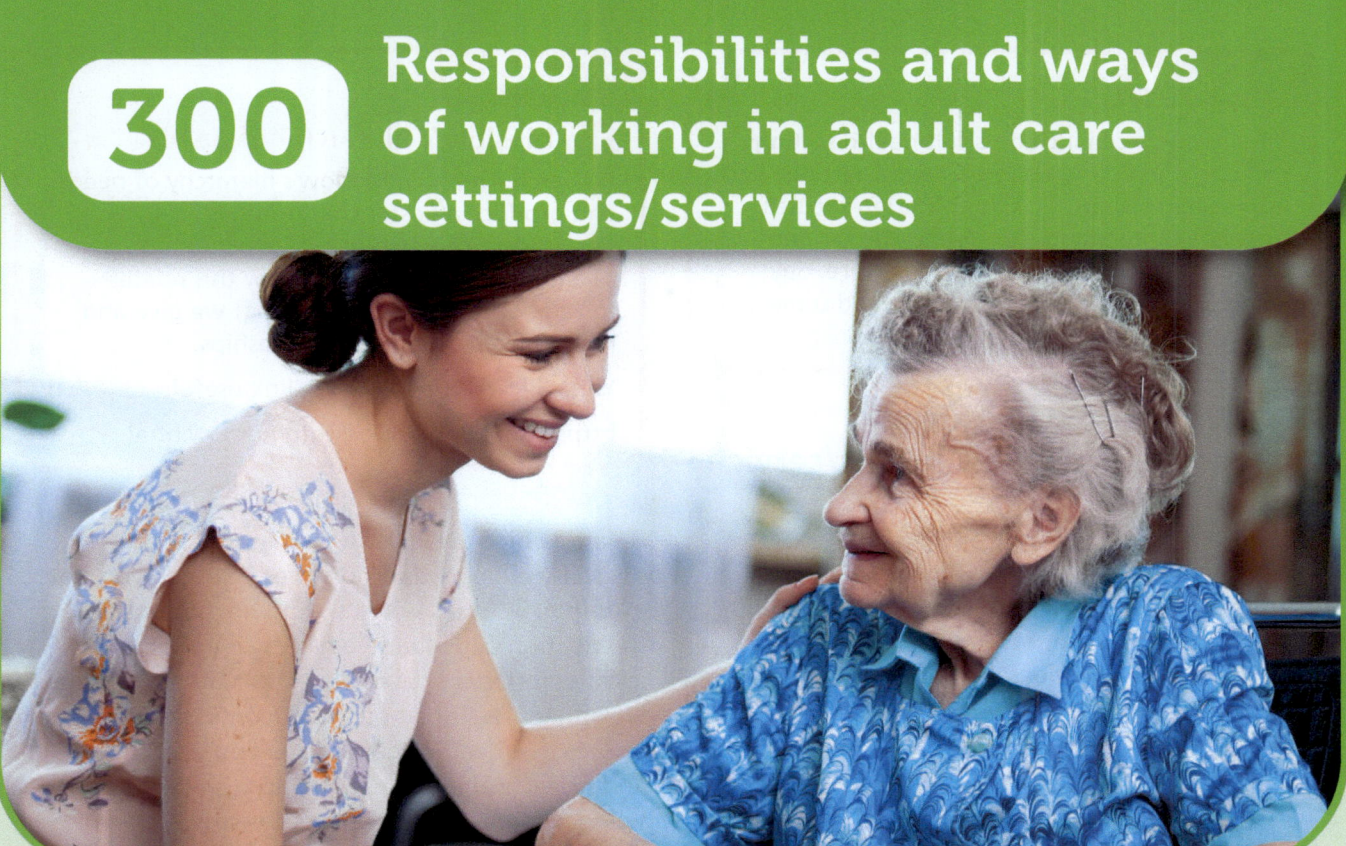

About this unit

Credit value: 2
Guided learning hours: 18

The best teamwork happens in **care settings** when there are good working relationships between individuals, their families, friends, advocates, team members, colleagues and other professionals, when everyone works in ways agreed with the employer and together in partnership as one big team.

In this unit, you will learn about what makes an effective working relationship, including the key differences between a working relationship and a personal relationship. You will also learn about what your employer expects of you, including the reasons why it is important to work in agreed ways with your employer and promote ways of working which contribute to efficient use of resources. In addition, you will be able to explore opportunities to contribute and make sure the experience for the individuals you care for is a positive one.

Finally, you will learn about the benefits of working in partnership with others, the different skills and approaches needed for resolving conflicts and the range of sources of support available to you about partnership working and resolving conflicts that may arise.

Learning outcomes

By the end of this unit you will:

LO1: Understand working relationships in care settings/services

LO2: Understand agreed ways of working

LO3: Be able to work in ways that are agreed with the employer

LO4: Be able to work in partnership with others

Key terms

Care settings can include adult health settings, children and young people's health settings and adult care settings. This qualification focuses on adult care settings. These include residential homes, nursing homes, domiciliary care, day centres, an individual's own home and some clinical healthcare settings.

LO1 Understand working relationships in care settings/services

Research it

1.1 Maslow's hierarchy of needs

Research Abraham Maslow's hierarchy of needs and produce a poster that outlines his five-tier model of human needs (often depicted as a pyramid). Think about how this relates to relationships in terms of what we give and receive from different relationships.

You will find the following link useful:

https://simplypsychology.org/maslow.html

Getting started

Think about the different people you work with. What different types of working relationships do you have? How does your role vary with each person you work with? Are there some people that you work more often or more closely with than others? Why is this?

AC 1.1 Explain how a working relationship is different from a personal relationship

Relationships feature in all our lives and develop throughout childhood and into adulthood. According to the psychologist Abraham Maslow, some of the basic human needs we must all fulfil are love and belonging. Maslow defines these as including:

- friendship, for example a best friend who has known you since school
- intimacy, for example a partner who knows you in a romantic and/or sexual way
- trust, for example a colleague at work who you can confide in and rely on
- acceptance, for example your sibling who accepts you for who you are
- receiving and giving affection and love, such as the relationship you have with your parents
- affiliating, in other words being part of a group, for example friends, family, colleagues at work.

These are the key ingredients of relationships and the reasons why relationships exist. They are the basis of our communications and interactions with others, they help us to get to know each other and form close bonds and they are the source of support through which the sharing of ideas takes place.

Relationships also play a crucial role in our overall wellbeing and how we see ourselves. For example, in times when we are not at our best, the relationships that we have can be a source of great emotional support; they can lift us up when we are not feeling at our most confident and can improve our self-esteem. Have you ever felt down and upset and had a reassuring conversation with a friend who has cheered you up? Does the feeling of being around people make you happier? As people, we like to feel included and part of a bigger group and meaningful relationships are a key part of that, both in and outside of work.

Relationships can also vary according to the people involved and the context in which they are created in terms of whether they are personal relationships or work relationships.

Key features of personal relationships

Personal relationships can be formed with family, friends and partners. Figure 1.1 identifies some examples of who these types of relationships can involve.

Family

Personal relationships with family can mean different things to different people and can depend on who you trusted and relied on as you grew up. Family may be the people that you feel most comfortable with and with whom you feel you belong. You may grow closer over time, or you may find that you are less close as time goes by. A family may be related to you:

- by birth, for example you may have biological parents, siblings, aunts, uncles, grandparents
- by marriage, for example your spouse or partner
- by adoption, for example your parents or guardian.

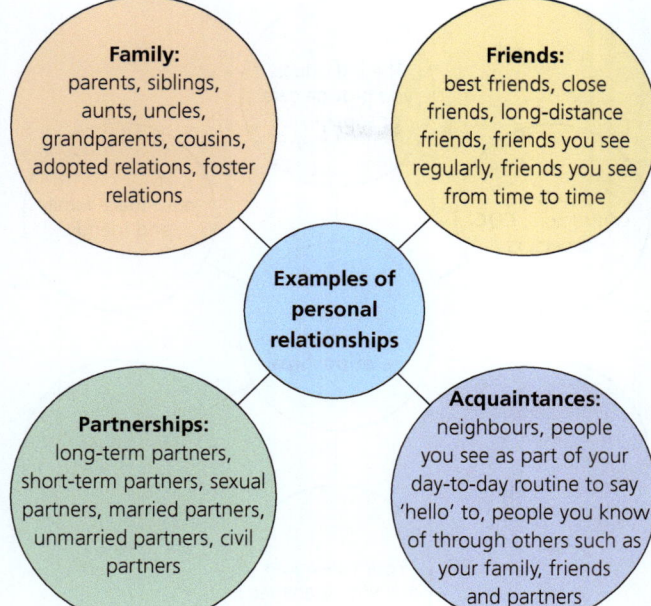

Figure 1.1 Personal relationships

The meaning of family can also differ as there are various structures. Family does not just refer to 'the nuclear family' consisting of a mother, father and children. Some families may be one parent families, or there may be step-families where one person may play the role of step-parent for example. There are also extended families that include grandparents, uncles and aunts who may also live alongside parents and children. You will find that you will work with a variety of family structures, so it is important that you understand the different relationships that exist.

6Cs

Care

Care involves putting others' interests before your own. This is because caring for someone involves being kind, thoughtful and approachable. A good carer does not just provide high-quality care as a one off – but consistently, over and over again. You can show that you care by doing something kind for someone else, that shows you have thought about their needs and want to make a difference to their situation. It is an important quality required in both personal and professional relationships and especially important if you want to build positive relationships.

Reflect on it

1.1 Your relationships with family members

Think about what family means to you. Who do you consider to be your family? Why? Think about what all your relationships with family have in common.

Friend

This refers to a personal relationship with someone with whom you have a close connection or bond. If you think about who your friends are, they are usually people who you like, have things in common with and perhaps you have shared similar experiences. For example, you may have a best friend who has known you since primary school and who you shared the same lessons at school with, went to each other's birthdays and other family celebrations, spent time with during the holidays and socialised together after work. Some friendships can last a long time, others come and go, but it is usually our close friends that have most impact on our general wellbeing. Making a connection with others can be a skill (which will come naturally to some people but not to others) and it is often a skill that we have learned through making the friends we have already. It is a skill you will need to draw upon in the care setting where you work.

Partnership

This refers to a personal relationship with a partner who you know intimately in a romantic and/or sexual way. Partnerships are therefore different to relationships with family and friends because they usually develop out of romantic affection and physical closeness.

Acquaintances

These are personal relationships that may be frequent but not develop into anything more than an acknowledgement. Your next-door neighbour may be someone who you see every morning and say hello to but apart from that (and perhaps seeing them out in the area where you live) you have no other contact with them. Some relationships with acquaintances can develop over time into friendships and even partnerships. For example, you may previously have only seen someone in the local shop every now and again

Key terms

CQC refers to the Care Quality Commission which is the independent regulator of health and social care services in England. They register care providers as well as monitor and inspect care services.

Social workers assess, commission and coordinate care services and seek to improve outcomes for individuals, especially those who are more vulnerable. They may work in multidisciplinary teams and can specialise in areas such as mental ill-health, learning disabilities, care for older people or safeguarding.

Professional refers to carrying out your job in a skilful and knowledgeable way, showing behaviour that is moral and acceptable for the role that you are in.

Agreed ways of working are your employer's policies and procedures that are set out to guide you in relation to your work activities, such as those in relation to safeguarding, health and safety. They may be less formally documented with smaller employers.

Boundaries are the limits that you must work within when carrying out your job role.

Policies and procedures may include other agreed ways of working as well as formal policies and procedures, such as in relation to handling comments and complaints.

Personal information that is recorded and held by an organisation may include contact details as well as information about the individual's health, care needs, and family background.

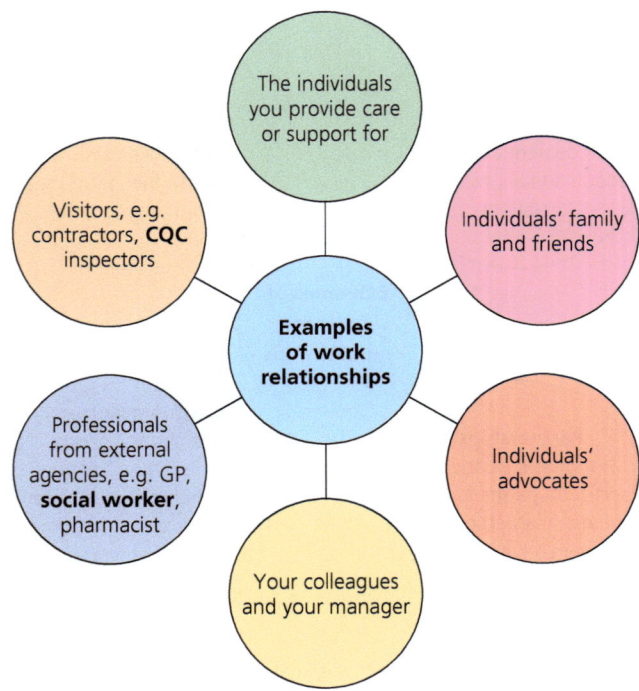

Figure 1.2 Work relationships

but you may get to know them a lot better over time and find that you share the same interests. Similarly, you may only ever 'see' someone you went to school with on social media, but a message may lead you to getting back in touch and this may develop into a friendship beyond social media.

Key features of work relationships

Work relationships, as the term suggests, are formed with the people you interact with as part of your day-to-day work tasks. In care settings, work relationships are formed between those who work there and others, as Figure 1.2 shows. How many of the work relationships identified in the diagram have you formed in the care setting where you work? Are there any others not featured in the diagram?

Why are good working relationships important?

Having good working relationships is essential for:

- **providing good quality care** and support because it means everyone works together to ensure individuals' needs are met
- **enjoying your work** and job satisfaction (there is nothing better than waking up in the morning and looking forward to going to work). In addition, others who you work with will feel your positivity and commitment to the job and you will therefore be contributing towards a nice atmosphere
- **encouraging mutual trust and respect** – working together as one team will encourage you and your team members over time to build trusting working relationships with each other and learn to respect each other's ideas and contributions. You will also learn how to support one other.

Companies tend to focus on improving relations between team members, and may even organise team-building days in order to encourage positive relationships between staff. This is because they recognise the importance of effective working and how it can lead to a happier, productive workforce and (in a care setting) how it can improve the quality of service and support that we provide to individuals.

How do work relationships differ from personal relationships?

There are some important differences between relationships at work and personal relationships. You need to be aware of these so that you can carry out your role in a **professional** way. Table 1.1 outlines the main differences between personal and professional working relationships.

Table 1.1 The differences between a work and a personal relationship

A working relationship	A personal relationship
Working relationships are planned. In your care setting, you work with individuals and within a team in order to provide individuals with care or support; you do not choose the people you work with. You will work with those that you need to in order to fulfil the requirements of your job and provide the best care possible.	Personal relationships by contrast, such as those with friends, develop naturally and you choose who you want to be friends with.
Working relationships are structured. In your care setting, you and the team will have rotas and plans for how work activities are to be carried out, including specific objectives and associated timescales for their completion. These are agreed before carrying out any work activities such as the support you provide to individuals in the mornings for their personal hygiene routines or during the day for eating and drinking, for example.	Personal relationships by contrast are not necessarily structured. The time you spend with family and friends will depend on your and their availability, it does not necessarily have to be planned. For example, you can be spontaneous and decide that you are going to give your friend a visit or decide during an evening visit to your family that you are going to stay overnight. You do not have to decide on a schedule or agenda for your meeting or how long the meeting will last.
Working relationships have clear boundaries in place. Your care setting will have guidelines (often written guidelines) that explain what is and what is not acceptable as part of your job role. This includes what is and what is not acceptable behaviour in the care setting where you work. You will be expected to demonstrate professionalism, work to a high standard to provide the best-quality support and fulfil your duty of care (see Unit 303 Understanding duty of care). You will also have to ensure that you adhere to the codes of conduct in your setting. You will be expected to turn up on time for work, it will not be acceptable for you to always be late; you will be expected to be polite to individuals' families when they visit, it will not be acceptable for you to be rude to them.	Personal relationships, by contrast (although there are unwritten rules of what is acceptable behaviour), do not have the same **boundaries**, i.e. ones that are written down that you must comply with. For example, you should not tell others anything that a friend has told you in confidence – but there is no contract to say that this is not allowed.
Working relationships are bound by agreed ways of working. In your care setting, you will have requirements set out by your employer including **policies and procedures** as well as codes of conduct which you must follow in relation to how you must behave when at work. ● The care setting where you work may have a gifts policy in place that prevents you from accepting gifts of any kind from the individuals that you provide care or support to and their families. This is because others may think the reason you are being given a gift is because you somehow favoured these individuals and their families over others when providing them with care or support and as a result they have given you a gift. ● The data protection policy and procedures in your care setting may prevent you from sharing **personal information** about the individuals that you work with outside of the care setting.	By contrast, in personal relationships you are not bound by any rules and can give a gift to anyone. This can be any type or monetary value of your choice, in other words it can be as expensive or as inexpensive as you like. You can also share personal information about your families and friends with other family and friends, if you choose to do so – you are not bound by any confidentiality rules, only by your own conscience.

Table 1.1 The differences between a work and a personal relationship *continued*

A working relationship	A personal relationship
Working relationships include unequal balances of power. In your care setting, you will know personal information about the individuals you provide care or support to, such as their date of birth, their likes and dislikes and their family background. However, they will not necessarily know any personal information about you. Individuals depend on you to have their care or support needs met, but you do not depend on them to have your needs met.	Personal relationships, by contrast, are more equal. Those involved in the relationship share personal information about themselves; this is one of the ways in which close bonds are built.

\	Dos and don'ts for maintaining professional relationships with the people you provide care and support to
Do	Try to keep things as professional as possible. Of course, it is good practice to be friendly, but you may be caring for a wide range of individuals, not just one, so making sure that you remain professional means that you will be able to provide equal care and support for all, and not be seen as favouring some over others. This can be a tricky task because it may be that while working together you feel rather close to the individual. However, remember that you are also a professional.
Do	Share information so that you are friendly and personable but do not overshare. It is important to share things with the individual that you care for, but being professional means that you do not go into too much detail. This oversteps the boundaries and means that you may be seen to favour some over others. Also, oversharing means that the relationship can become personal and there is a risk that it could be misinterpreted.
Don't	Accept gifts, money or anything in case it looks like you have favoured particular individuals. An individual may want to give you a gift as a thank you but it is important that you try not to accept these. An appropriate response may be 'Thank you very much, that is a lovely thought, but I really cannot accept. I'm sorry.' You could even say that you are not allowed to accept gifts and that you would be breaking the rules by doing so. Remember that providing the best possible care to some of the most vulnerable people is your top priority. You are there to provide care for them. Do not expect gifts or support in return for your work.
Don't	Tell the individual about your worries and problems. It is your responsibility to listen to them and help them with any issues they may have. Just because they tell you about their worries, do not use it as an opportunity to share your concerns. This is all part of maintaining a professional relationship.

Case study

1.1, 2.1, 3.2 Relationships at work

Aamna has worked as a senior support worker with five older individuals with learning disabilities in a residential care setting for ten years. Aamna has got to know every individual so well over the years that they always turn to her when they need support or advice; this even includes on her days off. This makes Aamna feel good about herself and gives her tremendous job satisfaction. Over the last few years Aamna has taken it upon herself to come in on one of her days off every two weeks to arrange outings with individuals to different places of interest including to the garden centre, cinema and bowling club. Aamna's manager is very impressed with Aamna's commitment to her job and sees her as a valued member of the team.

This week Aamna requested a meeting with her manager to inform her that, due to her husband being diagnosed with a serious illness, she will be resigning from her senior support worker role to care for her husband at home. Aamna's manager is shocked by her news and wonders how she is going to manage without her expertise. The individuals for whom Aamna provides support are very upset that she is leaving and do not want her to go – particularly because they liked her arranging their outings. One of the individuals is so upset that they have asked to meet with their social worker as they wish to leave the care setting if they will no longer be receiving support from Aamna.

> *Discuss:*
> 1 Have the boundaries between Aamna's working relationships become confused? If so, why have they become confused?
> 2 The individuals and colleagues in the setting have not taken the news of Aamna's departure well. Could this have been avoided? Suggest some different ways that the news could have been announced.

Evidence opportunity

1.1 Personal and working relationships

Identify two people that you have a personal relationship with and two people you have a working relationship with.

For each person you identify write down:
- how well you know them
- when you see them, how often and the reasons why
- what you do together when you see them, how often and the reasons why
- what you know about them
- what they know about you.

Read through your comments to the above points. Explain the differences between the working relationships and personal relationships you have with these people. Provide a written account.

AC 1.2 Describe different working relationships in care settings/services

Working together with others is part of your day-to-day role as a care worker. You will work with a variety of people from colleagues and individuals that you care for, to their families, their advocates, GPs and other people and organisations outside the setting. For example, in a typical day, you may work with a colleague to provide support to an individual with an activity or communicate with an individual's advocate about arranging to meet with them, or you may work alongside an individual's social worker and GP to protect the individual from harm. Every one of the working relationships you have in the care setting where you work will be different. See Table 1.2.

Table 1.2 Examples of working relationships and aspects of what will be involved

Working relationships	Aspects of what is involved
An individual who you support in your care setting	Providing support with daily tasks such as with personal hygiene, eating and drinking, moving and handling, cooking and shopping.
	Supporting the individual to understand information in relation to their home, daily activities, finances.
	Enabling the individual to be part of their community, for example by supporting them to visit family and friends, encouraging them to socialise with others, supporting them to access local facilities such as the gym, leisure centre or shops.
An individual's mother who visits their relative on a weekly basis	Supporting the individual's mother to ask their relative about their week and activities.
	Providing the individual's mother with information about the care setting in relation to the services it provides, how many individuals live at the setting, how many staff are on each shift.
	Enabling the individual's mother to participate in some of the activities being organised at the care setting, such as a summer fete open to all or a coffee morning open to individuals' relatives.
An individual's advocate	Discussing with the individual's advocate how an individual's communication needs have changed.
	Asking the individual's advocate for their advice on how to support an individual at a meeting about their care needs.
	Receiving information from the individual's advocate about the communication aids that the advocate uses to support the individual to communicate.

Table 1.2 Examples of working relationships and aspects of what will be involved *continued*

Working relationships	Aspects of what is involved
A volunteer from within the organisation you work for	Discussing with the volunteer how they can support the outdoor activity planned with an individual. Providing the volunteer with information about the individual, their needs and the plan for the outdoor activity, including its purpose. Agreeing with the volunteer how to work together as a team to encourage the individual to participate in the planned outdoor activity.
A colleague who works the same shifts as you in your care setting	Sharing with your colleague how you developed a successful group craft activity. Supporting your colleague who is having difficulties making themselves understood when communicating with an individual who has hearing loss. Agreeing with your colleague how to work together as a team to move an individual from a sitting to standing position.
Your manager	Discussing with your manager whether you can book some additional annual leave. Discussing with your manager your achievements at work and the areas you would like to improve on. Seeking guidance from your manager when you have witnessed a visitor speaking to an individual inappropriately.
An individual's GP	Telephoning the individual's GP to make an appointment. Providing the individual's GP with information about the individual's symptoms when they are feeling unwell. Finding out what support is available from the GP surgery for an individual who wants to stop smoking.
A contractor who has come to repair the sink in the staff room	Checking with the contractor before allowing them access to the premises – such as the purpose of their visit and their identity. Accompanying the contractor to the staff room to repair the sink in the staff room. Providing the contractor with all the necessary information in relation to the repair needed to the sink, i.e. where it is leaking, the length of time it has been leaking.
A volunteer from another organisation, such as a local charity	Finding out from the volunteer how they and their organisation can support a music session with a group of individuals. Asking the volunteer about the resources that will be required to facilitate the music session. Agreeing with the volunteer how to work together as a team to meet the needs of each individual in the group during the music session.

Team building and good working relationships

You cannot expect to understand how your colleagues work and how you can all work well together on day one. There will be times when you are able to all work successfully to meet an objective but there will also be times when you disagree with one another. This is all part of being in a team. In order to ensure that you work well with others, you should try and remember that good working relationships have key features, some of which you will explore in the other mandatory units, such as good communication (see Unit 304), good values (Unit 313), good understanding and good support (Unit 300).

	Dos and don'ts for supporting colleagues
Do	Support one another if a colleague is struggling with a task. Maybe they are struggling with a moving and handling procedure. If so, help them. If you don't know how, then find someone who can help them.
Do	Share best practice. If something has worked well in practice, then share this with colleagues so that they can also learn from you. Likewise, if you have undertaken some training and found this helpful, share what you learned and encourage them to go on the course. Support one another to be better care workers.
Don't	Undermine or belittle a colleague. If you feel that they have done something incorrectly, it is useful to give helpful constructive advice. It is important that colleagues feel that they are part of a team and you cannot be part of a team if you constantly seek faults in others. Remember, however, that you must always tell your manager if you observe a colleague carrying out unsafe working practices.
Don't	Underestimate the importance of your colleagues just because you are busy. Value them! If someone is not well, or feels overwhelmed about something at work (or outside work), then be there for them. You could ask if they want to talk about the problem. Everyone is busy at work, but if you make time for one another, it will lead to more positive and supportive working relationships and a better working environment.

6Cs

Communication

Communication in a working relationship is essential for ensuring that you all work together as a team towards ensuring positive outcomes for individuals. Without good communication, misunderstandings may arise that may lead to an individual's care or support needs being unmet.

You can show good communication in your working relationships by:

- only writing down accurate information in your daily reports about the care you have provided to individuals
- remembering that if you have agreed with a colleague to do a task, then communicate this to your colleague when you have completed it
- effectively communicating to support colleagues by being friendly and polite in your communications and by using encouraging and supportive language, such as 'I thought you handled the situation with Jones really well. I know it must have been hard for you especially because you have been really busy with other individuals, but you did really well.'

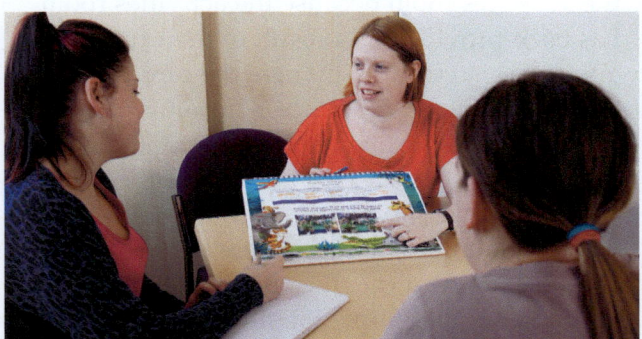

Figure 1.3 How can you tell if your working relationships are effective?

Evidence opportunity

1.2 Different working relationships

Building on your work from Evidence opportunity 1.1, develop an information handout about the different working relationships you have in the care setting. For each working relationship, provide some details about why it is important and what makes it effective.

AC 1.3 Explain own role in the quality assurance processes to promote positive experiences for individuals receiving care

What is quality in care?
Good-quality care means that:
- an individual's experience will be positive, caring and enabling
- an individual's experience will meet their expectations as well as those of their family, friends or advocates
- care services will be safe
- care services will be effective.

What is quality assurance in care and how can you contribute to it?
Quality assurance means to ensure a high quality of care in the setting. It is about offering the best care and service possible and meeting the needs and requirements of those who use the services. We cover some of the different aspects involved in quality assurance in the following text.

Fact finding
This involves finding out about the care individuals receive, and will include the aspects of care that are working well for an individual and the aspects that require further development. Finding out this information means you can further improve the areas that are not working so well to ensure that individuals receive the highest quality of care. For example, an individual may express that they are pleased that they can request their care worker to arrive a little earlier or later in the mornings depending on what their plans are for the day. This works well during the week but they may find that this does not work as well at the weekends because sometimes the care workers may arrive quite late in the mornings.

You have a very important role to play in contributing to the quality assurance process and your practices will be observed. It is through quality assurance that you too can be part of an individual's positive experience of care. The following are some tips for how you can do this.

- **Focus** – start by deciding what you want to find out – and the reason why. Think about whether there are a few specific aspects of individuals' care needing improvement or whether there is just one aspect. For example:

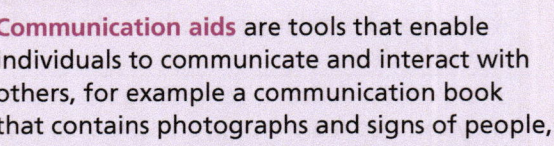

Key terms

Communication aids are tools that enable individuals to communicate and interact with others, for example a communication book that contains photographs and signs of people, places and objects familiar to the individual.

Risk assessment is a process used in work settings for identifying hazards, assessing the level of risk and putting in place processes for reducing the risk identified. See Unit 310 Promoting health and safety in adult care settings/services, LO3, for more information on the risk assessment process.

- care provided with eating (one aspect)
- care provided overnight or over weekends (multiple aspects).

Think about whether these aspects of care are specific to one individual or whether they apply to more than one individual. For example:
- providing support when communicating with a **communication aid** (one individual)
- **risk assessment processes** that are followed when supporting individuals on activities out in their local communities (more than one individual).

- **Work with others** – next, you need to decide who to involve in quality assurance processes and the reasons why. For example, if you are trying to find out why the new activities room in the care setting where you work is not being used as much as you thought it would be, you may want to involve the individuals who use the activities room because the activities room has been provided as a result of their request. You may also want to involve the care workers and Activities Co-ordinator who support the individuals to participate in the activities because they may also be able to share with you their observations about what individuals like or don't like about the activities rooms as well as what difficulties there may be such as not enough lighting, too much noise, or not enough space for individuals who use wheelchairs. You may be aware that from time to time some of the individuals' relatives will also provide support during activities; you may identify who these are and ask them too for their views.

- **Take action** – you need to consider the methods available and which ones you think will be most suitable to use to find out the information you want to know. For example, you will need to consider whether you want to have a discussion with individuals in pairs, in small groups, or on a one-to-one basis. You may opt to use questionnaires that can be completed over email or sent out in the post to relatives and others. Again, you will need to think about what kind of information you want to collate; for example, if you would like to hear the opinions and suggestions of the individuals then a discussion may be better, whereas if it is factual information you need, questionnaires that contain specific questions may be more suitable.

Contributing to quality assurance processes to promote positive experiences for individuals receiving care means having open discussions where there is an honest exchange of information and ideas, obtaining feedback from all those involved and reflecting on this. It also involves a high level of commitment from you to ensure that quality assurance processes continue to be maintained and are effective.

6Cs

Commitment

Commitment to quality assurance is necessary to ensure that you and others promote a positive experience for the individuals who receive your care. This means not being afraid to find out how effective the care or support you provide is and then make the improvements that are necessary to meet individuals' and others' expectations. You can do this by showing that you are genuinely interested in finding out about the experiences, the views and opinions from everybody involved and by taking on board all the feedback you receive. You can regularly review and monitor the care or support you provide to all individuals.

Taking action

This involves listening to what is being said or observing what is happening, using this information as the basis for making improvements to the care provided, discussing it with colleagues and putting this into action. For example, an individual's family may tell you that they have noticed that when their relative has their afternoon coffee in their room it often arrives lukewarm but that this never happens if the resident has their afternoon coffee in the lounge. You decide to take action by informing your manager as well as the chef in the kitchen. As a result, new coffee pots are bought so that when the coffee is served to residents in their rooms it retains its heat. It is also agreed for a team member to check 15 minutes or so after the coffee has been taken to the resident's room that it is to the individual's liking.

Monitoring

This involves assessing how well a service is running including how well the care being provided to individuals is working. For example, in the situation described above about the individual having a hot drink in their room, it will be important to check that the measures that have been put in place to resolve the situation are still working. For example, you may want to check with the individual and their family by asking them at regular monthly intervals directly about their experiences. You could speak with the chef and the care workers to find out their views about how the new coffee pots are working. You could

Key terms

Preferences refer to an individual's wishes, likes and own personal choices, for example for food, clothes, activities and wellbeing. These may be based on an individual's beliefs, values and culture.

Rights are legal entitlements to something, for example the right to have personal information held about you by an organisation kept secure.

Dignity in a care setting means respecting the views, choices and decision of individuals and not making assumptions about how they want to be treated.

Values are what you hold true and believe to be important to you, such as your independence, or your family. Often a person's beliefs can develop into their values.

Duty of care refers to the legal requirement that health and social care workers have to ensure the safety and wellbeing of individuals and others while providing care or support. This concept is covered in Unit 303 Understanding duty of care.

also take on board any other suggestions shared with you for further improving the situation.

Monitoring whether the CQC's fundamental standards are being met is a responsibility of all services that provide individuals with care. It is important that services are regularly checking on the quality of the care or support being provided, i.e. is it tailored to individuals' needs and **preferences**? Are individuals' **rights** to **dignity** and privacy being upheld? The safety of the care or support being provided also needs to be checked regularly. Does it promote individuals' health and wellbeing, and safeguard them from abuse – for example, by ensuring that risk assessments are completed, and that staff are trained, qualified and competent to provide care and support?

Quality assurance is not:

- **one size:** all individuals receiving care are different with their own **values**, beliefs, views and experiences.
    - For example, when finding out about individuals' experiences of care you may ask one individual directly by discussing this with them but you may have to make arrangements for another individual who has communication needs to have their advocate present so that they can ensure that the individual's views and preferences are expressed.
- **a one-off:** promoting positive experiences for individuals receiving care does not just happen once a year or on one occasion; instead it is an ongoing process.
    - For example, ensuring that the activities provided in the care setting where you work are safe is an ongoing process as it involves daily, weekly and monthly checks. You can't stop checking that they are safe or only assess activities for any risks they present once, it has to be done every time the activity is provided to ensure it does not place yourself, individuals and others in danger or at risk of harm. This is part of your **duty of care**.
- **an exercise:** promoting positive experiences for individuals receiving care is not about filling in questionnaires and about ticking boxes on forms; quality assurance is a process.

Following your employer's agreed ways of working is an integral aspect of your job role. For example, you don't assess how well you do this by answering a short questionnaire about your own working practices; you do this by discussing this with your manager in supervision meetings and by seeking feedback from your colleagues, the individuals you provide care to and their families, friends and advocates.

Case study 1.3 will help you consider the different factors you need to take into account when contributing to the quality assurance processes in the care setting where you work.

Reflect on it

1.3 Why is quality assurance important?

Think about the reasons why quality assurance is important for the care setting where you work. What are your expectations for providing quality care in your job role and care setting? Why do you think this is important?

Research it

1.3 Quality assurance processes in your setting

Carry out some research in the care setting where you work about the quality assurance processes that are in place for promoting positive experiences for individuals receiving care. Produce an information handout with your findings.

You will find it useful to speak with your manager and access the quality assurance policy and procedures that are in place in your work setting.

Case study

1.3 Contributing to quality assurance processes

Michael is a senior day care centre worker. As part of his role, he works in a team of four to support the activities provided for young adults with learning disabilities by encouraging and enabling the individuals to participate. The team met last week to discuss the activities being provided because they do not seem to be as well attended as before and the team are unsure as to the reasons why.

The team has agreed to involve all the members who attend the activities as well as those who used to attend but have stopped doing so. This also includes involving individuals' relatives who from time to time support the activities and also the activities worker who leads on the outdoor activities at the weekend.

Michael and his colleague will be interviewing the individuals who attend and have decided that due to their range of needs, they will interview them one by one. Michael has developed a set of questions that he plans to use with individuals; he has also adapted these to include photographs and signs as some individuals are unable to read and others prefer to communicate through signs. Michael's colleague has also arranged for an individual's advocate to be present during the interview as the individual feels less anxious in a one-to-one situation when someone he knows well and trusts is present.

Discuss

1. Why is it important for the team to find out the reasons why individuals are not attending the activities?
2. Why did Michael and his colleague take into account individuals' needs when making arrangements for interviews?
3. What other methods could be used by the team for obtaining feedback from all those involved?
4. How could Michael and the team continue to monitor how the activities are working?

Evidence opportunity

1.3 Quality assurance processes and positive experiences for individuals

Think about an individual you work with – how could quality assurance ensure their care is of the highest quality? Demonstrate to your assessor how you have put this into practice with an individual receiving care, showing how you contributed to quality assurance processes and how this influenced positive experiences for them.

Write an account about how your role in the quality assurance processes influenced and promoted a positive experience for this individual.

AC 1.4 Explain why it is important to work in partnership with others

Your job role in adult social care will involve working alongside a wide range of different people and organisations that have different roles and responsibilities. This may include the individuals you provide care or support to, their families, friends, advocates or others who are important to them, your colleagues, other team members such as your manager, and professionals from other organisations, such as social workers, mental health nurses, dieticians, dementia care nurses, GPs.

Working in partnership with others is more than just working alongside them. It involves becoming 'a team'. This can only happen when you are all committed to:

- sharing a common set of values – to support individuals' independence, to safeguard individuals from harm, to respect individuals' unique differences
- agreeing goals – to enable positive outcomes for individuals (which may be agreed over both short and long periods of time)
- communicating effectively – communications must be open and honest, timely and regular both with individuals and others, including both verbal and written communications. (You may find it useful to refer to Unit 304 Effective communication in adult care settings/services and Unit 305 Handling information in adult care settings.)

Working in partnership brings many benefits for you, the individuals who require care, as well as others both inside and outside the organisation.

> **Evidence opportunity**
>
> **1.4 The importance of working in partnership**
>
> Think about three case studies when you were required to work in partnership with a range of professionals. Develop a PowerPoint presentation that outlines who you worked with, what organisations they were from, how good this partnership working was and why partnership working was important. Ensure your reasons are specific to the people and organisations you identified.

Most importantly in a setting, working effectively as a team and in partnership means that you all have the shared goal of providing the best support possible for individuals.

Working in partnership and working effectively together can have the following benefits.

- You all improve and develop your understanding of different ways of working, sharing knowledge and best practice. For example, a colleague may show you a more effective way of communicating with an individual who has hearing loss.
- A stronger team creates a better working environment where you all feel supported. For example (similar to what we mentioned above), working in partnership with others involves sharing skills, knowledge and getting to know each other. This enables team members to learn from each other and share good ideas.
- Understanding one another's roles and responsibilities will avoid duplicating one another's work so that staff make better use of their time. You may also share resources, such as meeting venues, which can reduce costs and encourages everyone to meet together.
- You all work together to provide person-centred care. Individuals receive care that is coordinated and meets all of their individual needs (they will receive better services).

AC 1.5 Describe different skills and approaches used when working in partnership with others

Working in partnership in care settings with different people and organisations can at times be challenging. Although everyone is working towards agreed goals, disagreements may result over how to achieve these goals due to people's different ideas about how to deal with situations.

If conflicts are not managed effectively then this can be very damaging to how the team works together, communication can break down causing resentment and people may stop sharing information, which in turn may lead to the care and support not meeting individuals' needs.

> **Research it**
>
> **1.5 Conflicts**
>
> Carry out some research in the care setting where you work. Speak with your colleagues about some of the conflicts that have arisen in the team and how these have been resolved. Find out what happened for two of these conflicts. Why did they arise? Who was involved? How did they make everyone feel?
>
> Discuss your findings with your manager. Reflect on how you felt doing this activity. Did you feel uncomfortable or awkward about asking these questions? Why might you feel awkward?

> **Reflect on it**
>
> **1.5 Consequences of not resolving conflicts**
>
> Reflect on the two conflicts you researched earlier that arose and were resolved in the care setting where you work. Reflect on the consequences should these not have been resolved. Why would these have impacted negatively on the team working together, and the care and support provided to individuals?

Therefore, it is important that you are aware of the main skills and approaches needed when working in partnership with others. The main skill that you need to work in partnership with others is good communication. If someone disagrees with you, or if you disagree with them, the best way to resolve the issue is to have an open and honest discussion where you can both talk over your differences in a calm way.

You should openly state what the issue, conflict or disagreement is. Each of you should listen to what the other person (or people) have to say and put forward your thoughts and opinions. You may need to involve others who have more experience in the area that is the cause of the dispute.

You can then try to find a way to resolve the conflict. This should not be an argument or a debate. It should be a discussion where the **best interests** of the individual, the setting or best practice are at the heart of the matter. Good communication is essential.

Table 1.3 includes some examples of the main skills and approaches needed for working in partnership with others.

> ### Evidence opportunity
>
> **1.5 Skills and approaches used when working in partnership with others**
>
> Think of a time when conflict arose in the care setting where you work. Write down the skills that would need to be shown, and the working approaches that could be taken, in order to resolve this conflict and work in partnership with others.

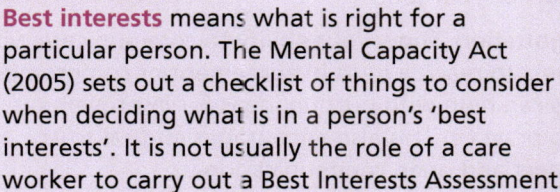

> ### Key terms
>
> **Best interests** means what is right for a particular person. The Mental Capacity Act (2005) sets out a checklist of things to consider when deciding what is in a person's 'best interests'. It is not usually the role of a care worker to carry out a Best Interests Assessment.
>
> **Empathy** is the ability to understand how someone else may be feeling, or understand another person's way of thinking.
>
> **Negotiation** means reaching an agreement through discussion.
>
> **Care plan** may be known by other names, such as a support plan, or individual plan. It is the document that sets out the agreed plan of care or support for an individual and where day-to-day requirements and preferences for care and support are detailed.

Table 1.3 Skills and approaches needed for working in partnership with others

Skills used when working in partnership with others	Approaches used when working in partnership with others
Empathy: Show that you are able to put yourself in someone else's shoes. This can help you gain a better understanding of others' views and feelings and it also encourages mutual respect as the other person knows that you are taking their view into account. **Assertiveness:** Show that you are confident and able to make clear your views and the reasons why. This will inspire confidence, as it will show that you are capable of making reasoned judgements and know what you are talking about. This also encourages mutual trust.	**Use effective communication:** For example, it is important to show that you are genuinely interested in what others are saying; you can do this by using positive body language such as nodding, smiling and maintaining eye contact, by actively listening and trying to understand others' views. This also encourages a willingness to work together. **Be positive:** It is important to show that you are being constructive and taking into account others' views and beliefs. You can do this by acknowledging what others are saying by repeating their views back (to show that you have understood) and by using respectful language. This encourages mutual respect.

Table 1.3 Skills and approaches needed for working in partnership with others *continued*

Skills used when working in partnership with others	Approaches used when working in partnership with others
Honesty: Be honest when sharing information and communicating with others. This will show that you have a genuine interest in individuals' wellbeing and promoting positive outcomes. This also encourages others to approach you and encourages open communications. **Enthusiasm:** Show your willingness to work in partnership with others. This can help with team building and will show that you genuinely care about working with them and not simply because it is part of your job. **Negotiation:** Show your ability to communicate with others to reach a mutual agreement or compromise. This can help with putting ideas for improvement into practice. This also encourages mutual trust, respect and open communications.	**Make the conflict the difficulty** rather than the individual or a member of the team. Focus on the conflict rather than on a person. This avoids making it personal and stops anyone feeling like they are to blame. (You can do this by not using negative language or making negative comments about specific individuals or members of the team.) This encourages positive teamwork as everyone knows that while you may disagree, you are still a team working together to resolve an issue.

AC 1.6 Outline how and when to access support and advice about a) partnership working b) resolving conflicts in relationships and partnerships

As partnership working and resolving conflicts involves working with many different people and organisations there may be times when you need to seek support or advice. This may be when:

- an individual's family wants you to disclose personal information about their relative that they do not have a need to know – this might mean that the individual's family is frustrated with you that you are not disclosing this information as they may feel they have a right to know as they are related to the individual and you are not
- you have been asked to complete a work activity that involves you working with a physiotherapist. You feel anxious as this is not something you have done previously. If you don't carry it out this may result in your employer thinking that you are not skilled enough for the job role you have been employed to carry out - but on the other hand you know that you also have a duty of care
- you have been asked to support an individual with accessing a college course where you will need to work alongside others including tutors.

For example, you may support the individual to find out what courses are available and what they involve and to ask any other questions they may have.

Being able to recognise the different types of situation and when you must ask for support and advice is just as important as knowing how to do so. There will be procedures in the care setting where you work for how to do this and you must ensure that you comply with these agreed ways of working when seeking support and advice about partnership working and resolving conflicts. If you have tried to resolve the issues with the people concerned or feel unable to approach those involved directly then there are other options available to you.

Sources of support and advice available within your **work setting** can include an experienced colleague who you trust, your manager or someone else in a senior position. These colleagues, due to their experience, may have come across a similar difficulty or conflict before and will also have the skills and expertise to be able to assess the best ways to resolve the situation quickly and satisfactorily.

It is important not to delay seeking support and advice because doing so may lead to these difficulties becoming worse, tensions increasing and the quality of care and support provided to individuals being affected negatively.

If you are unable to access the support you need or are dissatisfied with the advice offered by your manager then you must contact the next level of management within the care setting where you work. For example, this may be a more senior manager or the owner.

If you are still dissatisfied with the response you receive from senior management, then you may need to seek advice from independent external sources. Sources of support fall into two categories: those relevant to the care being given to an individual, and those that relate to employment issues. CQC is the regulatory body for care and would be able to assist with care-related issues; the Advisory, Conciliation and Arbitration Service (**ACAS**) would be able to assist with employment-related issues.

The reflective exemplar that follows will help to draw your attention to the importance of always taking action when there are difficulties with partnership working or resolving conflicts.

Key terms

Work settings may include one specific location or a range of locations, depending on the context of a particular work role, for example a domiciliary carer who may work in individuals' own homes and in residential care homes, or an activities worker who may work in residential homes, day centres, nursing homes or in an individual's own home.

ACAS is an independent organisation that provides impartial and confidential advice to employees for resolving difficulties and conflicts at work.

Research it

1.6 Policies and procedures in your setting

Research the procedures that are in place in the care setting where you work for seeking support and advice about partnership working and resolving conflicts. Develop a poster with your main findings.

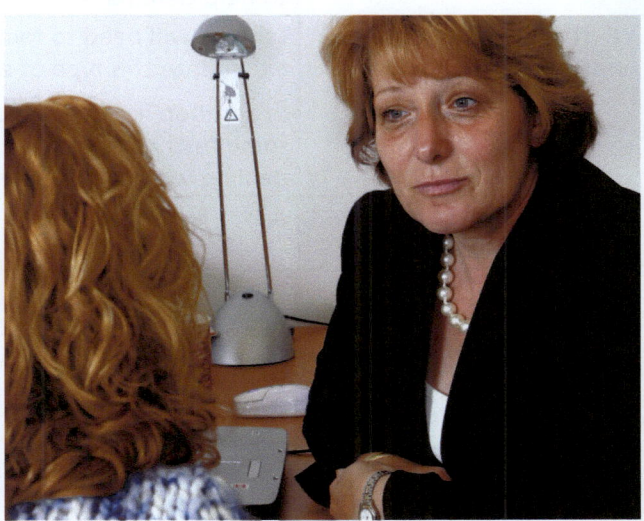

Figure 1.4 What support does your manager provide for resolving conflicts?

Reflective exemplar	
Introduction	I work as a Lead Personal Assistant to Gemma, a young woman who has cerebral palsy and episodes of depression. My duties involve supporting Gemma with personal care tasks such as showering, dressing, eating and drinking.
What happened?	Yesterday morning I arrived as usual to support Gemma with her personal hygiene and saw that she was smoking cannabis in bed. I asked Gemma what she thought she was doing smoking cannabis, an illegal drug, and she told me that she had been doing this for a while as it helped her physical body spasms and reduced the pain she was in.
	I explained to Gemma politely that I didn't think this was appropriate as it wasn't good for her health and wellbeing. Gemma told me that it was her home and she could do what she liked and that as she employed me as her personal assistant I would have to continue with assisting her with her personal hygiene routine.

Reflective exemplar	
	I explained to Gemma politely that I didn't agree and left immediately without telling anyone so as not to cause any more conflict.
	The next day I found out from the office that after I had left Gemma, she telephoned her advocate and her parents to tell them that she was very unhappy with me as her personal assistant because I did not treat her as an adult and did not respect her beliefs. I was also informed that Gemma had requested a different personal assistant.
What worked well?	I was polite and I communicated calmly with Gemma in this difficult situation.
What did not go as well?	I should not have left without telling anyone. I should have sought advice straight away and communicated that I was doing so to Gemma.
	Also, I should have explained clearly to Gemma my duty of care towards her and showed more compassion in understanding her situation, i.e. that she was in pain. Perhaps I could have suggested alternative remedies that are available to help Gemma.
What could I do to improve?	I think I will need to familiarise myself again with the procedures to follow if I experience this type of situation again.
	In addition, I plan to discuss this situation with my line manager and request some further training in how I can be more confident and assertive when dealing with conflicts at work.
Links to unit assessment criteria	ACs: 1.4, 1.5, 1.6

Evidence opportunity

1.6 How and when to access support and advice about partnership working and resolving conflicts

Write a reflective account of how and when you would seek support and advice in relation to a conflict or a difficulty with partnership working at work.

Ensure that you are able to show how you identified the most appropriate source of support and advice, what you reported and recorded, the reasons why as well as a positive outcome.

LO2 Understand agreed ways of working

Getting started

Think about an occasion when a work activity was not carried out to a high standard. Why do you think this happened? What could have been done differently to prevent this happening again? What was the outcome of the work activity not being carried out to a high standard? What are the potential consequences for individuals, the employer, you, your colleagues?

AC 2.1 Describe why it is important to work within the scope of own role, responsibility and training

Your job role

Developing effective working relationships with others can only be achieved if you carry out all the tasks that form part of your job role; this is commonly referred to as 'the agreed scope' of the job role. In the care setting where you work, you will have a **job description** that sets out all the responsibilities you have agreed to with your employer.

These will include the following:

- **the responsibilities, tasks or work activities** that you must carry out as part of your job role. These might include:
  - providing support to individuals with daily living activities to meet their needs
  - maintaining accurate records of the support provided to individuals
  - attending all training provided
  - as a Lead Adult Care Worker, you will provide guidance and support to care workers, supervise and monitor the work practices of care workers, lead on the care and support provided.

- **how you must carry out your work activities.** This might include:
  - promoting individuals' rights such as privacy, dignity, independence
  - maintaining detailed and accurate records while protecting individuals' confidentiality at all times
  - putting into practice all training attended by using person-centred ways of working
  - promoting people's rights to be treated fairly, supporting others to provide high quality care and support.
- **who you report to**, such as your manager, team leader or your employer, who may be the individual
- **who your supervisor is**
- **what your hours of work are**, for example flexible shifts, including evenings and weekends
- **how much you will be paid per hour**
- **where you must work**, for example in a variety of settings including in individuals' own homes, in residential care settings.

Job descriptions will vary depending on the job. They will also vary in detail; some may be brief with an outline of the job role and key responsibilities but good descriptions will detail the purpose of your role, responsibilities, different tasks you will be required to complete, and also the reasons for doing so. In this way you have a clear understanding of why you are doing what you are asked, and understand how it impacts on the individual and setting. For example, instead of saying in the job description 'assist in mealtimes', it would be more helpful to say 'assist in mealtimes and ensure that the meal meets the dietary requirements and needs of the individual.' Or instead of saying 'provide good care for individuals' it would be more helpful to say 'provide care that involves treating individuals with compassion, dignity and respect and ensuring that they are involved in their care'.

Adhering to the agreed scope of your job role also involves working within the boundaries or limits of the job role. The 'dos and don'ts' table provides tips to make sure you work within the boundaries. Basically, if it is not part of your job description, then you should not be expected to carry out the task.

Key terms

Supervisor refers to the person in your work setting that oversees your work and assesses your performance at work; this is usually your manager or, if you are a Lead Personal Assistant, your employer.

Job descriptions are documents that outline the purpose and responsibilities of your job role.

	Dos and don'ts for adhering to the scope of your job role
Do	Comply with the agreed lines of reporting. For example, if you have a concern about an individual's wellbeing, then you should report your concerns to your manager in the first instance rather than going straight to the individual. Your job description will outline whom you will report to and you must work within these boundaries and the scope of your job.
Do	Only carry out work activities within your agreed hours of work. Do not assist an individual who wishes to go to the shops after your shift has ended without first seeking permission to do so.
Do	Work in locations agreed with your employer. Again this will be outlined in your job description and the scope of your job so do not provide support to an individual in your house or in the home of one of the individual's relatives instead of the individual's own home, for example.
Don't	Take part in work activities that have not been agreed as part of your job role and that you are not trained to do. For example, if your job description does not mention assisting individuals with medication, reviewing care plans, or supervision of new members of staff, then you should not be expected to do this. You may of course receive training and as a result your job role and the scope of your role may change but this is something you should discuss with your manager before you undertake tasks that are not outlined in your job description.
Don't	Work in ways that are not person-centred. For example, by imposing your views and denying individuals their rights, or by documenting your opinions when recording the support provided to individuals.

> **Research it**
>
> **2.1 Your job description**
>
> Find your job description for the care setting where you work. Identify the responsibilities you have agreed to with your employer, including what you must not do as part of your job role.
>
> Discuss the scope of your job role with a colleague. How do your responsibilities compare to theirs?

The importance of adhering to the agreed scope of your job role, responsibility and training

Working within the agreed scope of your job role is essential for ensuring that you carry out your job responsibilities to the best of your ability. It is also very important for a number of other reasons set out below.

- **It ensures you are working at the correct level:** ensuring you adhere to the scope of your job ensures that you are working to your ability and doing the tasks that you are qualified to do. Doing tasks that you do not have any expertise or qualifications in risks the health and safety of those around you and yourself. You can of course gain knowledge and skills in those areas but it is best to stick to what you know before you start taking on responsibilities that are not outlined in your job description and those you have not discussed with your manager first.

- **It ensures you are only responsible and accountable for what you do:** all organisations need structures and a clear outline of what everyone does in the setting. That way, you are only accountable for those things that you are responsible for and not for others. It is also clear to management who is responsible for what tasks and so there are no misunderstandings (if you are all doing what you are responsible for). That is not to say you cannot assist colleagues; it just means you should not take on tasks that are not in the scope of your job.

- **It is how your employer will assess your competence:** during supervision meetings with your manager and as part of your appraisal at the end of the year, your employer will discuss with you how you have performed in your job role. You will discuss whether you have carried out your work activities to the best of your ability, in line with your job role's requirements and within your employer's expectations of you. By adhering to the agreed scope of your job role you will be more likely to show that you are doing what is expected of you and that you are doing this competently, to a high standard. You can find out more about supervision and appraisals in Unit 313 Continuous development when working in an adult care worker role.

> **6Cs**
>
> **Competence**
>
> Competence refers to your ability to apply the knowledge and skills you have learned to your day-to-day work activities. This is important because it means that you will only be carrying out work activities and working in ways that are set out in the agreed scope of your job role – activities that you have the knowledge and skills to carry out. You can show you are doing this by keeping a record of your professional development and discussing this with your manager during your supervision and appraisal meetings. You can also show your competence by obtaining feedback from the individuals and others you work with about how you carry out your work activities.

- **It is part of your duty of care:** you have a duty of care to ensure you provide the best possible care, and the support you offer is in the best interests of the individual. You can review your learning about this concept in Unit 303 Understanding duty of care. For example, assisting an individual to move from their bed to their chair on your own when the moving and handling guidelines specify that two staff should be present can have serious consequences for both you and the individual. You may lose your job for carrying out a task on your own that you do not have the agreement from your employer to do. You may also injure your back during the move. Your actions may cause the individual to fall and fracture one of their limbs. Adhering to the agreed scope of your job role is therefore essential for your safety as well as the safety and wellbeing of individuals.

- **It ensures the health and safety of everyone:** you have a responsibility to ensure the safety of everyone you work with. Your responsibilities with regard to health and safety are covered in Unit 310 Promoting health and safety in adult care settings/services and Unit 312 Implementing health and safety in adult care settings/services. Not adhering to responsibilities around health and safety, such as reporting concerns, can have serious consequences. For example, if you do not report concerns about a colleague's unsafe working practices when preparing food, it could result in illness such as food poisoning for those in the setting (as well as visitors). It could even prove fatal if they already suffer from other illnesses. If you do not report your concerns, your colleague will not be able to access the support and training they need. Both you and your colleague may also run the risk of losing your jobs. That is not to say you should spend your days worrying about what *might* happen, but it is a good idea to be mindful of the reasons why you should work within the scope of your job role and responsibilities.

- **It protects you from untrue allegations:** meeting with an individual on a one-to-one basis when it has been agreed that all meetings with this individual will take place in the presence of two members of staff can have serious consequences for everyone. You may be accused of something that you did not do, for example shouting at the individual. This will in turn mean that your employer will be required to conduct an investigation into what happened. The incident will also need to be reported to the individual's family and to CQC, the external agency who regulates the services provided at the care setting. This may result in the individual requesting a move to another care setting, you losing your job and could even mean an end to your career in the adult social care sector. Again, this example is not designed to scare you, but you should remember that your job description has important reasons for everything that it outlines including the working methods you should follow. You shouldn't need to be too concerned about the consequences if you are following the rules and guidelines in your job description.

If the individual is your employer/if you are a private carer

If your employer is the individual to whom you provide care or support, or you work on your own as a private carer to an individual, then it is important that you understand and read through the guidance provided to you by the person who is employing you; this may be written formally and included in your contract of employment, or may be in the form of a personal plan of work that the individual has prepared. Some individuals and their families may also brief you verbally, and may ask you to approach them if you have any questions or concerns. You could also seek support from other carers you know or other lone workers who you meet when you attend training or conferences.

> **Evidence opportunity**
>
> **2.1 Adhering to the scope of your job role, responsibility and training**
>
> Think about three work activities that you are required to carry out as part of your job role. For each work activity, describe to your assessor why it is important you carry it out competently and within the agreed scope of your job role. What happens if you do not follow the scope of the job role?

AC 2.2 Define what is meant by the term 'delegated healthcare task'

What is a 'delegated healthcare task?'

A delegated healthcare task is a health intervention or activity, usually of a clinical nature, that a registered healthcare professional delegates to a paid care worker and that forms part of an individual's care or support plan. For example:

- supporting skin integrity and wound healing by changing dressings
- supporting an individual's nutrition using a **PEG (Percutaneous endoscopic gastrostomy)**
- supporting an individual to manage their **diabetes** through insulin administration and monitoring
- supporting an individual who has difficulties mobilising using a bed hoist
- supporting an individual who has difficulties communicating to use **PECS**.

Key terms

Percutaneous endoscopic gastrostomy (PEG) is a small tube that is inserted through the skin into an individual's stomach when they are having difficulties swallowing so that they can receive food, fluid and medication without swallowing.

Diabetes is a health condition that occurs when the amount of glucose (sugar) in the blood is too high because the body cannot use it properly.

PECS (the Picture Exchange Communication System) is a communication system that uses visual symbols and is used with individuals who have communication difficulties and autism spectrum conditions.

Autism spectrum conditions (ASC) are lifelong conditions that affect how people perceive the world and interact with others. For example, they may have difficulties communicating, interacting and socialising with others.

Evidence opportunity

2.2 Delegated health care tasks

Take it in turns to discuss with a colleague the meaning of the term 'delegated healthcare task'. Agree on a written definition of this term.

AC 2.3 Explain own limitations and responsibilities when undertaking delegated healthcare tasks

A healthcare task will only be delegated by a registered healthcare professional once the paid care worker has been:

- assessed as being competent to carry it out
- trained to carry it out
- supported to carry it out safely and competently.

It is the employer's responsibility to ensure that assessment, training and support have been provided prior to the care worker carrying out the delegated healthcare task. It is the care worker's responsibility to comply with their employer's agreed ways of working and only carry out delegated healthcare tasks if they have been trained and feel competent to do so.

If a care worker has been delegated a task and they do not feel confident to carry it out because they may feel that they do not have sufficient knowledge about what the task involves, or because there are certain aspects of the training they received that they did not understand, then it is their responsibility to raise their concerns with their employer. The paid worker must not carry out the delegated healthcare task if they have any concerns about their ability to do so.

This is essential for:

- ensuring they're complying with their employer's agreed ways of working
- following up-to-date working practices
- carrying out safe practices
- avoiding putting themselves, individuals and others at risk
- carrying out their job role and responsibilities to the best of their ability

AC 2.4 Explain who might delegate a healthcare task and why

Who might delegate a healthcare task?

Healthcare tasks can only be delegated by a registered healthcare professional who is involved in the individual's care and support. Examples of registered healthcare professionals can include:

- registered nurses
- nursing associates
- occupational therapists
- **physiotherapists**

- radiographers
- **speech and language therapists**
- **dieticians**.

Key terms

Physiotherapists are trained professionals who help to restore the body's movement and function when an individual is affected by injury, illness or disability through mobility exercises, for example.

Speech and language therapists are professionals who support individuals who have communication difficulties. They might assist those who have speech problems or difficulties using language.

Dieticians are qualified health professionals whose role it is to assess, diagnose, and treat diet and nutritional issues.

Research it

2.3, 2.4 Registered healthcare professionals

Research the role and main responsibilities for two registered healthcare professionals you have learned about.

You will find it helpful to refer to the Health & Care Professions Council's (HCPC) website: www.hcpc-uk.org

What are the main differences and similarities between the roles and responsibilities of these two registered healthcare professionals? Write a report with your findings.

Why are healthcare tasks delegated?

Not all care workers will have healthcare tasks delegated to them, but it is important that you understand not only what these are but also their benefits in case you are delegated a healthcare task in the future. The delegation of healthcare tasks takes place because it benefits not only the individual but also you and the team you work within. The benefits to the individual include having a consistent level of care provided by people who know their needs and preferences, and improving the quality of the care and support that is provided because it is person-centred and focuses on the individual themselves thus giving them more choice and control. You will learn more about person-centred care in Unit 306 Promoting and implementing person-centred practice.

The delegation of healthcare tasks also brings a range of benefits to the care worker and the team they work within, such as increased job satisfaction from knowing that the care and support provided is of a high quality, enabling an individual to live their life fully, developing new skills and knowledge.

Reflect on it

2.3, 2.4 Delegated healthcare tasks

Reflect on the different healthcare tasks that may be delegated to care workers. What role do employers play in the delegation of healthcare tasks? What are the care workers' responsibilities if they have been delegated a task that they do not fully understand? What are the consequences of employers and care workers not following their responsibilities? Who benefits from the delegation of healthcare tasks?

Evidence opportunity

2.3, 2.4 Understanding delegated healthcare tasks

Identify two designated healthcare tasks you have undertaken in the care setting where you work. Explain to your assessor what your limitations and responsibilities were when undertaking these. Include in your explanation who delegated these tasks to you and the reasons why.

LO3 Be able to work in ways that are agreed with the employer

Getting started

Think of an occasion when you were part of a group and formed a team together. For example, this may have been in a social environment, to arrange a celebration on behalf of someone, or it could even have been when you were at school or college. How did it feel to be part of the team? How did you all work together? What different skills did each of you contribute? Why were these different skills important?

AC 3.1 Access full and up-to-date details of agreed ways of working

As you have learned, agreed ways of working refer to working practices that are used in the care setting where you work that have been agreed with your employer and set out how you will carry out your job role and its associated responsibilities.

Adult care settings are all different and therefore agreed ways of working vary between the different settings. However, all adult social care employers will have the following policies, procedures and guidelines in place.

- **Policies** are the general guidelines for the way you should work. Your setting will have many policies in place such as one for health and safety, one for handling information and one for dealing with visitors. The policies in your setting will comply with **legislation** and they will reflect the aims of the care setting. For example, in order to comply with the **Data Protection Act 2018** (see Unit 305 Handling information in adult care settings/services AC 1.1, for more details), your care setting must have in place a policy that describes how it will ensure that individuals' personal information will be kept secure at all times when being used, recorded, stored and shared.

- **Procedures** set out in detail how you should work and the ways of working that your employer expects you to follow on a day-to-day basis to ensure the policies are being put into practice. Basically, the procedures detail the processes to follow! For example, data protection procedures describe your responsibilities for handling individuals' and others' personal information. Procedures explain how to follow the data protection principles, what to do when an individual requests access to their personal information and the process to follow when you have issues or concerns. This includes the people you must report these to, such as your manager or the data protection officer who has overall responsibility for managing data when there are issues or concerns. In your setting, there will be procedures for nearly everything you do, from moving and handling, to giving medication to individuals, to how to deal with an emergency such as a fire.

- **Guidelines** set out *precise* ways of working that your employer will expect you to follow for the care of specific individuals and work activities. For example, data protection guidelines may be in place for one individual who has given strict instructions that you are not to tell their family every time they have a fall so as not to worry them. It is important that you respect the individual's right to not have this personal data shared with their family. Another example may include an individual who uses photographs to communicate with others. There may be specific guidelines in place to advise you on how to ensure that these photographs are kept secure and handled in such a way that others do not have access to them. It may be that you need to ensure that communications only take place in a private area where others cannot have access to the photographs or you may need to ensure that when the photographs are being used they are placed in a holder that can only be viewed by you and the individual.

Key terms

Legislation refers to laws that are made by the government and must be followed; these include Acts of Parliament as well as Regulations.

Data Protection Act 2018 is a set of data protection laws that protect individuals' personal information. This is the UK's implementation of the EU's General Data Protection Regulation (GDPR).

Agreed ways of working relate to many aspects of work in care settings, as Figure 1.5 shows.

Reflect on it

3.1 Your work activities and agreed ways of working

Reflect on the different work activities you carry out as part of your job role. Which 'agreed ways of working' are these related to?

Can you think of any other examples not mentioned in Figure 1.5

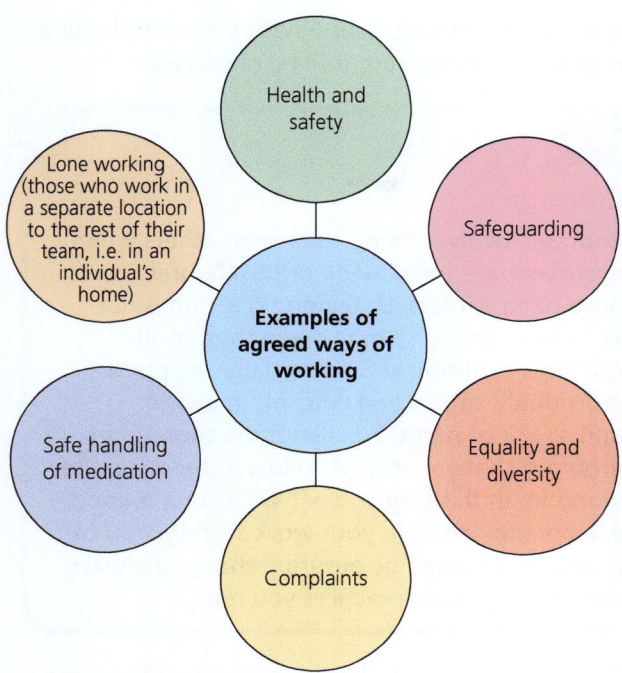

Figure 1.5 Agreed ways of working

Accessing agreed ways of working

Policies, procedures, guidelines and agreed ways of working are stored in adult care settings so that they can be accessed by workers. In this way workers can follow these when carrying out their work activities. You should remember that you will be observed while doing this as part of your assessment. In some care settings, they may be stored in the team leader's office, in others they may be stored in the staff room. In addition, there is usually a process that you must follow to gain access to them and although this varies across different care settings there are some general steps that you will be required to follow.

You should:

- request permission to access the documents from either your manager or your team leader
- read them in a private area so that others who do not need to have access to them cannot pry
- confirm that you have read and understood them by signing and dating them when you have finished.

If there are any aspects of your employer's agreed ways of working that you do not understand or are unsure about then you must seek advice from your manager. Do not sign them indicating that you have understood them if you haven't, as doing so will mean that you may not be following them as you are legally required to do. This may mean not only the loss of your job but also that you will be placing everyone's health, safety and wellbeing at risk.

Full and up-to-date details of agreed ways of working

Having access to full and up-to-date information with respect to agreed ways of working is essential for ensuring that your work practices are safe, legal and up to date. Agreed ways of working need to be updated when there are:

- **changes to legislation:** so that you can ensure that your work practices comply with legal requirements. For example, when the Data Protection Act came into force in May 2018, care settings' agreed ways of working needed to be updated to reflect this. It is important you are aware of these changes and what they will mean for your working practices so that your practices remain legal.
- **changes to best practice:** so that you can ensure that your work practices are up to date, safe and reflect current best practice. For example, first aid procedures and the actions to follow for different health emergencies are always being reviewed and updated on a regular basis depending on current research. It is important you are aware of these changes so that any actions you take are safe and do not put yourself or others in danger or at risk of harm.
- **changes to individuals' needs:** so that you can ensure that your work practices are safe and promote individuals' health, safety and wellbeing. For example, an individual's guidelines with respect to the support they require for eating and drinking may change if the individual has developed swallowing difficulties. They may require support with ensuring that they are in a comfortable position when eating and they may only be able to eat soft foods and have small sips when drinking (they may need to use a straw). It is important you are aware of the changes so that the support you provide is safe, meets the individual's needs and prevents the individual from choking.

> **Evidence opportunity**
>
> **3.1 Accessing full and up-to-date details of agreed ways of working**
>
> Your work practices will be observed for this AC.
>
> Find out who has the responsibility in the care setting where you work for maintaining and keeping the agreed ways of working complete and up to date.
>
> 1 Carry out some research in the care setting where you work. Find out where your setting's agreed ways of working are stored. Are they stored in one location? Find out the process you must follow for gaining access to them. Why is this process in place?
> 2 Produce a poster with your findings.

The information in your employer's agreed ways of working must be complete and up to date so that it provides a true and accurate picture of the requirements expected of you in your job role. You can check agreed ways of working contain full and up-to-date details by:

- checking the legislation that supports these; for example, legislation that supports the agreed ways of working may be included
- asking your manager; you could check with them whether you are reading and signing the most up-to-date version
- using your own knowledge of the individuals you provide care or support to, for example if there is a change to an individual's condition and you notice that this has not been updated on the individual's guidelines. In this situation, you would report your concerns to your manager immediately.

Your working practices will be observed to ensure that you know how to check that the agreed ways of working you access contain full details and are up to date.

AC 3.2 Demonstrate how to implement agreed ways of working within scope of own job role

Working in line with your employer's agreed ways of working, as you have learned, is an essential part of your job role and ensures that you are carrying out your work responsibilities lawfully, safely and in line with current best practice; your work practices for working in line with your employer's agreed ways of working will be observed.

> **6Cs**
>
> **Courage**
>
> Courage involves being clear with others when mistakes have been made or unsafe practices have been witnessed. Taking no action is not an option. Doing so may mean that unsafe practices continue and potentially can place individuals, others and yourself in danger and at risk of harm. You can show courage by ensuring that you always follow agreed ways of working; in this way you will be setting a good example to others in your work setting. You can also show courage by ensuring that you always report any unsafe practices you notice.

Below are some tips to help you work in line with your employer's agreed ways of working.

1 Ensure you find out where your work setting's agreed ways of working are, including how to gain access to them. Read them, and if there is something you do not understand, seek advice from your manager.
2 Ensure you only carry out work activities that have been included in the scope of your job role.
3 Attend all training and read all information updates provided to you by your employer. If you do not feel confident to carry out a work activity that you have been trained to do be honest with yourself and talk this through with your manager.
4 If you observe an unsafe working practice or if an individual, their family or a visitor brings something of this nature to your attention, ensure that you report it to your manager immediately. You will also need to make a record of these observations. Showing your **courage** in these situations will ensure that you promote your own and others' health, safety and wellbeing.
5 Be prepared to explain why you are carrying out your work activities in the way that you do, for example to the individuals who you are supporting with a daily activity or to a colleague you are working with, such as when you are both working together to assist an individual to mobilise.
6 Find out who you must report to when carrying out your work activities; ensure you do this and comply with any information or guidance that this person provides, for example this may be your manager or another senior member of the team.

7 Observe individuals, listen to their feedback (and the feedback of others) for how you carry out the work activities you are responsible for. Reflect on their feedback and use this to continue to improve your work practices.

Research it

3.2 Agreed ways of working and feedback

Carry out some research in the care setting where you work. Work with two colleagues, your manager and one other person; this could be an individual, another colleague, or a professional who visits the care setting.

Ask each person you have identified for their feedback in relation to the following:

- what they like about the way you carry out your work activities
- what work activities you carry out the best and why
- what work activities you carry out that could be improved and why.

Collate the feedback you have obtained and reflect on whether you always work in line with agreed ways of working. What could you do to improve?

Evidence opportunity

3.2 Work in line with agreed ways of working

You will be observed for this AC.

Identify two work activities you feel you are competent to carry out. Arrange for your assessor to observe you while carrying them out. Ensure that you can show that you are working within the scope of your job role and in line with your employer's agreed ways of working.

AC 3.3 Promote ways of working which contribute to the efficient use of resources by: a) reducing waste, b) managing waste to help protect the environment, c) recycling materials

Reduce, Reuse and Recycle contributes to reducing financial costs and harm to the environment. There are many different examples from adult care settings and services of ways of working that can contribute to the efficient use of resources; below are some examples of these.

Reducing waste

- In the NHS, 1.4 billion gloves are used every year. In 2018, Great Ormond Street Hospital launched their 'Gloves off' campaign which was very effective in reducing unnecessary glove use at the hospital. It then also promoted ways of working that encouraged staff to think about their apron usage too through risk assessing when aprons and gloves were needed and why they were being used, to avoid unnecessary usage. The campaign involved not just training and educating their nurses and healthcare assistants at the hospital but also other professionals who worked there such as porters, occupational therapists, physiotherapists and pharmacists. As a result of this campaign it has been estimated that in one year Great Ormond Street had saved 21 tonnes of plastic! You can read more about this campaign here: https://www.gosh.nhs.uk/news/gloves-are-off/
- Reducing waste can also be achieved by donating equipment that is no longer being used rather than disposing of it in landfill. In this way disposal costs can be reduced, for example hiring a skip or paying someone to dispose of old equipment. For example, Wrap It accepts donations of office furniture such as desks and filing cabinets as well as household furniture such as sofas and tables. Local charities in the area may also from time to time accept donations of furniture, providing it is in good condition, and may even come to collect it, saving you and others time.

Key terms

Infection refers to when germs enter the body and cause an individual to become unwell.

Managing waste to help protect the environment

- Managing waste involves using safe methods when disposing of different types of waste to help protect the environment through helping to prevent the spread of **infection**. This is achieved by implementing the colour-coded waste stream system. For example, the yellow colour waste stream is used for hygiene waste that includes items contaminated with urine,

faeces, vomit, sputum, pus or wound exudate, from individuals with no risk of known or suspected infection, such as aprons, gloves, continence pads and period products. The black colour waste stream is used for domestic waste that includes items which do not contain infectious materials, sharps or medicinal products, e.g. paper towels from hand washing, packaging, newspapers.
- How you dispose of waste is also important. Ensuring waste bags are no more than three-quarters full can prevent waste spillages by allowing sufficient space for the bag to be tied using a plastic tie or a secure knot. Similarly, placing a torn waste bag into another waste bag can prevent its contents from spilling over.
- If your role involves supporting individuals with care or support needs who live in the community you could encourage them to return any unused or old medicines to their local pharmacy for safe disposal instead of flushing them away. This will protect the environment by reducing water pollution and protecting aquatic life.
- Managing waste to help protect the environment also involves saving water. This can be achieved in the care setting or service where you work by for example only boiling the kettle with the amount of water you need, using a half flush instead of a full flush when flushing the toilet, not leaving the water running when it is not being used or immediately reporting a tap that you notice is dripping. The benefits to the environment of for example having shorter showers and only washing full loads in the washing machine as opposed to half loads could also be encouraged. These simple ways of saving water can be achieved by everyone in the care setting where you work. They could be encouraged as part of your day-to-day tasks by setting an example yourself and encouraging individuals and others you work with to do the same.
- Other ways of working which contribute to efficient use of resources and saving energy can include remembering to switch off electrical equipment no longer being used and the lights when you leave a room, and encouraging others to do the same. You could also discuss with your manager the benefits of using LED light bulbs that produce light up to 90 per cent more efficiently than other light bulbs.

Research it

3.3 Safe disposal of waste in care settings/services

Research methods for the safe disposal of waste in care settings and services. You may find the guidance produced below for care home settings useful: https://www.infectionpreventioncontrol.co.uk/content/uploads/2020/07/CH-18-Safe-disposal-of-waste-July-2020-Version-2.00.pdf

Discuss with a colleague the key safe methods you found out about.

Recycling materials

- When reducing waste isn't possible, recycling materials can contribute to protecting the environment by reducing the **carbon footprint** of the adult care setting or service you work in. Recycling services that come to the setting or service are offered by local councils and you can also take recycled materials to your local recycling centre. Materials that can be recycled can include: paper, cardboard, non-contaminated plastic, aluminium and glass. Ways to encourage recycling can include having designated recycling waste bins not just outside but in the setting/service too so they act as a reminder to recycle. You could also encourage individuals and others to take a walk down to the recycling centre to dispose of recycled materials.
- Adult care settings and services produce a lot of paper and much of it is shredded because it may contain personal, sensitive information. One way that paper waste can be reduced is by thinking about what needs to be shredded, in other words you could shred the page that contains sensitive information and recycle the rest. You could also consider setting your printers to default to 'double side' and photocopy double sided where possible to encourage full use of every page that is printed; the back of some pages may also be used for scrap paper providing they do not contain any personal or sensitive information.

Key term

Carbon footprint refers to how you measure the total greenhouse gas emissions caused by a person, organisation, service, event or product.

> **Reflect on it**
>
> **3.3 Recycling materials in your workplace**
>
> Keep a diary for one week and make a note of the materials that you recycled in the care setting or service where you worked. Reflect on how much you recycled and think about the following questions.
>
> - Could you have recycled more? If so, why didn't you?
> - How can you recycle more the following week when you're at work?
> - How can you encourage individuals and others to do the same?

> **Evidence opportunity**
>
> **3.3 Working to reduce waste and improve recycling**
>
> Through discussion with your manager, develop a plan for promoting ways of working that reduce waste, manage waste to help protect the environment and recycle materials.
>
> Agree with your manager to review your plan after you have put it into practice and discuss which ways of working were most effective and any areas where further improvements are needed.

LO4 Be able to work in partnership with others

AC 4.1 Demonstrate ways of working that can help improve partnership working

As you will have learned there are many benefits to partnership working and so it is important that you are able to recognise this and show you are able to demonstrate different approaches and methods that can help improve partnership working. For this assessment criterion you will be observed as part of your assessment.

Below are some useful tips to help you do this.

1. **Be clear about your own roles and responsibilities** and show your understanding of the role and responsibilities of all those who you work in partnership with. This encourages mutual trust and respect because it involves recognising and encouraging your own and others' contributions.
2. **Communicate well** and consistently by being honest, listening actively, showing a genuine interest. This also means making sure that the different 'partners' are kept informed of any information that they should know. This is essential for learning from one another, sharing ideas and working practices and ensuring your relationships are open and honest. You may find it useful to refer to Unit 304 Effective communication in adult care settings/services.
3. **Work to shared goals and objectives** so that everyone is working together to support individuals to achieve their goals. Working to shared goals and objectives also means that everyone will be working as one team consistently to provide good-quality care.
4. **Involve others in planning, discussions and decision making** so that partners feel included and everyone can come to an agreement about the best course of action together. This also means that you can draw on everyone's expertise and that the different areas of expertise inform the decision. For example, you may need to make decisions about an individual's medication with the help of your manager, the individual's GP and their family.
5. **Be a role model** to others by being professional and trustworthy, by using positive language and showing positive behaviours, such as open communication, being punctual and polite. This is essential for others respecting you and looking to you to lead by example.
6. **Be supportive** by showing you have a genuine interest in individuals' wellbeing and showing that you recognise and value others' contributions, values and beliefs which may be different to your own. Value the people you work with, what they bring to the team, draw on their knowledge and expertise, show that you value them in team meetings, or even during one-to-one meetings.
7. **Show your passion, commitment and enjoyment of working together** with other people to achieve positive outcomes for individuals. This is essential for enabling everyone involved to feel comfortable and motivated to work with you.
8. **Agree to work together as one team.** This is essential for achieving agreed goals and involves you obtaining and providing information about the progress of the goals,

whether there have been any difficulties in achieving them, and what needs to be done to resolve these difficulties. This involves sharing good practices as well as learning together from mistakes made.

> ### Evidence opportunity
>
> **4.1 Demonstrate ways of working that can help improve partnership working**
>
> Demonstrate to your assessor a situation that involves you working in partnership with others in the care setting where you work. For example, this may be working with a colleague when moving and positioning an individual, or meeting with an individual and their family to discuss the care the individual is receiving from you. Alternatively, it might be carrying out a group activity working alongside your colleagues and other professionals such as music therapists or drama teachers.

AC 4.2 Demonstrate different skills and approaches used when working in partnership with others

As you will have learned in AC 1.5 of this unit there are many different skills and approaches used when working in partnership with others. For this assessment criterion you will be observed as part of your assessment. In the following table are some questions about working in partnership with others that you could ask yourself and that will help you think about how you can demonstrate to your assessor the skills and approaches you have and use.

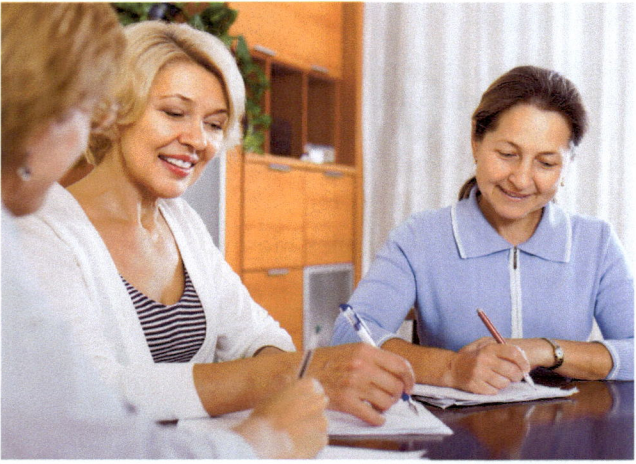

Figure 1.6 How do you work in partnership with others?

> ### Evidence opportunity
>
> **AC 4.2 Different skills and approaches used when working in partnership with others**
>
> Demonstrate to your assessor a situation that involves you working with others in the care setting where you work. For example, this may be supporting an activity or having a discussion with an individual and/or their family about their care and support. Show your assessor the different skills and approaches you have and use with others.

Table 1.4 Skills and approaches used for working in partnership with others

Working in partnership skills and approaches	How I can demonstrate this
Being an effective communicator	How do I communicate when I work with others? What communication skills do I use and why? Why do I adapt my communication skills with different people I work with? How do my communication skills impact on the relationships I develop when working in partnership with others?
Being honest	Am I honest with others? How do I do this and why? How does being honest impact on open and approachable communications when working in partnership with others?
Being empathetic	How do I show empathy when working with others? Why is this important? How does showing empathy impact on mutual respect when working in partnership with others?
Being assertive	How do I ensure all my communications with others are clear and confident? Why is this important? How does being assertive impact on mutual trust when working in partnership with others?

Table 1.4 Skills and approaches used for working in partnership with others *continued*

Working in partnership skills and approaches	How I can demonstrate this
Being enthusiastic	How do I ensure that I show I'm willing to work in partnership with others? How do I do this and why? How does being enthusiastic impact on team building when working in partnership with others?
Being able to negotiate	How do I ensure that I'm able to reach a mutual agreement or compromise with others? How does this benefit the team's working practices?
Being able to resolve conflicts and/or differences of opinion	How do I ensure I play my part in trying to work together with others to resolve conflicts and/or differences of opinion that may arise? Why is this important? How does this encourage positive teamwork?
Being positive	How do I ensure that I'm being constructive when working in partnership with others? How does this encourage mutual respect?

6Cs

Compassion

Working in partnership with others requires compassion because without it you would not be able to work alongside others effectively. Being compassionate involves being kind, polite and empathetic towards others and their situations. Showing compassion therefore is an essential skill to have.

Legislation	
Act/Regulation	**Key points**
Civil Partnership Act 2004	You can get married or form a civil partnership in the UK if you are: 16 or over, free to marry or form a civil partnership (i.e. single, divorced or widowed), not closely related. You need permission from your parents or guardians if you are under 18 in England, Wales and Northern Ireland.
Data Protection Act 2018 (the UK's implementation of the EU's GDPR)	Employers must ensure the secure handling of all information and data. Adult care settings therefore have policies, procedures and agreed ways of working in place to ensure that individuals' personal information is kept secure and handled lawfully when recorded, used, stored and shared.
	In May 2018, the Data Protection Act came into force. It provides detailed guidance to organisations on how to govern and manage people's personal information and this will need to be included in the care setting's policies, procedures, guidelines and agreed ways of working.

301 Safeguarding and protection in adult care settings/services

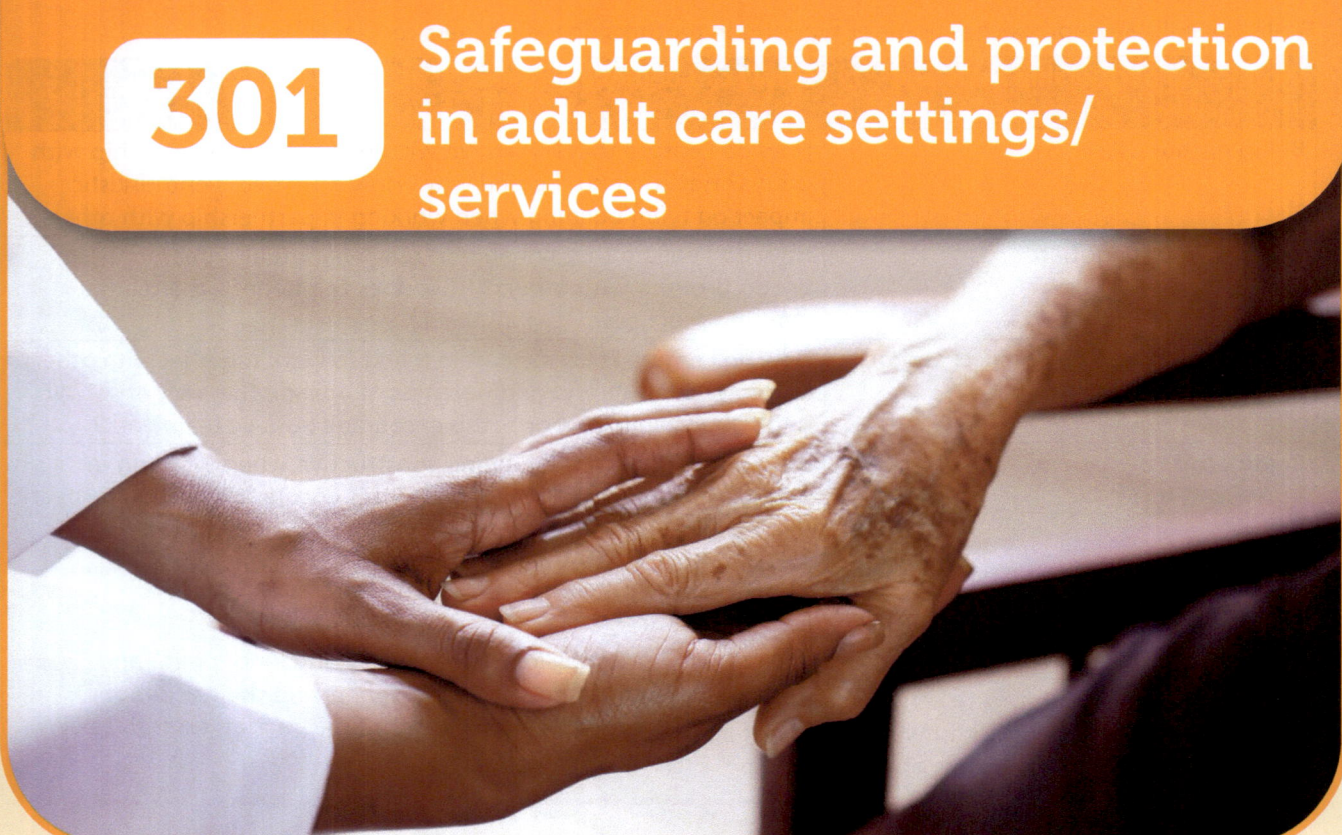

About this unit

Credit value: 3
Guided learning hours: 24

One of the most important aspects of your role as an adult care worker is to protect individuals with care or support needs. In this unit you will find out about the legislation, principles, national policies, frameworks and local systems that are in place to help safeguard individuals from abuse and improper treatment. This unit will also equip you with the principles that underpin safeguarding adults, including understanding and recognising the different types of abuse, as well as the factors that may contribute to making an individual more vulnerable to abuse and improper treatment.

You will explore your safeguarding role, and your responsibilities for responding to suspicions and disclosures of abuse and improper treatment, and understanding how to reduce the likelihood of abuse or neglect from happening.

Finally, you will learn about recognising and reporting unsafe practices, and you will see how understanding the principles of online safety will ensure that you carry out your duty of care.

Learning outcomes

By the end of this unit you will:

LO1: Understand the national and local context of safeguarding and protection from abuse and improper treatment

LO2: Understand principles of safeguarding adults

LO3: Know how to recognise signs of abuse and improper treatment

LO4: Know how to respond to suspected or disclosed abuse and improper treatment

LO5: Understand ways to reduce the likelihood of abuse or neglect

LO6: Know how to recognise and report unsafe practices

LO7: Understand the principles of online safety

LO1 Understand the national and local context of safeguarding and protection from abuse and improper treatment

> **Getting started**
>
> Think about a case of abuse you have heard about in the media. You may have read about a case in the newspaper or heard about it on television. What happened? Which organisations were involved in safeguarding the individual? For example, adult social care services or the police?
>
> Now think about the care setting where you work; who safeguards the individuals you provide care or support to in your care setting? What is your role?

AC 1.1 Outline relevant legislation, principles, national policies, frameworks and local systems that relate to safeguarding and protection from abuse and improper treatment

Abuse occurs when someone is mistreated in a way that causes them pain and hurt. This can mean physical, sexual, psychological or mental abuse. Neglecting an individual, not caring for their needs and improper treatment are also forms of abuse. Improper treatment may include degrading and humiliating treatment, rough treatment, disproportionate and unnecessary restraint and threatening behaviour. You will learn more about what these terms mean in LO2.

Safeguarding the individuals you work with from abuse and improper treatment involves learning about the current legislation, principles, national policies, frameworks and **local systems** that are in place for safeguarding adults. Legislation, policies and systems change and are updated so it is important that you keep your knowledge up to date. You can do this by attending updated training, reading through updated information provided by your employer and regularly referring to the government's website (www.gov.uk). You should also refer to Unit 313, AC 1.4 on personal development and LO2 about keeping up to date with your knowledge and work practices.

Legislation

Table 2.1 provides some useful information about the current legislation that exists in relation to safeguarding adults.

Table 2.1 Legislation and how it safeguards individuals

Legislation	How it safeguards adults
Modern Slavery Act 2015	• Aimed at tackling slavery, servitude and forced or compulsory labour in the UK • Addresses issues such as human trafficking and the exploitation of people
Care Act 2014	• Identifies the ten types of abuse and **neglect** that individuals may experience • States that individuals' safety and wellbeing must be promoted to safeguard them from abuse and neglect • States that organisations must work in partnership to keep individuals safe • States that effective safeguarding policies and procedures must be developed • Established the role of **Safeguarding Adults Boards (SAB)** • States that individuals must have access to representation during the safeguarding process, for example access to an **advocate**. The right to an advocate is one of the areas specifically covered in the legislation
Health and Social Care Act 2012	• States that services such as health and social services (now adult social care services) must work in partnership to improve the care provided to individuals • Established the role of **clinical commissioning groups (CCGs)** to safeguard individuals who access health and social care services, for example by responding to abuse and neglect that takes place, undertaking enquiries or reviews of services where abuse or neglect has taken place • Established the role of **health and wellbeing boards** to oversee the provision of services in each local area

Table 2.1 Legislation and how it safeguards individuals *continued*

Legislation	How it safeguards adults
Equality Act 2010	• Safeguards individuals from unfair treatment and **discrimination** • Makes it unlawful to discriminate against individuals based on one of the following protected characteristics: age, disability, gender reassignment, marriage and civil partnership, pregnancy and maternity, race, religion or belief, sex and sexual orientation
Safeguarding Vulnerable Groups Act 2006	• Established the **Vetting and Barring Scheme** that prevents people who are not suitable to work with individuals with care or support needs from doing so • Established the Independent Safeguarding Authority (ISA) which later merged with the Criminal Records Bureau (CRB) to become the **Disclosure and Barring Service (DBS)**

Mental Capacity Act 2005	• Safeguards individuals who are unable to make choices and decisions for themselves because they lack the **mental capacity** to do so, i.e. due to an illness or a disability
	• Based on five key principles:
	  1 Always assume that individuals are able to make their own decisions; never assume a **lack of capacity** to do so
	  2 Support individuals so that they can make their own choices and decisions
	  3 Respect individuals' rights to make decisions that others may not agree with
	  4 All decisions made on an individual's behalf, i.e. when they lack capacity, must always be in their best interests
	  5 Decisions made on an individual's behalf must be the least restrictive option, i.e. the option that promotes the individual's rights as much as possible

Mental Capacity (Amendment) Act 2008:	• Amends the Mental Capacity Act 2005 and introduces the Deprivation of Liberty Safeguards (DoLS). • The DoLS safeguards individuals from having their liberty deprived unlawfully. For example, a setting such as a care home is required to seek authorisation to deprive an individual of their liberty because they feel it is in the individual's best interests.
Mental Capacity Act (Amendment) Act 2019	• Replaced DoLS which was introduced by an earlier amendment to the Mental Capacity Act in 2008 with the Liberty Protection Safeguards (LPS). The LPS provided a streamlined process to authorise deprivations of liberty for persons who lack capacity.
Mental Health Act 1983	• Gives rights to individuals with mental health needs • Promotes individuals' rights when being assessed and treated in hospital, for example **consent** to medical treatment, and individuals' rights when being treated in the community, for example receiving aftercare
Human Rights Act 1998	• Gives rights to every individual who lives in the UK, such as the right to life, right to liberty and security, and prohibition of slavery and forced labour • Promotes individuals' rights to respect, freedom, privacy, **equality**, dignity and fairness • Includes individuals' rights to live safely, independently and not to be harmed or treated cruelly
Female Genital Mutilation Act 2003	• Made it illegal to perform **female genital mutilation (FGM)**, including assisting a child or adult to mutilate their own genitalia • Extended the previous legislation by making it an illegal act for UK nationals to perform FGM outside the UK
Data Protection Act 2018	• Promotes individuals' rights to security over the use of their personal information by others, for example restricts who can access their data, how long it can be kept for • Promotes individuals' rights to privacy over the use of their personal information by others, for example gives individuals rights to access their own data and ensure it is accurate and up to date • See Unit 305 Handling information in adult care settings/services, AC 1.1, for more information.
The Public Interest Disclosure Act 1998	• Protects workers who disclose information about malpractice, including abuse at their current or former workplace for example, by ensuring organisations have **whistleblowing** procedures in place • Promotes individuals' rights to be protected from abuse or harm by ensuring any suspicions or **disclosure of abuse** can be reported by workers free from fear or repercussions from their employers

Research it

1.1 Legislation

There are various other pieces of legislation that protect people from abuse. These include the Sexual Offences Act 2003, the Health and Safety at Work Act 1974, Mental Health Act 1983, Family Law Act 1996, Criminal Justice Act 1998, Care Standards Act 2000, Protection of Vulnerable Groups 2007, Protection from Harassment 1997, Fraud Act 2006 and Office of the Public Guardian.

Research three pieces of legislation that are relevant to safeguarding and protecting adults from abuse. For each one, identify the reasons why they are relevant. Produce a poster with your findings. You will find the UK Government's website a useful source of information: www.gov.uk

You may also wish to do some research into how health and social care policy has evolved over the years. You may find it useful to read 'Our Health, Our Care, Our Say'.

Key terms

Abuse occurs when someone is mistreated in a way that causes them pain and hurt. This does not just mean physical abuse but can also mean sexual or psychological or mental abuse. Neglecting someone and not caring for their needs is also a form of abuse. It is important to be aware of the different types of abuse because you will be working with vulnerable people.

Neglect means failing to care for someone so that their needs are not met. See Table 2.4 for more information on neglect. Also see AC 2.1 for a description of the term 'self-neglect'.

Local systems may include employers' safeguarding policies and procedures as well as multi-agency protection arrangements for your local area, for example a Safeguarding Adults Board.

Safeguarding Adults Boards (SAB) safeguard adults with care or support needs by overseeing local adult safeguarding systems and ensuring all organisations work in partnership. See AC 1.2 for more information on these.

Clinical commissioning groups are organisations that are responsible for the provision of NHS services in England.

Health and wellbeing boards are health and social care organisations that work together to improve the health and wellbeing of the people living in the local area they are responsible for.

Discrimination means treating people unfairly or unlawfully, because they have a disability, or are of a different race, gender or age, for example.

Vetting and Barring Scheme ensures that anyone who is not fit or appropriate to work with adults and children does not do so.

Disclosure and Barring Service (DBS) is a government service that makes background checks for organisations on people who want to work with children or adults with care or support needs.

Mental capacity refers to an individual's ability to make decisions and give consent.

Lack of capacity is a term used to refer to when an individual is unable to make a decision for themselves because of a learning disability, a condition such as dementia or a mental health need, or because they are unconscious.

Consent refers to informed agreement to an action or decision; the process of establishing consent will vary according to an individual's capacity to consent.

Equality refers to ensuring equal opportunities are provided to everyone irrespective of their differences such as ages, abilities, backgrounds, religions. In an adult care setting, this also means making sure that everyone is entitled to the same rights, and opportunities.

Female genital mutilation (FGM) refers to a practice where the female genitals are deliberately cut, injured or changed and might be done because of cultural beliefs.

Whistleblowing refers to when a person exposes any kind of information or activity that is deemed illegal, unethical or not correct, for example unsafe practices, abuse, harm.

Disclosure of abuse is when an individual tells you that abuse has happened, or is happening to them.

Principles for safeguarding are the basis for how best to safeguard adults from abuse and improper treatment, and they apply to all health and social care settings. There are six principles of safeguarding, and these form part of the Care Act. (You may find it useful to refer back to the legislation table on pages 33–34.)

Table 2.2 Principles for safeguarding

Safeguarding principle	How it safeguards adults
1 Empowerment	This principle states that individuals must be supported to make their own choices and decisions. If an individual lacks capacity to make their own decisions, due to an illness or disability, for example, then they can be supported to access advocacy services to ensure their views and feelings are known and are represented. Empowerment can be achieved, for example, by ensuring that individuals are provided with all the necessary information to make an informed choice, including all the options that are available, their potential benefits, consequences and any risks.
2 Prevention	This principle states that prevention of abuse and improper treatment can only happen if action is taken; doing nothing is not an option and may result in individuals being placed in danger and harmed. For example, by attending safeguarding training and raising awareness of how to recognise signs of abuse and improper treatment you can respond early to any signs that abuse and improper treatment may be happening. (You'll learn more about indicators of abuse and improper treatment in LO3 of this unit).
3 Proportionality	This principle states that the least intrusive method must be used when responding to a safeguarding concern, for example by assessing the risk presented by considering whether the individual's life is in danger. If it is, then the safeguarding concern needs to be responded to by, for example, informing the Police immediately. If it isn't, then reporting it to the Safeguarding Lead may be sufficient.
4 Protection	This principle states that individuals must be supported and their interests represented to ensure that they are protected from harm, for example by all those who work with them understanding how to respond to safeguarding concerns when they arise, including preventing the abuse and improper treatment from getting worse, and by supporting the individual through the safeguarding process.
5 Partnership	This principle states that organisations and local communities (which individuals are part of) must work together to safeguard individuals from abuse and improper treatment. For example, organisations raising awareness amongst local communities of the indicators that abuse and improper treatment may be happening, can mean that individuals are more likely to be protected from harm.
6 Accountability	This principle states that safeguarding is everyone's responsibility, because everyone is responsible for keeping individuals safe. For example, everyone should recognise that it is their duty to report any safeguarding concerns they have about an individual, irrespective of who they are, i.e. the individual's carer, physiotherapist, relative, friend or neighbour.

Reflect on it

1.1 Safeguarding principles

Reflect on the six safeguarding principles that you learned about. How can you embed them into your safeguarding practice? Why are these principles important?

National policies, frameworks and local systems

As well as legislation and principles there are also policies that apply nationally across England. There are also local systems in place for safeguarding adults who have care or support needs. Table 2.3 gives you some examples of both.

Table 2.3 National policies, frameworks and local systems, and how they safeguard adults

National Safeguarding Policies and frameworks	How it safeguards adults
Safeguarding Adults: A National Framework of Standards for Good Practice and Outcomes in Adult Protection Work 2011	It is published by the **Association of Directors of Adult Social Services (ADASS)**. It safeguards individuals by providing best practice guidance to those in leadership roles in services. This is so that individuals who have care or support needs can have access to (care and support) services that are more effective in terms of safeguarding them from abuse and neglect.
Safeguarding Strategy 2019 - 2025: Office of the Public Guardian	OPG set out how they plan to improve their safeguarding strategy by increasing awareness amongst their safeguarding partners of OPG's role and responsibilities, working more closely with safeguarding partners, dealing with all reported concerns, encouraging working practices that put individuals first and providing greater support for individuals.
A Vision for Adult Social Care: Capable Communities and Active Citizens 2010	Published by the Department of Health (DoH). It promotes individuals' rights to take control of their care by ensuring information about care services is made available to individuals, therefore making them less likely to be abused or harmed. Promotes working in partnership between individuals and other agencies to ensure individuals are active partners in their care, for example in care services, housing services, the NHS. This is to reduce individuals' risk of being abused or neglected.
Think Personal: Act Local 2010	Established as a national initiative that ensures individuals who have care or support needs are the focus in their care or support, for example by promoting person-centred ways of working. Promotes individuals and other agencies working in partnership to provide effective care and support services that are person-centred.
Dignity in Care 2006	An ongoing campaign that aims to improve the quality of care or the support individuals receive in adult care services. It promotes person-centred ways of working that include showing respect for individuals' rights to make their own choices and decisions thus reducing their risk of being abused or harmed.
Professional Registration and Standards	Requires professionals, for example doctors, nurses and social workers, to register with a professional body so that they can ensure they are practising to the current **standards** and continuing their professional development. Organisations such as **Skills for Care** publish codes of conduct and standards for adult care workers so that they can comply with best practice standards when carrying out their job role. For example, the Code of Conduct for Healthcare Support Workers and Adult Social Care Workers in England, The Care Certificate Standard 10 Safeguarding Adults. The Care Quality Commission regulates adult care services and sets the Fundamental Standards of Quality and Safety for all those organisations registered with them who provide care services. These Fundamental Standards are essential for preventing abuse, harm and neglect of adults.

➔

Table 2.3 National policies, frameworks and local systems, and how they safeguard adults *continued*

National Safeguarding Policies and frameworks	How it safeguards adults
Safeguarding Adults Boards (SAB)	Local authorities are responsible for setting up a SAB.
	Provide strategies to safeguard individuals but also to deal with issues that affect specific individuals. For example, they can decide that they need to increase awareness of abuse in the local area through publicity, or they may deal with complaints around abuse against a care worker in a setting.
	Made up, for example, of different agencies including the police, housing, transport all of whom can bring their expertise to a situation. This is what is meant by multi-agency working (see AC 1.2 for further information).
	A SAB is responsible for arranging a Safeguarding Adults Review (SAR) when an adult in its locality dies as a result of being abused or neglected or if there are suspicions that an adult may have experienced abuse or neglect because agencies such as care services, health services could have worked together more effectively.
Organisations' policies and procedures	All adult care services are required to have safeguarding policies and procedures in place – ones that define the different types of abuse and neglect, set out how individuals will be safeguarded, how to report concerns and arrangements for whistleblowing.

Key terms

The **Association of Directors of Adult Social Services (ADASS)** is a charity whose members are active directors of social care services and whose aim is to promote high standards of social care services.

Standards may include codes of conduct and practice, regulations, minimum standards, National Occupational Standards.

Skills for Care is the Sector Skills Council for people working in social work and social care for adults and children in the UK as well as for workers in early years, children and young people's services. It sets standards and develops qualifications for those working in the sector.

Evidence opportunity

1.1 Legislation, policies, frameworks

Research and reflect on the national policies, frameworks and systems that influence the safeguarding arrangements in place at the care setting where you work. Why are these important? How do they impact on your ability to safeguard and protect the individuals you provide care for?

Make some notes on your thoughts and then produce a one-page information handout that identifies examples of relevant legislation, national policies and local systems that are in place to safeguard and protect adults from abuse.

AC 1.2 Describe the roles of different agencies in safeguarding and protecting an individual's right to live in safety and be free from abuse and improper treatment

As you will know, safeguarding and protecting individuals from abuse is achieved by agencies working together in partnership. The important work of these agencies recognises that:

- all individuals must be supported to be in control of their lives and their care or support
- all individuals have a right to live their lives in safety and free from abuse or being at risk of abuse
- everyone has a role to play in preventing abuse from happening and responding to abuse when it occurs.

The following are some examples of the important roles different agencies play in safeguarding and protecting individuals from abuse.

The Police work with other agencies such as the local authority's adult and children's social care services health services and education services to safeguard individuals who may be at risk of abuse or improper treatment.

The **regulatory body**, the **Care Quality Commission**, is responsible for regulating the provision of health and care services by monitoring care and support services to ensure they safeguard and protect individuals from abuse and improper treatment. The Care Quality Commission also ensures that best practice is highlighted and shared with, for example, organisations and local Safeguarding Adult Boards (SABs). They can also raise their concerns with SABs if they find a service is placing individuals at risk of being abused.

The **Office of the Public Guardian (OPG)** helps individuals remain in control of their decisions about their health and finance by supporting people to make decisions on behalf of those who are unable to decide for themselves. The OCG also helps people to plan for others to make decision for them should they lose the mental capacity to do so.

Safeguarding Adults Boards (SABs) are responsible for working with agencies in each local authority to ensure they develop effective systems for safeguarding and protecting individuals from abuse. SABs ensure that agencies work in consistent ways, for example by sharing information about individuals who may be at risk of abuse. They can respond to abuse quickly and work in partnership to ensure individuals' rights, safety and wellbeing are protected by all agencies working with them. SABs also promote agencies working together to share good practice so that they can learn from one another.

Adult and children social care services are responsible for overseeing and co-ordinating how different agencies work in partnership to safeguard and protect children, young people and adults from abuse and improper treatment.

Local authorities are responsible for setting up Local Safeguarding Adults Boards, so that they can ensure that all agencies are working together in partnership to ensure individuals are being safeguarded and protected from abuse. They will ensure that agencies are working to the same consistent standards and ensuring positive outcomes for all individuals with care or support needs. For children, the Children and Social Work Act 2017 replaced local safeguarding children boards with multi-agency safeguarding arrangements that came into force in 2019.

The **Disclosure and barring service** provides organisations with information regarding criminal records and barring decisions of people who want to work with individuals with support needs. This agency safeguards individuals by preventing organisations from recruiting unsuitable people to work with individuals. The DBS provides free information, support and advice to employers to ensure that they recruit safely. For example, in April 2022, DBS and Skills for Care provided free training to social care providers across the Midlands, to support safer recruitment in adult social care by providing a better understanding of DBS checks and barring referrals.

Voluntary agencies are responsible for providing independent advice and support to individuals, their families and workers in relation to safeguarding and protection from abuse. These include Hourglass, ADASS, and whistleblowing helplines. Voluntary agencies can provide useful information and much needed support; for example, when an individual is being abused or an individual's family is worried that they may be at risk of being abused.

Health and social care settings are responsible for developing policies, procedures and agreed ways of working to ensure individuals are safeguarded and protected from abuse. Each service is also responsible for ensuring their care workers are fully trained in these areas. Care workers should inform the individuals they care for about what abuse is so the individual is in control of their own care and support, and is less likely to be abused.

> **Evidence opportunity**
>
> **1.2 Roles of different agencies**
>
> Research the safeguarding procedures in place for the local authority where your care setting is located. Find out about the different agencies that your local authority works in partnership with to safeguard adults from abuse. You will find your local authority's website a useful source of information. Discuss the roles of each agency with your manager and obtain a witness testimony.
>
> Produce a leaflet that explains the roles of these different agencies, the professionals who work for them and how the different agencies work together. Include the key responsibilities for safeguarding and protecting the individuals for whom you provide care.

AC 1.3 Evaluate how reports into serious failures in upholding an individual's right to live free from abuse have influenced current practice

When safeguarding systems and the agencies who work together to safeguard adults from abuse and neglect are not as effective as they should be then this has very serious consequences that can result in serious failures to safeguard and protect individuals from abuse. It is these serious failures that are reported in the media and through which the public becomes aware of how care and support services for individuals can fail them. You may have heard of some of the following examples where care has gone wrong and where settings failed to protect individuals from abuse:

- Wyton Abbey Residential Home – where an individual with dementia who was on a two-week stay at the care home did not receive the care and treatment they required, which resulted in their death
- Winterbourne View Hospital – where individuals with **learning disabilities** were abused and neglected by the staff who worked there
- Purbeck Care Home – where individuals at a care home were abused by staff.

After a serious failure in safeguarding to protect individuals from abuse has occurred a Safeguarding Adults Review will take place. It is a detailed process that reviews:

- the abuse that happened
- how it happened
- what allowed it to happen
- how it could have been prevented
- what needs to be changed in order to prevent it from happening again
- the key lessons learned.

Safeguarding Adults Reviews also review the services provided by each organisation.

Once the Safeguarding Adults Review (previously known as a Serious Case Review) is completed, a report of its findings is published and made public so that everyone can learn from its key findings and prevent abuse from occurring again. For example:

- The Safeguarding Adults Review report, published in 2021, concerned the deaths of three adults, Joanna, Jon and Ben, who had learning disabilities and had been patients at Cawston Park Hospital, a private hospital in Norfolk, registered with the Care Quality Commission for the assessment and medical treatment for people detained under the Mental Health Act 1983.
- Joanna, Jon and Ben had been admitted to the hospital under sections of the Mental Health Act (1983), and were all listed as people whose behaviour could challenge services and sometimes their families too. All three died between April 2018 and July 2020.
- During the review process, the families and friends of these three adults said that they were concerned about the way the hospital had worked with their relatives, and stated that the Hospital did not spend time trying to find out why their relatives were unwell or distressed.
- Their main concerns included: staff using **restraint** and **seclusion** too much and without the right training, putting individuals in groups which were not safe, giving individuals too much medication, leaving individuals often with no activities, and records not being kept about individuals. For example, information about Ben's care was not written down for more than a year.

> **Key terms**
>
> **Learning disability** refers to reduced ability to think and make decisions as well as difficulty with everyday activities which affects a person for their whole life. This may, for example, include difficulties with budgeting, shopping and planning a train journey.
>
> **Restraint** is when an individual is held to stop them from moving.
>
> **Seclusion** is when an individual is moved to a separate room or space, away from other people.

The Review influenced current practice by setting out recommendations for changes, as well as key areas for learning and improvement to prevent the abuse from happening again. Some of the main recommendations are outlined below:

- **Communication** – a very high number of the placements for individuals were commissioned by different providers, which meant that face-to-face reviews were rare and Norfolk agencies were often unaware of the individuals who lived there. Communication and information sharing needs to be improved for both day to day care and safeguarding issues.
- **Professional curiosity and challenge** – the quality of reviews and advocacy was poor. Visiting practitioners missed opportunities to ask questions on behalf of the individuals living there. Practitioners must not take things they are told at face value, they should ask for evidence and make sure they are listening to the voice of the person, not just the provider of the service.
- **Transitions** – some of the individuals had experienced a high number of moves in their lifetimes, sometimes at very short notice. The impact on individuals of moving from one setting to another, especially when poorly planned or rushed, must be considered by practitioners, including how it may influence their behaviour and the support that they may need.
- **Support for individuals with behaviours that challenge others** – physical interventions were used with many individuals with no consideration of the cause and potential triggers to prevent their presenting behaviours occurring in the first place. Practitioners must consider all behaviours as communication, and it is for practitioners to try and understand what the individual may be trying to communicate, without making any assumptions. In addition, the impact of the lack of meaningful activity on individuals' physical, emotional and psychological health must also be taken into account. Without activity, individuals can become bored, frustrated, gain weight and lose motivation.
- **Support for staff** – individuals living at the hospital racially abused staff on a regular basis. The hospital did little to address this and staff also did not report these incidents when they happened. It is important that all incidents are reported, irrespective of who is perpetrating them and who they are towards; not doing so can lead to difficult work environments and can impact on the quality of the care provided.
- **Taking action when the individual being abused doesn't want to complain** – individuals living at the hospital said they did not want to make a complaint and staff accepted this. Staff need to ensure that they take action when an individual does not want to complain, such as exploring why they may feel this way, i.e. perhaps the person feels things may get worse for them, or that there is no point because nothing changes. It is important that staff help individuals understand more about safeguarding, as well as their responsibility to protect them when they're being supported in the service. It is also important that staff are aware that in certain situations information may still need to be shared or action taken, especially if the individual may be a risk.
- **Prevention** – preventing abuse from taking place is very important and the review identified a number of areas where this could have been improved. For example, for providers to carry out regular risk assessments, for visiting practitioners to ask questions, staff to involve and listen to individuals' family and friends, staff to use individuals' family and friends' views and insights to inform how individuals' care and support is provided.

In 2019, The Safeguarding Adults Review report for the death of Jo-Jo was published. Jo-Jo was aged 28 and had Downs Syndrome and a learning disability. She lived with her mother and her step-father. Jo-Jo's mother was her main carer: she supported her with her personal care, nutrition and managing her finances.

- Jo-Jo had eczema when she was a child and she continued to have severe eczema into adulthood on her whole body. Jo-Jo's support plan of 2016 stated that she needed support to maintain her personal care, including in relation to her skin condition.
- In 2017, Jo-Jo died in hospital after being taken there by ambulance for an emergency dermatology appointment arranged by the GP who had visited Jo-Jo at home the day before.
- Jo-Jo's body was found to have been in a very neglected state and had the presence of a severe scabies infection.

The Review influenced current practice by setting out recommendations for changes, as well as key areas for learning and improvement to prevent the abuse from happening again. Some of the main changes are outlined below:

- **Communication** – Jo-Jo experienced poor standards of care, including poor co-ordination of her care. For example, there was little communication between those involved in Jo-Jo's care, i.e. her mother, the GP, the dermatologist, about how the care for Jo-Jo's skin was going to be managed and by whom. Jo-Jo's mother frequently suspended and then reinstated her engagement with practitioners and services. Support plans must set out clearly an individual's care and support needs, what they are, what the ongoing risks are, how the risks are going to be managed and by whom.
- **Continuity of care** – Jo-Jo did not have a regular social worker in 2016. Jo-Jo appeared to have seen numerous GPs at her practice. It's important that there is one named professional in every service who has responsibility for an individual's ongoing needs, including the monitoring of their health, thus ensuring the continuity of care for individuals who may be vulnerable, i.e. such as Jo-Jo, because she had a learning disability.
- **Taking action when the individual is at risk** – Jo-Jo was not sent to hospital when the GP visited, despite knowing that Jo-Jo was unwell, incoherent and unable to stand. Access to emergency care for individuals must not be denied when it is evident an individual is unwell and at risk.

- **Mental capacity (see Unit 302)** – Jo-Jo was not consulted and her wishes were not taken into account when her mother suspended her engagement with services. No-one questioned Jo-Jo's mother, everyone assumed she was acting in Jo-Jo's best interests. A mental capacity assessment must be carried out with an individual who has care and support needs.
- **Support for carers** – Jo-Jo's mother was not offered a carer's assessment of her needs and therefore no one asked her what support she needed. A carer's needs must be assessed and reviewed to assess whether more support is required at home. In addition, Jo-Jo's mother did not recognise the deterioration in Jo-Jo's health until it proved to be fatal. Support to carers to raise awareness of early warning signs of physical health deterioration and report on signs that they see must be provided through the practitioners and services they access.
- **Prevention** – preventing this type of neglect from taking place is very important, and the review identified a number of areas where this could have been improved. For example, ensuring that all individuals with learning disabilities have a named doctor involved in their care because of their increased vulnerability, having a follow up system in place for when an individual fails to attend their appointments so any health issues can be identified early, i.e. Jo-Jo failed to attend her annual health check at her GP practice and her dermatologist's outpatient appointments and there was no follow up.

Evidence opportunity

1.3 Reports into serious failures

Research a Safeguarding Adults Review that has been published following a case of an individual or individuals who have been abused.

Read through this and then produce a report on the different factors that featured in the abuse and neglect, including how it upheld the individuals' rights to live free from abuse and how it influenced current practice.

You will find the internet a useful source of information; each local authority will also publish all the reports that it has completed on its website.

> **Reflect on it**
>
> **1.3 Abuse reported in the media**
>
> Reflect on a case of abuse and neglect you have heard about in the media. For example, this may be one of the care settings listed in this section, or perhaps another example reported in your local area. How did the news report make you feel?
>
> Now imagine you were the individual, or a member of this individual's family – how do you think this made them feel?

Responding to abuse is everyone's responsibility and although we can all learn lessons from reports published into serious failures to protect individuals from abuse, it is important that you are able to recognise and respond to individuals at risk from abuse so that you can safeguard and protect them from being abused and neglected.

AC 1.4 Outline sources of information and advice about your own role in a) safeguarding and protecting individuals from abuse, b) whistleblowing, c) accountability for decision making, d) information sharing

Safeguarding and protecting individuals from abuse

To understand your role and responsibilities in safeguarding and protecting individuals from abuse you may need to seek further information and advice from the care setting where you work. This can include:

- **Your manager** will be able to guide you on how to carry out the job you are employed to do in ways that safeguard individuals and protect them from abuse. Your manager can guide you with any aspect you are unsure about or arrange extra training around safeguarding. (Your manager can also advise you on how your job role fits in with other professionals and the agencies you work with.)
- **Your colleagues** will be able to inform you of the procedures to follow if you have concerns about an individual or if you witness unsafe practices that may lead to an individual being abused or placed at risk of abuse. More experienced colleagues may also be able to provide you with advice about your responsibilities for safeguarding and protecting individuals from abuse.
- **Safeguarding policies and procedures** will provide you with information about the agreed ways of working that you must follow in your care setting. They will detail the process to follow if you have concerns that an individual is being abused or is at risk of being abused. They will also include information about the whistleblowing procedures in place including the external organisations you can seek support from if your concerns are not taken seriously.
- **Safeguarding training** provided to you will ensure that you keep yourself up to date with how to ensure that your working practices reflect best practice and current legislation for safeguarding and protecting individuals.

Other sources of information and advice can also be accessed through external organisations, such as from the Care Quality Commission who will be able to respond to any concerns you have relating to an individual being abused or at risk of being abused. Similarly, if you believe that there are failures within the care setting where you work and they are *not* being taken seriously or *not* being responded to effectively, then you can report your concerns to them. They also issue guidance on how to be a whistleblower. The Care Quality Commission's website frequently publishes reports of both good practices and serious failures in the provision of care and support services to individuals.

- **The police** will be able to provide you with information and advice about what to do if an individual is being abused or is at risk of being abused, including whether a criminal act has been committed and whether any unsafe practices you may have concerns about are unlawful.
- **The local authority** adult care services department will be able to provide you with information and advice about what to do if you have concerns that an individual is being abused or is at risk of being abused. Each local authority will also have information on their website about the role and purpose of their Safeguarding Adults Board (SAB), good practice guidance for safeguarding individuals from abuse to be shared with all agencies as well as the reports

based on the findings from Safeguarding Adults Reviews completed within the local area.
- **Independent organisations** can provide information and advice on best practice when safeguarding individuals from abuse, including the most effective ways of working for achieving positive outcomes for individuals. For example, the Social Care Institute for Excellence (SCIE), the Carers Direct Helpline and whistleblowing helplines.

Whistleblowing

To whistleblow means to report any unsafe or illegal working practices used in your setting. One of the key concepts of whistleblowing is that you must have reasonable belief that disclosure is in the interest of the public. Remember, sources of information and advice about whistleblowing can be obtained – from both your place of work and sources outside of work as mentioned above.

Whistleblowers receive protection. For example, the employment rights or career of a whistleblower will not be affected as a result of them reporting unsafe practice. Legislation is also in place to protect a whistleblower. Your care setting will have a whistleblowing policy and procedures in place for advice on what to do.

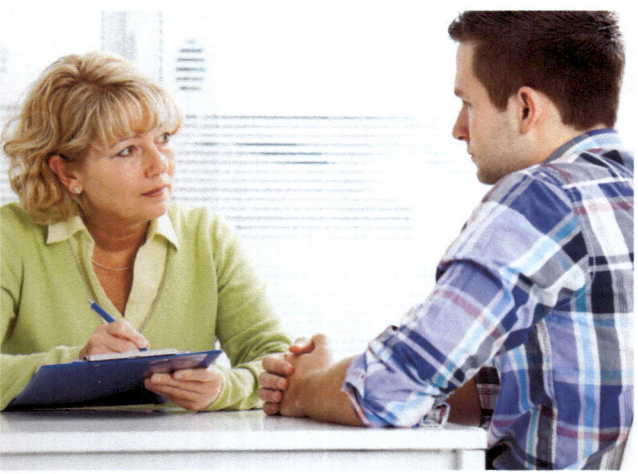

Figure 2.1 How can you raise your concerns about unsafe practices at work?

Remember that you have a duty of care to report any unsafe and illegal practice, even though it may seem scary to report the people you work with. If you feel you are unable to speak to the manager in your care setting then you can report your concerns to someone more senior or go directly to the Care Quality Commission. You can do this by telephoning them or emailing them with your concern(s). All information you share will be treated as confidential – and if you prefer, you can do this anonymously (this means that you do not have to leave your name or contact details when you email or telephone).

Anything you suspect that is of a criminal nature should still be discussed with your manager first, but you must then contact the police about this.

If your report is about the setting where you work and not just a colleague, then you may need to go directly to the CQC. Obviously, if there are minor concerns that you feel you are able to speak to your manager about, then you should discuss these with them first. If, however, the concerns are of a more serious nature such as failures to care for individuals on the part of the setting, you may need to go directly to the CQC. You should also refer to organisational abuse in AC 2.3.

> **Research it**
>
> **1.4 Whistleblowing guidance**
>
> Research the guidance: 'Whistleblowing: Quick guide to raising a concern with CQC' which can be accessed from the CQC's website:
>
> www.cqc.org.uk/contact-us/report-concern/report-concern-if-you-are-member-staff
>
> Discuss the key points from this document with a colleague.

Accountability for decision making

As you learned earlier, safeguarding individuals from abuse and improper treatment is everyone's business and therefore everyone, including you, your manager and the organisation you work for are responsible for making decisions. You can be responsible for your actions by following your employer's agreed ways of working, because these will set out what your role is in relation to safeguarding individuals, including the actions you must take in relation to reporting and recording when you have any safeguarding concerns. You can also ensure that you follow all best practice guidance in place, such as the six principles for safeguarding in your work practices, i.e. empowerment, protection, prevention, proportionality, partnership and accountability.

Accountability for decision making means not only being able to respond effectively to safeguarding concerns, it also involves being open and honest about the decisions you make, and placing the individuals' safety and wellbeing at the centre of all the decisions you make. Your manager and colleagues at work can prove to be useful sources of information and advice when sharing best practice with you and discussing different situations that may arise. You will also find it useful to learn more about the principles for effective information-sharing that follow in the next section.

Be willing to account for your actions

You will need to take your role and responsibilities in safeguarding individuals seriously. This means accepting that you must account for all your actions. You can do this by ensuring that you attend safeguarding training and apply what you have learned in your day-to-day practices when working alongside individuals and others, as well as by spending time and making the effort to get to know the individuals that you care for and support. This is important because in this way you are ensuring that you are maintaining your expertise in safeguarding and recognising its importance as part of your role.

When handling disclosures of abuse, it is really important that you know how to do this both professionally and sensitively, as doing so will make an enormous difference to the experience that the individual has sharing this personal information with you. Showing good practice when an individual alleges that they are being abused is very important.

Information sharing

Safeguarding individuals from abuse and improper treatment will involve sharing personal information about individuals, and at times this information may be sensitive and/or confidential. For this reason, you may need to seek further information and advice about how and when to do this in your role, so that it can be done in a lawful and professional way. Sources of information and advice can include:

- Your work setting's policies and procedures. These can provide more information about what information to share if you have safeguarding concerns about an individual, including how and when to report your concerns.
- Your manager. They can also be a good source of information and advice in helping you to understand your role in sharing information about an individual during the safeguarding process, such as with other agencies who may request information, e.g. the hospital, the police, and/or they may know what to do if you have concerns about an individual's wellbeing or suspect that they may be at risk of abuse or improper treatment.
- Training provided by your employer. This can help you to keep your knowledge updated in relation to your role in information sharing when safeguarding individuals, including how much information to share with whom and when. For example, you can find out more about how the Data Protection Act 2018 support the sharing of information to keep individuals safe from abuse and improper treatment.
- External organisations such as the **ICO** and **SCIE**. These organisations can also provide up-to-date information and advice about information sharing. For example, SCIE has produced a guide for practitioners, 'Safeguarding adults: sharing information' that includes information and advice about how confidential, personal information can be shared lawfully when there are safeguarding concerns, when an individual's wellbeing is at risk or their life is in danger, including the principles and seven golden rules for information-sharing:

1. Use the legislation in place, i.e. the Data Protection Act 2018, as a guide on how to share personal information about individuals, and remember it does not act as a barrier to do so.
2. Always be open and honest with the individual and/or their representative (unless it's unsafe or inappropriate to do so) about the information you will be sharing, including what information, why, how and with whom.
3. Seek advice from others if you are unsure or have any doubts.
4. When sharing information about an individual, seek their consent where possible. If the individual does not give you their consent it is still possible to share information about them if it's in the public interest to do so, i.e. if the individual's life is in danger, or if others' lives may be placed in danger.

5. Prioritise safety and wellbeing when sharing information, i.e. the individual's safety and wellbeing and the safety and wellbeing of others who may be affected.
6. Necessary, proportionate, relevant, accurate, timely, secure. Ask yourself these questions: is it necessary for me to share this information? Am I sharing the information only with those people who need it? Is it accurate? Is it up-to-date? Am I sharing this information in a timely manner? Am I sharing it securely?
7. Keep a record of the decision you make and the reason for it, i.e. whether you decide to share information or not. If you do make the decision to share information, then record what you have shared, with whom and the reason why.

Reflect on it

1.4 Safeguarding and information sharing

Reflect on how the six safeguarding principles you learned about in AC 1.1 link to the seven golden rules for information-sharing. Discuss your thoughts with a partner.

Key terms

ICO refers to the Information Commissioner's Office, which is the independent authority that upholds rights with regards to people's information, and promotes openness by public bodies and data privacy for individuals.

SCIE is a UK charity and improvement support agency that shares knowledge of best practice across the whole social care sector, and works closely with both adults and children care services.

Evidence opportunity

1.4 Sources of information

Develop a poster that identifies your role in safeguarding and how to source information and advice when protecting individuals from abuse. Use examples of both internal (in the work setting) and external (an organisation separate to your work setting) sources of information.

LO2 Understand principles of safeguarding adults

Getting started

Think about a story you have heard or read about in the media that involved adults being abused and not being kept safe. For example, you may have read or heard about care homes where older individuals died as a result of poor quality care.

How did these news stories make you feel? Why?

AC 2.1 Explain what is meant by the terms a) safeguarding, b) abuse, c) harm

Everyone, including the individuals you care for, has a right to live their lives safely and free from hurt, abuse and neglect. To safeguard individuals means to protect them from harm and abuse. In your role, you will be working with some of the most vulnerable people in society, not only because of health issues, but because they may have suffered harm and abuse. It may be that the individuals you care for are being abused by the people who should be protecting them from abuse such as family members, friends, neighbours, other individuals in the setting and even care workers – all the people that are supposed to care for the individual. Abuse and neglect can occur in individuals' own homes, at work, in care settings, medical settings – again places where individuals should feel safe!

In order to safeguard individuals, you will need to know about the signs to look for, identify when someone is being abused and know the actions to take. Safeguarding also means promoting individuals' rights to good health and wellbeing. This involves providing individuals with good quality care and support.

Abuse

Abuse occurs when someone is mistreated in a way that causes them pain or hurt, such as physical, psychological or sexual abuse. You will learn more about all the different types of abuse in AC 2.3. Individuals may experience one or several types of abuse at the same time, or at different times. Abuse can be done by people who are supposed to care for the individual. Abuse can happen in all sorts of places (including places that are supposed to provide care); not only in their own homes and care settings, but also at the home of someone they know, outside in a public area or in an office or place of work. Therefore abuse can happen anywhere, by anyone and at any time.

Harm

The term 'harm' refers to any type of abuse or neglect, whether intentional or not, that can have a negative effect on an individual's physical, emotional, social health and wellbeing.

Self-harm

Harm may not always be caused by others, but can be caused by the individuals themselves. Others involved in the care of the individual, such as GPs and their family, will be able to tell you if they have a history of, or are currently self-harming and are a risk to themselves, or are likely to self-harm. Self-harming may include individuals physically abusing themselves by cutting for example.

Whatever form the self-harm takes, you should follow the policies and procedures in your setting for working with someone who self-harms and make sure that their care plan and your practice is informed by this. You may also need to seek advice from organisations and charities that have specialist knowledge in this area.

Research it

2.1 The Care Act 2014 and safeguarding

Research what the Care Act 2014 says about the meaning of safeguarding adults who have care or support needs. Produce a poster with your findings.

You will find it useful to access Skills for Care's resource about the Care Act and its role in safeguarding adults:

www.skillsforcare.org.uk/resources/documents/Developing-your-workforce/Care-Certificate/Care-Certificate-Standards/Standard-10.pdf

Evidence opportunity

2.1 What do 'safeguarding', 'abuse' and 'harm' mean?

Identify an individual who has care or support needs. Write down a definition of the terms safeguarding, abuse and harm. How can this individual be safeguarded and protected from harm and abuse? Think about the different aspects of the terms 'safeguarding', 'abuse' and 'harm'.

AC 2.2 Explain your role and responsibilities in safeguarding individuals from abuse and improper treatment

Everyone involved in the lives of individuals who have care or support needs has a responsibility to safeguard them from abuse, neglect and improper treatment. This includes you and your colleagues, their families, friends and neighbours and other professionals such as GPs and social workers.

Your role and responsibilities

Discovering that an individual you care for is being abused can be one of the most challenging situations you face in your role, but you must remember that protecting and safeguarding individuals is your responsibility and part of your duty of care. (You may want to refer to this concept in Unit 305 Duty of care in care settings.) As we mentioned earlier, as a care worker, you will need to know about the signs to look for and what to do if you think that someone you care for is being abused. It is important to follow the agreed ways of working in your care setting as these will set out what is expected from you in the safeguarding process.

However, there are some important ways of working that you must follow to support individuals to remain safe from abuse, neglect and improper treatment.

Understand different situations where abuse or improper treatment may be occurring and stay alert

This will mean knowing the different signs to look for, which we will discuss in LO3. You should constantly be mindful of these. Individuals you care for may be vulnerable and may not disclose or tell you about abuse or improper treatment that they are suffering. It may be that they fear what may happen if they do. It may even be that they do not realise they are being abused or think that they are the problem and so deserve what is happening to them. It may also be that they cannot communicate abuse to you as they are either too weak given health issues or because of their age.

Therefore, you should constantly look for signs or clues that may suggest they are being abused. That is not to say you should be suspicious of everyone the individual comes into contact with. However, you will need to consider it as a possibility if individuals you care for have an injury that they cannot explain to you or are behaving differently to how they normally do or behave differently around different people.

If you are aware of the signs, dangers and risks that individuals face, whether they are physical dangers in the setting (such as a spillage on the floor), or abuse from people (such as family members), then you will be well placed to identify abuse and can act immediately to investigate the situation and to protect the individual.

Your first port of call should be to consult your agreed ways of working in your setting. Your manager will also be able to advise you on what to do. Make sure that you accurately record details of why you suspect abuse, or if someone has disclosed it to you, then accurately record this so that you can clearly communicate this to your manager.

Prevent individuals from being subjected to any danger, abuse, neglect or improper treatment

You can do this by developing an individual's knowledge and understanding about the meaning of danger, abuse, neglect or improper treatment and what they must do if this happens to them. Reassure them that they will always be supported if they are being abused or neglected or if they report that they are being abused, neglected or subjected to improper treatment. You may need to seek support from the individual's advocate and adapt the information you provide so that it can be understood – by using pictures or signs if needed. This is to make sure the information is accessible. This is important, because in this way you will supporting the individuals to learn how to safeguard themselves and as a result make them less likely to be abused by others, or if they are already being abused, then you will be able to stop it from happening. There is more on the ways to reduce the likelihood of abuse in LO5.

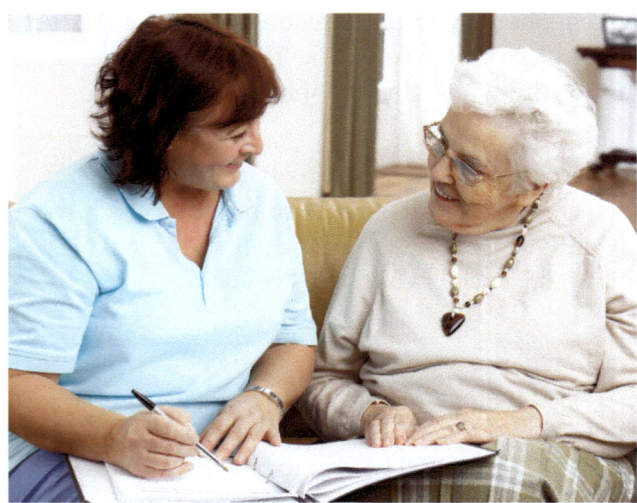

Figure 2.2 How can you be an effective partner in care?

Evidence opportunity

2.2 Safeguarding roles and responsibilities

Carry out some research in the care setting where you work and find out what your employer's agreed ways of working for safeguarding individuals say about your role and responsibilities. For example, they may include your reporting and recording responsibilities as well as how you must support individuals. Discuss this with your manager, decide on the key points and make detailed notes.

AC 2.3 Outline what is meant by different terms

As we discussed right at the start, abuse can take place by people who are supposed to care for the individuals. Abuse can happen in all sorts of places (including places that are supposed to provide care); not only in their own homes and care settings, but also at the home of someone they know, outside in a public area or in an office or place of work. Therefore, abuse can happen anywhere, by anyone and at any time.

When you think about abuse, consider the questions outlined in Figure 2.3.

The Care Act 2014 defines abuse as falling into ten different categories. You will have had an opportunity to learn more about this in LO1.

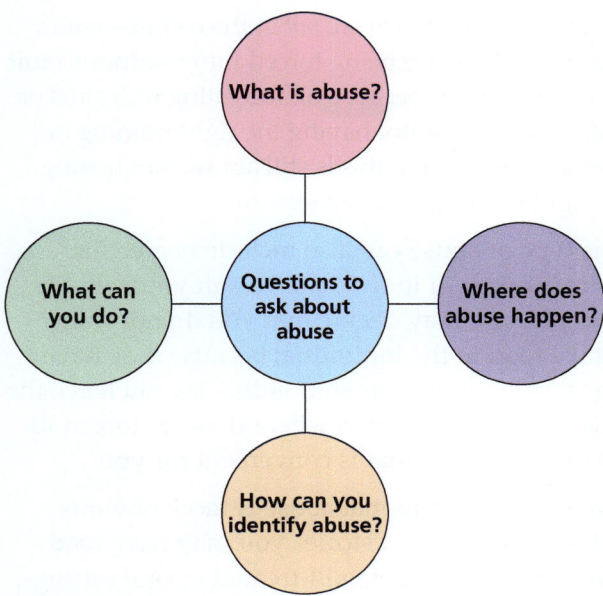

Figure 2.3 Questions to ask about abuse

Different types of abuse and what they mean

a) Physical abuse

Physical abuse is unwanted contact leading to injuries or pain. This can include hitting, hair pulling, scalding, slapping, pinching and other physical actions that can cause harm.

However, some other forms of physical abuse are less obvious. Physical abuse can also include over use of medication, withholding food, unlawful isolation such as locking an individual in their room, or unlawful restraint such as not allowing an individual to get up from their bed by keeping the bed rails up.

b) Domestic abuse

Domestic abuse can include controlling and coercive or bullying behaviour between family members and partners. This can include threats, humiliation, isolation (such as from their friends), **honour-based violence** and female genital mutilation (FGM).

> **Key terms**
>
> **Honour-based violence** refers to domestic violence because the individual is perceived as having brought shame to their family or community.

c) Sexual abuse

This includes individuals being subjected to unwanted sexual contact and involvement in sexual activities and relationships. This can include rape, sexual assault, sexual harassment, making an individual watch pornography or sexual acts and indecent exposure.

There will be situations where individuals you care for will be in sexual relationships, ones they have consented to, but you will need to recognise the difference between this and ones where individuals are being abused by partners, family members or even care staff. (See AC 3.1 Identify indicators that an individual may be being abused.)

Basically, any sexual activity that the individual has not consented to, was forced to consent to, was unable to consent to or tricked into consenting to can be defined as sexual abuse.

The issue of consent is a very important one here as many of the vulnerable individuals you work with will not have the capacity to consent or make informed decisions.

d) Emotional/psychological abuse

These are abusive actions that make an individual feel worthless and humiliated. This can include bullying, threatening harm or intimidation, or controlling and denying an individual's right to privacy, dignity and choice. It can also include isolating people from others or from accessing services, or being verbally abusive by swearing or shouting at them. This type of abuse underpins all the others because individuals will of course experience emotional pain when they are being abused in other ways. It is hard not to be emotionally hurt when you are physically abused.

Remember that not all abuse may be so obvious or it may not be actual abuse but it still causes distress. Often behaviour that is harsh and unacceptable can be offensive and cause emotional hurt. This can include belittling someone, treating them like a child, patronising them, or bullying them. You should also be aware of this and the potential for this to cause harm. It could also lead to further and different types of abuse.

e) Financial and material abuse

This is the unauthorised use (without permission from the individual) of a person's finances. This can include theft, fraud, misuse of benefits or direct payments, threats or manipulation in relation to wills and inheritance. It can include abusing and exploiting them to benefit financially.

It may result in vulnerable individuals who are not able to look after their finances becoming victims of theft and fraud and losing their homes in extreme cases. For example, think about the news stories you have either heard or read about in relation to people being the victims of fraud. It is happening more and more now as technology is being used to exploit people.

f) Modern slavery

This means the exploitation of a person in order to serve others (domestic servitude) without being paid. This includes slavery – human trafficking where individuals are exploited by others and sold as slaves. Enslaved people do not have a choice, they are forced to work. It is forced and compulsory labour.

You will have learned that slavery has occurred throughout history. However, this is something that still occurs today, not just in other countries, but also in the UK. The Modern Day Slavery Act 2015 is in place to prevent the enslavement and trafficking of people. See AC 1.1 for more information on legislation.

g) Discriminatory abuse

This is the unequal treatment or denial of a person's rights based on a protected characteristic (that is, as defined in the Equality Act 2010). This can include discrimination because of their age, disability, gender reassignment, marriage and civil partnership, pregnancy and maternity, **race**, religion and belief, sex or sexual orientation.

When people are discriminated against, they may also be harmed physically or emotionally, neglected or harassed. It is therefore important to understand how different types of abuse are connected and linked to others.

h) Organisational abuse

Institutional or organisational abuse occurs when the setting focuses the service on the needs of the organisation and the workers rather than on the needs of the individuals who access the service. This might include rigid routines and systems such as specific times for individuals to get up or go to bed, isolating individuals from families and friends, or disrespectful behaviours towards individuals such as swearing and being patronising.

You may not even realise that you and the setting are being abusive in this way. It may be that you think your setting is being efficient by specifying routines and times for meals and bed, or think that it is in the best interest of the individual. However, in this way, the individuals' needs are *not* at the centre – yours are! Individuals are being forced into routines to suit you. This may be because of budgeting restraints or staff shortages, or not having the right training but the fact remains that this is still abuse. Not having the right training is not an excuse!

This type of abuse can also include neglecting the care needs of individuals to suit yourself. For example, you may decide that you do not want to take food to the individual because they have requested it after your shift ends – so you leave the individual in a situation where they are forced to eat food at a time that is convenient for you.

Sometimes institutional abuse is more obvious. Think about some of stories you may have read about individuals being ill-treated in care settings, where they have been neglected or handled in an aggressive way. This is a serious breach of duty of care and abuse not only of the individuals but also of the care worker's responsibility.

i) Neglect/acts of omission

Neglect is a failure by others to care for and meet an individual's needs, which results in harm being caused to the individual. Neglect can be intentional or unintentional and can include, for example, ignoring an individual's emotional, physical or medical care needs by not providing them with access to food, water, heating and clothes, or not taking into account their cultural or religious needs. Acts of omission can also be intentional or unintentional, and involve not doing something, for example not providing an individual with support to take their medication, or with regular meals or access to physical activity. Neglect and acts of omission also involve leaving individuals in unsafe environments, generally not supporting them with their individual needs and simply leaving them to be alone.

> **Key terms**
>
> **Race** refers to the common physical characteristics associated with a group of people from the same culture and/or shared history such as skin colour, nationality, ethnic or national origins.
>
> **Lifestyle** refers to the way a person lives their life; this can be related for example to their health, morals and/or finances.

You should refer to the earlier section on organisational abuse, but remember that families and friends and others who are supposed to care about individuals can also be guilty of neglect. This may be because they are finding it difficult to care for the individual alongside other things in their life, or it may be a very deliberate and even cruel type of neglect.

Many of the types of abuse that we have discussed above are criminal offences which means those committing the acts can be prosecuted by police. Whatever form of abuse you suspect is happening, do not ignore it. Follow your agreed ways of working so that you can stop any abuse that may be happening and safeguard and protect the individual.

You should also remember that a lot of abuse spans several of the categories we have discussed, and so often the category is less important than actually identifying that abuse is taking place.

j) Self-neglect

This is the failure of individuals to care for themselves and meet their own needs. This can result in them causing harm to themselves. Self-neglect can include showing no care for one's own personal hygiene, not eating or drinking healthily, or perhaps not taking prescribed medication, not accessing care and support services available. They may do this because of health reasons, disabilities or simply because it is their choice to follow a certain **lifestyle**.

Research it

2.3 Abuse reported in the media

Research two cases of abuse that have recently been reported in the media. You can, for example, choose cases in relation to domestic abuse such as honour-based violence and modern slavery. You will find newspapers, the television and the internet useful sources of information. Produce an information handout about each case. You may find it useful to look at the following stories as a starting point:

www.bbc.co.uk/news/uk-england-london-59123551

www.bbc.co.uk/news/uk-england-cumbria-60043132

Case study

2.3 Different types of abuse

Wood Green is an established supported living scheme where three men with autism and other complex needs live together. One afternoon, all three individuals are sitting in the lounge. A senior care worker asks Jonas, one of the individuals with care needs, whether he is ready to cook his evening meal. Jonas kicks the care worker hard on the leg and runs upstairs. The senior care worker runs up after Jonas and shouts at him angrily, telling him that she will not tolerate him abusing her and for that reason instructs him to remain in his room for the rest of the evening. The senior care worker goes back downstairs and tells the two other individuals in the lounge that Jonas will not be eating this evening and will remain in isolation until he apologises to her.

Discuss:

1 What types of abuse are taking place in this care setting?
2 Why do you think these types of abuse occurred?
3 How could these types of abuse have been prevented?

Evidence opportunity

2.3 The different types of abuse

Produce a leaflet for an adult care worker who has never worked in a care setting. Include the meanings of the following different types of abuse: physical, domestic, sexual, emotional/psychological abuse, financial/material abuse, modern slavery, discriminatory abuse, institutional/organisational abuse, neglect/acts of omission, self-neglect.

LO3 Know how to recognise signs of abuse and improper treatment

> **Getting started**
>
> Think about someone you know well. How can you tell if this person is not being their usual self? For example, do they act differently? Perhaps they are unusually quiet when usually they are very chatty. Perhaps they appear different; they may look unwell or unhappy. Perhaps they tell you how they are feeling. Are they anxious, worried, angry? Perhaps you notice changes in their personality. Do they suddenly become very irritable or withdrawn?
>
> Recognising these signs means that you know when there is something wrong. Knowing there is something wrong means you can take action to put it right.

AC 3.1 Identify indicators that an individual may be being abused

You can only carry out your role and responsibilities to safeguard individuals from abuse, harm and neglect fully if you are able to recognise the indicators that may suggest an individual is being abused.

Table 2.4 lists the different indicators of abuse. You should remember, however, that these are not evidence of abuse. It may be that there are other reasons for a visible injury that the individual cannot explain.

The most effective way that you can safeguard individuals and protect them from harm or abuse is by getting to know every individual so that you notice and act upon any unusual changes that they do show, however small.

Working with colleagues and other professionals will also help you to understand any wider context; for example, the individual's medical history will inform you of any bruising and injury in the past. Therefore, you will need to look at the indicators in the wider context of the individual's life and care. You may also need to observe and communicate with the individual to understand any injuries better.

It is important to remember that because all individuals are unique, the way they may experience abuse or harm will also be unique. This means that individuals will not necessarily show the same signs and symptoms associated with each type of abuse.

Nonetheless, Table 2.4 will provide you with a good understanding of common indicators of abuse and ones that you should look out for and be mindful of. Although the table does not cover all the possible indicators, it will give you an idea of the major ones to look out for.

Table 2.4 Types and indicators of abuse

Type of abuse	Indicators of abuse
Physical abuse	Unexplained or unusual bruises, cuts, scratches, burns, frequent unexplained injuries, fractures, rashes or pressure ulcers, weight loss, general worsening of their health and mood.
	There may be some signs in their behaviour like flinching in the presence of the abuser, wearing long sleeves in hot weather to cover up bruises, or they may not want to see visitors.
	Some more obvious ones might include cigarette burns, black eyes that indicate violence, repeatedly falling or repeated overdosing.
	Individuals may also be unable to explain the injuries.
	Being in pain and discomfort, showing fear, being withdrawn particularly in the presence of another person.
Domestic abuse	Unexplained or unusual bruises, cuts, burns, broken bones, (see signs of physical abuse above), being humiliated in front of others.
	Others showing controlling behaviour, or behaviour that challenges, can also be an indicator.
	Other signs can include those associated with physical, emotional/psychological, sexual and financial abuse.

Table 2.4 Types and indicators of abuse *continued*

Type of abuse	Indicators of abuse
	Low self-esteem, fear of socialising with others or being reluctant to let others come to the house, increased isolation from family and friends.
	Other symptoms can include those associated with physical, emotional/psychological, sexual and financial abuse.
Sexual abuse	Physical signs include unexplained or unusual bruises around the thighs, buttocks, breasts and genital area. There may also be burns or scratches and even bite marks, unexplained bleeding, stained or torn underclothing, difficulty in walking or sitting. The individual may have (repeated) urinary infections or genital infections, they may be pregnant.
	There may be some signs in their behaviour, they may seem more withdrawn, they may attempt suicide, they may be unable to explain where they have been.
	Others showing aggression or suggestive sexual behaviour may also be an indicator.
	Poor concentration, inability to sleep, being withdrawn, fear of relationships with others, fear of being alone in the presence of the other person/people, aggression, anxiety, withdrawal of care and support services; they may, for example, refuse assistance with personal hygiene.
Emotional/ psychological abuse	A change in eating habits, i.e. leading to weight loss or weight gain, being uncooperative, displaying behaviours that challenge towards others.
	Remember that being teased or humiliated, belittled, treated like a child by others with no regard for them as an individual with their own opinion is also a sign that someone may be abused or that this could lead to abuse.
	If you care for someone in their home, it may be that neighbours have reported shouting or you may see that people living in the area are continually parking outside their home so that the individual is unable to park.
	It may even be that someone is using language that is not obviously racist, but still stereotypical.
	Often people experience emotional distress from things that may not be obviously abuse, but are still hurtful and could lead to abuse.
	Disturbed sleep, low self-esteem, very underconfident, distressed, becoming upset easily, withdrawn particularly in the presence of the other person, feeling unwell, feeling anxious.
Financial/ material abuse	Unexplained lack of money and withdrawals of money, unexplained living conditions, i.e. personal possessions disappearing or insufficient food.
	The individual may not be kept informed of what is happening with their finances, nor be allowed to manage this aspect of their life.
	Their property may be sold without their knowledge. They may be unable to pay for their care or relatives may be reluctant to pay. Their will may be changed.
	Feeling anxious about paying bills, not wishing to pay for essential food shopping items, fear of not being able to manage financially.
Modern slavery	Appearing malnourished, looking unkempt, i.e. appearing dirty, not wearing clean clothes.
	Other signs can include those associated with physical, emotional/psychological abuse.
	Becoming isolated from others, fear of speaking to others, appearing fearful or withdrawn in the presence of the other person/abuser.
	Other symptoms can include those associated with physical, emotional/psychological abuse.

Table 2.4 Types and indicators of abuse *continued*

Type of abuse	Indicators of abuse
Discriminatory abuse	Displaying behaviour that challenges towards others, not being supported or being offered support or services that do not meet the individual's needs.
	Individuals may be denied access to care, places, people and activities. They may not be given information on how they can be supported to tackle discriminatory behaviour. See signs of emotional abuse as well.
	Becoming isolated, feeling fearful, frustrated, anxious, withdrawal from services. They may also have low self-esteem.
Organisational abuse	Poor care standards, for example individuals being hungry, dehydrated, lack of management, inadequate staffing, rigid routines, lack of choices and individuality, e.g. lack of access to personal possessions, lack of individual care plans, denial of individuals' rights, e.g. dignity, privacy, independence, absence of visitors. Individuals may not be allowed to go outside; medication is not properly or appropriately administered.
	Low self-esteem, feeling frustrated, anxious, angry, upset.
Neglect by others/acts of omission	Malnutrition, dehydration, living in dirty or unsafe conditions, pressure sores, wearing inappropriate clothing, for example items that are worn or inappropriate for the weather conditions, untreated injuries and illnesses.
	There may be general worsening of health and the individual may be deprived of access to medical and healthcare needs. Some of the physical signs of abuse will also apply here.
	Feeling confused, low in mood, fear of involvement from others such as professionals, services, withdrawal from socialising with others such as family and friends.
Self-neglect	Malnutrition, dehydration, weight loss, poor personal hygiene, looking unkempt, living in dirty or unsafe conditions, failure to access care or support services, or ignoring their health and medical needs. They may need emergency medical treatment for an injury or illness. General apathy for their own wellbeing.
	Feeling confused, low in mood, anxious.
	Becoming withdrawn and isolated from others.

You have a duty of care to inform individuals of any dangers, but not to make decisions for them, unless they lack the capacity to do so. However, make sure you consider the different factors you have learned about with regard to consent and capacity. You will find it useful to refer to Unit 303 Understanding duty of care, as well as Unit 306 Promoting and implementing person-centred practice.

Feelings that individuals may experience

Individuals may experience a range of feelings and emotions when they have suffered from abuse. This can include a range of emotions including anger, frustration, depression and sadness, and suicidal feelings. These feelings can arise whether the abuse is fairly recent and has only occurred once or if the abuse has been going on for a long period of time.

Abuse can change a person significantly, it can change the way they view others and the world generally. You will need to ensure that you try to understand what the individual may be going through. Learn from them, learn from the experience you may have had, learn from the experiences of people you know and the experiences of your colleagues so that you can empathise with individuals and provide appropriate and long-lasting care. You may need to draw on the expertise of others such as therapists where this is beyond your experience.

Taking care of yourself

While it is important to look for signs of abuse, you must also remember to be aware of your own feelings when you are dealing with someone who has been abused. This is a tricky situation to go through as a care worker, one that may cause you upset and distress. The situation may cause you to become angry for the individual. However, remember to take care of yourself and ask for support from others. Speak to your manager, speak to others in the setting or others you know, remembering not to be too specific when it comes to the individual's personal and confidential details. It is normal to want to tell others and remember that you are not alone in dealing with this situation. Your setting will be able to provide you with appropriate support and you should make use of this. There are also support organisations that will be able to help you such as The Care Workers Charity.

Taking care of the person committing abuse

Remember to always remain professional. Do not confront the person committing the abuse, remain calm and try to keep the safety of the individual as your priority. Confronting the individual will not help matters. At the same time, the person who has committed the abuse may also require help and, if this is the case, you should discuss this with your manager and find out if it is appropriate to suggest support for them. Of course, this will depend on the nature of the situation but you should be considerate of their situation too.

> **Evidence opportunity**
>
> **3.1 Indicators of abuse**
>
> Produce a written account detailing the indicators of each of the following types of abuse: physical, domestic, sexual, emotional/psychological, financial/material, modern slavery, discriminatory, organisational, self-neglect, neglect by others and acts of omission.

AC 3.2 Identify indicators of perpetrator behaviour

A perpetrator of abuse is someone who deliberately harms another person or deliberately allows another person to be harmed. Perpetrators of abuse usually behave in demeaning, controlling and manipulative ways and may hide their behaviour from others by appearing friendly and kind when in fact they're not. Knowing about some of the indicators of perpetrator behaviour is very important, as it can help you to recognise when an individual is being manipulated so that they become isolated, withdrawn, dependent and therefore vulnerable to being abused, harmed and neglected. This is very important, particularly as you will have learned that some individuals may not have the mental capacity to understand that they are being manipulated, or be too afraid to tell anyone. Some of the indicators of perpetrator behaviour can include:

- preventing the individual from developing and maintaining relationships with others including seeing their family and friends, so that they become isolated and dependent on them.
- encouraging the individual to spend all their time with them so that the individual gives up their education, job and other social activities they may have been participating in.
- making the individual believe that the perpetrator is their friend or partner, although the individual does not really know anything about them.
- giving the individual gifts, such as items of clothing and jewellery that the individual would not usually buy for themselves.
- placing pressure on the individual to, for example, hand over money or carry out sexual acts. This may result in the individual being worried about having sufficient funds to pay for day-to-day items, or becoming unusually withdrawn or angry.

> **Research it**
>
> **3.2 Perpetrator behaviour**
>
> For one case of abuse that you have heard or read about in the media, find out how the abuse happened and what the indicators were of the perpetrator's behaviour. Complete a written account with your findings.

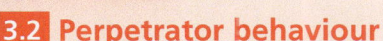

> **Evidence opportunity**
>
> **3.2 Indicators of perpetrator behaviour that have featured in cases of abuse**
>
> Identify two cases of abuse of adults. For each one, discuss the indicators of the perpetrator's behaviour.
>
> Which of the indicators were the same? Were any indicators different?

AC 3.3 Describe factors that may contribute to individuals being more at risk from abuse and improper treatment

The individual

Some of the factors that may contribute to an individual being more vulnerable to abuse and improper treatment are associated with the individual. For example:

- **Individuals who depend on others for their care or support** may be reluctant to report an abuser because they may fear they will lose their care or that the abuser may lose their job.
- **Individuals who have specific communication difficulties** because of a disability such as a learning disability or an illness such as a **stroke** may not be able to express what is happening or communicate any abuse that may be happening to them to others.
- **Individuals who have specific conditions** such as **dementia**, poor mobility, mental health needs, a history of substance misuse may have memory difficulties for example and therefore may not be able to recall what has happened. An individual with poor mobility may be frail and physically unable to defend themselves from others who may try to harm them.

> **Key term**
>
> **Stroke** refers to a life-threatening medical condition that occurs when the blood supply to part of the brain is cut off. Depending on the part of the brain it damages, it can affect how your body works, your communication and how you think and feel.
>
> **Dementia** refers to a group of symptoms that affect how a person thinks, remembers, problem-solves, uses language and communicates, and their ability to carry out tasks and activities. They occur when brain cells stop working properly and the brain is damaged by injury, or by disease such as Alzheimer's.
>
> **Stress** is the body's physical and emotional reaction to being under too much pressure. It can have positive as well as negative effects, but in this unit the word is used to refer to negative stress.

An individual with mental health needs may have experienced (as part of their illness) hallucinations (when a person sees, hears and/or senses things that are not there but they feel strongly that they are) and false beliefs and therefore may not be believed by others about what has happened. An individual with a history of substance misuse may be targeted by an abuser particularly if they have a history of violent behaviour as they may not be believed about what is happening to them and could also be taken advantage of while they are abusing substances.

The carer

Some of the factors that may contribute to an individual being more vulnerable to abuse and improper treatment are associated with the carer. These can include families, the care worker and others involved in the care of the individual. For example:

Other priorities: the carer may have a family, children and others that they care for, or need to be home at certain times for. They may have a job which they need to manage alongside caring for the individual. Such strains can be a contributing factor for abuse. Not always, but significant **stress** can affect the care given and abuse and neglect can occur.

The individual may be seen as a 'burden': The carer may experience difficulties in terms of financing the care of the individual; they may have issues around space and accommodating the individual in their home. Job pressures mean that their time is also limited and they may have their own health issues to deal with. They may also find that their social life is affected as a result of caring for the individual.

Difficulties in relationship with the individual: The carer and the individual may already have a difficult relationship and the individual may even be aggressive or violent towards the carer. It may be that the carer has a history of violent behaviour, or is easily agitated or angered.

Lack of support: The individual may feel unsupported, or they may be inexperienced because of their age. This may lead to inadequate care and abuse of the individual even though it may not be intended.

Case study

3.2, 3.3 At-risk individuals

Carlos is 28, has learning disabilities and lives with his brother Pepe. Carlos goes out every day with his brother to the local shops and to visit other family members and family friends. When Pepe works at night, he is worried about Carlos going out and being taken advantage of or coming to harm by others, and so he locks him in his room to keep him safe until Pepe returns home in the morning. Yesterday, Carlos tried to leave his room by trying to kick the door down, and now Pepe has threatened that he will no longer let Carlos see his friends and family if he does not do as his brother says.

Discuss:
1. Is abuse taking place?
2. If so, what type and in what way?

Research it

3.3 Legislation

Research legislation that is in place to support carers, such as The Care Act 2014. How does the Work and Families Act for example support individuals? What does it say about the protection that is available for carers?

Remember carers can experience abuse too

Remember that carers can also be victims of abuse. It may be that they suffer verbal abuse from the individual that they provide support for. They could be suffering physical and emotional abuse, for example the individual may refuse support and lash out. There is legislation such as the guidance in the Care Act 2014 to protect carers. Go to LO1, AC 1.1 for more information on this.

The environment or setting

Other factors that may contribute to an individual being more vulnerable to abuse and improper treatment are associated with the environment the individual lives, works or socialises in. For example, individuals who:

- **live in a remote location** such as at the end of a quiet road, on the top floor of a building (where few visitors are received) may become separated from the people who know them well such as family and friends. Families may be unable to visit regularly and individuals are isolated. This may make them a target for abuse because there is less likelihood that anyone will recognise the signs or symptoms that they are being abused.
- **receive care or support in settings that are poorly managed** may be abused because there will be a lack of monitoring of care workers to check that they are following the procedures for keeping individuals safe. The abuse may be intentional, or it may be accidental if care workers follow poor practice as a result of a lack of support or training.
- **receive care or support in settings that lack resources.** Care workers who have large and stressful workloads may feel under-valued and over worked. This may leave them feeling frustrated and stressed with the individuals they provide care and support to. There may be a shortage of staff and emphasis may be placed on the needs of the setting rather than those of the individual, all resulting in poor quality care, lack of time made for the individual and general disregard for the individual's needs.

Evidence opportunity

3.3 Factors

Read through the research report produced in November 2015 by Age UK, 'Financial Abuse Evidence Review', which explores why older people are more likely to experience financial abuse. It can be accessed here:

www.ageuk.org.uk/globalassets/age-uk/documents/reports-and-publications/reports-and-briefings/money-matters/financial_abuse_evidence_review-nov_2015.pdf

Discuss the findings with a colleague and outline your findings by producing a written account that describes the factors that may make older people more vulnerable to financial abuse. Ensure you summarise in your own words.

As before, with the signs and symptoms, these factors are not evidence of abuse. For example, just because a family member is under stress, does not mean that they are abusing the person they care for.

Case study 3.1, 3.2, 3.3 provides you with an opportunity to consider how to recognise the signs and symptoms of abuse in an individual as well as know the factors that may make them more vulnerable to abuse.

Case study

3.1, 3.2, 3.3 **Recognising abuse**

Elsie is 70, has a learning disability and lives in a residential care home; you work there as a senior care assistant. Elsie's family and friends have spent all Sunday afternoon with her as it was her birthday. As soon as everyone leaves, Elsie appears unhappy and tells you she is going to stay in her room this evening. Later, you go up to Elsie's room and ask her how she's feeling. She shakes her head and in a tearful voice tells you she has a stomach ache and doesn't want anything to eat this evening. You respect Elsie's wishes and leave. At the end of your shift, you record your observations of Elsie, including what she told you.

The next morning when you arrive at work Elsie appears her happy, usual self. You ask her how she is and she tells you she is fine and is about to watch a film with the others in the lounge. A half hour or so later the doorbell rings. It is Elsie's brother, who says he just thought he'd visit Elsie again to ask her about whether she enjoyed her birthday yesterday. You ask Elsie's brother to come in and, at the same time, notice that Elsie looks up from the lounge, sees him, looks shocked and shouts out that she's got another stomach ache, is going to her room and doesn't want to be disturbed.

Discuss:

1. What are your immediate thoughts, after reading this Case study about Elsie's behaviour? Why?
2. Identify any potential indicators that may indicate that Elsie is being abused.
3. What factors do you think make Elsie more at risk of abuse?
4. Have you come across a situation like this in your setting? How did you respond? Were the indicators different? Was the individual at risk in other ways?

LO4 Know how to respond to suspected or disclosed abuse and improper treatment

Getting started

Think about how you would feel if you were verbally abused by someone in a busy place such as in a high street and no one did anything to help you. Why do you think you would feel this way?

Now imagine you witnessed someone you did not know being verbally abused out in public. Would you intervene or not? Explain why.

AC 4.1 Describe the actions to take if there are suspicions that an individual is being abused or being subject to improper treatment

Recognising the signs and symptoms of abuse is not enough on its own to protect individuals from abuse because you will also need to know what to do when you suspect an individual is being abused or subjected to improper treatment. In addition, it could be that someone else shares their **suspicions** with you, or an individual tells you that they are being abused or being subjected to improper treatment.

Key term

Suspicions of abuse occur when you notice indicators or are told by someone about indicators that make you think or suspect abuse is happening.

It can often be difficult to accept that abuse may be happening, because you may worry that you could be incorrect or raise concerns unnecessarily and it may be the first time that you have come across it. However, if you have any **suspicions** that an individual is being abused or being subjected to improper treatment, you must always act on it; doing nothing is not an option. You must show **courage** because it is your legal duty of care to protect the individuals that you care for. Your agreed ways of working will detail the actions you will be expected to take in line with the agreed scope of your job role if there are suspicions that an individual is being abused or being subjected to improper treatment.

6Cs

Courage

Courage means standing up for what you believe in when you know it is the right thing to do. When you suspect that abuse is happening, you can be courageous by showing that abuse will not be tolerated and any suspicions that an individual may be at risk of being abused or harmed will be acted on straight away. You can show your courage by ensuring you discuss your suspicions, however small, with your manager as soon as you have them so that individuals will be kept safe and protected from being abused or harmed.

Actions to take

Figure 2.4 explains the key actions to take if you suspect that an individual is being abused or being subjected to improper treatment and each of the points are explained in a bit more detail below.

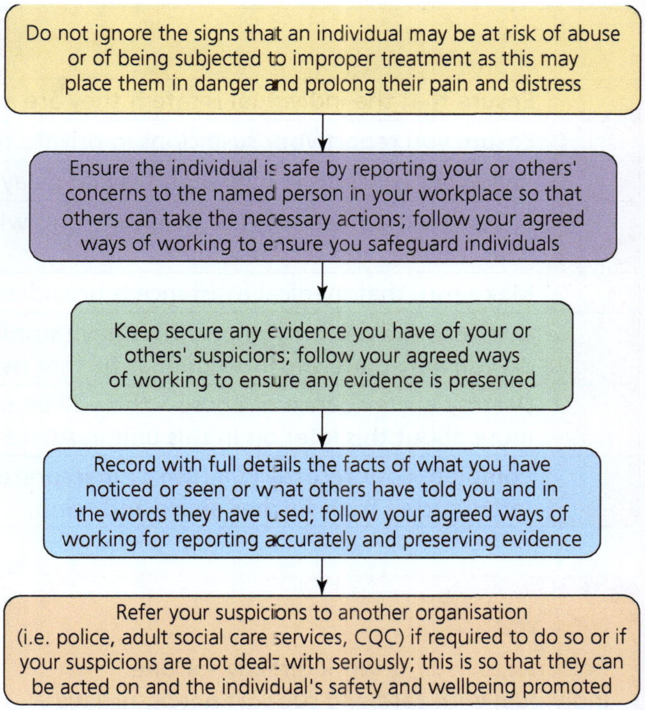

1. Do not ignore any signs that an individual may be at risk of abuse or of being subjected to improper treatment, as this may place them in danger and prolong their pain and distress. Even if it is a suspicion and the individual has not made a **disclosure**, you should still act immediately and follow the next step.
2. Ensure the individual is safe by reporting your concerns to your manager or the named person in your setting so that others can take the necessary actions and safeguard individuals. They will be able to advise on what action to take and whether you will need support and further advice from anyone else, such as the individual's family or medical assistance from a GP.
3. Keep evidence secure. If you or others have suspicions, follow your agreed ways of working to ensure any evidence is preserved (see AC 4.6 for more information).
4. Record, in full, the facts with details of what you have seen (or what others have told you) and in the words they have used – follow your agreed ways of working for reporting accurately and preserving evidence. This may take the form of a written report, or if you need to, make an audio recording ensuring you back this up with a written report afterwards. Make sure that you record what your suspicions are with clear reasons for these. Suspicions should not be your opinions – they should be based on evidence and observation. Suspicions that others have told you about should also be clearly and accurately recorded. Detail is very important – remember to not confuse other people's opinions with facts. Record other people's suspicions at the earliest opportunity so you do not forget the exact details.
5. Refer all your suspicions to another organisation (that is, the police, adult social care services, or the CQC) if your manager suggests that you should do so, or if your suspicions are not treated seriously. This is so that they can be acted on and the individual's safety and wellbeing is promoted.

Do not ignore the signs that an individual may be at risk of abuse or of being subjected to improper treatment as this may place them in danger and prolong their pain and distress

↓

Ensure the individual is safe by reporting your or others' concerns to the named person in your workplace so that others can take the necessary actions; follow your agreed ways of working to ensure you safeguard individuals

↓

Keep secure any evidence you have of your or others' suspicions; follow your agreed ways of working to ensure any evidence is preserved

↓

Record with full details the facts of what you have noticed or seen or what others have told you and in the words they have used; follow your agreed ways of working for reporting accurately and preserving evidence

↓

Refer your suspicions to another organisation (i.e. police, adult social care services, CQC) if required to do so or if your suspicions are not dealt with seriously; this is so that they can be acted on and the individual's safety and wellbeing promoted

Figure 2.4 Actions to take when there are suspicions of abuse

Make sure that all safeguarding decisions are proportionate. You can do this by weighing up how low or high the risk is that an individual may be abused or subjected to improper treatment. In this way, all safeguarding decisions made will be relative to the risk posed to the individual.

When the individual is the employer

Not all workers are employed by organisations. Sometimes individuals and/or their representatives directly employ their own **personal assistant** and therefore the individual is also the employer. Where this is the case, you will need to familiarise yourself with the roles and responsibilities that are set out in your contract of employment, as well as the local authority's procedures that are in place for where you work.

	Dos and don'ts when taking actions if there are suspicions that an individual is being abused or subjected to improper treatment
Do	Ensure that the individual is safe if they are at risk of immediate danger, harm or abuse.
Do	Ensure you report your suspicions in private to maintain individuals' confidentiality and privacy.
Do	Raise your concerns immediately – avoid delay because it may prolong an individual's distress and pain.
Do	Follow your agreed ways of working – this will ensure you are safeguarding individuals in line with your job role and responsibilities.
Do	Make sure that medical assistance is provided if there are signs of injury and abuse.
Don't	Confront the person you or others have suspicions about because it is not your role to do so – if you do you may place the individual at further risk of abuse.
Don't	Destroy any evidence of abuse – this will be needed if an investigation takes place. (You will learn more about this later on in this unit in AC 4.6.)
Don't	Complete your records in a rush or inaccurately – doing so may mean that individuals are not safeguarded from further abuse and harm.

Key term

Personal assistants work directly for one individual with care and support needs, usually within the individual's own home.

People you may suspect

The actions you will take when you have suspicions will generally be the same whoever you suspect is committing the abuse against the individual. However, there may be subtle differences when someone you know or work alongside commits the abuse.

A colleague: it is important you do not confront your colleague or talk about your concerns with another colleague. You must report this to your manager.

Someone in the individual's personal network: the information discussed above relates to the people that may be in their 'network.' In other words, they may be family and friends. You must report this to your manager.

Your line manager: it is important that you do not ignore your suspicions or worry about reporting this simply because it is your manager that you suspect; you must follow your organisation's whistleblowing procedures. (See AC 6.3 for more information about whistleblowing.)

Others: others may refer to other professionals such as an individual's tutor or physiotherapist. Again, you must report your suspicions immediately to your manager and you could follow their organisation's whistleblowing procedures. (See AC 6.3 for more information on whistleblowing.)

Reflect on it

4.1 Recording suspicions of abuse or improper treatment

How can you ensure all suspicions of abuse or improper treatment are recorded fully, in detail, factually and clearly? Why is this important? What are the consequences of not doing so? Reflect on your learning in Unit 305 Handling information in adult care settings/services (if you have already covered this unit) about completing records fully and accurately.

Evidence opportunity

4.1 Actions to take if you suspect abuse or improper treatment

Research the safeguarding procedures and agreed ways of working for the care setting where you work if there are suspicions that an individual is being abused or subjected to improper treatment. Discuss the key actions to take with your manager and obtain a witness testimony from them for evidence.

Produce a factsheet that explains the key actions to take if you suspect that an individual is being abused or subjected to improper treatment in the care setting where you work.

AC 4.2 Explain the actions to take if an individual discloses that they are being abused

When working with individuals, you will get to know them and develop good working relationships with them and their families over time. This means that their trust and confidence in you will grow which may in turn lead to them confiding in you when things go wrong. For example, an individual may disclose to you that they are being abused, or someone they know, such as a family member, may disclose that another person is abusing their relative. When this happens it is very important that you are compassionate towards them because the individual may be concerned that they are not going to be taken seriously or believed, or that they may be blamed for what has happened, and so making a **disclosure of abuse** has taken a lot of courage and determination on their part.

The care setting where you work will have in place procedures and agreed ways of working for the actions to take if an individual alleges they are being abused. It is also important, as well as knowing what actions to take, that you understand the reasons why it is important to take these actions and the consequences of not doing so. Figure 2.5 will help you with developing your understanding of the key actions to take and why these are important.

Believe them if they report abuse

Individuals may not report abuse because they worry about what will happen, or worry that no one will believe them. It is important that you listen carefully when someone tells you about any abuse they are suffering. Reassure them, be compassionate and make sure that they know you believe them. If they do not want you to tell anybody else, then remember that this is one area where you may not be able to keep information confidential. You should politely and calmly explain that you will need to speak to and tell your manager first and foremost about what they have told you, but reassure them that they will be kept informed, they will be asked before information is shared with anyone else and will be kept part of the process for safeguarding them.

Explain that you will need to pass on in confidence what the disclosure is

By doing this, you can show that the individual knows you are taking them seriously and doing something about this. As we discussed above, you should explain that you will need to tell your manager. Reassure them that you will all help to protect them.

Confidentiality may be an issue here as the individual may have shared some very private information and it has taken a long time to report the abuse to just one person and so sharing information beyond telling you may be a big ask of them. The basic rules to remember around confidentiality when someone has disclosed abuse are as follows:

1 Always tell the individual who you will need to share disclosures of abuse with – you should do this before you share the information.
2 Only share information with your manager in the first instance.
3 Check with the individual first that it is okay for you to tell others who will be able to provide support and advice. You will find it useful to refer to Unit 304 Effective communication in adult care settings/services, ACs 6.1 and 6.2 about sharing information on 'need-to-know' terms.
4 If the individual does not consent or give you permission to share information with anyone besides your manager, tell your manager who will advise on the next course of action.
   - Sometimes there is simply nothing you can do if the individual has said 'no' to sharing information.
   - Or, it may be that you need to breach confidentiality if the individual's life is in danger, or if a serious crime has taken place that puts the lives of others in danger. However, you must tell the individual who you will need to tell and why.

Also see Unit 305 Handling information in adult care settings/services, AC 1.1, on the Data Protection Act 2018.

There may also be issues around capacity that you will face here, for example if an individual lacks capacity to make decisions. Also see Unit 302 Understanding mental capacity and restrictive practice.

Empower individuals in the safeguarding process

If abuse is identified, you can empower individuals in the safeguarding process by discussing the different options for tackling the issue, including the benefits and potential risks. This is important because in this way individuals can make their own informed choices and remain in control.

[Flowchart: Actions to take when there are disclosures of abuse]

- Listen to the individual and reassure the individual that you believe them – try not to show shock or disbelief so that the individual is made to feel comfortable and not humiliated
- Ensure the individual is safe and explain that you will need to pass on in confidence what the disclosure is so that the individual knows you are taking them seriously and doing something about it
- Report to the named person in your workplace the disclosure of abuse happening; they are trained and will therefore know what to do next
- Keep secure any evidence that there may be of the abuse in order to preserve it for any future investigation that may take place
- Record with full details the facts of the disclosure you have been told about and in the words used by the individual – this will help preserve the evidence and ensure a true and accurate record of what happened
- Refer the disclosure to another organisation (i.e. the police, adult social care services, CQC) if required to do so or if the disclosure is not dealt with seriously; this forms part of your care setting's whistleblowing procedure so that all disclosures are reported and acted on

Figure 2.5 Actions to take when there are disclosures of abuse

Protect individuals during the safeguarding process

You can do this by ensuring that individuals have access to support and representation during the safeguarding process when they require it. For example, this may include an independent advocate and can be before or after they have reported abuse or neglect. This is important because in this way individuals will feel supported during the safeguarding process and are less likely to withdraw from the process or feel anxious.

Report the disclosure of abuse

First, you will need to tell your manager or the named person in your workplace who is trained and therefore knows what to do next. Your setting will have its own policies and procedures for the recording and reporting of information. Normally there will be a report form you need to complete which will include very precise information about the disclosure, such as, who made the disclosure, when, how and to whom. It will also require details of any actions taken such as a medical examination and whether anyone else has been consulted, for example a GP. You will also need to include any information or actions that may not have been taken and still need to be taken.

Keep any evidence secure

This is in order to preserve it for any future investigation that may take place. See AC 4.6 for more information on this.

Record with full details the facts of the disclosure

As we discussed in AC 4.1, make sure you record what you have been told about and in the words used by the individual – again this will help preserve the evidence and ensure a true and accurate record of what happened.

As with suspicions, remember to record with full details the facts of the disclosure – what you have been told, in the words they have used. You can record the details in written form or make an audio recording. If recorded verbally, then make a written report afterwards. Remember not to confuse facts of what you have been told with any opinion. Accuracy and detail are key. It may be that you cannot get all the facts and information when the individual first makes the disclosure, but either way, you will need to accurately record what you have been told and then follow up these points once you have more information. Make sure you record information at the earliest opportunity so that you do not forget the exact details. This will be especially important if you need to make a statement to the police or in court later on.

Refer the disclosure to another organisation

If required to do so, you may need to refer a disclosure to the police, adult social care services, or the CQC. You may need to do this if the disclosure is not dealt with seriously by the care setting. This forms part of your care setting's whistleblowing procedure so that all disclosures are reported and acted on. When referring the disclosure, you should make sure that you provide as much information as possible. Your setting may have their own referral form but usually this will include details of the disclosed abuse, actions that have been taken, information around consent and capacity, whether the individual knows you have referred them and background information. You should, however, refer to your own setting's referral form for a better idea of what one looks like.

6Cs

Compassion

Compassion is essential when an individual discloses that they are being abused because without it the individual will be left feeling devalued, humiliated and at worst may even feel that what has happened to them is all their fault. Compassion involves putting yourself in the place of the individual and considering how you would feel if you shared a very intimate detail about something that happened to you with someone you trust and you were not believed or taken seriously. You can show your compassion when an individual discloses they are being abused by acknowledging what they tell you, giving them reassurance that they have done the right thing and telling them what you are going to do next so that they know that they have been listened to and taken seriously.

Care

Good care involves working in ways that are consistently positive and supportive. In relation to safeguarding individuals, working together with others to provide good care ensures that individuals' rights and safety are promoted in a consistent way by everyone. Care also promotes the wellbeing of individuals. Telling them about what safeguarding means, and what abuse is, can even help to prevent abuse or neglect as well as create awareness of the actions that can be taken if their rights to live safely are violated or disrespected.

	Dos and don'ts for when an individual discloses abuse
Do	Show that you believe what an individual is saying.
Do	Listen to what the individual is telling you without interrupting or questioning them. Give the individual time to talk to you and share with you how they are feeling and make sure they can see that you are listening. Refer to Unit 303 Promote communication in care settings.
Do	Let the individual lead the conversation.
Do	Reassure the individual that they have done the right thing by telling you. Sit with them and explain what actions you are going to take next.
Do	Inform the individual why you must report the abuse and to whom. Reassure them that all information shared will be in strictest confidence. It is also important that you ask your care setting to keep you informed of what actions have been taken and decisions reached so that you know it has been dealt with appropriately and the individual is protected.
Do	Encourage the individual to allow you to share information if they say they do not want you to. Calmly explain the reasons and benefits for sharing information.
Do	Ensure the individual is not left alone with the person they are disclosing they have been abused by. This will usually involve the person accused of the abuse not being able to visit the individual until the investigation into the abuse is complete.
Do	Record all disclosures of abuse made to you fully and accurately. The care setting where you work will have a form that you will be required to complete; it is important that you do so and that you keep it confidential so that the correct information is provided on which actions can be taken quickly to ensure the safety of the individual. The information you record must also be documented legibly and only contain the facts of what was disclosed to you; again, this will help with establishing what happened to the individual.
Don't	Look shocked – as this may be misinterpreted by the individual as you not believing them.
Don't	Ask lots of questions.
Don't	Tell the individual that you will not share information when you know you have to. Be honest in your interactions to maintain trust in your relationship.
Don't	Include your opinions when recording disclosures of abuse. You can ensure your records are accurate by only recording the facts and using the words the individual used when they made the disclosure.

> **Research it**
>
> **4.2 Recording abuse**
>
> Carry out some research in the care setting where you work to find out about the records that you are required to complete when an individual makes a disclosure of abuse.
>
> Discuss with your manager the information that you are required to document as well as the reasons why and how you should do this in line with your care setting's agreed ways of working.

> **Evidence opportunity**
>
> **4.2 Actions to take when abuse is disclosed**
>
> Discuss with your assessor the actions to take if an individual in your care setting discloses that they are being abused. Remember to explain the reasons for your actions.

AC 4.3 Describe the potential tensions relating to consent to share information

Consent

You may come across issues around consent here. For example, your suspicions may be based on indicators of serious abuse, but the individual may not actually allege abuse, or may refuse to make any sort of statement against the abuser. This poses a dilemma for you and the setting.

As we discussed earlier, your role here will be to provide as much information as possible, or to simply be there for the individual. For example, if you see a bruise, or notice bleeding, you could help the individual by asking them if they would like any treatment: 'I notice a bruise on your arm, is it sore? Would you like a bandage for it?' Avoid asking too many questions at this point, however. Remember that if the injury is of a more serious nature, you must report this to a doctor so that they can decide on the best course of action.

Capacity

You will also need to consider issues around capacity and whether the individual has the ability to make their own decisions. Much of your action and intervention, and those of your manager, will depend on whether the individual has the capacity to make decisions and refuse treatment. See AC 4.4 for more information on confidentiality and consent. Also see AC 5.1 for more information on working in partnership.

These examples we've discussed are all potential tensions, because by you safeguarding and protecting the individual from potential and/or actual abuse or improper treatment, you are in direct conflict with their right to share personal information about themselves with whom they want to. However, when you believe that someone is at risk of abuse or improper treatment, you have no choice but to fulfil your duty to promote the safety of individuals and others, by protecting them from danger and abuse. You will learn more about having a duty of care in Unit 303, Understanding duty of care.

Effective communication of information about the next steps and the reasons for these will be key. Remember to provide lots of reassurance, remind the individual that they are not at fault and that you will do everything you can to help and protect them. You will have to explain procedures carefully if individuals need to be medically examined, or you could ask medically trained colleagues to speak to the individuals, as they may be best placed to provide advice here. Also, as we discussed in the section on suspicions, there will be questions around capacity.

You will need to explain to the individual that it is your legal duty and professional responsibility to share the information they have disclosed to you so that you can ensure that they continue to live safely and free from abuse.

> **Reflect on it**
>
> **4.3 Sharing information**
>
> Reflect on what you would say to an individual in your work setting who discloses to you that they have been abused, but insists that you keep it a secret as they are worried that the person may get into trouble and lose their job. What do your work setting's policies say about what you should say? Why is this important?

> **Evidence opportunity**
>
> **4.3 Potential tensions**
>
> Write a case study about the potential tensions relating to consent to share information for one individual with care and support needs. Remember to detail what the potential tensions are.

AC 4.4 Describe how to share information about suspicions or disclosures of abuse or improper treatment

Confidentiality

All information about suspicions or disclosures of abuse or improper treatment that is shared verbally or in writing must be treated as confidential and sensitive. This means that the privacy of the individual's information must also be respected. You can do this by ensuring that:

- all verbal and written reports of safeguarding concerns you make are completed in private, i.e. where others who do not have authorisation cannot overhear or see them.
- the information shared will only be passed on to others who need to know.
- only the information required will be shared with others who need to know.

You will find it useful to refer to Unit 304 Effective communication in adult care settings/services, LO6 that provides additional information about confidentiality in care settings/services.

Consent

All individuals have the right to be asked whether they agree to having their personal information shared. You will be more likely to obtain consent from individuals if you are open and honest with them and if you:

- explain why you want to share information about them, what information you are going to share, with whom and how, so that they feel in control.
- explain the benefits of sharing the information, as well as the consequences of not doing so, so that they understand.
- explain that it is their right to withdraw their consent at any point during the safeguarding process.

If an individual does not give you their consent, or if you are unable to obtain consent from an individual, then, as you have learned, you can still share information about an individual with the relevant professionals and agencies if there are safeguarding concerns, because it is in the public interest for you to do so. This means that protecting an individual from abuse or improper treatment outweighs the need to maintain confidentiality. Your responsibility to do this will also be set out in your work setting's policies and procedures. If you are unsure about what to do, you must seek advice and further guidance from your manager.

You should record in writing whether an individual has given their consent or not, so that it is clear what you and the individual discussed and agreed. You should document the actions you took to obtain consent from the individual, the individual's reasons for not giving their consent (if applicable), as well as your reasons for why you felt it was necessary to share the individual's information without their consent. All written records are permanent records, which means that they can be referred to at a later stage if there are any complaints made about you sharing an individual's information without their consent. In this way, you can show that you are being accountable for the actions you have taken to safeguard and protect an individual from potential and/or actual abuse or improper treatment.

> **Evidence opportunity**
>
> **4.4 Sharing information about abuse or improper treatment**
>
> Your manager has asked you to design a leaflet for the staff team about how to share information about suspicions or disclosures of abuse or improper treatment. Provide details of the key steps to take.

AC 4.5 Describe ways to keep an individual and others appropriately informed and involved about their safeguarding concern, in line with policies and procedures

The care setting where you work will have safeguarding policies and procedures in place that will detail how to keep the individual and others appropriately informed and involved regarding their safeguarding concern. It is important that you familiarise yourself with these policies so that you know and understand how you can support the individual and others with their safeguarding concern.

Below is a list of some tips for informing and involving the individual and others about their safeguarding concern:

1. Be open and honest with the individual and others about how they will be informed and involved regarding their safeguarding concern, including the reasons why, how this will happen and with whom.
2. Be clear with the individual and others about the agreed ways of working that you are required to follow in relation to their safeguarding concern.
3. Seek advice from your manager if you are in any doubt about informing and involving the individual and others about their safeguarding concern.
4. Consider the wellbeing and safety of the individual and others when informing and involving them regarding their safeguarding concern.
5. Ensure the information you share with the individual and others is accurate, up-to-date and shared securely.
6. Keep a record of how you have informed and involved the individual and others regarding their safeguarding concern, including any advice you sought and from whom.

Research it

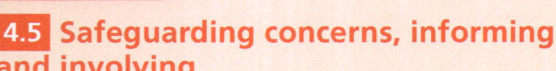

4.5 Safeguarding concerns, informing and involving

Carry out some research in the care setting where you work. Find out what the agreed ways of working are, with regards to keeping the individual and others appropriately informed about and involved with their safeguarding concern.

How does this relate to your job role and responsibilities?

Evidence opportunity

4.5 Safeguarding concerns and the wellbeing of the individual and others

Reflect on the benefits of the individual's and others' wellbeing when you inform and involve them about their safeguarding concern.

Produce an information leaflet on how to keep the individual and others appropriately informed and involved regarding their safeguarding concern, in line with the policies and procedures of the care setting where you work. Include the benefits of doing so.

AC 4.6 Outline ways to ensure that evidence of abuse is preserved

You will also have a role to play in ensuring all evidence related to a suspicion and disclosure of abuse is preserved.

Why is preserving evidence of abuse important?

Preserving evidence is important:

- so that an investigation into what happened can take place (you may need this for further investigation in the setting or you may need to pass this on to the police)
- because evidence can support any suspicions you have and disclosures that have been made
- so that the person carrying out the abuse can be prosecuted and brought to justice.

What evidence of abuse can be preserved and how?

- **Body fluids:** in the case of sexual abuse, body fluids that can be used as evidence include blood and semen left on the individual, on clothing and on bed linen. You can ensure the individual does not have a bath or shower, or have contact with other people and ensure that the affected items are not touched or washed. It may even be that the individual should not remove the clothing if the abuse has just taken place. In this way, this evidence can be preserved. If possible, others should not be allowed to enter the area where the abuse has taken place.
- **Broken items or personal possessions** can be used as evidence. You should make sure that there is no attempt to clean or remove these. They should be left exactly as you found them and you should not allow anyone else to clean or remove these items.
- **Photographs:** photos of people's living environments can be used as evidence of neglect.
- **Witness testimonies:** these may be used as evidence for physical abuse that may not necessarily have left a visible injury.
- **Records:** previous records that you have made about suspicions or disclosures can also be shared as evidence. This is why it is very important to record, sign and date any details of this nature straight away – as you will be less

likely to forget what you have been told, the record will be more accurate and it cannot be altered later.
- **Prints:** in the case of financial abuse (fraud or theft), financial documents such as bank statements, or statements of transfer can be used. Fingerprints and footprints on items can also be preserved by ensuring that people are not allowed to touch anything or to enter the area where the abuse is suspected or disclosed to have taken place.

> **Evidence opportunity**
>
> **4.6 Preserving evidence**
>
> Discuss with your assessor your role and responsibilities when preserving evidence of suspicions and disclosure of abuse. What are your employer's expectations of you when putting these into practice? Why?

AC 4.7 Describe both how and when to seek support in relation to responding to safeguarding concerns

Safeguarding and protecting individuals from abuse is part of your duty of care and responsibility as an adult care worker. At the same time, you cannot expect to know everything about abuse. There may be times when you just do not know how to respond to a situation. Doing nothing is not an option; therefore, should a situation arise in which you have no experience (or if it is outside your area of expertise), it is important to seek help.

Table 2.5 provides you with examples of situations when you will need to seek further support from either, or both, internal and external sources.

You must always follow your work setting's agreed ways of working, as these will describe how you can seek support in your work role, i.e. directly from an external source, such as a professional, or through an internal source first, such as your manager.

Table 2.5 Situations where you may need to seek support

When to seek support	How to seek support
You are dealing with a situation where a crime has been committed.	You will need to seek support from police when a crime is committed, for example when an individual has been burgled and has had their property damaged. You may not have expertise in how to handle this situation and how to preserve evidence.
You are dealing with a situation which requires a medical procedure which you have no knowledge of or skills in.	You may need to contact a medical professional when you do not know how to carry out a procedure or administer medication, for example when an individual is bleeding from the head. This will ensure the individual receives appropriate medical care and is not placed in danger.
You are dealing with an individual with an illness you have no medical expertise in, such as dementia.	You may need to contact a medical professional, or a charity such as Alzheimer's Society for more information on supporting an individual with dementia.
You witness an individual's family member shouting at their relative during one of their visits.	Seeking support from your manager will ensure the appropriate actions can be taken and the individual can be protected from any further abuse. By doing this, you are practising your duty of care to safeguard this individual. You can ensure that your safety is also maintained by seeking the support of your manager.
You report your concerns of an individual in your care setting being at risk of abuse from a colleague and your manager is too busy to deal with this.	Seeking support from an external organisation such as CQC will ensure that the individual is no longer at risk of abuse. By doing this, you will be protecting this individual's safety as well as others who may be at risk in the care setting where you work.
A colleague asks you to use unsafe practices when supporting an individual being hoisted.	Seeking support from your manager will ensure that you will be supported to not carry out these unsafe practices. This will also raise your colleague's awareness of unsafe practices and the consequences of these. This will ensure the safety and wellbeing of the individual you are supporting as well as you and your colleague's safety.

> **Evidence opportunity**
>
> **AC 4.7** How and when to ask for support
>
> Discuss with your manager the agreed ways of working you should follow when seeking support with two safeguarding situations in which you have no experience, or that are beyond your area of expertise. Write a written explanation of how and when you asked for support. Remember to include the reasons why in your explanation.

AC 4.8 Describe how to respond to a suspicion or disclosure that a child or young person is being harmed or abused

Safeguarding children and young people from abuse and harm involves:

- protection from maltreatment
- promotion of their health and development
- provision of safe and effective care
- enabling them to have the best outcomes in life.

The safeguarding of children and young people is underpinned by the following two principles:

1. **Safeguarding is everyone's responsibility**: this means that everyone who works with children and young people has a responsibility to keep them safe. You can do this by identifying and raising their concerns, working closely with other practitioners and services, ensuring you are aware of your role in safeguarding them and others from abuse and neglect, and they are aware of their role in safeguarding themselves and others.
2. **A child-centred approach**: this means the interests, needs and views of the children and young people in care must be put first. For example, you can do this by listening to children and young people's concerns, taking what they say or express seriously, providing them with reassurance about what they have disclosed and working with them to decide how best to meet their needs and keep them safe.

The care setting where you work will have procedures in place for how to respond if a child or young person discloses that they are being abused or harmed, or when there are suspicions that abuse or harm may be happening. It can be overwhelming when an individual discloses such information, even more so when the individual concerned is a child or young person, because of their vulnerability and the way they may express or tell you about the abuse or harm. The child or young person may become very distressed or be very fearful of their perpetrator. To avoid causing them any further distress, how you respond to suspicions and disclosures of abuse and harm is very important. Below are some of the key points to remember:

- **Provide support**: Remember to show your support of the child or young person by listening to what they are saying, believing what is being said, not showing shock and remaining calm. It is important that you support them in this way so that they continue to tell you about the abuse or harm that they have experienced, otherwise they may stop and withdraw everything they have said.
- **Provide reassurance**: Remember to reassure the child or young person by telling them you believe them, you are taking what they told you seriously and that they have done nothing wrong. Acknowledge that you realise how difficult it must be for them to tell you about the abuse or harm, reassure them that they are showing their courage for speaking out and are not at fault.
- **Don't make promises you can't keep**: Remember to only promise what you can do. For example, don't promise that you are going to make sure the abuse or harm stops or that you're not going to tell anyone about the abuse or harm they've disclosed. Explain to the child or young person that it is your duty to report what they have told you so that they can be kept protected from further abuse or harm; explain what you are going to do and what is going to happen next.
- **Communicate appropriately**: Remember to listen and be patient when a child or young person is disclosing information; let them explain to you in their own words and in their own time, don't rush them. Communicate with them in a way that is appropriate to their age and understanding, by using language they understand and the communication methods they prefer.

- **Report and record**: Remember to report any suspicions or disclosures to the person designated in the safeguarding procedures of the care setting where you work, and do not discuss this with anyone else. Make sure you record the actual words used by the child or young person, your observation of how they appeared, as well as the date, time and place where the disclosure took place. Record only the facts, not your interpretations.

Reflect on it

AC 4.8 Suspicions and disclosures of abuse and neglect

Reflect on the differences that there may be between an adult and a child or young person disclosing that they are being abused or harmed. How might they express themselves differently? Why? How might you have to respond differently? Why?

Evidence opportunity

AC 4.8 How to respond to suspicions or disclosures of abuse and neglect of children or young people

Read through the safeguarding procedures and agreed ways of working for the care setting where you work, and make some notes of what they say about responding to suspicions or disclosures or abuse or neglect of children or young people.

Produce a one-page information handout that explains how to respond when a child or young person has disclosed that they are being abused or neglected.

LO5 Understand ways to reduce the likelihood of abuse or neglect

Getting started

Think about someone you know that has care or support needs. This may be because of an illness or disability. Why do you think that they are more likely to experience some form of abuse? What do you think makes them vulnerable to abuse?

Now think about what you could do to reduce their likelihood of being abused. For example, how does the way you treat them impact on how they feel about themselves? Does it make them feel confident in themselves and valued? What else could you do to promote their safety and wellbeing?

AC 5.1 Explain how the likelihood of abuse may be reduced

You can explain how the likelihood of abuse may be reduced by:

- working with **person-centred values**
- enabling **active participation**
- promoting choice and rights
- supporting individuals with awareness of personal safety
- working in partnership with others.

The relevant safeguarding legislation, principles, national policies, frameworks and local systems you have learned about are what underpin your working practices in the care setting where you work. These, together with the way you carry out your day-to-day role and responsibilities, can reduce the likelihood of individuals being abused or neglected.

Key term

Person-centred values refer to ensuring that care provided places individuals at the heart and fits around them. Person-centred values include individuality, rights, choice, privacy, independence, dignity, respect, partnership, care, compassion, courage, communication and competence.

Active participation means enabling individuals to be involved in their care and support and can mean that people feel in control of their day-to-day choices.

Working with person-centred values

Working with individuals with care or support needs involves working in ways that embed person-centred values. This concept is covered in more detail in Unit 306 Promoting and implementing person-centred practice. Working with person-centred values can reduce the likelihood of abuse. Some examples are listed below.

- **Treating individuals with respect** and **showing that you value their individuality** will reduce the likelihood of an individual being discriminated against and abused. Respect for individuals and their differences promotes confidence in those that you care for; they are more likely to challenge and speak up about abuse if they are more confident in themselves.
- **Promoting an individual's dignity** means taking precautions to ensure that they do not feel humiliated or intimidated. For example, you can promote an individual's dignity **and respect their privacy** when they are having a bath by closing the door and placing a towel over them. Working in this way will reduce the likelihood of an individual being abused and make the individual feel comfortable about being supported with intimate care by workers. They will also become more aware of how care workers should support them and they will notice in future (and report) when the support they receive does not promote their dignity and rights. This will help individuals to **understand what their rights are** and what to do when their rights are being denied or ignored.
- **Showing compassion** when working with individuals and their families means that you are **showing genuine care** and concern for their wellbeing. For example, you can make time to understand why an individual may find it difficult to settle into their new care setting after living previously in their family home all their life. Working in this way will reduce the likelihood of an individual being abused because they will learn to trust and respect you and therefore be more likely to share any experiences of abuse or neglect from others. The individual's family will also feel able to approach you with any concerns they might have.
- **Supporting an individual's independence** means that you are enabling an individual to do as much for themselves as possible, including **making their own informed choices** by providing them with the information about what options are available, and helping them to assess any risks that they may face. **Supporting an individual's independence takes courage**, because it means you may have to change the way you work in order to do the right thing for the individual. It also includes speaking up for an individual who is being abused and is too scared to report it, because they fear their perpetrator.
- **Effective communication** is essential for **working alongside and together in partnership** with individuals and others, to safeguard individuals from abuse and improper treatment. Effective communication involves actively listening to what individuals say and do; doing so means that you will be more likely to recognise any indicators of abuse or improper treatment when they occur, and therefore you can prevent the abuse from continuing or getting any worse. Effective communication and working in partnership requires you to **have competence in your job role**, and to have the necessary knowledge, skills and expertise to care for individuals and safeguard them from abuse and improper treatment.

Enabling active participation

Active participation is a way of working that encourages individuals to be active participants in their care or support rather than passive recipients. It is a way of working that recognises that individuals with care or support needs have the right to participate in day-to-day activities as independently as possible. Encouraging active participation can reduce the likelihood of abuse happening in different ways. Some examples of this are included below.

- Supporting an individual's independence means that you are encouraging individuals to be actively involved in day-to-day activities at home and in their local communities. You can do this by supporting them to develop their skills in managing their money, learning how to cook, going shopping and socialising. Working in this way will reduce the likelihood of an individual being abused because they will not be seen as someone who can be exploited by others. It will also make the individual feel confident in their own abilities and believe in themselves.
- Encouraging individuals to be active in their care or support means working alongside them and letting them guide you with what is important to them and how they want to be cared for. For example, you can develop an

individual's care plan with them; this may mean providing them with all the information they need to decide what activities they would like to participate in – and those that they would not. Working in this way will reduce the likelihood of an individual being abused because using their care plan will ensure that the individual's history, preferences, needs and beliefs are taken into account. Both the setting and the individual will recognise when those needs are not met. Their care or support will be led by the individual rather than the care workers and will therefore make them feel in control of their own care or support. It makes the individual feel empowered rather than someone who is always dependent on others.

> **Research it**
>
> **5.1 Active participation**
>
> Carry out some research in the care setting where you work about how you can enable active participation. You will find it useful to speak to your colleagues and your manager.
>
> Discuss the techniques used, the reasons why these are effective and how they meet individuals' needs.

Promoting choice and rights

Promoting individuals' choices and rights underpins all person-centred ways of working and is effective when reducing the likelihood of abuse happening because it encourages workers to put individuals' needs first and to focus on individuals' best interests rather than on what the workers think may be best. Some examples of how promoting individuals' choice and rights can reduce the likelihood of abuse are included below.

- Promoting an individual's choices means that you are encouraging individuals to think about the options available so that they can make their own choice. For example, by providing them with relevant information about the different ways they can travel to visit a friend, such as by rail, bus or taxi, they can then consider all the information available to them and then make a decision based on what they prefer to do. Working in this way will reduce the likelihood of abuse because it encourages individuals to be more bold and assertive not just in their behaviour but confident in themselves.
- Promoting an individual's rights means treating individuals as you would like to be treated, that is, on equal terms with all the same rights that you have. Working in this way will reduce the likelihood of abuse because you will be informing and raising individuals' awareness about what is fair and equal treatment (in terms of their care or support), empowering the individual to feel in control and know when their treatment is not fair and equal.

Actively supporting individuals to fulfil their rights in your day-to-day working, for example by supporting their safety at home when mobilising, and supporting their wellbeing at all times, will reduce the likelihood of abuse because you will be supporting their rights to be safe. In this way, they will develop their own understanding of their rights, how to stay safe and how they can be supported by those who work around them.

Supporting individuals with awareness of personal safety

Awareness of personal safety can be a very effective way of supporting individuals to be in control of their own safety and therefore reduce the likelihood of them being abused. Some examples of how supporting individuals with awareness of personal safety are set out below.

- Promoting personal safety when working alongside individuals can be a very effective way to increase an individual's knowledge about how to stay safe. You can do this by providing information leaflets about the dangers that exist in the home, such as: not opening the door to people they do not know, checking that the gas is turned off after using the cooker in the evening, not blocking fire escape routes with furniture and not leaving the windows open when leaving home. You can warn them of the dangers that exist in the community, for example remind them not to walk on their own late at night. Working in this way will reduce the likelihood of abuse because you will be informing individuals about **hazards** so that they can take precautions to reduce the potential **risks** these may cause. There is more information about risk assessment in Unit 307 Promoting choice and independence in adult care settings/services.

> **Key term**
>
> **Hazards** are dangers with the potential to cause harm, for example a spillage on the floor or a broken wheelchair.
>
> **Risk** is the likelihood of hazards causing harm, for example slipping over on a spillage on the floor, an individual falling out of a broken wheelchair.

- Supporting an individual's personal safety by involving them in working in safe ways will increase their awareness of personal safety by ensuring they always consider the dangers associated with different activities and the potential risks these pose. They can then use this information to make decisions that do not compromise their safety. Working in this way will reduce the likelihood of abuse because you will be actively supporting individuals to think about and make decisions that put their own safety first.

Working in partnership with others

Working together in partnership means working with an individual's family, friends and advocates, as well as your colleagues, manager and other professionals for the benefit and wellbeing of the person you are caring for. For example, you can ensure that you share information so that you can all work to protect the individual in the most efficient way, and only use ways of working that are person-centred. This concept is covered in Unit 306, Promoting and implementing person-centred practice. This is important, because in this way, you will all be working together to care for and support the individual, therefore making it less likely that the individual will be abused or neglected.

As you get to know the individual, you will also be more likely to notice any unusual changes that may indicate that something is wrong. Working in partnership will also help with this, as you will be able to learn more about the individual from others who know them well.

Working in partnership with others also means working alongside different agencies that safeguard and protect individuals from abuse or improper treatment. You will find it useful to refer back to AC 1.2 in this unit for more information about the roles of these different agencies. Working in partnership with these agencies will mean that you:

- will be part of a team with extensive knowledge of and expertise in the safeguarding and protection of individuals
- will be able to share best practice in safeguarding and protecting individuals
- have a support network in place if you have any safeguarding concerns.

Working in partnership with others is very important, because it means that you are able to understand an individual's holistic needs, rather than just the aspect of the individual's life that you see or know about. In turn, this means you will be more likely to identify any risks of abuse or neglect.

> **Evidence opportunity**
>
> **5.1 Ways to reduce likelihood of abuse**
>
> Produce a leaflet that describes how:
>
> - working with person-centred values
> - promoting choice and rights
> - supporting individuals with awareness of personal safety
> - enabling active participation and
> - working in partnership with others
>
> can all reduce the likelihood of individuals in the care setting where you work being abused.

AC 5.2 Explain the importance of an accessible complaints procedure for reducing the likelihood of abuse

All organisations that provide care or support services are required to have a procedure in place to respond to complaints. A complaints procedure that is accessible means one that can be:

- available in different formats, for example Braille for individuals with vision loss with signs and symbols for individuals with learning disabilities; in audio for individuals unable to read; in different languages to meet individuals' preferences
- available to all and located in places that can be accessed easily and without having to ask for permission to do so, for example in the entrance hall to a care setting

- explained and reinforced by the care staff on an on-going basis in relation to its purpose, what it can be used for and how confidentiality will be maintained when it is used
- reviewed alongside the individuals and others it is aimed at to ensure its effectiveness.

An accessible complaints procedure can reduce the likelihood of abuse because:

- it empowers individuals to respond to concerns they have about themselves and others
- it brings complaints out into the open so that they can be acted on through effective and clear communication
- it increases the confidence of individuals and others in the quality and safety of the care or support being provided – everyone knows that there is a way to report abuse if they need to do so
- it raises individuals' awareness of their rights to good quality care or support.

Being able to raise concerns over safety or any risk of being abused is an effective and important way of ensuring that health and social care services or other agencies involved in safeguarding individuals are alerted to the potential of abuse happening so that they can act to prevent it.

6Cs

Communication

Communication is essential for developing good complaints procedures. Effectively communicating your setting's complaints procedures involves ensuring that they can be used effectively by those who need them. You can ensure that this is communicated effectively by reporting when you have any concerns that an individual or someone else may not have understood your care setting's procedures. In this way these procedures can be adapted to meet the individual or someone else's needs and they can access the additional support they require to understand them. This will also increase the likelihood of them using it and decrease the likelihood of them not doing so, which may result in them continuing to be abused or neglected.

Evidence opportunity

5.2 Consequences of not having an accessible complaints procedure

Reflect on the consequences of not having an accessible complaints procedure. What impact may this have on the likelihood of abuse happening? Why? Make notes to evidence your reflection. Remember to think about the impact that accessible formats, such as Easy Read, can have.

Then develop a flow diagram that explains how each stage of an accessible complaints procedure can reduce the likelihood of abuse taking place.

AC 5.3 Outline how the likelihood of abuse can be reduced by a) managing risk and b) focusing on prevention

Risk enablement is a way of working that reduces the likelihood of abuse happening by using techniques that encourage risk to be managed and focuses on the prevention of abuse.

Reflect on it

5.3 Managing risk and preventing abuse

Reflect on the consequences of not being able to manage risk effectively. How could this lead to abuse? Reflect on the importance of early prevention of abuse. What are the consequences of not doing so?

How can you reduce the likelihood of individuals being abused by managing risk and focusing on prevention?

In AC 5.1, we discussed the different ways in which you can work to reduce the likelihood of abuse happening.

Risk enablement can reduce the likelihood of abuse because it involves using the following techniques and approaches, which you should implement.

- **Encourage individuals to do what they can to protect themselves from being abused and harmed.** Empower them to be active participants and in control of their own care or support. For example, if an individual wants to move freely around their house on their own but has mobility difficulties, risk enablement would support the individual to mobilise safely around their home.

You can do this by ensuring the individual has a walking aid and access to a personal alarm (that they can wear and use when on their own) in case of an emergency. Risk enablement enables individuals to do what they want safely; this makes individuals feel listened to and valued while maintaining their safety, thus reducing the likelihood of abuse taking place.

- **Empower individuals to complain when care or support goes wrong.** For example, if an individual knows that care workers must treat him or her with respect at all times then they will be more likely to complain when a care worker does not treat them with respect. As a result of risk enablement, the risk of them not having their rights respected or them being abused is less likely to happen.
- **Support individuals to understand and take managed risks.** For example, risk enablement can mean that an individual is supported to identify any risks that may be associated with an activity that they want to do and then decide, having assessed the benefits and consequences of the activity, whether they still want to do it or if they need to consider other safety precautions. They can also understand how to manage risks.
- **Enable care settings to focus on the managing of risks and the prevention of abuse.** Risk enablement means that you promote the protection of individuals in your setting, for example undertake safeguarding training (on the potential signs and symptoms that an individual is being abused) which can help identify abuse early on. You will become more aware of the factors that increase the likelihood of an individual being at risk of abuse and be able to help the setting focus on how the individuals' rights, safety and wellbeing can be promoted.

Caring for carers

Remember, you can reduce the risk of abuse happening by trying to prevent abuse before it starts and by spotting potential signs of abuse. If you see that carers are under immense pressure to support the individuals, then you should offer support and advice to them. Stress and pressures do not mean that abuse will always happen, but spotting it means you are able to address it early on and be there for carers as well as individuals. Be empathetic and if your own work pressures mean that you cannot offer them support daily, then make sure that you tell them about support and services they can access. Not only could this reduce and prevent the likelihood of abuse, but it also means that you are able to build a good empathetic relationship with the carer, one where they feel supported.

Research it

5.3 Support carers in a practical way

Research the support that is available for carers. You could ask your manager about the sorts of practical support you could offer carers. For example, how can carers be supported with any practical equipment they may need? Do they need a stair lift in their home? Do they need help with daily tasks such as their shopping? Do they need any training for any tasks they do not have the skills to do?

How can you support them with this? How will this support the carer and the individual? How can this help to prevent abuse?

Evidence opportunity

5.3 Managing risk and preventing abuse

Read the Risk Enablement Policy in place in the care setting where you work.

Produce a one-page information handout or a poster that outlines how the likelihood of abuse can be reduced by managing risk and focusing on prevention.

LO6 Know how to recognise and report unsafe practices

Getting started

Think about an occasion when you witnessed something that was unsafe and made you feel uncomfortable. This may have happened at work or outside of your work setting. For example, you may have witnessed one of your colleagues not putting on gloves when supporting an individual to get washed and dressed.

How did this make you feel? Why? Did you do anything about it? Why?

Think about the benefits of reporting unsafe practices immediately. Now think about the consequences of not doing so. What will you do next time if this situation arises again and why?

AC 6.1 Describe unsafe practices that may affect the wellbeing of individuals

Being able to recognise unsafe practices when they occur and understand the procedures your care setting has in place for reporting these will help you to ensure that your ways of working focus on the prevention of abuse.

Unsafe practices are those that may lead to an individual, you, a colleague or visitor being placed in danger or at risk of being injured or harmed.

Table 2.6 includes examples of three different types of unsafe practice that may occur in a care setting due to poor working practices, resource difficulties and operational difficulties.

All three types of unsafe practice can lead to an individual being subjected to abuse and neglect and therefore have the potential to affect their safety. Table 2.6 includes how unsafe practices may affect the different aspects of an individual's wellbeing. (See Unit 308 Supporting individuals with their health and wellbeing for more information.)

Table 2.6 Unsafe practices and how they affect an individual's wellbeing

Unsafe practices	Examples of how the wellbeing of an individual is affected
Poor working practices	Poor health and safety practices may lead to accidents in the care setting and have the potential to cause both physical and mental harm to those involved.
	Not taking suspicions of abuse seriously may mean that individuals continue to be abused which can in turn affect their physical, emotional and mental wellbeing. If the abuse is financial then it will impact on their economic wellbeing and their trust in others. They may withdraw and become isolated thus having an effect on their social wellbeing.
	Unsafe practices when moving and handling may lead to individuals, you and your colleagues being injured or harmed physically. In turn, this will impact on the confidence of individuals and others and will have a negative effect on their emotional and mental wellbeing too.
Resource difficulties	Insufficient or a lack of equipment will mean that individuals' needs will remain unmet. For example, they may be injured, or their independence may be restricted which may in turn mean that their emotional and social wellbeing is affected because they may have to be more dependent on others.
	Insufficient workers to care for individuals will mean that individuality will not be recognised as there will be insufficient time to attend to every individual's personal needs. This may mean that the support provided does not take into account their intellectual abilities, cultural and spiritual needs.
	A lack of regular training will mean that a carer's way of working may not reflect current best practice or legislation. They may fail in their duty of care to safeguard individuals, which will have a direct impact on their social, emotional and physical wellbeing.
Operational difficulties	A lack of effective management means that no one is monitoring the care and support provided by workers. This means that the individuals may be subjected to abuse more easily which will impact negatively on their wellbeing physically, emotionally and socially.
	A lack of support for workers may mean that they cannot respond effectively to situations where they have insufficient expertise. As a result, abuse of an individual may go unnoticed. This can change how an individual feels about themselves, their confidence and their identity, e.g. in terms of their spirituality.
	Poor communication systems with other agencies may mean that the signs that an individual is being abused are not recognised or reported, thus enabling the abuse to continue causing a detrimental effect to the individual's wellbeing; this could be physically, culturally, emotionally and socially.

Reflect on it

6.1 Unsafe practices

Reflect on how unsafe practices can affect an individual's wellbeing. How do you think an individual may feel? Why? How do you think you would feel if that were you? Why?

Evidence opportunity

6.1 Unsafe practices and wellbeing

Develop two case studies for two different individuals who have different care or support needs. For each one write a description about how unsafe practices may affect their wellbeing.

Being able to recognise unsafe practices is essential for maintaining the safety and wellbeing of the individuals, your colleagues and others you work with. Not doing so can lead to individuals being abused, the likelihood of accidents increasing, and the safety and wellbeing of individuals being affected, which can in turn increase the likelihood of abuse happening.

AC 6.2 Explain the actions to take if unsafe practices have been identified

The care setting where you work will have procedures in place for reporting unsafe practices that have been identified. It is your responsibility to ensure that you are familiar with these and to report any unsafe practices that you observe or are told about.

Research it

6.2 Your job description

Research your job description, your job role and responsibilities. What does it say about your responsibilities towards the individuals you provide care or support to? What does it say about your responsibilities towards others who you work with?

Discuss how you can ensure that your ways of working are safe and fulfil your responsibilities to individuals and others. Make notes about your discussion.

Below is a list of some tips for the actions to take.

1. Follow your employer's procedures and agreed ways of working when unsafe practices have been identified so that the necessary action can be taken to prevent the unsafe practices from continuing to take place or injury or harm to individuals or others.

2. Constructively challenge (in a way that will be useful and beneficial) all unsafe practices so that the person that is carrying these out can understand the reasons why their ways of working are unsafe and how these could lead to the abuse and neglect of individuals or others. It is possible that they are not aware that their way of working is unsafe. Challenge the person constructively, in a calm way because you do not want them to react aggressively, or for them to feel embarrassed because they did not know their practice was unsafe.

3. Do not continue or carry out an activity that you think may be unsafe as this will place individuals at risk of abuse or put you and others in danger. Changing your practice will mean that your safety and those of others will be protected; individuals' wellbeing will also be protected.

4. Discuss your concerns with your manager so that your manager is made aware and so that the necessary actions can be taken. Your manager will be experienced in this area and so will be able to provide you with some useful advice and guidance as well as reassurance that you have followed the agreed ways of working of your care setting.

5. Record the concerns you have so that there is a permanent account on file of your concerns. This record will be particularly useful if at a later stage there is an investigation into a case of abuse of an individual or a review of the care setting's procedures for safeguarding individuals. Your record shows the actions you have taken when unsafe practices have been identified.

> **Evidence opportunity**
>
> **6.2 Actions to take**
>
> Reflect on how the list of tips above compares to the actions you are required to take in the care setting where you work should you witness or be asked to carry out unsafe practices.
>
> Produce a wall display to illustrate different examples of unsafe practices that may arise in care settings, what the outcome will be for the wellbeing of individuals, and the action that should be taken to eliminate the unsafe practice.

AC 6.3 Describe the actions to take if suspected abuse or unsafe practices have been reported but nothing has been done in response

You should ensure that your concerns about unsafe practices or suspected abuse that you have reported are followed through and addressed. This is very important and an essential part of your duty of care. Your care setting will have whistleblowing procedures in place that will set out what you can do. It is important that you show your **commitment** when following these through.

You could in the first instance discuss your concerns again with your manager and ask them to tell you what has been done in response. If your manager is unable to explain what has been done in response or you find out that your manager is also involved in the suspected abuse or unsafe practices identified, then you could report these to the next level of management in the organisation.

If you have reported your concerns to the next level of management and still nothing has been done, then you must persist and contact an outside agency such as the **regulator** of health and social care services, the Care Quality Commission (CQC) or the safeguarding team in adult social care services. See Unit 301 AC 1.2 for more information about the CQC. If you are member of a trade union then you could also seek advice from your representative.

Following through your concerns about suspected abuse or unsafe practices when nothing has been done in response is essential for ensuring the safety and wellbeing of individuals. Case study 6.1, 6.2, 6.3 provides you with an opportunity to think about the impact of doing so and complying with your care setting's whistleblowing procedures.

> **6Cs**
>
> **Commitment**
>
> You can show commitment to protecting individuals by speaking up for them to ensure their safety and wellbeing. You can do this by always following your agreed ways of working for whistleblowing. In this way, individuals will know that they can count on you to take the necessary action when they have been subjected to abuse or unsafe practices.

> **Key term**
>
> **Regulators** are bodies that supervise a particular sector.

> **Reflect on it**
>
> **6.3 Reporting concerns**
>
> Reflect on how you may feel reporting your concerns to the next level of management in the organisation. How do you think you may feel about doing this? Why? Do you think this will make you feel uncomfortable?

> **Evidence opportunity**
>
> **6.3 Actions to take**
>
> Consider what further action you would take if you had reported suspected abuse or unsafe practices in your care setting but nothing had been done in response.
>
> Produce a flow diagram detailing the key actions to take when you have to follow up your report of suspected abuse and unsafe practices in your setting for a second time.

Case study

6.1, 6.2, 6.3 Unsafe work practices

Emma is a residential care worker who supports individuals with learning disabilities to live independently. Emma's work shift partner is Dave who is a senior residential care worker. During the morning shift, Emma observes Dave restrict an individual from leaving his room while explaining to him that this is in his best interests (because he had injured his leg and he had been told by his GP to rest). Emma notices that the individual looks frustrated.

Emma feels uncomfortable about Dave's actions and so discusses her concerns with Dave. Emma constructively explains to Dave that she doesn't feel that it was necessary to physically restrict the individual as it was his right to leave his room and not be confined in it. Emma also explains that she thinks that this individual is able to make his own decisions.

Dave thanks Emma for her concerns and reassures her that there is nothing to worry about. He tells her that she should trust him, as he is the senior colleague, and work with him as she has done for many years.

Discuss:
1. Emma's approach to challenging Dave
2. Dave's response to Emma
3. The actions Emma should take next and why.

LO7 Understand the principles for online safety

Getting started

Think about all the online activities you and your friends participate in. For example, this may involve using a mobile to text your family and friends and/or surf the internet, using a tablet or PC to buy items online or accessing social networking sites such as Facebook or Twitter. Have you ever experienced any problems with your safety online? If so, what happened? If not, what could happen?

Now think about an individual you know who has care or support needs. How can you make sure that you keep them safe while they participate in online activities?

AC 7.1 Explain the importance of balancing online safety measures with the benefits that individuals can gain from accessing activities online

Promoting online safety does not mean that individuals are prevented or deterred from accessing activities online, but rather that they are informed of the risks, and are involved in assessing them and in making their own decisions about how to use these activities safely. **Competently** working in this way is part of risk enablement (a way of working you learned about in AC 5.3) and also embeds person-centred values.

6Cs

Competence

Competence in relation to promoting online safety refers to applying your knowledge and skills to ensure that you are able to communicate to individuals the risks and benefits that they face when using electronic systems and devices. You should tell them about how they can take control when doing so and keep themselves safe. You can also give them information leaflets, take the time to discuss the different risks with them and encourage them to ask you questions or share any concerns they have with you.

Reflect on it

7.1 Person-centred values when promoting online safety

Reflect on the person-centred values you have learned about. How can you instil these in your working practices when promoting online safety? Why is it important to do so? What are the consequences of not doing so?

The benefits to individuals of using electronic systems and devices are numerous and can include some of the following:

- **making new friends** – there can be more opportunities for meeting new people and being part of a group of friends. This can make individuals feel like they belong to a social group and can share their common interests with others.

- **learning new skills** – there are opportunities for developing new skills such as being able to communicate with others verbally and in writing. They can also be creative and express themselves through writing blogs, and posting pictures and online videos.
- **developing your knowledge** – there are opportunities for developing your knowledge about a range of different topics, and interests and study skills can be developed in this way.

Striking a balance between the risks associated with online safety and the above benefits means that the rights of the individual are promoted and their wellbeing enhanced. The reflective exemplar below provides you with some additional information about the importance of balancing the risks with the benefits of accessing activities online.

> **Evidence opportunity**
>
> **7.1 Balancing measures**
>
> Discuss with your assessor the importance of balancing measures for online safety against the benefits to individuals of accessing activities online. Remember to think about how personalisation is relevant here.

Reflective exemplar	
Introduction	I work as a Lead Personal Assistant to John who has learning difficulties. I visit him once a week to support him to visit one of his best friends who lives locally.
What happened?	Last week, while supporting John to visit his friend he had a video call with another friend on his mobile phone. His friend began to tell him how unwell she was and also shared with him the personal difficulties she was having at the time with her family. I was aware that everyone on the bus was looking at us and could hear what John's friend was saying to him. I quietly pointed this out to John and told him not to 'FaceTime' his friend. John got very upset and when the bus stopped, he got off the bus suddenly and accused me of treating him like a child, and not an adult.
What worked well?	I raised my concerns with John discreetly. I identified the risks of video calling another person in public.
What did not go as well?	Telling John about my concerns while we were still on the bus. I should have suggested to John that we get off at the next stop because I wanted to talk to him about something important. This way I could have talked through with him my concerns and supported him to understand the risks.
What could I do to improve?	I think I will need to put John's needs first rather than my own; it was my embarrassment on the bus that prevented me from handling this situation sensitively. I think I will need to reflect on the benefits that video calls have for John. I will suggest some suitable locations where he can have video calls. I will explain to him the reasons why I have identified these locations so that he can make his own decisions by choosing which one he prefers.
Links to unit assessment criteria	ACs: 7.1, 7.2, 7.3

AC 7.2 Explain why it is important to uphold an individual's rights to make informed decisions about online safety

Upholding an individual's rights to make informed decisions about online safety involves doing everything you can to support individuals to make their own choices and decisions, and to be independent without compromising their or others' safety. This is important, because it means that individuals can be supported to take risks by assessing what the potential dangers are online and by considering what can be put in place to reduce those risks and protect individuals from danger, harm, abuse and neglect. It does not prevent individuals from doing what they want, but rather helps individuals, and you, to manage these risks effectively by considering what can be done to reduce them. In this way you will be exercising your duty of care by supporting individuals' rights to live how they want to, and to make their own informed choices and decisions after giving careful consideration to the associated benefits, risks and consequences.

Taking risks is also a key aspect of providing person-centred care, because taking risks is part of everyday life and an essential part of upholding an individual's rights to make informed choices and be in control of their safety online. This approach is also known as positive risk taking and involves weighing up the benefits and harms of different choices and decisions. It is linked to promoting individuals' rights and responsibilities because it involves:

- enabling individuals to grow in confidence and make their own decisions based on information available on a range of options
- promoting individuals' strengths and abilities
- supporting individuals to take opportunities
- supporting individuals to understand their responsibilities and those of others
- supporting individuals to understand the benefits of taking risks
- supporting individuals to understand the consequences of taking risks
- supporting individuals to learn from their mistakes
- developing good working relationships with individuals and others
- being positive about taking risks.

You can also refer to Unit 303 Understanding duty of care for more information on risk taking and risk management.

Upholding an individual's rights to make informed decisions about online safety is therefore part of working in a person-centred way and involves working in partnership with the individual to reduce the likelihood of them becoming a target to be abused online. You will also find it useful to refer to Unit 300 Responsibilities and ways of working in adult care settings/services, AC 1.4, that explains the importance of working in partnership with others.

Reflect on it

AC 7.2 Consequences

Reflect on the consequences of not upholding an individual's rights to make informed decisions about online safety. What would be the consequences for the individual, you and your work setting?

Evidence opportunity

AC 7.2 Upholding individuals' rights to make informed decisions

Provide a written account explaining how you promote individuals' rights to make informed decisions about online safety in the care setting where you work and why this is important. How can you use positive risk taking to promote individuals' rights to make informed decisions about online safety? Why is this important?

AC 7.3 Describe the potential risks to individuals using a) electronic communication devices, b) the internet, c) social networking sites, d) online financial transactions

Potential risks for individuals with care and support going online include:

- the use of electronic communication devices
- the use of the internet
- the use of social networking sites
- carrying out financial transactions online.

Whether you are an online expert or not, it is important that you are aware of the potential risks presented by individuals with care or support needs going online so that you can fulfil your duty of care to maintain their safety and promote their wellbeing.

The use of electronic communication devices

Individuals may increasingly use their mobile phones and tablets when they are out and about. It is important that individuals are made aware of the risks of others obtaining their security passwords to commit fraud or even being subjected to theft of their electronic devices.

Individuals are able to access websites and download apps such as Facebook, Instagram and Snapchat that enable them to comment and share images with others. While these are ways for them to connect with others, they may also be subjected to unwanted comments, offensive images or be subjected to bullying online. Apps such as these also send information out about the individual's location, so others can see where the individual is; again, this may make them the target for abuse.

The use of the internet

The internet can be a great place to connect with others and share our lives whether it is through our updates, blogs, or photos. However, because we may be sharing so much information, there is a danger that some of this may be abused or used dishonestly. Some of the potential risks that the internet poses are listed here.

- Individuals may use the internet and search engines such as Google to search for information about what is happening in their local communities and so that they can find out more about places to shop or eat out in. However, this sometimes requires sharing your location to find good spots to eat – and the location is made public to others.
- Individuals need to be made aware of the risks of searching for information on unofficial sites that may contain offensive language. They must also be aware about the risk of finding or being exposed to information that may be of a sexually explicit nature.
- Sharing financial details about their bank account – even if this is on a well-known or trusted website – can leave people open to fraud and theft (having their banking details stolen) if someone else is able to gain access to these details. See the section on 'Carrying out financial transactions online', on page 82, for more information on this.
- Individuals can also play games online and may interact with their friends in this way. It is important that individuals understand that these games could become addictive and can lead to them spending many hours on these sites (becoming increasingly socially isolated from family and friends). They should also be informed about the risks that gambling websites pose as this too can become an addiction.

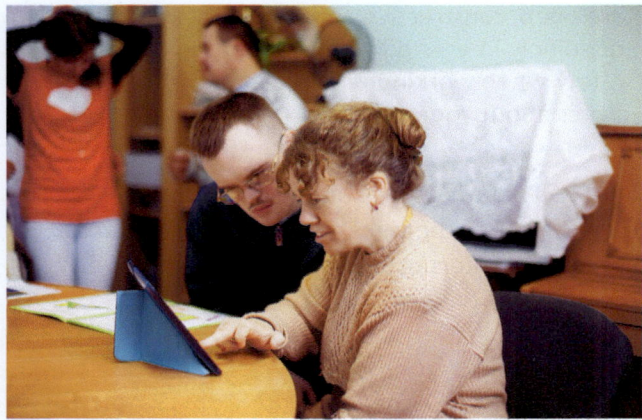

Figure 2.6 How do you support individuals to stay safe when they are online?

> **Research it**
>
> **7.3 Online safety in your setting**
>
> Carry out some research in the setting where you work. Find out how individuals use the internet. What sites do they use? How often? Produce a table with your findings.
>
> Have the results surprised you? Say why you are surprised – or not.
>
> For more information about data protection, see Unit 305 Handling information in adult care settings/services.

The use of social networking sites

Social networking sites such as Facebook and Twitter can be a source of positivity and enable individuals to keep in touch with family and friends. However, social networking sites also pose risks that individuals must be made aware of. As you will know, these sites can be a forum for people to share all the different things that are happening in their lives, such as marriages, births and parties. The list is endless. It is human nature to compare our lives with those of others, but this can be harmful to people's health if they compare their lives too seriously. Individuals may also be excluded from certain online activities, such as 'live streaming' videos sent by some friends, and this could make them feel devalued and upset. Of course, individuals may make new friends on these sites but it is important that they are aware that not all information friends share is true. They should also be made aware of the security measures and privacy settings that they can put in place to ensure that they are not exploited by people who do not know them.

Social networking sites such as those mentioned above also mean that individuals can keep up to date with people in the public eye who they may admire such as their favourite group or actor. It is important that individuals remember, what is reported on these sites is not always true and therefore they must not let this influence who they are and how they live their lives.

Moreover, 'fake news' has become more of an issue in recent years where news stories with incorrect and biased information are available on various websites including social media. This means that people are reading news that may not be based on fact and may have incorrect information. In some cases, the stories may be completely made up. This can influence a person's view of the world and the people they interact with, so it is important that individuals are made aware of 'fake news' as it is also a potential risk presented by the internet and social media.

> **Reflect on it**
>
> **7.3 Social media**
>
> Reflect on the benefits to individuals with care or support needs of using social networking sites. Do you use social networking sites? If so, why?

> **Research it**
>
> **7.3 Misuse of personal data**
>
> In 2018, it was widely reported in the media that data and personal information belonging to millions of people was misused.
>
> You can read news stories about this online.
>
> After you have read a bit more about this, think about your setting. How can such developments and breaches around online data affect vulnerable individuals? How can you help to ensure you protect individuals that you support? How does this highlight the importance of keeping up to date with issues around adult care, and online safety?

Carrying out financial transactions online

Online shopping and banking have made our lives a little easier as we no longer need to visit the shops to buy clothes, or visit the bank to make a transfer. However, this too can pose risks for you and those you care for.

Individuals may pay bills, buy items and pay for their transactions online. The risks associated with this include unauthorised organisations (people and websites pretending to be lawful and asking for money) trying to commit fraud and steal from the individual. This can also happen via email. How many times have you read about email or internet scams where people have thought they were sending money to a trusted source or person, but later found out that this was a lie and had their money stolen as a result?

Often a password is required to carry out a financial transaction and people are usually required to confirm this if they are carrying out financial transactions online. If these are shared with others or obtained fraudulently by others, they can then be used to access individuals' money.

AC 7.4 Describe ways of working inclusively with individuals in order to reduce the risks presented by online activities

Ways of working inclusively that promote online safety are underpinned by the following key principles.

- **Educate individuals about online safety and be open** – speak to individuals and tell them about the risks presented by using devices and internet sites.
- **Be constructive** – encourage individuals to assess the risks presented by using devices and internet sites and suggest ways for how these can be overcome and how they can stay safe.
- **Be interested** – show individuals that you have a genuine interest in promoting their safety and wellbeing while they participate in online activities.

> **Reflect on it**
>
> **7.4 Promoting online safety**
>
> Reflect on how you can work in ways that are open, constructive and show that you are genuinely interested when promoting online safety when working with individuals. Write up notes about your reflection.

Table 2.7 includes some suggestions for how you can reduce the risks presented by electronic devices and internet sites. Can you think of any others?

Table 2.7 Promoting ways of working inclusively with individuals for online safety

Online activities	Promoting ways of working inclusively with individuals for online safety
The use of electronic communication devices	Inform individuals about the privacy settings that their electronic devices have and that can be switched on to protect their privacy to restrict the information that can be accessed by others.
	Inform individuals about the privacy settings that their electronic devices have and that they can switch on so that others are unable to access their device or contact them.
	Ensure individuals use passwords when using their electronic devices so that if they leave them unattended or forget them in a public place, it will be more difficult for others to access the device and the personal information it contains.
The use of the internet	Inform individuals that when using the internet they may meet people who are not who they claim to be, for example when playing games online.
	Remind individuals that they can block these people and report them.
	Remind individuals that they can also tell you.
	Also, inform individuals that if they receive emails from people that they do not know – perhaps asking for money or asking to meet them, then they should always tell someone about this. The people emailing may sound convincing or intimidating; so it is always best to check with someone else.
The use of social networking sites	Ensure individuals remain on official social networking sites only and do not have private 'chats' with others away from these sites.
	Remind individuals not to give out any personal information about themselves including photographs that they do not want to be shared publicly.
	Remind individuals that they do not have to accept 'friend requests' or 'follow requests' and invitations from people that they know – or do not know – if they do not want to.
	Remind individuals that they can tell you about any concerns they have if they are being made to feel uncomfortable by any person on these sites.
Carrying out financial transactions online	Inform individuals that all financial transactions online should only be completed on official sites. Often official sites will start with 'https' and there will sometimes be a security certificate that appears on screen.
	Inform individuals that all financial transactions should be completed in privacy and not in public places, so that others cannot see their personal information.
	Inform individuals of how to check whether organisations are who they say they are, i.e. by checking they are registered with professional bodies.

6Cs

Communication

Working with individuals for online safety involves communicating with them clearly about how to use electronic devices, including providing them with the necessary information and support they may need to operate these safely while protecting their privacy at the same time. Keeping the channels of communication open with individuals in relation to their online activities will mean that they will be more likely to come to you for advice and further support.

> **Research it**
>
> **7.4 Agreed ways of working for online safety**
>
> Research your employer's agreed ways of working for online safety. Find out whether there are any training and development opportunities available so that you can provide support to the individuals you care for in the care setting where you work.

> **Evidence opportunity**
>
> **7.3, 7.4 Risks**
>
> Produce an information leaflet showing the potential risks presented by the use of electronic communication devices, the internet, social networking sites and carrying out a financial transaction online. Make sure you also include information about the different ways you can reduce these risks.

Legislation	
Act/Regulation	**Key points**
The Care Act 2014	There are ten different types of abuse that individuals may experience. It also defines safeguarding as individuals living safely, free from harm and abuse.
The Health and Social Care Act 2012	Health and social care services must work in partnership together to safeguard individuals effectively.
The Equality Act 2010	A person must not be treated unfairly or discriminated against in relation to their protected characteristics. These are defined by the Equality Act as age, disability, gender reassignment, marriage and civil partnership, pregnancy and maternity, race, religion and belief, sex or sexual orientation.
Safeguarding Vulnerable Groups Act 2006	It established the Vetting and Barring Scheme that prevents people who are not suitable to work with individuals with care or support needs from doing so; DBS checks are required from all those who work with individuals with care or support needs.
Mental Capacity Act 2005	It safeguards individuals who are unable to make choices and decisions for themselves because they lack the capacity to do so.
Modern Day Slavery Act	It is aimed at tackling slavery, servitude and forced or compulsory labour in the UK. It addresses issues such as human trafficking and the exploitation of people.
The Human Rights Act 1998	Everyone in the UK is entitled to the same basic human rights and freedoms. This includes individuals who have care and support needs. The Act supports individuals' rights to make their own choices and decisions, dignity, respect, and rights to be treated fairly when accessing care or support services and to live safely and free from harm or abuse.
The Data Protection Act 2018	It promotes individuals' rights to security over the use of their personal information by others and safeguards them from others infringing their rights to privacy over their personal information. This came into effect from May 2018 and introduced some new and different requirements for data protection. See Units 303 and 304 for more information.
The Public Interest Disclosure Act 1998	It established whistleblowing procedures so that concerns over individuals' safety and wellbeing can be reported by workers free from fear or repercussions from their employers. You may make a disclosure about unsafe work practices or a crime.

See AC 1.1 for more information on legislation.

302 Understanding mental capacity and restrictive practice

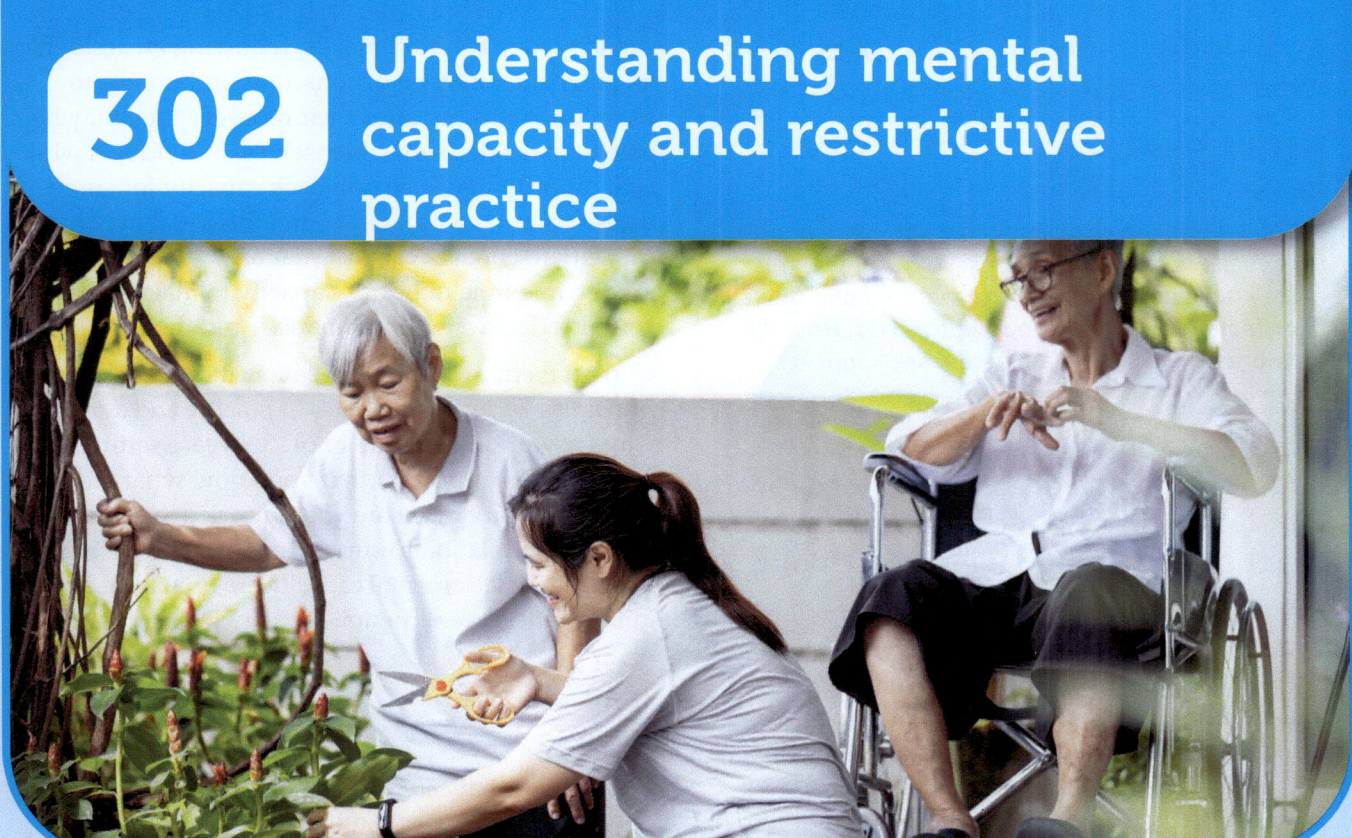

About this unit

Credit value: 2
Guided learning hours: 18

Providing care and support to individuals in care settings/services involves working with individuals who can and can't make decisions for themselves. It is important that you understand what you can and can't do when making decisions on individuals' behalf when they do not have the mental capacity to do so themselves.

In this unit you will learn about the principles of mental capacity, including relevant and current legislation, codes of practice and agreed ways of working. You will also find out more about what factors can influence an individual's mental capacity and their ability to consent.

Understanding your role and responsibilities in supporting the rights of individuals in relation to establishing an individual's consent, as well as when informed consent cannot be readily established, will also be explored in this unit. You will also learn about the strategies and skills that could be used to maximise individuals' capacity to make their own decisions.

Finally, you will consider the range of restrictive practices that may occur within a care setting/service and the policies and procedures that must be followed when using these in line with your working role.

Learning outcomes

By the end of this unit you will:

LO1: Understand the principles of mental capacity

LO2: Understand the application of the principles of mental capacity and consent

LO3: Understand restrictive practices

LO1 Understand the principles of mental capacity

> **Getting started**
>
> Think about an occasion when you were unable to make your own decisions. For example, this may have been because you were feeling unwell or feeling confused about what to do. How did you feel? Why? Did you access any support?

AC 1.1 Describe how the main purpose and principles of current mental capacity legislation are reflected in codes of practice and agreed ways of working

Mental capacity refers to an individual's ability to understand information and make decisions about their life, such as in relation to their care and support. If an individual is unable to make a decision about their care, i.e. because they do not understand the information that has been provided to them because of a learning disability or a condition such as dementia, then they are seen as lacking the capacity to make decisions about their care. An individual's lack of capacity can, however, also be temporary because they may only lack capacity for a certain time; i.e. following an accident an individual may be unconscious and unable to make decisions but after their recovery they may be able to make decisions themselves. Individuals who lack capacity may also only lack capacity for some decisions but not others, i.e. an individual may have capacity to choose what to wear and what to eat and at the same time may lack capacity to make more complex decisions about finances and their future.

Current mental capacity legislation and its associated principles underpin the **codes of practice** and agreed ways of working that are in place in care settings/services. It is important that you know what these are so that you can ensure your knowledge and work practices in relation to supporting individuals who may have or lack mental capacity are up to date and in line with current mental capacity legislation.

> **Key term**
>
> **Codes of practice** refer to the guidelines and standards that care workers are expected to follow when carrying out their roles.

Legislation

Table 3.1 provides some useful information about the current legislation relating to mental capacity.

Table 3.1 Purpose and principles of mental capacity legislation

Mental capacity legislation	Purpose and principles
Liberty Protection Safeguards 2019	• The Liberty Protection Safeguards (LPS) were introduced in the Mental Capacity (Amendment) Act 2019 and replaced the Deprivation of Liberty Safeguards (DoLS) and came into force in April 2022. All the key principles of the Mental Capacity Act 2005 (see below) will apply in full. • The LPS apply to everyone of 16 years of age and above who is cared for/supported in a care setting/service who is or needs to be deprived of their liberty for their care or treatment and lacks the mental capacity to consent. • They provide protection for individuals who lack mental capacity including people with dementia, autism and learning disabilities. • Local authorities and NHS bodies are responsible for organising the assessments required to justify that a deprivation of liberty is needed. Three assessments will form the basis for authorising a deprivation of liberty: 1) a capacity assessment, 2) a medical assessment to determine if the person has a mental disorder and 3) a necessary and proportionate assessment to determine if the deprivation of liberty is necessary to prevent harm to the person and proportionate to the likelihood and severity of that harm. • Local authorities and NHS bodies will have a duty to consult those involved in the individual's care and who have an interest in the individual's welfare. Family members and others who are close to the individual can represent and support the individual through the process as an 'appropriate person'. Source: Gov.uk (2021) Liberty Protection Safeguards Factsheets, 'Liberty Protection Safeguards: what they are'

Table 3.1 Purpose and principles of mental capacity legislation *continued*

Mental capacity legislation	Purpose and principles
Mental Capacity Act 2005	The Mental Capacity Act (MCA) 2005 protects and empowers individuals who lack the mental capacity to make their own choices and decisions about their care and treatment. The MCA is based on five key principles: 1 Always assume that individuals are able to make their own decisions; never assume that they do not have the capacity to do so. 2 Support individuals so that they can make their own choices and decisions. 3 Respect individuals' rights to make decisions that others may not agree with. 4 All decisions made on an individual's behalf; i.e. when they lack capacity, must always be in their best interests. 5 Decisions made on an individual's behalf must be the least restrictive option; i.e. the option that promotes the individual's rights as much as possible. The 'Best interest' principle: If a person has been assessed as lacking capacity then all decisions taken on behalf of that person must be in their best interests. To do so, the following factors must be taken into consideration: - Do not discriminate or make assumptions about what is a person's best interests, i.e. based on their age or condition. - Take into account the circumstances, i.e. the person's situation at the time. - Consider whether the person's lack of capacity is temporary, i.e. due to an accident, and if so, whether the decision can wait. - Involve and consult the individual as fully as you can. - Ensure you take into account the individual's wishes, feelings, views, values, beliefs, preferences. - Consult with as many people as you can who know the individual and/or have an interest in their welfare.
Human Rights Act 1998	- Protects the rights of every person who lives in the UK including those who lack mental capacity and may be denied their human rights. - The right to liberty, Article 5 of the Human Rights Act 1998, protects a person's right to not be detained or have their movement restricted unreasonably. - If a person has to be detained or their movement restricted under the Mental Health Act, then the legal safeguards as set out under the LPS must be followed.
Equality Act 2010	- Protects people from discrimination and gives people the right to challenge it. - The Equality Act 2010 makes it unlawful to discriminate against people who have a protected characteristic and therefore protects individuals who lack mental capacity. - The nine protected characteristics are: age, disability (which can include mental health problems), gender reassignment, marriage and civil partnership, pregnancy and maternity, race, religion or beliefs, sex and sexual orientation.
Mental Health Act 1983	- Promotes the rights of people with mental health problems e.g. **depression, anxiety, schizophrenia, bipolar disorder**. - Promotes individuals' rights in relation to assessment and treatment in hospital and also when they have left hospital and are living in the community, e.g. being given information about why they have been detained under the Mental Health Act (also known as being **sectioned**), the treatment that is going to be provided in hospital, how to get support from an advocate, the care that will be provided after they leave hospital.

Table 3.1 Purpose and principles of mental capacity legislation *continued*

Mental capacity legislation	Purpose and principles
Health and Social Care Act 2012	• This Act emphasises the importance of improving the physical and mental health of people living in England by improving the prevention, diagnosis and treatment of mental illness and physical illness. For example, it establishes the role of health and wellbeing boards to oversee the provision of services in each local area. • It promotes the rights of individuals who may have mental capacity as well as individuals who may lack or lose mental capacity because of, for example, an accident or illness. For example, individuals who have the capacity to consent to treatment must give their consent before treatment is provided; individuals who have given their consent to treatment have a right to withdraw their consent at any time, and this includes those individuals who may lose their capacity to consent.
Care Act 2014	• This Act promotes the rights of individuals who are 18 years of age and over and who access services and support. For example, it promotes the right to advocacy for individuals with mental health problems that need support in accessing the services and support that they need. • The Act also recognises and promotes the rights of carers who provide care and support to individuals who are 18 years of age and over, such as to their partner, a close relative or friend. For example, it promotes the right of carers to have their caring needs assessed by completing an assessment and to receive support from the local authority for any eligible needs they have.
Data Protection Act 1998 and 2018	The DPA 1998 protects individuals who may lose their capacity due to a condition such as dementia or due to mental illness because it sets out the rights people have in relation to how information about them can be legally accessed, used, recorded, stored and shared and so minimises information about them being misused or abused when they lack capacity. The DPA 2018 is the UK's implementation of the EU's General Data Protection Regulations 2018 (GDPR) and builds on the principles of the DPA Act 1998 and the rights people have under the DPA. For example, it places more emphasis on how organisations, businesses and the government share people's personal information. The DPA 2018 sets out strict rules referred to as the data protection principles that must be followed when using personal data to ensure it is: • used fairly, lawfully and transparently • used for specified, explicit purposes • used in a way that is adequate, relevant and limited to only what is necessary • accurate and, where necessary, kept up to date • kept for no longer than is necessary • handled in a way that ensures appropriate security, including protection against unlawful or unauthorised processing, access, loss, destruction or damage.

> **Key terms**
>
> **Depression** is a medical condition causing low mood that affects your thoughts and feelings. It can range from mild to severe but usually lasts for a long time and affects your day-to-day living.
>
> **Anxiety** is a feeling of fear or worry that may be mild or serious and can lead to physical symptoms such as shakiness.
>
> **Schizophrenia** is a mental health problem where people may experience some of the following symptoms: feeling disconnected from your emotions, difficulty concentrating, hallucinations that include hearing voices and/or seeing things others don't.

> **Key term**
>
> **Bipolar disorder** is a mental health problem that in the main affects people's mood and where they experience feeling high (referred to as manic episodes) and feeling low (referred to as depressive episodes).
>
> **Sectioned** means that being detained in hospital under the Mental Health Act 1983.

> **Reflect on it**
>
> **1.1 'Best interests' in the Mental Capacity Act 2005**
>
> Reflect on what the Mental Capacity Act 2005 means when it talks about 'best interests'. You will find it useful to read through section 5 of the Code of Practice for the Mental Capacity Act 2005 which can be accessed via this link:
>
> https://assets.publishing.service.gov.uk/government/uploads/system/uploads/attachment_data/file/921428/Mental-capacity-act-code-of-practice.pdf

Codes of practice and agreed ways of working

Codes of practice provide guidance on how to implement legislation, and agreed ways of working include policies and procedures that explain what employers expect from their employees. The purpose and principles of mental capacity legislation are reflected in codes of practice and agreed ways of working that are used on a day-to-day basis in care settings and services. The table below gives you some examples of both. Do you know of any others?

Table 3.2 Codes of practice and agreed ways of working

Code of practice	How it reflects the purpose and principles of mental capacity legislation
Code of Practice for the Mental Capacity Act 2005	This provides guidance for how to put the MCA 2005 into practice when working or providing care and support to individuals who lack mental capacity to make their own decisions. It also applies to those who work and care for individuals such as an attorney appointed under a lasting power of attorney or an independent mental capacity advocate or a carer. For example, it describes how to support individuals to make their own decisions, the responsibilities that people have when acting or making decisions on behalf of individuals who lack the capacity to do so for themselves and provides guidance on what people must do. The COP also describes the full best interests checklist as set out by the MCA which must be followed when making a best interests decision: 1 Will the person regain capacity? 2 Involve the person. 3 Consult all relevant people. 4 Consider all the information. 5 Do not make any assumptions. 6 Consider past, present and future wishes. 7 Always pick the very least restrictive option.
Code of Practice for the Mental Health Act 1983	This provides guidance to professionals on how to put the MHA 1983 into practice. It also provides guidance on the rights of individuals, their families and carers. For example, it describes how to put into practice the five principles of the MCA when making decisions about care, support or treatment such as in relation to using the least restrictive option, maximising independence, empowerment and involvement, promoting respect and dignity.

Table 3.2 Codes of practice and agreed ways of working *continued*

Agreed ways of working	How it reflects the purpose and principles of mental capacity legislation
Mental capacity – procedure for supporting individuals to make decisions	This provides guidance on how to support individuals to make decisions themselves before deciding that an individual lacks capacity and reflects the four key points included in the MCA Code of Practice: 1 provide relevant information 2 communicate in an appropriate way 3 make the person feel at ease 4 support the person. For example, providing relevant information includes ensuring that the individual has all the information they need to make a decision including the different options that are available to them. For example, communicating in an appropriate way includes ensuring the information being presented to the individual involves using their preferred communication methods to aid their understanding including the use of others such as an advocate or speech therapist.
Mental capacity – procedure for supporting individuals who may lack capacity to make decisions	This provides guidance on how to support individuals who may lack mental capacity to make decisions themselves and reflects the principles of the MCA and its associated Code of Practice. For example, check whether the individual has capacity for some decisions but not others, check whether the individual may regain their capacity in the future with support and therefore may be able to wait to make a decision until another time, review all capacity decisions on a regular basis to ensure that they still reflect the individual's ability to make decisions. For example, involve others who know the individual and are involved in their life to ensure all decisions made truly are in the individual's best interests and reflect their preferences and wishes.

Case study

1.1, 1.2 The rights of individuals

Elsie is 64 years of age, has a learning disability and schizophrenia and has just returned home from a stay in hospital having experienced an episode of schizophrenia. Elsie lives in a shared house as a supported housing tenant and receives support to live there.

One morning, Elsie's advocate, Jenny, visits her at home and finds out from Elsie that she is feeling frustrated because her support workers are not letting her use the communal areas in the house where she lives or the garden, in case she has another episode of schizophrenia and becomes aggressive to the other tenants who live there.

Jenny and Elsie discuss Elsie's situation with the supported housing manager and explain that Elsie has full capacity to make her own decisions and has rights as a tenant to access the communal areas and garden. Jenny then puts forward some suggestions for how Elsie would like to be supported following her schizophrenic episode including being reminded to take her medication and being accompanied by one of the support workers when she is accessing the communal areas or garden.

Discuss

1 How did Jenny, Elsie's advocate, promote Elsie's 'best interests'?
2 What mental capacity legislation is relevant to Elsie's situation? Why?
3 What could the consequences be if the supported housing manager does not action Jenny's suggestions for how Elsie would like to be supported?
4 If you were the supported housing manager, what would you do? Why?

> **Evidence opportunity**
>
> **1.1 Mental capacity legislation and codes of practice**
>
> Research two pieces of mental capacity legislation and two codes of practice you have learned about. Discuss with a colleague the main purpose and principles of each one. How do they promote the rights of individuals who lack **mental capacity**? How do they relate the agreed ways of working in your care setting/service? Make notes of your research and discussion to add to your portfolio.

AC 1.2 Describe factors that influence an individual's mental capacity and ability to express consent

What is consent?

You will already know that person-centred care involves respecting individuals' choices and decisions. To do so also requires you to provide the individual with sufficient information to be able to understand the choices and decisions they are making. Similarly, before providing individuals with any form of care and support, you must ensure that you have their agreement to do so and that you have provided them with sufficient information about their options, the benefits, risks and consequences of not doing so to ensure their understanding – this is referred to as 'informed consent'. You will need to answer their questions as best you can and, if you don't know the answer, to check with someone who does or refer them to someone who does. Make sure the person who needs this information receives it, so they can make an informed decision/consent, whether this is the individual or their family, for example.

> **Reflect on it**
>
> **1.2 Consent**
>
> Reflect on an occasion when you gave your consent to something, for example when you were asked where you wanted to go on a night out or what you wanted to eat. How did this make you feel?
>
> Now imagine how you would feel if you were not asked for your consent.

Factors that influence mental capacity and consent

As you will have learned, obtaining an individual's consent is important but sometimes you may come across an individual that may not be able to express their consent. This may be because:

- **The individual lacks capacity** and is therefore unable to make a decision for themselves. This may be due to a learning disability, a condition such as dementia, a mental health need, because they are confused, drowsy or unconscious or because they have misused a substance such as an illegal drug or alcohol.

  An individual who lacks capacity will be unable to express their consent. In other words, they will not be able to do one or more of the following: understand or retain the information they have been given, evaluate the information they have received to make a decision, or make a decision and express their decision to someone else.

  It is also important to take into consideration that an individual's **lack of capacity** may vary and/or may be temporary. An individual with dementia may lack capacity on some days but not others, similarly some individuals with a learning disability may lack capacity to make some major decisions such as about their future care but not minor decisions such as what to eat or wear. It is important to be aware of all these factors that can influence the capacity of an individual to express consent.

  Remember that when an individual does not have capacity for one decision this does not mean that they lack capacity for every decision.

- **The individual is undecided over whether to give their consent** and is therefore unable to express their wishes. This may be because the individual requires more time to make a decision. This may be the case particularly if the decision they have to make is an important one such as changing the type of support they receive or moving house, or because they are anxious about it. For example, in relation to having some medical treatment they may be concerned about going into hospital or the side effects of the medications they will be taking.

- **It is unclear whether an individual has given their consent** and therefore it cannot be assumed that the individual has expressed their consent. This may be because the individual has specific communication needs and it is difficult to understand what the individual is trying to express, or because an individual is feeling anxious or becomes withdrawn and therefore makes it unclear whether they are expressing their consent.

- **It is unclear whether an individual has understood the information provided to them** and therefore again, it cannot be assumed that the individual has expressed their consent. This may be because the information provided to the individual is not in a suitable format that meets their needs; the language used may be too complex or the photographs used may not be easily recognisable by the individual. It could also be due to poor working practices that mean that the information provided is done in a rush or in a way that does not meet the individual's specific communication and language needs and preferences or causes offence to the individual, for example if it is not respectful of their **culture** and beliefs. You can refer to Unit 304 Effective communication in adult care settings/services for more information about effective working approaches for meeting individuals' specific communication language needs and preferences.

> **Key term**
>
> **Culture** refers to particular ideas, traditions and customs practised and shared by a group of people, usually from a particular country or society.

- **The environment** can influence an individual's mental capacity and ability to express consent if the individual does not feel comfortable. For example, a room that is too hot or too cold can act as a barrier because this can make the individual feel uncomfortable and not at ease and therefore less likely to be able to understand information being given to them and make decisions. Similarly, asking an individual who has dementia what they would like to eat in a busy kitchen area may mean that as there are too many distractions the individual may not be able to focus on what they are being asked and may feel confused and, as such, may not respond or may withdraw from the situation by leaving the area.
- **Noise**, like the environment, can also be an unwelcomed distraction that may result in some individuals not being able to express consent. For example, an individual may find it difficult to discuss their plan for their care and support and make decisions if the discussion is being held in an area where there is a lot of noise, because they may mishear what is being discussed or may find the level of noise too distracting. The individual may also feel that that they are unable to speak their mind because they may have to speak more loudly and therefore risk others overhearing what they are saying; the individual may also feel that their rights to privacy and respect are being denied.
- **The time of day** can have a significant impact on an individual's mental capacity and ability to express consent. For example, asking an individual about their hopes for their future early in the morning when they have just woken up can be detrimental because the individual may not be fully awake and therefore less likely to understand information being presented to them and make decisions for themselves. Similarly, asking an individual to make a decision about for example their housing late one afternoon when they are in a rush to go to the shops would not be conducive as the individual will not have the time to consider the different housing options available to them. Choosing the correct time of day is therefore very important when establishing an individual's mental capacity and their ability to express consent.
- **Coercive/controlling behaviour from others** can make individuals fearful of making their own decisions and therefore more likely to let others make decisions for them or make decisions that they feel others would approve of. Coercive/controlling behaviour from others can make individuals withdrawn, feel less able to think independently and express what they want. This is not because individuals do not have the mental capacity to express their consent but because they are anxious about what may happen if they do. For example, an individual who has been told by their sibling repeatedly that there is no point in them learning to swim because they have a learning disability and will find it too difficult to do so and will embarrass themselves in front of others may decline the opportunity of having swimming lessons, not because they don't want to but because they think they haven't got the ability to do so as a result of their sibling's behaviour.

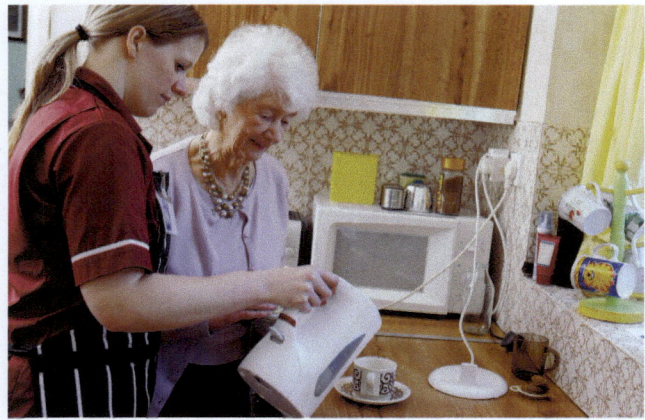

Figure 3.1 Seeking consent is also important when you are carrying out an activity with an individual, such as cooking, mobilising or going out

> ### Evidence opportunity
>
> **1.2 Factors influencing mental capacity of individuals and their ability to express consent**
>
> Develop a case study of an individual who has care and support needs and who at times lacks the capacity to express their consent for care and support. Discuss the factors that can influence their capacity to consent. Remember that you cannot include personal details about the individual and you must maintain confidentiality.

AC 1.3 Explain the link between an individual's mental capacity and a) consent, b) choice, c) safety

Consent

As you will have learned in AC 1.2, an individual's mental capacity will determine their ability to express their consent. If an individual lacks mental capacity due to for example a mental-health condition, dementia, a learning disability, loss of consciousness due to an accident, brain damage such as from a stroke, or the effects of substances such as alcohol or drugs, then this will affect their ability to express their consent because they will be unable to provide it:

- verbally (e.g. by saying to a nurse 'Yes I agree to have a blood test')
- non-verbally (e.g. by the individual holding out their arm to have their bloods taken)
- in writing (e.g. by signing a consent form that indicates that the individual agrees to having further tests including blood tests).

Choice

The individual making choices over, for example, their care and support or treatment must have the mental capacity to make that choice, i.e. they must be able to not only understand the information that has been given to them but they must also be able to use it to make their own choice. This is more commonly referred to as making an **informed choice**. For example, if an individual is asked whether they would like to go to hospital and have an x-ray of their hand that is hurting, they will only be able to make an informed choice if they understand:

- the reasons why their hand may be hurting, i.e. they may have sustained a sprain or a fracture
- the purpose and pros of having an x-ray, and what this involves, i.e. to determine if they have sustained an injury that needs to be treated and can prevent the injury from worsening, to go to hospital and have an image taken of their hand by a specialist health professional called a radiographer, a painless procedure
- the cons of having an x-ray, i.e. they may have a long wait when they arrive at A&E, they may not agree with the fact that x-rays involve radiation passing through their body
- the consequences of not having an x-ray, i.e. the pain in their hand may worsen, their hand injury may become more difficult to treat successfully the longer it is left without treatment.

Safety

An individual's mental capacity is also linked to their safety because there may be occasions where the individual's safety is paramount. For example, if the individual is:

- unconscious due to a road traffic accident – the individual will lack capacity to make a choice over whether to have treatment but if emergency treatment is needed to save their life then this will be provided to the individual. Once the individual regains consciousness then the treatment provided as well as the reasons why can be explained to the individual.
- refusing treatment for a mental health condition that involves the individual self-harming and being violent towards others – the individual may lack the mental capacity to understand that they are a danger to themselves and others and therefore their consent to obtain treatment for

their condition is overridden by the necessity to keep them and others around them safe and free from danger and/or harm.

AC 1.4 Outline what is meant by 'valid consent'

An individual's mental capacity is closely linked to their ability to consent, make choices and promote their safety.

What is valid consent?

For consent to be valid it must be given:

- voluntarily by the individual, i.e. it must be the individual's own decision to consent or not to, the decision must be made freely by the individual and they must not have been pressurised or persuaded by others such as their family or carers.
- by an appropriately informed individual, i.e. the individual must be given all the information they require to make an informed decision including the options available, the benefits and risks as well as the consequences of not giving their consent. This is more commonly referred to as informed consent.
- by an individual who has the capacity to consent, i.e. the individual must have the mental capacity to understand and use the information provided to them to make an informed decision and then express their decision to consent or not to.

If an individual has the capacity to consent and makes a voluntary and informed decision to, for example, consent to or refuse medical treatment, then their decision must be respected. If an individual does not have the capacity to give their consent to medical treatment then the situation must be discussed by the healthcare professional with others who know the individual such as their family and carers to ensure that any decisions that are taken by the healthcare professionals in relation to the medical treatment are in the individual's best interests. You may find it useful to review your previous learning in AC1.1 of this unit around the Mental Capacity Act 2005 that sets out what factors to consider when making best interests decisions on behalf of an individual who lacks capacity.

Reflect on it

1.4 Valid consent

Reflect on the meaning of obtaining valid consent in relation to the care and support you provide to individuals in the care setting/service where you work. Do you have any agreed ways of working in place? Why?

Evidence opportunity

1.3, 1.4 The link between capacity and consent, choice and safety

Produce an information handout for new team members to explain the link between an individual's capacity and consent, choice and safety. Ensure you also include the meaning of the term 'valid consent'.

LO2 Understand the application of the principles of mental capacity and consent

Getting started

Reflect on your current job role and responsibilities. How do you uphold the rights of individuals you provide care and support to? Think about an occasion when you promoted an individual's best interests. Why did you do this?

AC 2.1 Describe own role and responsibilities when upholding the rights of individuals following principles of mental capacity legislation and codes of practice

Upholding the rights of individuals following principles of mental capacity legislation and codes of practice involves working within the scope or limits of your job role and responsibilities. It is essential that you do this, so that you can carry out your role and responsibilities to the best of your ability.

It is also very important because it ensures that you are:

- providing the best care and support you can to individuals
- working at the correct level and only carrying out the responsibilities you have been trained and qualified to do
- carrying out out your responsibilities safely
- doing what is expected of you and you are doing it well and to a high standard
- following working practices that are used in the care setting/service where you work and that have been agreed with your employer.

You will find it helpful to review your previous learning around how to work in ways that are agreed with your employer in Unit 300 Responsibilities and ways of working in adult care settings/services and the concepts of competence and duty of care in Unit 303 Understanding duty of care.

> **Reflect on it**
>
> **2.1 Not following agreed ways of working**
>
> Reflect on the consequences of not following your employer's agreed ways of working when upholding the rights of individuals. How do you think this would impact on individuals, you, others you work with, the organisation you're employed by? Why?

Job roles and responsibilities will vary between different adult care settings but upholding the rights of individuals by following the principles of mental capacity legislation and codes of practice will not. Below are some tips to help you ensure that you uphold the rights of individuals in your day-to-day work responsibilities:

1. Ensure you know and understand the scope of your job responsibilities and agreed ways of working in relation to upholding individuals' rights. If there is something you do not understand it is your responsibility to seek additional advice and guidance from your manager and/or your employer.
2. Attend all training and read all information updates provided to you by your employer about the Mental Capacity Act, its associated principles and code of practice.
3. Follow principles 1-3 of the Mental Capacity Act to support individuals to make their own decisions by not assuming an individual does not have capacity because they have a condition or disability (principle 1), doing everything you can within the limits of your job role to support and empower the individual to make their own decisions and involve the individual as much as possible (principle 2), and not assuming an individual lacks capacity because the decisions they make are unwise or eccentric; everyone is a unique individual with their own unique values and preferences (principle 3).
4. Follow principles 4 and 5 of the Mental Capacity Act to support individuals' decisions when they are lacking mental capacity by ensuring all decisions made on behalf of the individual are in their best interests (principle 4) and the least restrictive option is being put forward (principle 5).
5. Follow the guidance included in the associated mental capacity codes of practice in relation to how to make an assessment of capacity before carrying out any care, support or treatment by considering whether the individual is able to do one or more of the following four things: understand the information given, retain the information given, weigh up the pros and cons of the information given, communicate their decision. If they cannot then they are lacking capacity.
6. Follow the guidance included in the associated mental capacity codes of practice in relation to how to make a best interests decision by asking yourself the following questions: Will the individual regain capacity? Has the individual been involved? Have all relevant people been consulted? Has all the information gathered been considered? Have any assumptions been made? Have the individual's past, present and future wishes been considered? Has the least restrictive option been chosen?
7. If you observe an individual's rights not being promoted or being denied because of

their mental capacity or lack of it, or someone brings this to your attention, do not ignore it; raise your concern with your manager or another senior member of the team as soon as you can. Remember to also ensure you record your observations.

8 Be a good role model for others you are working with when providing care and support to individuals by being prepared to explain the importance of upholding an individual's rights and following mental capacity legislation and codes of practice.

9 Reflect on how you carry out the day-to-day work activities you are responsible for and use your reflections, including any feedback you receive to continue to improve your work practices.

6Cs

Care

Upholding individuals' rights must always be at the heart of the care you provide to individuals and forms part of your responsibilities. For example, following principles of mental capacity legislation and your employer's agreed ways of working will ensure that you provide the very best care that you can to individuals because you will be upholding their rights and providing care that is in their best interests.

Commitment

Showing commitment involves showing your dedication to providing individuals with high-quality care so that you can support them to improve their lives. For example, you can show your dedication when supporting individuals by ensuring you always follow the principles of the Mental Capacity Act and work in a person-centred way.

Evidence opportunity

2.1 Upholding individuals' rights

Keep a diary of how you uphold the rights of individuals following principles of mental capacity legislation and codes of practice in the care setting/service where you work.

AC 2.2 Explain why it is important to establish an individual's consent when providing care and support

Why is obtaining consent important?

Obtaining an individual's consent when providing care or support is important because:

- **it is a legal requirement:** to comply with legislation, such as the Mental Capacity Act 2005, the individual must give their consent for the provision of care or support. When an individual is unable to give their consent because they lack the capacity due to having a condition such as dementia then a representative may decide on their behalf but only if they act in the individual's best interests at all times. The 'best interests' principle in the Mental Capacity Act 2005 means that all decisions made on behalf of an individual who lacks capacity must benefit the individual – this may be in relation to the individual's health, care or support. You will learn more about what to do when consent cannot be established in AC 2.6. Obtaining consent also means that the individuals you care for have given their agreement for their care and as a result you and your setting are protected legally.

- **it is necessary for working in a person-centred way:** obtaining an individual's consent when providing care or support means that you are respecting the individual's right to agree or refuse and promoting their dignity by not assuming that you know what care or support the individual wants, needs or prefers.

Remember it is the individual who knows best. It is the individual or their representative who decides what care or support is needed and/or preferred. The care and medical professions are able to advise on care and medical treatment but individuals and their representatives must be able to decide what happens to them.

Research it

2.2 Mental Capacity Act 2005

Research what the Mental Capacity Act 2005 says about the importance of establishing consent when providing care or support and promoting individuals' rights. Find out more about the five principles:

1. A person must be assumed to have capacity unless it is established that they lack capacity.
2. A person is not to be treated as unable to make a decision unless all practicable steps to help them to do so have been taken without success.
3. A person is not to be treated as unable to make a decision merely because they make an unwise decision.
4. An act done, or decision made, under this Act for or on behalf of a person who lacks capacity must be done, or made, in their best interests.
5. Before the act is done, or the decision is made, regard must be had to whether the purpose for which it is needed can be as effectively achieved in a way that is less restrictive of the person's rights and freedom of action.

Source: Mental Capacity Act 2005, Part 1, Section 1 The principles (www.legislation.gov.uk/ukpga/2005/9/section/1)

There is a useful link below:

www.mind.org.uk/information-support/legal-rights/mental-capacity-act-2005/overview/

Evidence opportunity

AC 2.2 Establishing an individual's consent

Discuss with a colleague the importance of establishing an individual's consent when providing care and support. Remember to consider in your discussion the consequences of not doing so for the individual, you and others.

AC 2.3 Explain how personal values and attitudes can influence perceptions of situations and of individuals' mental capacity

It is important to be aware that personal values and attitudes can also influence perceptions of situations and individuals' capacity, and this is why it is very important that you do not let these **prejudice** your perceptions of situations you may come across and of individuals' capacity. You may also find it useful to review your previous learning around values, attitudes and prejudices in Unit 309, Promoting equality, diversity, inclusion and human rights in adult care settings/services.

Key term

Prejudice refers to your bias towards something as a result of your beliefs and values and can include, for example, believing that someone with a mental health condition is at risk of being violent (which may be based on media stories or hearsay, but not on any actual experience of your own).

Table 3.3 describes examples of how personal values and attitudes can influence perceptions of situations and of individuals' capacity.

Table 3.3 Examples of how personal values and attitudes can influence perceptions of situations and of individuals' capacity

Examples of personal values and attitudes	How personal values and attitudes can influence perceptions of situations and of individuals' capacity
Believing that an individual with a mental health condition is at risk of being violent because of hearsay	Holding this personal value/attitude can influence how you perceive situations that arise. For example, if the individual gets frustrated that they cannot go out to the shops as planned because there isn't a staff member available you may perceive this as the individual showing aggression towards you, when the individual may just be expressing how they are feeling about the situation.

Table 3.3 Examples of how personal values and attitudes can influence perceptions of situations and of individuals' capacity *continued*

Examples of personal values and attitudes	How personal values and attitudes can influence perceptions of situations and of individuals' capacity
	It can also influence how you perceive individuals' capacity. For example, you may make an assumption that the individual's mental health condition means that they are unable to make decisions for themselves because they are unaware of how their actions may affect the safety of themselves and/or others, when the individual may just require support to make decisions.
Believing that an individual with dementia lacks capacity to make decisions because of their condition	Holding this personal value/attitude can influence how you perceive situations that arise. For example, you may not ask the individual who they would like to invite to their care review because the day before they appeared confused for most of the day. The individual may have just been confused yesterday but not today. This attitude can also influence how you perceive individuals' capacity. For example, you may assume because the individual experiences confusion on some days that they lack capacity, when the individual may just lack capacity to make decisions on some days but not others.
Believing that an individual with a learning disability lacks capacity to make decisions because of their condition	Holding this personal value/attitude can influence how you perceive situations that arise. For example, you may not involve an individual who has a learning disability in decisions about what activity they would like to participate in because it has already been established that they lack the capacity to make decisions in their life such as where they want to live. However, the individual may have just been unable to make a decision about their housing but they still have the ability to decide what activity they would like to participate in. This personal value/attitude can also influence how you perceive individuals' capacity. For example, you may make an assumption that because the individual lacks capacity to make decisions about their life, they also lack capacity to make other decisions, when the individual may lack the capacity to make major decisions but not minor decisions.

> **Evidence opportunity**
>
> **AC 2.3 How do personal values and attitudes influence perceptions of situations and mental capacity?**
>
> Think about two individuals you provide care and support to in the care setting/service where you work. Develop a presentation that explains how personal values and attitudes can influence perceptions of situations and both individuals' mental capacity.

AC 2.4 Describe strategies and skills that may be used to maximise individuals' capacity to make their own decisions

You and others who care for and support individuals will know them best and it is yours and others' knowledge of them that forms the basis of helping individuals to make their own decisions. There are also a range of strategies and skills to provide practical support that may also be used to maximise individuals' capacity to make their own decisions. For example:

- Effective communication skills – providing information to individuals in different formats and using communication aids can enable individuals to understand you, make themselves understood and be able to communicate their decisions. You will also find it useful to review your previous learning around using a range of different communication methods, skills and styles with individuals in Unit 304 Effective communication in adult care settings/services.

> **6Cs**
>
> **Communication**
>
> Being an effective communicator is an essential skill to have when supporting individuals to make their own decisions. For example, it involves communicating with individuals in a way that they can understand; you can only do this if you know individuals' preferred communication methods and styles. Communication also involves giving individuals the time and space to express how they think and feel so that they can make their own decisions and feel good about doing so.

- Effective engagement skills – enabling individuals to engage with you involves ensuring individuals remain at the heart of your communication with them, as doing so will make them feel that you respect them and therefore that they can trust you. To engage individuals effectively you will need to address any environmental barriers that may exist (see AC 1.2 in this unit for more information) as well as ensure that you listen attentively to what individuals are communicating and can recognise and respond appropriately to coercive/controlling behaviours from others. Again, you will find it useful to review your previous learning around the use of communication skills to build relationships and how to overcome barriers to effective communication in Unit 304 Effective communication in adult care settings/services.

> **6Cs**
>
> **Compassion**
>
> Treating individuals with compassion involves showing kindness and empathy. Placing individuals at the heart of all communications and decisions will ensure that they feel respected and that you are upholding their rights to be treated with dignity. Showing compassion is also essential for building relationships with individuals that are founded on trust.

- Using agreed ways of working – maximising individuals' capacity to make their own decisions can also be achieved by using agreed ways of working such as risk assessment processes. Carrying out a risk assessment with an individual is a useful and practical method of helping the individual to consider the available options and weigh up the pros and cons including the potential risks and how these can be reduced or eliminated. You will find it useful to review your previous learning around the use of support mechanisms, guidance and risk assessment methods in Unit 307 promoting choice and independence in adult care settings/services.
- Supporting individuals' independence – empowering individuals to be independent involves encouraging them to make their own decisions and not rushing in and making decisions for them. It also involves respecting individuals' decisions even when you do not agree with them and giving them the time and space to take risks and make their own mistakes while maintaining their safety and wellbeing. This means it is absolutely essential that you do not let your personal values, beliefs or attitudes influence individuals (see AC2.3 in this unit).
- Being a positive role model – setting a good example for others involves being able to explain to others the reasons why individuals have the right to make their own decisions, supporting individuals to question and challenge any decisions made about them that they do not agree with, offering to share good practice ideas with others as well as having the courage to report any concerns you have when you do not think that individuals' rights to make their own decisions are being promoted.

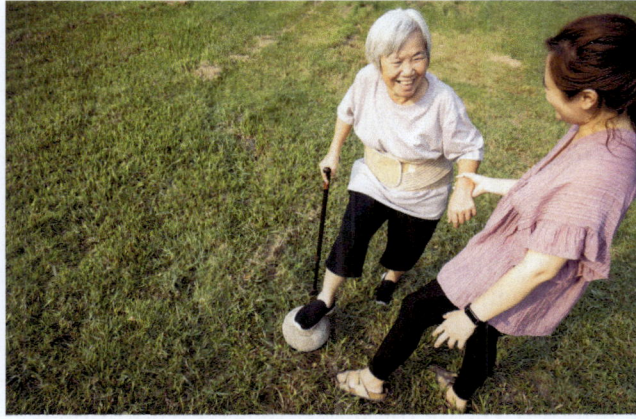

Figure 3.2 Are you a good role model for maximising individuals' capacity to make their own decisions?

> **Evidence opportunity**
>
> **2.4 Maximising individuals' capacity to make their own decisions**
>
> Develop a case study of two individuals with different care and support needs and describe the strategies and skills that you can use to maximise both individuals' capacity to make their own decisions.

AC 2.5 Explain own role in identifying when an assessment of capacity may be required

As you will have learned in LO1 of this unit the Mental Capacity Act 2005 is the piece of legislation that protects individuals who lack the mental capacity at a specific time to make a decision and also states who can make decisions for individuals. You may find it helpful to review your previous learning of the Act including the five key principles it's based on.

When an individual has mental capacity it means that they are able to make specific decisions at specific times and this involves the individual:

- understanding the information they are given to make the specific decision
- retaining the information they are given to make the specific decision
- being able to weigh up the pros and cons of the information they are given to make the specific decision
- being able to communicate the decision using their preferred communication methods, e.g. verbally by saying it, non-verbally by using sign language, in writing, or using assistive technology.

If you are working with an individual and they are unable to carry out one of the above, then you must try and support the individual as best you can to make the decision themselves. For example, you may try and present the information you give the individual in a different way by using different communication methods, breaking down the information into smaller chunks or by seeking additional help from someone else such as the individual's advocate.

If after providing the individual with additional support they are still unable to make a decision for themselves, then it is important to not ignore or keep this to yourself because doing so may mean that the individual's right to have decisions made in their best interests is denied. You must follow your organisation's policies and procedures and take the necessary steps within the scope of your role to raise a concern that an assessment of capacity may be required. Depending on your role this may involve you reporting this directly to your supervisor or manager and/or seeking further advice from the individual's social worker or GP. It is also important to record the specific decision at the specific time the individual lacked capacity and the support you provided to help them make the decision themselves so that this can inform the assessment at a later date.

> **Evidence opportunity**
>
> **2.5 Identifying the need for an assessment of capacity**
>
> Write an account that describes your role in the care setting/service you work in for identifying when an assessment of capacity may be required for an individual.

AC 2.6 Outline the steps to take when informed consent cannot be readily established

As you will have learned in AC 1.2, sometimes it may not be possible to establish informed consent with an individual for various reasons.

If informed consent cannot be readily established take the following steps:

- Always adhere to the principles of the Mental Capacity Act.
- Always follow your organisation's policies and procedures including when making best interest decisions.
- Always work within the scope of your job role and responsibilities and follow agreed ways of working and codes of practice.
- Try explaining the information to them again. This is so that they understand what the procedure entails, the benefits, risks and consequences.
- Seek advice from, for example, your manager. It is your duty to not ignore the concerns you have

but to report that the individual has not given consent, seek further guidance and discuss your concerns. Settings will have their own policies and procedures in place in case of such situations. Doing so reflects your competence for providing good care and support and ensuring that the best outcome for the individual can be reached.

- Consult with the individual's representative. In some cases you may be able to seek further clarification from a person who knows the individual well, for example the individual's advocate. Discussing this with someone else may help. You must always check before doing so with your manager as this information is personal to the individual and is therefore protected data.
- Record your findings in relation to the actions you took to establish consent with an individual and the actions you took when you were unable to establish consent with the individual. Include what happened, what the individual said/expressed, the guidance you were given, by whom and when.

If, after trying all these options, consent can still not be established with an individual then it may be that you are unable to do anything. However, this will depend on a number of things, such as the individual's capacity and whether refusal means their health will be in danger. Advice may need to be sought by your manager from external agencies, such as the Courts, who can provide legal clarification, and **Professional Councils** who can provide additional support.

Key term

Professional Councils are organisations that regulate professions, such as adult social care workers who work with adults in residential care homes, in day centres and who provide care in someone's home. They can provide advice and support around working with individuals who lack capacity to make decisions.

Reflect on it

2.6 When an individual lacks capacity

Reflect on your previous learning in AC 1.2. What is the meaning of the term 'lacks capacity'? How can this impact on how consent is established with individuals?

Case study

2.6 The Cheshire West case

Mr P, a 39-year-old man with cerebral palsy and Down's syndrome, lacked the capacity to make decisions about his own care. He was living at home with his mother but when his health deteriorated, Cheshire West and Chester Council placed him in the care of the local authority. Mr P's mother successfully argued that her son's care should be regularly reviewed to ensure that he was not being deprived of his liberty, because once placed in care he was under constant supervision and was not free to leave.

The outcome of the case was that Mr P would have regular independent care reviews to ensure that the care provided was appropriate and met his needs.

Discuss

1 'A gilded cage is still a cage.' What does this phrase mean? Reflect on how this is relevant to individuals who lack the capacity to make decisions.
2 How can independent care reviews mean that individuals who lack capacity have their human rights upheld?
3 What do you think of individuals who lack mental capacity being equated to birds trapped in cages?

> **Evidence opportunity**
>
> **2.6 Steps to take when informed consent cannot be established**
>
> Think about an occasion when you or someone you work with found it difficult to establish informed consent with an individual. What happened and why was it difficult?
>
> Produce a step-by-step diagram that shows the steps you or your work colleague could take if this situation arose again. Remember to explain the reasons why each step is necessary and how these are in line with your employer's agreed ways of working.

LO3 Understand restrictive practices

> **Getting started**
>
> Reflect on what the word 'restrictive' means to you. What kind of images does this conjure up? Why? Have you heard about or read about the use of 'restrictive practices'? If so, in what context was this?

AC 3.1 Describe what is meant by restrictive practice

Restrictive practice includes actions that deliberately limit an individual's movement or freedom. As we will discuss, there are times when you may need to use restrictive practice. However, there are times when restrictive practice may cause abuse, harm and neglect if it is used inappropriately or unlawfully. This might include physically restraining an individual for no reason by tying them to a chair so that they are unable to move, or using medication to make an individual drowsy. It could also include locking an individual in the house so that they are unable to leave their home on their own.

Restrictive practice denies an individual their basic human right of freedom and movement and can have serious consequences including pain, harm, suffering and even fatalities if not used correctly.

> **Research it**
>
> **3.1 Safeguarding Adults Boards (SABs)**
>
> Research the inappropriate use of restrictive practice by looking at your local SAB's website for recent reviews.
>
> Discuss the effects on the individuals with care and support needs with a colleague.

AC 3.2 Outline how the following restrictive practices within a care setting/service may occur: a) physical, b) mechanical, c) chemical, d) seclusion, e) segregation, f) psychological and g) restraint and the threat of restraint

As you will have learned, restrictive practice means restricting someone from doing something that they want to do and involves restricting someone's rights or freedom of movement. Restrictive practices limit the rights of an individual and include actions that are intended to restrict and restrain them as well as practices that do so inadvertently. This might include for example the following practices:

- Physical restraint that involves physically preventing, restricting or subduing movement of the body, or part of the body of an individual – e.g. holding an individual down on the floor when they become physically aggressive so they are unable to get up and harm themselves and/or others.
- Mechanical restraint that involves using a device to prevent, restrict or subdue movement of the body or part of the body of an individual – e.g. placing an individual's arms in splints when they become restless at night to restrict them shaking and moving their arms and harming themselves.
- Chemical restraint that involves using medication to control or subdue behaviour – e.g. using medication to make an individual drowsy so that they relax, become less anxious and are able to go to sleep.
- Seclusion that involves isolating and confining a person, in an area where they are prevented from leaving – e.g. locking an individual in their room so they are unable to leave the building.

- Segregation that involves isolating an individual, in an area where they are kept away from others – e.g. preventing an individual from participating in a group activity by placing them in a separate room away from others.
- Psychological restraint and the threat of restraint involves controlling an individual by not allowing them to make their own choices, making them do something they do not want to do or restricting what they can do by using threats and coercion – e.g. threatening an individual that they will not have anything to eat every time they become verbally aggressive.

Reflect on it

3.2 Restrictive practices in your workplace

Reflect on the use of restrictive practices in the care setting/service where you work. What restrictive practices, if any, are used? Why? Do you know what your organisation's policies, procedures or agreed ways of working say about the use of restrictive practices?

Evidence opportunity

3.1, 3.2 Restrictive practice

List two examples of appropriate restrictive practice and two examples of inappropriate restrictive practice. Describe how the appropriate practices can be used to safeguard individuals. Explain why the inappropriate practices are inappropriate. Keep a copy of your list and make notes to evidence this.

AC 3.3 Explain the reasons for seeking the least restrictive option for individuals

When restrictive practice may be needed

Restrictive practice must only be used legally and when necessary. It is important to seek the least restrictive option for individuals because you will be complying with the Mental Capacity Act 2005 and:

- keeping the individual safe
- restricting the individual's rights as little as possible
- restricting the individual's freedom as little as possible
- respecting the individual's rights such as to dignity and respect.

Restrictive practice should only be used as a last resort, when there are no other options. This point cannot be stressed enough. For example, it may be that other more proactive practices that encourage discussion and reassurance to diffuse situations that may arise have broken down. It may only be legal and necessary for restrictive practice to be used by trained professionals in the following situations (although all settings will be different and you should check with your manager about the policies and procedures in your setting).

- In an emergency, for example when an individual with mental health needs is self-harming by biting their arms. In this situation, it may be necessary for trained professionals to physically restrain the individual so they do not continue to harm themselves.
- When an individual requires life-saving treatment, for example when an individual with dementia is having a heart attack and prevents hospital staff from administering medical treatment because they are very anxious and physically hitting out. It may be necessary for trained professionals to use medication to calm them down so that their condition does not deteriorate.
- When escaping violence, for example this might be when an individual who is dependent on alcohol and drugs physically abuses another individual or adult care worker and causes damage to the setting, or displays threatening behaviour. Here, it may be necessary for trained professionals to use physical restraint to prevent the individual causing further harm to others and further damage to the environment.

Seeking the least restrictive option for individuals can have a positive impact on them and on you because this will be an opportunity to work closely with the individual and others involved in their life, such as their family or advocate, to find ways of respecting the individual's rights while maintaining their safety.

6Cs

Competence

Seeking the least restrictive option for individuals involves demonstrating your competence so that you can carry out your job role effectively. For example, it means being knowledgeable about when restrictive practices may be needed and what practices you are required to follow in your work setting. It also involves understanding the importance of seeking the least restrictive option for individuals. To do this effectively you must also know the individuals you are supporting and their unique needs.

Case study

AC 3.3 Seeking the least restrictive option – Part 1

Jessika is a support worker providing support to individuals who have mental health needs and is currently supporting Sam who has anxiety and panic attacks when he feels worried or afraid. Sam's anxiety usually manifests itself when he leaves the house, particularly in unfamiliar or different places, and he can become physically and verbally abusive towards others; as such he is meeting up with his friends less and is spending more and more time alone at home.

Discuss

1. What imaginative ways could Jessika use to support Sam when he leaves the house?
2. How could Jessika's support impact on Sam? Why?

Reflect on it

3.3 When to use restrictive practice

Reflect on the importance of restrictive practice only being used when absolutely necessary and legal to do so. What are the consequences of you not doing so? What are the consequences for you? What are the consequences for the individual? What are the consequences for the care setting where you work? What about the individual's setting?

Evidence opportunity

3.3 Seeking the least restrictive option

Write an account that describes the importance and impact of seeking the least restrictive option for individuals.

AC 3.4 Describe how to raise concerns when restrictions appear out of proportion with evident risk

As you will have learned, seeking the least restrictive option for individuals is important and can benefit individuals in different ways. It is therefore also important that you understand how to raise concerns when restrictions appear to not be proportionate to both the behaviour of the individual to be controlled and the nature of the harm likely to be caused. Avoiding saying anything is not an option because it is your responsibility to put an individual's wellbeing first.

6Cs

Courage

It is really important that you have the courage to speak up for individuals if you have concerns over restrictions being used. For example, you may think that the restriction being used is not the least restrictive option for the individual. If this is the case then it is important that you have the courage to say this so that you are upholding individuals' rights and promoting their wellbeing.

Below are some main points to remember about how to raise concerns if restrictions for an individual appear too restrictive and not proportionate to the risk of harm to the individual:

1. Do not ignore concerns you or others may have if restrictions for an individual appear too restrictive and not proportionate with the evident risk.
2. Familiarise yourself with and follow your organisation's policies and procedures for raising concerns in relation to who you should report your concerns to, how and when.

3 Depending on the concern it may be appropriate in the first instance to raise it informally by for example having a discussion in confidence with your manager or as part of a team meeting. At other times, it may not be appropriate to raise your concerns informally, i.e. because it is having a significant impact on the individual and you will then have to raise them formally as per your organisation's policies and procedures.
4 All concerns you raise must be done while respecting confidentiality, i.e. verbally and in writing.
5 If you have taken these actions and you still have concerns, i.e. because your concerns have not been acted on, then you must speak to someone more senior in the organisation. If you still have concerns after doing so then you may need to refer your concerns to another organisation such as adult social care services or CQC so that they can be acted on.

Case study

3.4 Raising concerns about restrictive practice – Part 2

Jessika has concerns about the restrictive practices being used with Sam by the team to ensure he comes to no harm when outside as he is at risk of becoming anxious and having panic attacks when away from his home. Jessika is not sure that restricting Sam's movements when he goes out to only his local shops in his immediate area is benefiting him, as Sam repeatedly says that he doesn't look forward to leaving home because he often doesn't meet anyone and the local shops don't have anything for him to buy.

Discuss

1 What actions could Jessika take about her concerns over Sam? Why?
2 How could Sam's wellbeing be promoted?

Evidence opportunity

3.4 Raising concerns about restrictive practices

Discuss with your assessor how to raise concerns about restrictive practices in the care setting/service where you work.

AC 3.5 Describe policies and procedures in relation to restrictive practices that govern own role

The care setting/service where you work will have in place policies and procedures in relation to restrictive practices. It is important that you familiarise yourself with these so that you can understand your role in putting these into practice and why the actions you take are important.

Organisational policies and procedures in relation to restrictive practices will typically provide you with information about the different types of restraint that there are, how they are used where you work, including the working approaches to take and how to record and report all restrictive practices used. It is important that your work practices comply with these and with any training your organisation provides you with to implement these because inappropriate use of restrictions may be viewed as abuse. Your work practices must also take into account the principles of dignity and respect when implementing restrictive practices; not doing so may also be viewed as a safeguarding concern.

Organisational policies and procedures for restrictive practices are based on the following principles:

- Restrictive practices must only be used as a last resort.
- Restrictive practices must be the least restrictive option for individuals.
- Restrictive practices must be reviewed regularly with the aim of reducing or removing the restriction.
- Restrictive practices must only be used when there is a real risk of harm to the individual or to staff or others if no action is undertaken.
- Restrictive practices must be proportionate to the risk of harm.
- Restrictive practices must meet the needs of individuals and where planned must form part of their support plan and risk assessment.

> **Evidence opportunity**
>
> **3.5 Policy and procedures for restrictive practices**
>
> Research your organisation's policy and procedures for restrictive practices. What do they say about your role in implementing restrictive practices? What are the key principles they're based on? Why are these principles important? Present your findings in a presentation to the team.

Legislation	
Relevant Act	**What it states**
The Care Act 2014	The rights of individuals who are 18 years of age and over and who access services and support as well as the rights of individuals' carers who provide care and support must be recognised and promoted.
The Health and Social Care Act 2012	Improving the physical and mental health of people living in England is important. The rights of individuals who have mental capacity as well as those who may lack or lose mental capacity must be promoted.
The Equality Act 2010	It is unlawful to discriminate against people based on one of the following nine protected characteristics: age, disability (including mental health problems), gender reassignment, marriage and civil partnership, pregnancy and maternity, race, religion or beliefs, sex and sexual orientation.
Liberty Protection Safeguards 2019	It protects individuals who lack mental capacity including people with dementia, autism and learning disabilities. It applies to everyone of 16 years of age and above who is cared for or supported in a care setting/service who is or needs to be deprived of their liberty for their care or treatment and lack the mental capacity to consent. To justify that a deprivation of liberty is required an assessment must be carried out; local authorities and NHS bodies are responsible for organising these.
Mental Capacity Act 2005	It protects and empowers individuals who lack the mental capacity to make their own choices and decisions about their care and treatment. It is based on five key principles, including the 'best interest' principle.
Mental Health Act 1983	It promotes the rights of individuals with mental health problems in relation to assessment and treatment in hospital and when they've left hospital and are living in the community.
The Human Rights Act 1998	Everyone in the UK is entitled to the same basic human rights and freedoms such as in relation to making their own choices and decisions, being treated with dignity, respect and fairly. This includes individuals who have care and support needs and those who lack mental capacity.
The Data Protection Act 1998 and 2018	It promotes individuals' rights to security over the use of their personal information by others and sets out how information about them can be legally accessed, used, recorded, stored and shared to minimise misuse or abuse from happening.

303 Understanding duty of care

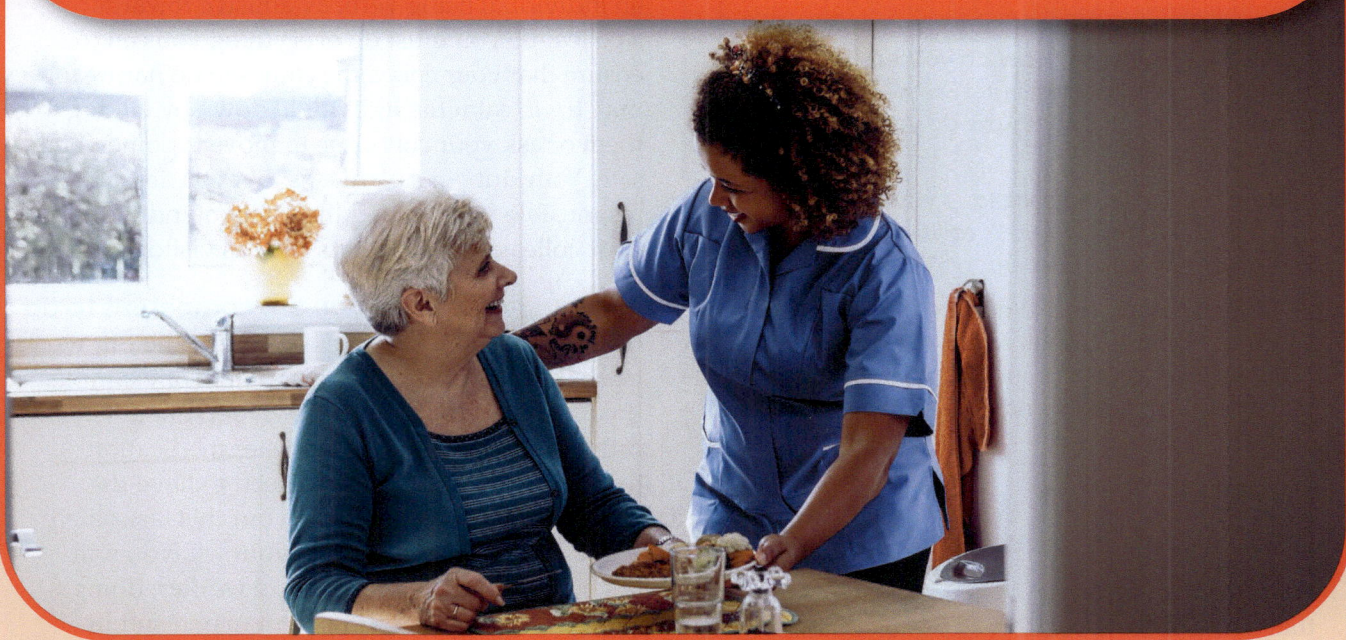

About this unit

Credit value: 2
Guided learning hours: 15

As a Lead Adult Care Worker or Lead Personal Assistant you have a duty of care to work safely in care settings with individuals with care and support needs and with others, including all those you work with and whose work practices you are responsible for supporting and monitoring.

In this unit you will develop your understanding of how duty of care contributes to safe practice in your work role and the reasons why this must underpin everything you do. This unit will also provide you with an opportunity to think about the links that exist between the duty of care and the duty of candour, including how they contribute to keeping individuals safe from **abuse** and improper treatment.

Fulfilling your duty of care while at the same time supporting an individual's rights can be difficult at times. This unit will guide you in identifying conflicts or dilemmas that may arise, understanding how to address conflicts and dilemmas to achieve positive outcomes for individuals, and the additional support and advice that you can access to resolve them. As part of your duty of care you must be ready to take action when care or support goes wrong and make the necessary changes and improvements to your practices, so this unit will also provide you with how to respond to comments, suggestions and complaints effectively. Finally, the unit will equip you with the knowledge to recognise and respond to adverse events, incidents, errors and near misses.

Learning outcomes

By the end of this unit you will:

LO1: Understand how duty of care contributes to safe practice

LO2: Know how to address conflicts or dilemmas that may arise between an individual's rights and the duty of care

LO3: Know how to respond to concerns and complaints

LO4: Know how to recognise and respond to adverse events, incidents, errors and near misses

LO1 Understand how duty of care contributes to safe practice

Getting started

Think about an individual that you provide care or support to. How do you ensure that you put their interests first? How do you respect their dignity? How do you maintain their safety?

Now think about a colleague you work with. How do you support your colleague to provide high quality care and support?

Why do you do this? What are the consequences of not doing so? Think about the benefits and consequences for the individual, their family, your colleague, you and your employer.

AC 1.1 Explain what it means to have a duty of care in own work role

A duty of care refers to the legal requirement that all health and social care professionals have towards the individuals that they provide with care or support and others they work with, including their employer, colleagues and other professionals such as doctors, nurses and individuals' families. Your duty of care underpins all your responsibilities and day-to-day work tasks set out in your job description, such as ensuring that you protect individuals from danger, harm and abuse, and ensures that you are able to provide high quality care and support to all the individuals you work with. This is essential for ensuring individuals' wellbeing and upholding their rights to, for example, privacy, dignity and independence.

Act in the best interests of individuals and others

Exercising your duty of care involves acting in the best interests of individuals and others you work with to ensure they are kept safe from harm. This means that you must ensure individuals are made aware of both the benefits and drawbacks of any decisions and are supported to make their own decisions.

Promote safety and protect others from danger and abuse

Your duty of care also involves promoting individuals' and others' safety by protecting them from danger and abuse. For example, if you observe an individual being verbally abusive towards a colleague you must do everything you can to ensure that your colleague comes to no harm. You may try to calm the individual down by talking to them or ask your colleague to move to somewhere safe. Your duty of care means that you are responsible for ensuring the safety of individuals, your colleagues and others such as visitors.

Only carry out tasks you are competent to do

Being responsible involves only carrying out work tasks that you are competent to do. For example, if you are asked to train a newly recruited care worker in how to administer medication to individuals then you will need to have the knowledge and skills to carry out this task safely. If you have not been trained yourself, you will not be able to train another care worker; doing so when you are not competent may result in you demonstrating unsafe practices. This could result in individuals being administered an incorrect dose or the wrong medication that in turn could lead to an adverse reaction and even fatal consequences. Your duty of care requires you to work with everyone safely and effectively.

If the individual to whom you provide care or support is also your employer, then the agreed ways of working will have been developed by the individual and/or their representative. You will be informed of this through your contract of employment, which will set out the agreed ways of working, as well as through any specific guidance that the individual and/or representative provides you with; this may be in writing and/or verbally explained.

Code of Conduct for Healthcare Support Workers and Adult Social Care Workers in England

Skills for Care and **Skills for Health** have jointly developed a Code of Conduct for Healthcare Support Workers and Adult Social Care Workers in England that sets out the standards that all healthcare and social care professionals are expected to meet to exercise their duty of care. It is voluntary, but it is seen as a sign of good practice. It states that to exercise your duty of care you must, for example, be able to work within the agreed scope of your work role, know how to behave responsibly, promote individuals' wellbeing and ensure that you protect individuals and others you work with such as their families, your colleagues and the wider public from harm, abuse and injury.

The Code of Conduct includes seven standards that you are expected to follow to exercise your duty of care:

1 Be accountable by ensuring you can answer for your actions or omissions
2 Be able to promote and uphold at all times the privacy, dignity, rights, health and wellbeing of people who use health and care services and their carers
3 Be able to work with your colleagues to ensure the delivery of high quality, safe and compassionate healthcare, care and support
4 Be able to communicate in an open and effective way to promote the health, safety and wellbeing of people who use health and care services and their carers
5 Be able to respect a person's right to confidentiality
6 Be committed to improve the quality of healthcare, care and support through **continuing professional development (CPD)**
7 Be able to uphold and promote equality, diversity and **inclusion**.

Source: *Skills for Care and Skills for Health (2013) 'Code of Conduct for Healthcare Support Workers and Adult Social Care Workers in England'*

For more information, see the Skills for Care (www.skillsforcare.org.uk/resources/documents/Support-for-leaders-and-managers/Managing-people/Code-of-conduct/Code-of-Conduct.pdf) or Skills for Health websites.

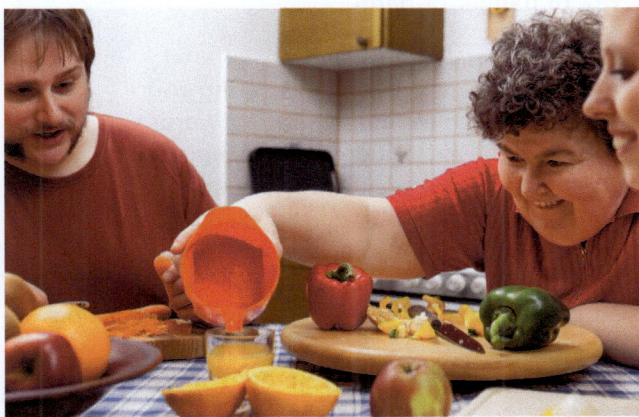

Figure 4.1 How well are you exercising your duty of care towards the individuals and others you support?

Key terms

Skills for Health is the Sector Skills Council for people working in healthcare.

Inclusion means being included or involved, for example being part of a wider group, or a group of friends. In an adult care setting, this means ensuring that all individuals are able to be included or partake in everyday life regardless of any differences. This can create a sense of belonging.

Continuing professional development (CPD) refers to the process of tracking and documenting the skills, knowledge and experience that you gain both formally and informally as you work, beyond any initial training. It is a record of what you experience, learn and then apply.

Reflect on it

1.1 Have you met the guidelines in the Code of Conduct?

How far do you think you've met the seven standards for exercising your duty of care included in the Code of Conduct described above? Are there any areas where you need to improve? How could you go about making these improvements? Discuss this with your employer.

6Cs

Competence

Competence involves having the knowledge and skills to carry out your work role effectively and supporting others to do the same. This includes, for example, carrying out your role safely and to the standard expected of you. You can acquire competence through training provided by your employer and by reflecting on how to further develop your knowledge, skills and practice and those of others. Remember that you have a duty of care to only carry out activities you are competent in, which you have been trained to do, and so ensure that your work practices are safe and do not place individuals and others at risk of danger or harm.

Compassion

Compassion involves demonstrating your empathy, kindness and warmth towards individuals. This includes, for example, taking the time to involve individuals in decisions about their care or support. You can exercise your duty of care while showing compassion by ensuring you always uphold individuals' rights and support others to do the same, and by reporting any discriminatory practices to ensure that individuals remain free from harm or abuse.

The Code of Conduct for Healthcare Support Workers and Adult Social Care Workers in England is commonly used alongside the Care Certificate. The Care Certificate is an agreed set of 15 standards that set out the knowledge, skills and behaviours expected of those who work in the health and social care sector, including Personal Assistants, Senior Home Care Workers and Reablement Officers and should be covered as part of an **induction** programme to ensure the provision of safe and compassionate high-quality care and support. The Care Certificate was developed jointly by Skills for Care, Health Education England and Skills for Health.

For example, Standard 3: Duty of Care requires you to understand why your duty of care is important and how it contributes to safe practice and impacts on your work role, how to manage dilemmas that may arise between the duty of care and an individual's rights, how to respond to comments and complaints and make improvements to the quality of the care and support provided, how to handle incidents, errors and **near misses** and how to manage difficult situations that may arise. This standard must underpin everything you do to ensure that your work practices are safe, compassionate and respectful. For more information, refer to www.skillsforcare.org.uk/Documents/Learning-and-development/Care-Certificate/Standard-3.pdf

Evidence opportunity

1.1 What it means to have a duty of care

Produce a verbal presentation that explains what having a duty of care in your work role means. Think about why it is important and relevant to your day-to-day work tasks. Include examples of how you are meeting the standards expected from you in your current work role. You could provide a written explanation detailing what it means to have a duty of care.

Key terms

Induction is the process of introducing a worker to an organisation and work setting by showing them round and explaining the agreed ways of working, for example.

Near misses refer to incidents that have the potential to cause harm, such as a delay in administering an individual's medication or a hoist battery that runs out just before an individual is about to be moved from one position to another. It may be that the individual is not actually harmed, but they could have been, and so it is a 'near miss.'

Duty of candour refers to the standards that adult care workers and professionals must follow when mistakes are made and an individual's care goes wrong. This will include being open and honest.

Candour refers to a way of working that involves being open and honest with individuals, your employer and others in the care setting where you work when something has gone wrong, such as incidents or near misses that may have led to harm.

AC 1.2 Explain how duty of care relates to duty of candour

All those who work in health and social care have a professional **duty of candour** towards the individuals they provide with care and support or their representative. This means that they must be open and honest with individuals when something has gone wrong with the care or support provided and harm or distress has been caused, or potentially could be caused. For you to exercise your duty of candour you must be:

- **honest:** for example, by telling the individual or their representative such as their family or advocate what has gone wrong with their care or support, or raising your concerns with CQC if necessary.
- **empathetic:** for example, by acknowledging how an individual or a member of their family feels about something that has not worked well for them.
- **supportive:** for example, by suggesting how what has gone wrong can be put right (if that is possible), supporting them to do this and participating in discussions and meetings with your employer if requested to do so.
- **open:** for example, by explaining fully to the individual and/or their representative the impact of what has gone wrong with their care or support and by being open with your colleagues about the effects of what has gone wrong, thus encouraging learning to take place.

Under Regulation 20 of the Health and Social Care Act 2008 (Regulated Activities) Regulations 2014, the Care Quality Commission (CQC) put in place a requirement for all registered organisations in England who provide healthcare and social care services to be open and transparent with individuals who use their services and to apologise when things go wrong. This means that organisations must ensure all those who work for them understand how to put into practice this duty of candour and why this is important. The regulation also sets out some specific requirements that providers must follow when things go wrong with individuals' care or support, such as informing individuals about what happened, providing support and apologising. If providers do not uphold their duty of candour, then the CQC can take action against organisations and prosecute them for breaching this regulation; organisations can also face closure and heavy fines for breaching their duty of candour.

Being open and honest with individuals and/or their representatives

You can be open and honest by ensuring that you always fully involve individuals or their representatives in decisions about their care or support; this involves exploring both the risks and the benefits of different options and ensuring their understanding of these before any decisions are made. For example, for an individual with a learning disability who wishes to travel independently for the first time you have a duty of care to ensure that you discuss the different travel options available to them, such as train, taxi and the Underground, and their associated benefits and risks. In addition, you must ensure that you provide this information to the individual in a format they can understand, for example by using signs, photographs or short sentences. You must then immediately check with the individual that they have understood the different options available to them.

If, for example, the individual chooses to travel via taxi and you realise on the morning that you forgot to book the taxi, then as soon as you realise this you must tell the individual you have made a mistake. You should also inform their representative if they have one. You must explain why you forgot to book the taxi – perhaps it was a very busy shift, or you had to deal with an emergency and therefore forgot. You should also explain what the likely consequences of your actions will be, give the individual and/or their representative the opportunity to ask questions and answer them honestly. If an individual shows no interest or prefers to not know why you forgot to book the taxi, then you must respect their wishes. Always record what information you have provided and not provided, as well as the reasons why, because this will then become a permanent record of how you exercised your duty of care and candour when things went wrong and could be referred to again in the future. For more information about handling information you will find Unit 305 Handling information in adult care setting/services useful.

You must also apologise to the individual for the mistake. Think carefully about how to do this so that the apology is received in the way you intend. It is important you choose a private place to apologise to the individual so that you can show empathy and be respectful of the individual's rights to privacy and dignity. Again, record that you have apologised to the individual. Your employer may require you to provide the individual with an apology in writing; the actions to take will be included in your agreed ways of working, so make sure you refer to these.

When apologising to an individual's representative pay careful attention to ensuring that you show warmth and compassion when conveying that you are sorry for the mistake. Choosing what you say and how, allowing sufficient time to do so and answering their questions honestly are all different ways that you can do this. You should also ensure that you provide them with contact details of who they can approach, and when, if they have any questions they would like to ask at a later date. For more information about communicating effectively you will find Unit 304 Effective communication in adult care settings/services useful.

By being open and honest with individuals and/or their representatives you will be fulfilling your duty of care because you will be promoting individuals' rights to safety and to be free from harm. In this way, you will be promoting individuals' best interests as well as complying with your employer's agreed ways of working. Providing individuals and/or their representatives with full and accurate information means that you will upholding their rights to being informed and communicated with – by treating them respectfully as an equal partner in their care or support.

Learning from mistakes made

Being open and honest when things go wrong means that you and others can learn from your mistakes to try to ensure that these never happen again. It is important to report and record mistakes as soon as they happen, so that you can fulfil your duty of care and ensure that individuals and others are safeguarded from possible further harm.

For example, if an error is made when administering medication to an individual – perhaps you realise at 8 pm that you forgot to give an individual an additional paracetamol at 4 pm – you must report this quickly and record it as soon as possible. Not doing so may mean that the individual continues to experience pain and will be unhappy that you did not uphold their request to have additional pain relief. Remember, you must always follow your organisation's agreed ways of working as they will have a duty to support those who work for them to report incidents such as these and may specify that additional actions must be taken such as reporting the incident to the regulator (i.e. the CQC). If you work in a team and the error is not made by you but by a colleague, then you are responsible for ensuring that you support them to do the same. You must never discourage them from reporting any errors – by openly discussing errors, agreeing on lessons learned and how to avoid making these errors again you will be leading by example and showing them how they must exercise their duty of candour and duty of care.

By learning from mistakes made you will also be fulfilling your duty of care by showing your commitment to being a professional and working in line with your employer's agreed ways of working. Learning from mistakes means you will be doing everything you can to ensure that the same mistakes are not made again; by doing so you will be exercising your duty of care towards individuals.

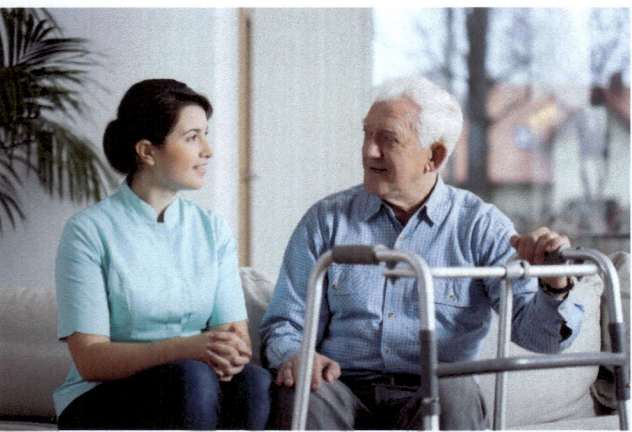

Figure 4.2 How open and honest are you with the individuals you care for and support?

Reflect on it

1.2 Learning from mistakes

Reflect on an occasion when you or someone you know made a mistake that resulted in the care or support provided to an individual going wrong. What happened? Why? What lessons were learned? How were these applied? How did the learning gained enable a duty of care and a duty of candour to be exercised?

Evidence opportunity

1.2 Duty of candour and duty of care

Imagine you are inducting a new member of staff. Provide a written account explaining how duty of care relates to duty of candour in their day-to-day working role.

AC 1.3 Explain how duty of care contributes to the safeguarding and protecting of individuals' right to live in safety and be free from abuse and improper treatment

Exercising your duty of care can also contribute to both the safeguarding and protection of individuals. If we think about the meaning of each of these concepts you will see why they are closely linked to your duty of care. Safeguarding adults involves:

- **protecting individuals' rights to live in safety, free from abuse and improper treatment:** your duty of care involves keeping individuals safe and free from harm such as illness, abuse and improper treatment. Your duty of care also means that you must do everything you can to ensure that individuals are not abused or neglected. This involves recognising when both abuse and improper treatment are occurring and when individuals may be at risk of both so that you can prevent individuals from being harmed and ensure that their pain and suffering are not prolonged.
- **working together with others to prevent the risk of abuse or improper treatment from arising and to stop them from happening:** your duty of care involves protecting individuals from potential abuse or improper treatment. You can do this by ensuring that you and your colleagues work in ways that empower individuals which will not only promote their wellbeing but will also make them less vulnerable to being abused or neglected. Developing an open and honest environment when working with individuals and others will mean that they will be more likely to approach you if they have concerns about safety. Safeguarding training will ensure that you keep up-to-date with current best practice. You can also work with other professionals and organisations such as the local council by taking the time to understand their roles and responsibilities, observing current best practice shared and by learning from any mistakes made.

Research it

1.3 Agreed ways of working for safeguarding

Research your employer's agreed ways of working for safeguarding. Produce a one-page written account that explains how it is underpinned by your duty of care.

- **promoting individuals' health and wellbeing by taking their views, preferences, wishes, beliefs and feelings into account:** your duty of care involves always acting in individuals' best interests and promoting their wellbeing. You can do this by actively involving individuals and/or their representatives in decisions about their care or support and providing them with all the information they require to make their own decisions. In this way you can ensure that you are not influencing their choices, you are simply facilitating the process by, for example, supporting them to explore the benefits and drawbacks of care or support options, and the impact different options may have on their lives.

Protecting adults involves:

- **knowing what to do when an individual has been abused, harmed or subjected to improper treatment:** your duty of care involves responding to situations where abuse, harm or improper treatment have taken place and doing this quickly and appropriately. You can do this by always complying with your employer's agreed ways of working for responding to abuse, harm or improper treatment. For example, this will involve you reporting and recording what has happened accurately and as soon as possible because this will act as a permanent record and may be referred to by others such as the police or Adult Social Care Services. You must also ensure that the individual is in a place of safety and cannot be abused, harmed or neglected again. See Unit 301 Safeguarding and protection in adult care settings/services for more information on responding when abuse, harm or improper treatment have taken place.

- **knowing what to do when there are concerns that an individual may be at risk of abuse, harm or subject to improper treatment:** your duty of care involves always acting in an individual's best interests. For example, if an individual with dementia who is at high risk of falling wants to go for a walk on their own, it is important that the benefits and drawbacks are considered carefully so you ensure that any decisions made are in the best interests of the individual and do not deny their rights to independence and control of their own life but at the same time do not put their safety in danger. Balancing individuals' rights against your duty of care can be difficult; you can learn more about how to manage risks associated with these types of situations in this unit in AC 2.2.

- **preventing further abuse, harm or improper treatment from taking place:** your duty of care involves keeping individuals safe from abuse, harm or improper treatment. You can do this by ensuring that your ways of working are in line with your employer's agreed ways of working in relation to health and safety; you will then be setting a good example to those others you support and work with. For example, by only carrying out moving and handling activities that you are competent in you will ensure individuals and staff are not harmed; by reporting unsafe practices immediately you will ensure that individuals do not suffer abuse or neglect, and by wearing PPE you will ensure that individuals' and others' health, safety and wellbeing are protected. See Unit 310 Promoting health and safety in adult care settings/services for more information.

Case study 1.1, 1.2, 1.3 provides you with an opportunity to think about the learning you have undertaken in LO1 in relation to how your duty of care contributes to safe practice.

Reflect on it

1.3 Your role in protecting individuals

Reflect on how your current job role involves protecting individuals who have care or support needs. What different ways of working do you use to ensure their protection? Can you ensure their protection at all times? Why?

Case study

1.1, 1.2, 1.3 Duty of care, candour and safeguarding and protection

Marcel is a Lead Support Worker and is overseeing the shift today in the Able supported living scheme (where people access support to assist them to live independently in their own home) where three individuals with learning disabilities live. Working alongside Marcel are two support workers and one volunteer.

Marcel begins by meeting with all three team members and outlining the plan of work for today's shift, including the work tasks and activities that have been allocated to them.

Discussions then continue, with Marcel updating each member of the team with the following items of information in relation to the three individuals who live at Able: 1) Simone woke up feeling a little unwell this morning and stated that she had a stomach ache, 2) Monica has requested to go swimming, unaccompanied by her sister, and 3) Chanelle has indicated that she is looking forward to her friend visiting her this afternoon.

In relation to Simone, Marcel explains that Simone has indicated that she does not want to go to the GP but would rather just stay in bed all day. Marcel explains that he has explained to Simone that, although it is her right to not go to the GP and to stay in bed all day, it is also the staff's duty of care to ensure her condition does not worsen and to explore with her the different options available to her that may make her feel more comfortable and reduce her pain.

With respect to Monica, Marcel explains that he would like to find out a little more about the reasons why Monica would like to go to swimming unaccompanied by her sister and plans to speak to Monica about this himself. Perhaps, Marcel explains, Monica would like to increase her independence from her sister or is not enjoying going swimming with her sister. Marcel adds that once he understands Monica's reasons, a plan to support her will be put in place.

Marcel informs the team that the friend that Chanelle is awaiting a visit from tends to not turn up. Given how upset Chanelle was last time this happened, he suggests that it would be a good idea to have other options for afternoon activities that Chanelle will enjoy participating in that may help distract her if her friend does not turn up again. Marcel adds that it will be important to give Chanelle the opportunity to talk about how she is feeling, if she wishes to do so.

Discuss:
1. How is Marcel exercising his duty of care as a Lead Support Worker?
2. How is Marcel supporting others to exercise their duty of candour?
3. How is Marcel contributing to the safeguarding and protection of Simone, Monica and Chanelle?

Evidence opportunity

1.3 How duty of care contributes to the safeguarding or protection of individuals

Think about two individuals with care or support needs who you work with. For each individual explain how your duty of care contributes to their safeguarding and protection. Provide a written account. You could also explain this to your assessor and provide a written account of your discussion.

LO2 Know how to address conflicts or dilemmas that may arise between an individual's rights and the duty of care

Getting started

Think about an occasion when you were faced with a dilemma that involved doing something you felt uncomfortable with. For example, perhaps you were asked by someone close to you to support them with something that you didn't agree with, such as something that was against your beliefs or views. How might you feel in this situation? Why? What's more important, supporting someone close to you or your beliefs and views?

AC 2.1 Describe conflicts or dilemmas that may arise between the duty of care and an individual's rights

When exercising your duty of care to the individuals you care for and support, you may find that acting in individuals' best interests may sometimes be in direct conflict with their rights to make their own choices and decisions. Your duty of care involves empowering individuals to be in control of their lives and therefore you cannot prevent them from taking risks or doing something that is not in their best interests. Your duty of care is to enable individuals to understand the potential benefits, risks and consequences of their actions. By doing this you can ensure that balanced decisions are made that enable you to exercise your duty of care and individuals to exercise their rights to lead their lives as they want to.

Conflicts and dilemmas

As a Lead Adult Care Worker or Lead Personal Assistant you may find that conflicts or dilemmas may arise between exercising your duty of care and individuals' rights. Table 4.1 includes examples of the different conflicts or dilemmas that may arise. For examples of ways in which you might address each of the situations, see Table 4.2.

Table 4.1 Examples of different conflicts or dilemmas that may arise

Conflicts or dilemmas	Why are these conflicts or dilemmas?
Eating a healthy, balanced diet: Mila is obese and suffers with lower back pain. She finds it difficult to use the stairs without getting out of breath. She refuses to change her diet as she enjoys having takeaways most nights of the week and eating out with her friends at the weekend.	Mila's reluctance to eat a healthy, balanced diet is a concern as it is your duty of care to promote her health and wellbeing. By continuing to have takeaways and eat out at the weekends, Mila's weight will continue to increase, which may lead to her back pain getting worse because of the additional strain her bones, muscles and joints will be under. Mila is already experiencing shortness of breath, a sign that her lungs and heart are not working as effectively as they should – this also may worsen if she continues to have an unhealthy diet. However, it is Mila's right to eat what she wants; she is able to make her own choices and decisions about how she lives her life.
A lack of finances: Rosie is 84 years old and lives in her own home. Rosie discloses to you that this week she will not go to the hairdresser because it is her grandson's birthday and she wants to buy him something nice. Rosie asks you not to say anything to her daughter who will be visiting her this afternoon as she'll offer to pay for her hair. Rosie doesn't want her daughter to do this as she says she has always managed by herself.	Rosie's lack of finances is a concern because she is putting her grandson's needs before her own and it is your duty of care to ensure she is not placed at risk of abuse or neglect. This time she has decided to go without a haircut but next time she may decide to go without buying herself some food or clothes that she needs. This could result in Rosie neglecting her own needs over those of her family. There is also a concern that her family are unaware of her situation. However, it is Rosie's right to ask you to not inform her family about her personal finances as these are private and confidential to Rosie. It is Rosie's right to be independent, to manage by herself and not depend on her family. It is Rosie's right to feel valued, and doing things for her family such as buying her grandson a birthday present can enable her to continue to have a valued role within her family.

> **Evidence opportunity**
>
> **2.1 Conflicts or dilemmas**
>
> For two individuals with care or support needs you know, describe the conflicts or dilemmas that may arise between the duty of care and the rights of both individuals. Think about specific examples you have come across. Provide a written/reflective account.

AC 2.2 Explain how to work effectively with individuals and others to address conflicts and dilemmas related to duty of care in order to achieve positive outcomes for individuals

Balancing your duty of care and an individual's rights involves doing everything you can to support individuals to make their own choices and decisions without compromising their or others' safety in order to achieve positive outcomes for individuals. The risk assessment process involves supporting individuals to take risks by assessing the potential dangers and considering what can be put in place to reduce those risks and protect individuals from danger, harm, abuse or neglect. The risk assessment process does not prevent individuals from doing what they want but rather helps individuals and you to manage these risks effectively by considering what can be done to reduce them. In this way, you will be exercising your duty of care by supporting individuals' rights to live how they want to and make their own choices and decisions after giving careful consideration to the benefits, risks and consequences that are associated with these.

Reflect on it

2.2 Supporting individuals with their rights

Reflect on how it would make you feel if you were prevented from doing something in your life that you really wanted to do. Perhaps you want to go to university, pursue a career in social care, go travelling, learn a new skill? Now think about how it would make you feel being supported to do what you want to do in your life, to pursue your goals and dreams.

Now put yourself in the shoes of an individual with care and support needs who would like to pursue their goals and dreams. How do you think they may feel if they were prevented from doing so? And if they were supported to work towards these? Why is it important that you show the individual your **compassion**?

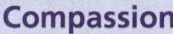

Do these ways still enable you to exercise your duty of care and support individuals' rights at the same time? What can you do if they don't?

6Cs

Compassion

Compassion refers to taking a genuine interest in how an individual may be feeling by putting yourself in their situation and thinking about how you may feel when not being supported, for example to make your own choices and decisions. Showing compassion also shows that you understand the reasons why individuals make choices and decisions. Being compassionate goes hand in hand with being empathetic and this is important because without this quality you will not be able to see things from others' perspectives and will find it harder to build effective working relationships.

You can show your compassion when conflicts or dilemmas arise between your duty of care and an individual's rights by getting to know an individual and observing what they are expressing so that you can then respond with kindness and consideration to their wishes, views and preferences. Being compassionate involves putting your views and preferences to one side so that you can fully understand those of individuals and ensure positive outcomes can be achieved.

Read through again in AC 2.1 the examples of conflicts or dilemmas that may arise between exercising your duty of care and individuals' rights, then look at the potential ways described in Table 4.2 that can be used to manage these risks and achieve positive outcomes for individuals. Can you think of other ways of managing these risks?

Table 4.2 Examples of how to manage risks associated with conflicts or dilemmas in order to achieve positive outcomes for individuals

Conflicts or dilemmas	How to manage risks associated with conflicts or dilemmas to achieve positive outcomes for individuals
Eating a healthy, balanced diet: Mila is obese and suffers with lower back pain. She finds it difficult to use the stairs without getting out of breath. She refuses to change her diet as she enjoys having takeaways most nights of the week and eating out with her friends at the weekend.	You could begin by exploring with Mila why she enjoys having takeaways most nights of the week. Perhaps this is because she finds it easier than cooking or likes the variety of foods she can buy. Together you could explore the benefits of having takeaways most nights (no need to cook, no washing up, saves on electricity and hot water), the drawbacks (expensive, unhealthy as high in salt, sugar and fat) and the potential consequences (will lead to an increase in weight, puts more pressure on the joints and back, may lead to increasing health difficulties). Similarly, you could then explore with Mila why she enjoys eating out with her friends at the weekend. Perhaps this is because she likes meeting up with them and enjoys going out to different places. Together you could explore the benefits of eating out with her friends at the weekend (socialising opportunity, feeling like she belongs), the drawbacks (expensive, difficult to make healthy choices when in a group with friends) and the potential consequences (will lead to an increase in weight, puts more pressure on the joints and back, may lead to increasing health difficulties).

Table 4.2 Examples of how to manage risks associated with conflicts or dilemmas in order to achieve positive outcomes for individuals *continued*

Conflicts or dilemmas	How to manage risks associated with conflicts or dilemmas to achieve positive outcomes for individuals
Eating a healthy, balanced diet *continued*	After assessing the benefits, risks and potential consequences carefully you could then discuss and agree how Mila could be supported to do what she wants by reducing the risks to her health and wellbeing. For example, perhaps Mila could have takeaways twice a week instead of nearly every night and could learn how to develop her cooking skills by learning how to cook easy meals with her favourite ingredients that are healthy and that she enjoys. In terms of eating out with her friends at the weekend, perhaps she could make healthy choices when eating out by reading through the menu carefully when at a restaurant. Some weekends she could also suggest to her friends that they try a different activity, for example rather than eating out perhaps they could go bowling or to the cinema. Mila could also try inviting her friends to her house; perhaps she could show off her newly learned cooking skills for healthy eating. Managing these risks in these ways will enable you to support Mila to continue to do what she wants while putting in place measures that will protect her health and wellbeing.
A lack of finances: Rosie is 84 years old and lives in her own home. Rosie discloses to you that this week she will not go to the hairdresser because it is her grandson's birthday and she wants to buy him something nice. Rosie asks you not to say anything to her daughter who will be visiting her this afternoon as she'll offer to pay for her hair. Rosie doesn't want her daughter to do this as she says she has always managed by herself.	You could begin by exploring with Rosie why she doesn't want her family to know about her personal financial situation. Perhaps she feels that she looks after her family, not the other way around, or perhaps she is embarrassed about her personal situation and uncomfortable about others paying for her. Together you could explore the benefits of not saying anything about her personal finances to her family (her family will not be worried, Rosie retains her pride, Rosie feels valued and continues to be financially independent), the drawbacks and potential consequences (she may run out of money, she may no longer be able to buy anything for her family, she may no longer be able to meet her own needs). After assessing the benefits, risks and potential consequences carefully you could then discuss and agree with Rosie how she could be supported to do what she wants by reducing the risks of abuse and neglect. For example, perhaps she could find other ways of increasing her finances, perhaps she has things that she no longer needs and wants to sell; the income from these could be used to pay for presents. If she has a skill such as painting or crafting she could make presents rather than buy them – homemade gifts are always appreciated just as much as bought presents. Perhaps she could review how she is managing her money on a day-by-day basis and put a plan in place to save up for presents as well as do the things she wants such as going to the hairdresser.

The key ways of effectively managing risks associated with conflicts or dilemmas between an individual's rights and your duty of care in order to achieve positive outcomes for individuals involve being knowledgeable about the individual, being respectful towards them, being open and honest with them and following your agreed ways of working.

Capacity

All the examples of conflicts or dilemmas between the duty of care and an individual's rights you have learned about so far involved people who had the capacity to make their own decisions and choices about what they want to do in their lives to achieve positive outcomes. But what happens if an individual lacks the capacity to make their own choices and decisions and therefore may not fully understand the benefits versus the risks and potential consequences of different wishes and goals they may have? This may be because the individual's mental health has deteriorated, or because an individual has a learning disability or dementia.

In 2005 the Mental Capacity Act (MCA) was introduced, which aimed to protect and give some power back to individuals who lacked capacity. It was also designed so that those working in health and social care could assess whether individuals have capacity. It outlined ways in which those who worked with individuals with care and support needs could support them to make decisions. The Act outlined five principles which are important for you to know and understand in your role as you have a duty of care to comply with this.

The five principles state that:

1. You must presume capacity
2. Individuals have the right to be supported to make their own decision
3. Individuals have the right to make unwise decisions: you may disagree with a decision and feel it is unwise, but individuals have the right to make such decisions
4. Best interests of the individual must be considered
5. Least restrictive option must be taken.

There is also a two-stage functional test of capacity that you should undertake to decide whether an individual has the capacity to make a decision:

- **Stage 1:** Is there an impairment of or disturbance in the functioning of a person's mind or brain? If so;
- **Stage 2:** Is the impairment or disturbance sufficient that the person lacks the capacity to make a particular decision?

These two questions are taken from SCIE's 'Mental Capacity Act 2005 at a glance' (www.scie.org.uk/mca/introduction/mental-capacity-act-2005-at-a-glance)

The MCA also introduced the Lasting Power of Attorney (LPA) which allows people over the age of 18 to formally choose someone to make decisions for them if they are unable to make decisions in the future. The MCA also introduced a Public Guardian to ensure that people who lack capacity are not abused and it also states that it is a criminal offence to neglect or ill-treat someone who lacks capacity. The Act is accompanied by a code of practice that provides guidance to people who act or make decisions on another person's behalf. All of this stresses the importance of maintaining your duty of care to individuals and doing all you can to ensure that you empower individuals to make their own choices and decisions and not prevent them from doing so, but to follow best practice when they are unable to.

Advance Care Plans

If an individual has an Advance Care Plan in place and the individual's decision is to refuse treatment and their family disagree with their decision about this then, providing the Advance Care Plan is valid, the individual's wishes must be respected.

However, the individual's family also has a right to explain why they think the decision is not valid or incorrect, and so this could be discussed with the family. If agreement with the family can still not be reached, an advocate could be sought and ultimately the individual's family could make a formal complaint to the care provider; if agreement can still not be reached then this could be referred to the Court of Protection.

> **Research it**
>
> **2.2 Mental Capacity Act**
>
> Research the Mental Capacity Act here: www.scie.org.uk/mca/introduction/mental-capacity-act-2005-at-a-glance
>
> Discuss how relevant it is to the individuals with care or support needs you work with. How does it impact on managing the risks associated with conflicts or dilemmas between individuals' rights and your duty of care?

Other circumstances

Other situations that arise while carrying out your work role may mean that are unable to support an individual's rights because your duty of care requires you to take alternative action:

- If the individual's decision will harm them or put others at risk of harm then you may not be able to support the individual to do what they want. For example, an individual may insist that they want to continue to drink alcohol heavily at night even though they know this makes them very aggressive. You may decide that you cannot let them do this because not only does it place their health in danger, it also means that the other individuals they live with and the team members that may be present will be put at risk of being harmed. You can try to speak to the individual about this first, but if the individual ignores you then you may need to speak to your manager. If the individual is also your employer you may need to seek assistance from outside, perhaps from the individual's family or an external organisation such as Alcoholics Anonymous.
- If the individual's decision means that they will be taking part in something that goes against your employer's agreed ways of working, then you may not be able to support the individual to do what they want. For example, an individual may insist that they want to go for a walk on their

own in the garden without their walking aid even though they recently had a fall, have only just recovered and using their walking aid was agreed as part of their plan of care and support. You may decide that you cannot let them do this because they may fall and injure themselves again. You can try to speak to the individual about this first to find out why they don't want to use their walking aid, but if the individual still insists on not using it then you may need to speak to your manager. If the individual is also your employer then you may need to seek assistance from someone else, perhaps from a health professional such as their physiotherapist or someone close to them such as a friend or family member.

- The individual's decision means that they will be taking part in something that is morally wrong, illegal or criminal. For example, an individual may tell you that they want to try drug taking with a new group of friends they've recently met in college. You have a duty of care to not ignore this and you must report your concerns immediately to your manager. If the individual is also your employer, then you may have to report your concerns directly to the police. It is important that the individual is aware of the actions you plan to take and that you explain to the individual why you have to take these actions as you have a duty of care towards them.

Evidence opportunity

2.2 How to address conflicts or dilemmas between an individual's rights and the duty of care, to achieve positive outcomes

Describe to your assessor how you work with individuals and others to address conflicts or dilemmas related to duty of care. Provide a written account describing this.

AC 2.3 Outline where to access additional support and advice about addressing conflicts and dilemmas in a care setting/service

At times, because the conflicts and dilemmas that arise between your duty of care and an individual's rights can be quite difficult to resolve, it will be necessary for you to ask for additional support and advice about how these can be resolved satisfactorily. Getting additional support

6Cs

Care

Care is not just about meeting an individual's needs and preferences. Care is about showing your genuine interest in ensuring that the care and support you provide makes a positive difference to an individual's life. This is important because without good care and support you and others in the team will not be able to support an individual's rights and preferences. You can show you care by thinking carefully about why you are providing care and support to an individual, how you are doing this and how it is being received. Ensuring you obtain feedback from individuals and others who you may work with, including your manager (if you have one, or from your employer who may also be the individual) and colleagues who know you well, ensures that you continue to assess how well you are caring for individuals and supporting others in the team to do the same.

and advice is a must so that any dilemmas that arise can be dealt with quickly, potential conflicts will be limited and individuals' and others' safety protected. Getting additional support and advice will also show individuals that you genuinely **care** about respecting and promoting their rights and that you have considered how the care you provide impacts them as you have gone to the effort to seek advice. As a Lead Adult Care Worker you will also ensure that you are setting a good example to others in your team; they will feel reassured that anything they report to you will be acted on, even if you have to seek advice yourself.

You can seek additional support and advice about conflicts and dilemmas that may arise both from within the setting where you work and externally from people and organisations outside.

Internal sources of additional support and advice

If you are unsure about how to resolve a conflict or dilemma that has arisen between your duty of care and an individual's rights, you should first approach your manager, if you have one, who will be able to advise you on what to do. If you are unable to approach your manager, then you could contact another senior person who works in the same organisation for their support and advice. If you work on your own and the individual is also your employer, you may need to seek additional support and advice from an external organisation – which organisation is most appropriate will depend on the nature of the dilemma or conflict. For example, if it relates to an individual with dementia then an organisation such as the Alzheimer's Society may be appropriate, or a dementia nurse if they have one. If it relates to supporting an individual who has depression, an organisation such as MIND or a mental health advocate if they have one would be appropriate. You should refer to your employer's agreed ways of working for who the most appropriate person or organisation to approach would be.

Other internal sources of additional support and advice are your employer's agreed ways of working; these can be useful to reference when you are unsure about what to do in terms of resolving dilemmas and the process to follow. Sometimes experienced colleagues or colleagues you trust can be useful sources of additional support because they may have come across these types of dilemmas previously and would therefore be able to offer you advice and support based on their own experience.

External sources of additional support and advice
Whistleblowing

Sometimes it may be necessary to seek additional support and advice from external bodies and organisations because, as you will have already learned, there are some circumstances where doing nothing is not an option (you may find it useful to refresh your knowledge about these circumstances by re-reading the relevant section in AC 2.2 of this unit). Reporting your concerns to external organisations when required is also part of your duty of care and you have a legal right to do this without being penalised by your employer for doing so – this concept is known as whistleblowing. Your employer will have in place agreed ways of working for whistleblowing and so it is very important that you familiarise yourself with and follow these.

The reflective exemplar provides you with some additional information about the benefits of following whistleblowing procedures about resolving conflicts or dilemmas that may arise.

> **Reflect on it**
>
> **2.3 Support and advice from others**
>
> Reflect on an occasion when you had to access advice or support from someone in the setting where you work. Who did you go to? Why? Was their advice or support useful? Was there anyone else you could have approached if this person wasn't available?

> **Research it**
>
> **2.3 Agreed ways of working for whistleblowing**
>
> Research your employer's agreed ways of working for whistleblowing. Do you know how to whistleblow if you need to? Do you feel confident in doing so? Do you feel confident in supporting others to do the same? Draw a flowchart of the steps to take if you had to report concerns you had about an individual's safety.

Reflective exemplar	
Introduction	I work as a Lead Personal Assistant with Marta, a young adult who has a physical disability. Marta lives on her own and is very independent.
What happened	This morning upon my arrival at Marta's home, Marta explained that as she was my employer and I was working in her home, she wanted me to carry her up the stairs rather than use the hoist because she felt that this was quicker and more convenient for her. I felt anxious about what Marta had requested of me because I knew that this was an unsafe practice, so I asked Marta to give me a moment to think about what she had asked me to do. I took the opportunity to step aside into the lounge and in private noted down what I had been asked, when and where. I used Marta's words so that I could keep it as factual as possible. I then decided to approach Marta with my concerns about the risk to her and to myself if I was to carry her up the stairs rather than use the hoist that had been provided. Marta reiterated that it was her home and therefore her rules. I tried again to explain calmly that doing this would be unsafe and also explained my duty of care towards her. Marta then stated that her other personal assistants have been doing this and no one has complained apart from me.

Reflective exemplar	
What worked well	As I felt that I could not resolve this with Marta I decided to speak to her social worker in the first instance about this.
	I positively challenged the unsafe practice of carrying Marta up the stairs.
	I decided that I would report this to Marta's social worker after not being able to resolve this with Marta, my employer.
What did not go as well	I did not explain to Marta what would happen next.
	I should have also challenged the unsafe practices that Marta told me about that other personal assistants had been using.
	I did not refer to my employer's whistleblowing procedures about the next steps to take in situations such as this where I identified unsafe practices. Was Marta's social worker the appropriate person to speak to or should I have approached someone else first with my concerns?
What I could do to improve	I think I will need to familiarise myself with my employer's whistleblowing procedures and ensure that I am following these when raising concerns I have about unsafe or illegal practices.
Links to unit's assessment criteria	ACs: 2.1, 2.2, 2.3

Specialist organisations

Seeking advice from specialist organisations and professionals may be necessary when dilemmas or conflicts are in relation to individuals' care or support needs or they involve specialist areas of knowledge and expertise. Specialist professionals may include social workers, mental health nurses, dementia nurses and advocates; specialist organisations may include MIND, Alzheimer's UK, local charities and support groups.

Friends and family

Involving individuals' family and friends needs to be decided on a case by case basis as this will be appropriate for some individuals but not for others. For example, an individual may have chosen a family member or friend to represent their views on their behalf or you may have observed that an individual often refers to a family member or close friend for advice. Another individual may not have a close relationship with their family, or they may request that their family is not involved in decisions about their care and support and therefore it would not be appropriate to involve them.

CQC, Skills for Care, HSE, trade unions

Other useful sources of support may be the regulator (CQC) for more specific advice on how to promote your duty of care, or Skills for Care for guidance on how to maintain good standards of care and support others to do the same. Your trade union, if you belong to one, is another source you could go to for advice on maintaining your legal duty of care or you could go to the **Health and Safety Executive (HSE)** for advice on how to carry out risk assessments effectively.

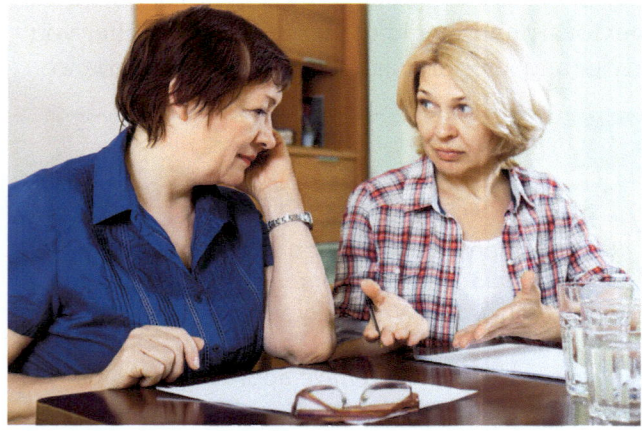

Figure 4.3 How do you use your communication skills to access additional support and advice about conflict and dilemmas?

Key term

Health and Safety Executive (HSE) is the independent regulator in the UK for health and safety in work settings.

6Cs

Communication

Communication is crucial to getting additional support and advice on how to resolve conflicts or dilemmas that may arise between your duty of care and an individual's rights. Communicating effectively and clearly explaining the details around the conflict or dilemma will mean that you are able to source relevant advice and support, enabling you to resolve the dilemma. In other words, if you seek advice from your manager, you will need to ensure you know and communicate:

- the details around the dilemma
- what you would like the individual to do and your reasons
- what the individual would like to do and their reasons
- why these are in conflict.

All these points are important to communicate so that your manager has a clear understanding of the situation, the 'different sides' or viewpoints and can advise you.

Communicating clearly and being open and honest with individuals means that they will trust and respect you; this in turn will enable you to maintain good working relationships with them and resolve conflicts or dilemmas. Good communication will avoid misunderstandings and delays in resolving such dilemmas, and will involve you:

- explaining clearly to the individual why there is a dilemma
- explaining what action you are going to take to resolve it
- reporting and recording information about the dilemma fully and accurately.

Evidence opportunity

2.3 Additional support and advice about resolving conflicts or dilemmas about duty of care and individuals' rights

Produce a written account that explains where to get additional support and advice on how to resolve conflicts or dilemmas that may arise between the duty of care and an individual's rights.

LO3 Know how to respond to concerns and complaints

AC 3.1 Explain own role in identifying and responding to comments and complaints

Getting started

Think of an occasion when you were unhappy or dissatisfied about a service you received. For example, this may have been in relation to the attitude of a shop assistant who was serving you – perhaps the shop assistant rushed you or appeared indifferent while they were serving you. How did this make you feel? Why? Did you say anything? Why? If so, how did you say it and why? How did the shop assistant respond? How did their employer respond? Why? What improvements to the service do you think are needed?

All organisations that provide health and social care services are required by law to have a process in place to respond to comments and complaints. We will look in more detail at what the law says about the main points that should be included in agreed procedures for comments and complaints in AC 3.2.

What is a complaint?

A complaint refers to when a person is not satisfied with an action or a lack of action by an employee or organisation and seeks to express their unhappiness so that the issue can be addressed. In adult care settings, complaints may be made in relation to many different issues, and by many different people such as individuals, family members or team members. A complaint may be made by an individual in relation to their care and support, or a team member in relation to their work rota, for example.

Complaints should not be seen as something negative; instead they are an opportunity to make changes and improvements to services. In fact, if your employer never received complaints about the service provided this may be more worrying than if they did! It could be an indicator that people are being discouraged from expressing their dissatisfaction, are too worried or afraid to do so, or that complaints are being ignored, not dealt with or are not being reported and recorded as they should be. Complaints will reveal if care, interactions, ways of working or anything about the setting is of a low quality and requires improvement; they will highlight bad or incorrect practice and they will also highlight anything that is lacking, for example any services that are not currently offered.

How to respond to comments and complaints

Every health and social care organisation will have developed their own process to follow when responding to comments and complaints and this must be followed every time a complaint is made. As a Lead Adult Care Worker responsible for other staff, you have a central role to play in creating a fair, open and honest working environment where individuals and others including individuals' families and friends, team members, other professionals and visitors feel able to raise any concerns they have, knowing that these will be acted on quickly and addressed fully. It is therefore important that you feel confident about how to respond when a concern or complaint is brought to your attention as this forms part of your duty of care. You can feel confident by:

- knowing what your employer's agreed ways of working say about your role in responding to comments and complaints
- discussing with your employer and asking questions about any aspect of the complaints process you are unsure about
- understanding how to respond to different types of comments and complaints received.

It is important that all comments and complaints are responded to fairly so that the complainant feels that their comment or complaint is being treated seriously and quickly, any issues or concerns can be resolved and improvements made. Responding to comments as soon as they are received can also at times prevent them developing into a complaint, because sometimes people prefer to make their views known informally rather than formally. To do this you need to view comments and complaints as an important way to improve the service rather than as a negative criticism of the service being provided. Viewing and responding to comments and complaints in this way will encourage mutual trust and respect between the complainant and the setting where you work and inspire confidence that the care setting is genuinely sorry for what has gone wrong and is doing its very best to put things right, promote best practice and improve their service.

Responding to comments and complaints effectively is important and requires you to be:

- **a good listener:** this means listening to what the complainant is telling you about what happened without interrupting them so that you can ensure that you understand what happened and you can identify what their complaint is about. You will find it useful to refer to Unit 304 Effective communication in adult care settings/services in relation to how to communicate effectively
- **fair:** this means remaining non-judgemental and non-biased towards the complainant. Being fair means not making assumptions about why the complainant is raising their concerns and includes completing full and accurate records. You will find it useful to refer to Unit 305 Handling information in adult care settings/services in relation to how to complete records fully and accurately
- **supportive:** this means both directly and indirectly providing the complainant with support such as by explaining the complaints process to them yourself, or by ensuring they have the support they need to follow the complaints process. For example, they may need an advocate to support them through the process or require it in another format that they understand, such as pictures. You should be professional and sensitive and show your **courage** when handling comments and complaints
- **assertive:** this means taking action quickly and confidently and may include directly handling a comment or and complaint yourself or passing this on to someone more appropriate. You will need to be polite at all times while remaining assertive, calm and professional
- **a good communicator:** this involves explaining the complaints process to the complainant clearly so that they can understand it, and keeping the complainant informed of the progress made with their complaint. You will find it useful to refer to Unit 305 Handling information in adult care settings/services.

6Cs

Courage
Courage relates to doing the right thing when you are handling comments and complaints. This is important because you will then be complying not only with your employer's agreed ways of working but also with the legislation that is in place. You can show your courage by not ignoring any comment or complaint, however small, be it informal or formal, and by ensuring you always respond to all comments and complaints respectfully and sensitively.

Commitment
Commitment relates to your determination to ensure that your ways of working make a positive difference to individuals' lives. This is important when handling comments and complaints so that complainants feel they can approach you with any concerns they have and not be deterred from complaining about any aspect of their care or support that they are unhappy about. You can show this by following your agreed ways of working and keeping the complainant informed about how their complaint is being handled throughout the whole process.

Reflect on it

3.1 Skills for responding to comments and complaints
Reflect on the skills you have that are useful for identifying and responding to comments and complaints. Why are these skills useful? Are there any other skills you need to further develop and/or improve? What difference would these additional skills make to the manner in which you respond to comments and complaints? What potential impact could they have for you, your employer, the individuals and others you work with?

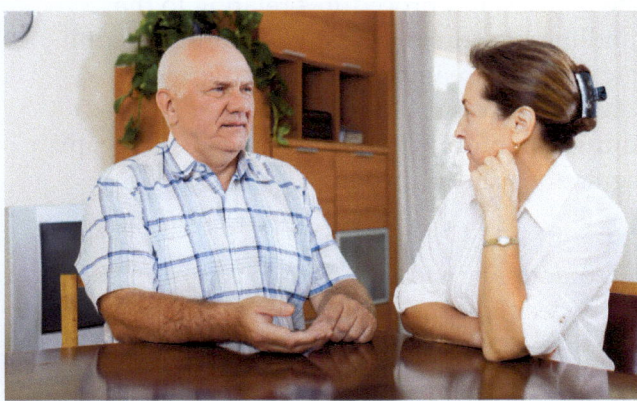

Figure 4.4 Can you respond to complaints effectively?

The process
When responding to comments and complaints you must follow your employer's agreed ways of working. Any process for responding to complaints must include the following key stages:

1. **Acknowledge the complaint when you receive it.** The complainant may make an informal complaint verbally to a care worker or a formal complaint in writing to the manager of the service or organisation. Both types of complaint must be acknowledged; this is usually done by writing to the complainant. In this way you will be able to clearly identify what the complaint is and the complainant will know that their complaint has been taken seriously.

2. **Acknowledge the complaint quickly, in writing and within the agreed timescale.** For example, acknowledgement should be made within three days of the complaint being received. In this way the complaint can be acted upon quickly.

3. **Make a decision over how to handle the complaint.** This could involve arranging for the complainant to meet with the manager of the service to discuss the issues raised or for a formal investigation to take place.

4. **Reach a decision on how to handle the complaint and discuss this with the complainant.** The reasons why a meeting or a formal investigation is required must be communicated to the complainant as well as how long it will then take to reach an outcome; this could be done verbally first but then must also be documented in writing. Again, this must be communicated within the agreed timescale, for example within ten days of the complaint being acknowledged.

5. **Contact the complainant and any others involved for further information.** If a formal investigation takes place, the person conducting the investigation will be impartial and may request to interview the complainant and/or any others involved.

6. **After reaching a final outcome, document a formal response and send this to the complainant.** This may be in the form of a full report of the investigation that has taken

place, its findings and any suggestions for improvements that will be made as a result.

7 **If the complainant thinks that their complaint has not been responded to fairly or by following the correct process, they will be informed that they have a right to contact an external organisation who will investigate their concerns**. This may be the **ombudsman** if the complaint is about the council, or the CQC if the complaint is about an independent provider of adult care services.

Key term

An **ombudsman** is a free independent service that investigates complaints against an organisation.

Note that an ombudsman can only look at certain complaints from agencies. The Local Government and Social Care Ombudsman (LGO) only looks at local authority complaints, the Parliamentary and Health Service Ombudsman (PHSO) looks at NHS and government departments. There is no ombudsman for private or voluntary care services.

Research it

3.1 CQC guidance

Research the guidance the CQC provides regarding making a complaint about a health or social care service:

www.cqc.org.uk/contact-us/how-complain/complain-about-service-or-provider

Discuss the key points to remember when supporting others to make a complaint.

Evidence opportunity

3.1 Describe how to respond to comments and complaints

Referring to your employer's agreed ways of working, produce a written account that describes how to respond to informal and formal comments and complaints received in the setting where you work. Include a list of dos and don'ts.

In addition, check that the complainant understands how to use the complaints procedure, explain how it works and what each stage involves including likely timescales. Inform your manager that the complaint has been made and follow your agreed ways of working for handling complaints, as how complaints are received and responded to will be analysed as part of service reviews.

AC 3.2 Outline the agreed policies and procedures for handling comments and complaints

As you have learned, following a process when responding to comments and complaints aims to ensure that comments and complaints are dealt with fairly, responded to fully and resolved as quickly as possible. Your employer will have in place a complaints policy and procedures as well as agreed ways of working that set out how to respond to comments and complaints; this will include the roles and responsibilities of yourself and others. Handling comments and complaints forms part of all care workers' training and is updated on a regular basis to ensure all care workers are following best practice when handling comments and complaints.

Legislation/regulations/guidance and how it relates to handling of comments and complaints

The policies and procedures relating to the handling of comments and complaints in adult care settings are informed by regulations, guidance and legislation. Below we discuss additional information about the most relevant regulations and legislation.

Care Act 2014
- Promotes individuals' right to complain about any decisions the local authority makes relating to their care or support, for example how much care or support they need, where it will be provided and by whom, what they have to pay for and what services they can access.
- Places a duty on the local authority to have in place clear information and a clear process for handling comments and complaints that can be accessed easily.

Health and Social Care Act 2008 (Regulated Activities) Regulations 2014: Regulation 16
- It states that all complaints received must be taken seriously and investigated.

- It states that all complaints must be acted on and action taken to make improvements when there are serious failures.
- It states that there must be an effective system in place for handling comments and complaints including identifying, receiving, recording, handling and responding to comments and complaints by individuals and others.
- It states that the complaints process must be managed by the person with overall responsibility for the adult care setting, such as the registered person at the setting.
- It states that the registered person must provide to the regulator (the CQC), when requested, a summary of all the comments and complaints made as well as the registered person's response to these and all related correspondence in relation to the complaints made.

CQC's 2014 guidance document 'How to complain about a health or social care service'

- It states that all complaints must be investigated and responded to promptly and fully.
- It states that all services must make available a copy of their complaints procedure. This must include information about who to contact, how complaints will be handled and the improvements that will be made as a result of the complaint made.
- It states that complaints can be received in person, over the telephone, by letter or by email.
- It states that if a complaint is made in person or over the telephone then the service must provide the complainant with a written copy of their complaint. They must let the complainant know how long they think it will take to investigate the complaint and provide them with a response.

Data Protection Act 2018

- It states that all personal information about individuals must be handled safely.
- This includes personal information that may be shared by complainants, for example in relation to how its security will be maintained when recorded and how it will be used, stored and shared during the complaints process.
- It states that individuals have the right to make a complaint if data held about them by an organisation is not in line with the Act. The organisation must keep the individual up to date with the progress made with their complaint, their findings and the proposed outcome to resolve their complaint.

You can find more information about the Data Protection Act in Unit 305 Handling information in adult care settings/services.

Comments and complaints policies

Comments and complaints policies in adult care settings are statements that set out how settings are complying with regulations and legislation relating to the handling of comments and complaints. All comments and complaints policies will include the following main points and principles:

- **Being open to receiving comments and complaints:** comments and complaints are welcomed and seen as a way of making changes, learning and improving services.
- **Making the comments and complaints process accessible to all:** comments and complaints are easy to make and can be done so by everyone; awareness of how to do so is reinforced with everyone.
- **Taking comments and complaints seriously:** all comments and complaints are taken seriously.
- **Handling comments and complaints effectively:** comments and all complaints, if handled professionally, sensitively, promptly and fairly can be resolved; a named person for handling comments and complaints is made available.
- **Inspiring confidence:** all comments and complaints if handled openly and honestly will instil confidence in the process and enable complainants to be listened to.

Comments and complaints procedures

Comments and complaints procedures in adult care settings describe how adult care settings will handle comments and complaints when received, and set out the (step by step) process that will be followed by all staff, for all comments and complaints. All procedures will include the process to follow for both informal and formal comments and complaints. These may vary across different care settings but the key steps to take will be the same.

Case study 3.1, 3.2 provides you with an opportunity to review your learning about best practice points when responding to comments and complaints.

Research it

3.2 Comments and complaints procedures

Research the comments and complaints procedures used in the care setting/service where you work. If you work in an individual's home and the individual is your employer, they will have in place a comments and complaints procedure.

Now research the comments and complaints procedures used in another adult care setting. How do these compare with your setting? Discuss their similarities and differences.

Case study

3.1, 3.2 Responding to comments and complaints

Chen is a senior support worker. As she is about to leave at the end of her shift she sees Bobby, an older individual, sitting at the front of the entrance hall.

Chen: 'How are you Bobby?'

Bobby: 'Good thanks, just had lunch.'

Chen: 'Was it nice?'

Bobby: 'Excellent as always.'

Chen: 'Pleased to hear it.'

Bobby: 'I'm not moaning, but I wish they'd remember the salt and pepper pots when staff bring me my lunch in my room. Nothing wrong with my legs. I went downstairs and got them myself!'

Chen: 'Good, pleased to hear it.'

Bobby (mumbling quietly): 'Not really because by the time I sat down again, my lunch was cold.'

Chen: 'What was that?'

Bobby: 'I don't want to moan or complain, forget it.'

Discuss:
1. What action should Chen take and why?
2. Is Bobby making a complaint?
3. What are the consequences of Chen not responding to Bobby?

Evidence opportunity

3.2 Policies and procedures relating to the handling of comments and complaints

Develop a flowchart that explains the main points included in policies and procedures relating to the handling of comments and complaints.

AC 3.3 Explain the benefits of empowering individuals and others to express their comments, suggestions and complaints

As a Lead Adult Care Worker responsible for other staff, you have a central role to play in creating a fair, open and honest working environment where individuals and others including their carers, loved ones, family and friends, colleagues and peers, managers and supervisors, professionals from other services, visitors to the work setting, members of the community and volunteers feel able to express their comments, suggestions and complaints, knowing that these will be acted on quickly and addressed fully.

Empowering individuals and others to express their comments, suggestions and complaints is important for:

- developing trust and respect, because individuals and others will feel that you are genuinely interested in listening and responding to what is important to them.
- demonstrating that you are genuinely committed to providing high quality care by striving to continuously improve your practices to achieve positive outcomes for individuals.
- safeguarding and protecting individuals and others from abuse and improper treatment, because doing so will mean that they will feel confident in identifying and expressing their concerns rather than letting the abuse or improper treatment continue and get worse.

- enabling individuals and others to have their voices heard in relation to the care provided and build on their skills to be able to shape their care to meet their expectations.
- enabling individuals and others to become more confident so that they can work together with you in making improvements and/or changes that are required.
- enabling individuals and others to be at the heart of the care and support provided and the services they access; this is essential for person-centred care and you will learn more about what this involves in Unit 306 Promoting and implementing person-centred practice.

You can empower individuals and others to express their comments, suggestions and complaints by:

- being open and approachable so that they will be more likely to share with you what they are thinking and feeling.
- making time to ask questions so that you can find out their opinions and ideas.
- getting to know them so that you can identify early whether they are dissatisfied with any aspect of their care, support or service they access.
- feeding back to them the actions that have been taken following their comments, suggestions and complaints, so that they know they have been taken seriously and changes/improvements have been made.

Reflect on it

3.3 Voicing your concerns or suggestions

Think about an occasion when you were empowered to voice your concerns or suggestions. How was this done? How did it feel to be empowered to do so?

Evidence opportunity

3.3 The benefits of empowering others

Write a short reflective account of an occasion when you supported an individual to express their comments, suggestions or concerns. Include how you empowered the individual.

LO4 Know how to recognise and respond to adverse events, incidents, errors and near misses

AC 4.1 Describe what is meant by: a) an adverse event, b) an incident, c) an error, d) a near miss

Handling adverse events, incidents, errors and near misses

Although safe working practices are everyone's priority in the workplace, things can still go wrong and mistakes can happen. Mistakes that occur can include adverse events, incidents, errors and near misses. It is your duty of care to ensure that when mistakes do happen you are able to recognise them as such and know what to do. Below are some examples of the different types of mistakes that may happen at work:

- Adverse events occur when actions taken or omitted lead to harm being caused. The harm caused is usually unintentional and preventable. For example, not reporting a spillage on the floor may lead to a visitor slipping over and harming themselves. Although the harm caused is unintentional it is preventable.
- Incidents occur when negative events cause harm or damage to individuals or an organisation. For example, a cyber attack by a third party can cause harm and damage to individuals and organisations as it may result in personal data being accessed by unauthorised others.
- Errors occur when a task was either not completed or was completed incorrectly, for example not recording that an individual has taken their medication as soon as it has been administered. This is important to ensure that the individual's medication records are accurate and so that they are not given another dose mistakenly.
- Near misses occur when an action had the potential to harm an individual but harm was avoided, for example not checking that a hoist battery is fully charged before moving an individual from one position to another. This could have resulted in the hoist suddenly stopping working and an individual being harmed while being moved but this didn't happen and so it is referred to as a near miss.

> **Reflect on it**
>
> **4.1 Mistakes**
>
> Reflect on some of the mistakes that you know about that have happened in the setting where you work. What category do they fall under?

> **Evidence opportunity**
>
> **4.1 An adverse event, an incident, an error, a near miss**
>
> Discuss with your assessor your understanding of the meaning of the following: an adverse event, an incident, an error, a near miss.

AC 4.2 Explain own role in recognising, reporting and responding to: a) an adverse event, b) an incident, c) an error, d) a near miss

Knowing about the different mistakes that may happen at work is the first step to recognising that something has gone wrong. Your employer will provide you with the necessary training that will help you. Always trust your instincts; if something doesn't feel right then it probably isn't and could mean a mistake has happened. Doing nothing is not an option; it is always best to raise any concerns you may have with a senior colleague or manager and discuss them together to establish whether an adverse event, incident, error or near miss has taken place.

It is not sufficient to simply recognise that something has gone wrong; it is also your legal responsibility to know how to report and respond. Your employer will have in place policies, procedures and agreed ways of working that set out who you must report mistakes to, when and how, including the actions you must take. How you report and respond to adverse events, incidents, errors and near misses will vary. For example, you may be required to call for help and complete an accident form in the event of an individual injuring themselves or raise the alarm in the event of a fire. It is your responsibility to ensure that you know what your employer's policies and procedures say about responding to and reporting different situations and mistakes that may occur at work and attend all training provided to you by your employer.

Although employers' agreed ways of working will vary, reporting mistakes that occur in your work setting will usually require you to make a verbal report to a named person, i.e. usually to someone in a more senior position to you, and/or a written report, i.e. by filling in a specific form, by only writing down the facts of what happened, and by including all relevant details. Responding to mistakes that occur in your work setting will usually require you to report these as soon as is practically possible, to avoid further harm or damage and within the limits of your role and responsibilities.

AC 4.3 Describe how effective practice may prevent further occurrences and improve quality of care

Recognising and responding to adverse events, incidents, errors and near misses in line with your legal responsibilities and your employer's agreed ways of working can prevent further occurrences by reducing the likelihood of the mistake occurring again and at the same time improving the quality of care. For example, it could be that, as a result of you recognising that a medication record has been completed incorrectly by a colleague and then reporting this to your manager, your colleague is provided with additional training, support and monitoring in their role, thus preventing them making the same error again and improving the quality of care provided to individuals when administering medication.

> **Reflect on it**
>
> **4.2, 4.3 Learning from mistakes**
>
> Think back over an occasion when a mistake happened in your work setting and you responded to it. What actions did you take? Why? How did this improve the quality of care? Is there anything you would have done differently?

> **Evidence opportunity**
>
> **4.2, 4.3** Recognising, reporting and responding to an adverse event, incident, error or near miss
>
> Research your role in your work setting in relation to recognising, reporting and responding to an adverse event, an incident, an error, or a near miss. Write an account with your findings that explains your role and details how effective practice can prevent further occurrences and improve the quality of care.

Legislation	
Act/Regulation	**Key points**
Mental Capacity Act 2005	Arrangements for individuals with care and support needs who lack capacity must be put in place so that they can be supported to make decisions. It was also designed so that those working in health and social care could assess whether individuals have capacity. The Act outlined five principles which are important for you to know and understand in your role as you have a duty of care to comply with these when supporting individuals to make decisions that are in their best interests.
The Human Rights Act 1998	Everyone in the UK is entitled to the same basic human rights and freedoms. This includes individuals who have care and support needs. The Act supports individuals' rights to dignity, respect, to be treated fairly when accessing care or support services and to live safely and free from harm or abuse.
The Care Act 2014	Individuals have a right to make a complaint about their care and treatment if they are unhappy. It requires the local council to provide clear information about how to complain about their services.
Health and Social Care Act 2008 (Regulated Activities) Regulations 2014: Regulation 16	Individuals have a right to make a complaint about their care and treatment if they are unhappy. It requires health and social care providers to have an effective system in place for identifying, receiving, handling and responding to complaints from individuals using the service and others. It requires that all complaints are investigated thoroughly, and action taken in response to any failures identified. It also requires providers to make available to CQC a summary of the complaints made along with all relevant correspondence.
Health and Social Care Act 2008 (Regulated Activities) Regulations 2014: Regulation 20	All CQC registered health and social care organisations must be open and transparent with individuals and others such as their families or advocates in relation to individuals' care and treatment. It also requires providers to act when things go wrong with care and treatment, including informing those involved about the incident, and providing support, true and accurate information and an apology when things go wrong.
Data Protection Act 2018	All individuals' personal information, including that shared during the complaints process, must be kept secure and handled lawfully when recorded, used, stored and shared.
	In May 2018 the Data Protection Act came into effect. It provides detailed guidance to organisations on how to govern and manage people's personal information and this will need to be included in care settings' policies, procedures, guidelines and agreed ways of working.

304 Effective communication in adult care settings/services

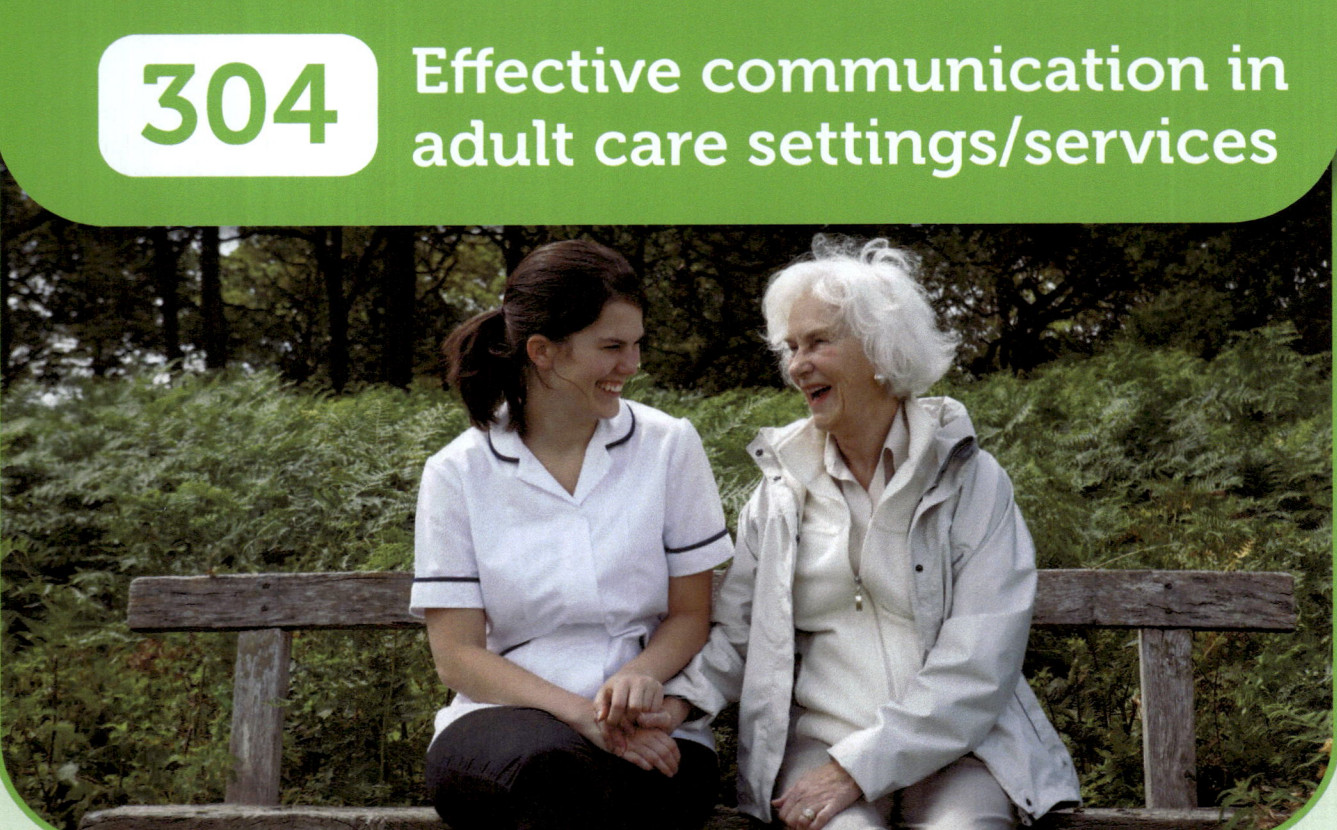

About this unit

Credit value: 3
Guided learning hours: 25

Communication involves exchanging and understanding information with others and is one of the key ingredients for building trust and caring relationships. Effective communication in care settings is essential for getting to know individuals and their families and being able to work in a caring and successful way with them and others, including your colleagues and other health and social care professionals.

In this unit, you will understand why effective communication is so important in your work, how you can meet the communication and language needs, wishes and preferences of individuals, how you can overcome barriers to communication as well as the role of independent advocacy services. You will also learn how to apply principles and practices relating to confidentiality.

Learning outcomes

By the end of this unit, you will:

LO1: Understand why effective communication is important in care settings/services

LO2: Understand the variety in people's communication needs and preferences

LO3: Be able to communicate effectively with others

LO4: Be able to meet the communication and language needs, wishes and preferences of individuals

LO5: Understand the role of independent advocacy services in supporting individuals to communicate their needs, wishes and preferences

LO6: Understand confidentiality in care settings/services

LO1 Understand why effective communication is important in care settings/services

> ### Getting started
>
> Think about where you work and the different people you communicate with on a daily basis. Why do you communicate with these people at work? What might happen if you didn't communicate with these people and why?
>
> What skills do you have as a communicator? What are your strongest? Your weakest? How could you improve these? Why is it important that you improve your skills of communication?

AC 1.1 Summarise the different reasons why people communicate

What does communication mean in your role?

In adult care settings communication is central to the quality of the care and support you provide and to the relationships that you develop with the **individuals** you care for, their families, carers, as well as your colleagues and other professionals that you may work with.

Ultimately, if you want to be a good care worker, you will need to have good communication skills. This will be key in helping you to build relationships and provide the best possible care and service for the individuals you care for.

Different reasons for communicating

People communicate in care settings for many different reasons. This may be to share information, to find out information, to enable others to express themselves, to develop relationships with those you provide care for and with those you work with, or to express thoughts and feelings. Ultimately, good communication will allow you to create connections. It will allow you to be understood and to understand others.

Communication can occur between those who work in adult care settings, for example:

- a senior support worker may need to speak to their manager about an individual's care
- care workers may need to communicate with those who work for external organisations
- a senior carer may need to communicate with an individual's social worker via email
- team members may need to communicate at a staff meeting or with an individual, their family and advocate at a **care review**.

6Cs

Communication

Communication in care settings is essential because without it you would not be able to build good, meaningful working relationships with the individuals you provide care and support to, your colleagues who form part of your team and others who you work alongside as part of your day-to-day role such as individuals' families, advocates, social workers, nurses, GPs and pharmacists.

Communication can include both verbal and non-verbal communication. The messages that we convey without words such as eye contact, gestures and body language are just as important as verbal communication for understanding those we care and work for.

Without communication you wouldn't be able to get to know the individuals you provide support to and find out their unique needs and preferences, including their different backgrounds and how they prefer to communicate. Without good communication skills you will not be able to encourage individuals to express how they are feeling, and building that trust means they may share information with you that will allow you to offer better, more informed care. Without communication you would find it very difficult to do your job, in fact it would be impossible! How would you be able to discuss individuals' needs with them, meet with their families, support others in the team and work with other professionals if you couldn't communicate?

Effective communication is very important in the work setting and an essential skill to have when working in care settings. This unit will help you to understand how to put principles of good communication into practice, and gain a good understanding of why communication is one of the '6Cs' in Health and Social Care.

Here we explore in more detail other reasons why people in adult care settings communicate.

To exchange information: Good communication allows us to share and obtain information to allow us to effectively carry out our duties as care workers. Exchanging information could mean providing facts when reporting at the end of a shift about the care provided to individuals and the skills they have developed in relation to maintaining their personal hygiene or developing their daily living skills in relation to cooking, budgeting and shopping. Information may also be exchanged between **adult care workers** and individuals on a regular basis when discussing what support they would like or when you may need to ask individuals to choose what they would like to eat or wear. Information is exchanged not only between team members and individuals but also when communicating with other professionals such as nurses, GPs, pharmacists, social workers and activity workers. For example, a **rehabilitation worker** communicates with an individual's social worker and housing support officer about how to support the individual to live independently. Having the information we need in turn allows us to fulfil our duty of care to individuals as well as the requirements of our job roles.

To express feelings: Good communication allows us to express how we feel, and also to enable others to express themselves. This might include an individual who expresses their happiness when being supported by an advocacy worker to communicate their wishes and preferences about their future care needs. It might include an **Enhanced Care Worker** who expresses their concerns about an individual with dementia who appears to be feeling anxious over remaining in hospital for another week. A senior care worker may express their frustration over the lack of staff available to work weekends at the **residential care home** where they work. Expressing our feelings, allowing others to and empathising or understanding how they may feel means we can really get to know the individual, build meaningful relationships, understand any changes in their behaviour and offer person-centred care.

Key terms

Day centres are settings that provide leisure, educational, health and wellbeing activities during the day.

Care review refers to a regular meeting where individuals and others discuss whether the individual's care and support are effective and how to further meet their needs and preferences, for example.

Rehabilitation worker refers to a person who supports individuals to live independently following an accident or illness.

Enhanced Care Workers are care workers who have been upskilled and trained to provide, for example, increased clinical support to registered nurses in nursing homes or improve the quality of dementia care to individuals with dementia who are hospital patients.

Residential care homes are homes that individuals live in. Care workers will provide meals and assistance with personal care tasks such as washing, dressing, eating.

Research it

1.1 Enhanced Care Workers and communication

Research the role of the Enhanced Care Worker in the adult care sector. Then develop a poster to identify the reasons why Enhanced Care Workers may communicate in the work setting. The links to the Care Management Matters and the International Longevity Centre (ILCUK) websites below provide useful information about this newly developed job role:

www.caremanagementmatters.co.uk/innovate-enhanced-care-worker-role/

https://ilcuk.org.uk/wp-content/uploads/2018/10/ILC-UK-Innovate-to-Alleviate.pdf

Produce a written account showing your findings.

To advise and guide: As part of your role, it is important that you are able to clearly advise and guide those who you work with, whether it is one individual who you care for in their own home, an individual you care for in a residential care home, your colleagues, or families and advocates of the individual. Good communication skills will allow you to clearly and effectively convey the relevant information that others need in a constructive way, one that will be most helpful to them. This might include a senior support worker completing an induction with a support worker on their first day at work so that they understand their day-to-day work activities; they may need to convey the support available for them and the aims of the organisation they work for. It might include an activities worker who guides an individual with a learning disability so that they can participate in a group quiz. It could also include an experienced senior carer who provides advice to one of their colleagues who may be finding it difficult to have regular communication with an individual's family.

Reflect on it

1.1 Advice and guidance

Reflect on a situation when you provided advice and guidance to someone, perhaps a friend or family member. How did you feel about doing this? Why? How do you think it made your friend or family member feel? Why? What did you communicate and why?

Key term

Domiciliary care is where health and social care workers provide care and support to individuals who live in their own home but require additional help such as support with household tasks or personal care.

To form and maintain working relationships: Another reason for communicating in care settings is to create meaningful relationships so that we can get to know those who we care for and work with. Good communication skills are also key to this. This could include a senior support worker who works in **domiciliary care** and forms and maintains good working relationships with individuals and their families, their colleagues and other professionals so that they get to know each other and learn to trust and respect each other. An activities worker may form and maintain working relationships not only with the individuals participating in activities but also with the individuals' families and staff who provide support. A rehabilitation worker may, for example, form and maintain working relationships with the individuals they are supporting with learning new skills and also with others who are involved in individuals' lives such as their partner, their children, or their physiotherapist.

Evidence opportunity

1.1 Reasons for communicating

Identify an individual who you provide care or support to in your work setting, or if you are a personal assistant, think about the individual that you provide care for. Now provide a summary of the different reasons why you and other team members communicate with this individual. Think about other people who this individual communicates with such as their friends, family, other professionals; why does this individual communicate with them? Why do they communicate with the individual?

Write down your responses. Remember to consider rules around confidentiality, so make sure you avoid including their name or details that may give away who they are.

To interact: Another reason for communicating with others is simply to interact with others. This could be a senior carer who wants to get to know an individual who has recently moved in to the residential care home where they work; they may want to find out more about the individual's family, background, culture and interests, for example. Teams of workers who work in adult care settings may interact with each other informally over coffee breaks and lunchtimes to relax but also more formally during staff meetings to communicate the care and support they are providing to individuals. An advocacy worker who wants to represent the views of an individual who has mental health needs in relation to his current housing situation must first interact with the individual to build up trust and find out from the individual how best to support them. The relationships we build are as a result of interactions with others. The more effective the interactions we have, the more effectively we can support individuals and fulfil our roles.

AC 1.2 Explain how communication affects relationships in a care setting/service

What is a good, effective relationship in a care setting?

As you have learned, communication is integral to the many different working relationships you will have formed and developed in the setting where you work. A good, effective relationship is one where:

- People trust and respect one another and can build effective professional relationships through mutual trust, respect and honesty.
- People can rely on each other and help one another with their tasks and workloads.
- People value the opinions, knowledge and expertise that others bring, and work as a team, share their knowledge and skills and learn from each other. They value and take an interest in the roles that others play in the setting.
- There is good co-operation, and it is quicker, easier and more efficient to complete tasks.
- Everyone is treated fairly and heard if there are any disagreements or conflict.
- People do their best to provide high quality care and support and have the best interests of the individual at the heart of what they do.

Effective relationships are key to doing your job to the best of your ability and working well together to provide the best support to some of the most vulnerable people, and having a positive, friendly outlook will help you to create rapport with colleagues, individuals and others. Good communication, however, is essential to building these effective relationships.

> **Research it**
>
> **1.2 Communicating with an individual who has dementia**
>
> Research how you can communicate effectively with individuals with dementia. Dementia UK, a national charity that provides information, advice and support to individuals with dementia and their families has produced an information leaflet, 'Tips for better communication'. The link below will direct you to this:
>
> www.dementiauk.org/wp-content/uploads/2017/07/Tips-for-communication.pdf
>
> Produce your own leaflet that explains how communicating effectively with individuals with dementia can affect your relationships with individuals and their families.

How effective communication impacts relationships in the setting

Communication can affect relationships both positively (if it is effective) and negatively (if it is poor). Table 5.1 provides examples of effective communication. The dos and don'ts table that follows will give you useful advice on communicating effectively.

Table 5.1 Examples of effective communication

Effective communication
Speaking to an individual who has a hearing impairment in a room that is well-lit and has no background noise: In a situation like this, the individual will be able to participate fully in the conversation with you as they will be able to hear and lip-read what you are saying and clearly see your facial expressions and body language. The individual will feel that you understand their needs and have taken a genuine interest in ensuring these are met. This in turn will have a positive impact on your relationship with the individual.
Meeting with an individual's family who have concerns that their relative is not settling in the nursing home where they now live. In your meeting, you ensure you actively listen and adopt an open posture when communicating with them: By **actively listening** to their concerns, the family will feel that you are taking their concerns seriously and are genuinely committed to addressing these. By adopting an **open posture**, you will create an impression that you have nothing to hide and that the individual's family can trust you to resolve their concerns. The individual's family will feel more relaxed and comfortable with you thus building their trust and respect for you; they will also feel reassured and feel that you have genuinely **empathised** with them. This in turn will have a positive impact on your relationship with the individual's family.

Table 5.1 Examples of effective communication *continued*

Effective communication
Speaking to an individual who has learning disabilities using Makaton, their preferred form of communication: The individual will feel that they are able to express what they want to communicate to you and feel that you have considered their needs and preferences. The individual will also feel comfortable with communicating in this way and will therefore be more likely to share with you want they want to say. This in turn will enable you to get to know them better, understand their views and preferences and will therefore have a positive effect on your relationship with the individual.

	Dos and don'ts for communicating effectively
Do	Speak clearly so that the person you are speaking to can understand you. If an individual cannot understand you then you will need to adapt the way you speak to ensure the individual can respond and communicate with you.
Do	Be patient and understanding so that the individual does not feel rushed and so that you can build trust.
Do	Show a genuine interest to get to know the individual. This will help you to understand their needs and preferences.
Do	Empathise by seeing things from someone else's point of view. This will allow you to understand how the individual may be feeling and will help to develop an open, honest and, most importantly, compassionate working relationship.
Do	Be aware of the other person's body language and what is being expressed so that you can understand how the individual may be feeling and adapt the way you communicate accordingly.
Do	Maintain good eye contact to show you are listening and understanding. This will also show that you are interested in what the individual is saying. You should be careful, however, as too much eye contact may make the individual feel uncomfortable. Try to assess the situation. Once you have a better idea of how the individual is feeling, you will know how much eye contact is necessary.
Do	Actively listen, not only to what is being said but to the meanings behind what is being said so that you can respond appropriately. For example, an individual may say that they agree with you but at the same time look unhappy; in this situation you could offer the individual another option so that you can check whether they really do agree with you.
Do	Be open and honest in all your communications. This will help with building trust and will ensure that misunderstandings are avoided.
Don't	Forget that you may need to alter the way you communicate with individuals from different cultures because some behaviours can convey different messages in different cultures. Not respecting individuals' communication preferences, needs or strengths will mean that individuals will not be able to express what they are thinking or feeling and will be less likely to communicate with you.
Don't	Look uninterested or allow interruptions as doing so will act as a distraction and it will be more difficult to find out about the individual.
Don't	Rush an individual or speak *at* them as this will make it harder to communicate and for them to trust you. Not making time to communicate effectively is disrespectful and can lead to misunderstandings.
Don't	Impose your views and preferences on an individual or use communication skills to control or take ownership of an interaction that puts down or patronises individuals. This will not enable you to build up a good working relationship with individuals.
Don't	Mumble, or speak very quietly, as the person you are speaking to will not hear properly and it could lead to misunderstandings.
Don't	Forget to pay attention to the non-verbal communication used by individuals and what it can mean.
Don't	Ignore the words being spoken or placate an individual. Try not hearing what you want to hear, and remember to actively listen (as mentioned above), otherwise the individual may feel ignored and confused.
Don't	Ignore an individual's feelings, or the different ways an individual may express how they are feeling.

How to build relationships through effective communication

Being an effective communicator therefore is essential for developing positive working relationships in the adult care setting where you work and ensuring individuals and others you work with feel valued and respected. It involves having a range of skills and personal qualities; you will, for example, need to show respect, be patient, actively listen, be honest and positive and show sympathy and compassion.

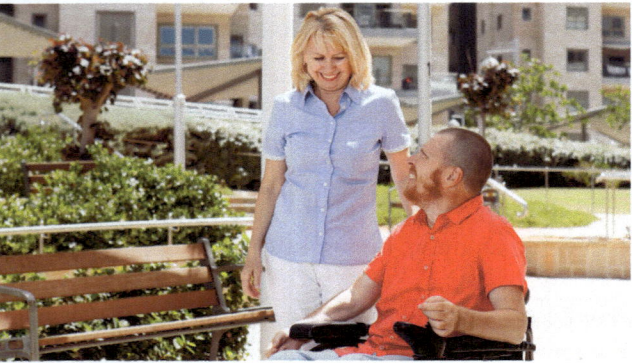

Figure 5.1 Are you an effective communicator? How could you improve your communication skills?

Key term

Open posture means not crossing your arms or legs in front of you, which avoids you appearing defensive.

Reflect on it

1.2 Personal qualities for communicating

It is important that you take time to reflect on your communication and interactions with others. You should think about what went well, what did not go well, and the things you could do to improve your communications that will help you to build relationships.

Reflect on the personal qualities that you think you have in relation to communicating with others; write these down. Now ask someone who knows you well such as a family member, a friend or a colleague what personal qualities they think you have in relation to communicating with others; write these down too. How do the lists compare? What similarities and differences are there?

For two of the personal qualities identified, reflect on how they affect your relationships at work.

6Cs

Compassion

Good communication requires that you work in a compassionate way, are aware of the feelings of others and are kind and supportive towards individuals, their families and the care workers you manage. This will show them that you care and as a result they will be more likely to work with you and trust you. Showing compassion also involves showing respect for others' feelings and views and treating them in a dignified way. This is essential when you communicate with others so that they know that your intentions are honest, and, in this way, they can approach you and learn to trust you with what's important to them. You can show this by, for example, taking time out to sit down with an individual or a colleague and listen to what is worrying them and then reassuring them that they have your support.

Care

Care involves providing individuals and your colleagues in care settings with a consistent good quality level of support. This means you need to take a genuine interest in them so that they know you care about them. Doing so will enable you to make a positive difference to their lives. Good communication is essential in order to provide the best possible care, to build these relationships, so that you can actively work to achieve what is important to them. You can show this by asking them questions about their communication and language needs and preferences and then ensuring that you remember and take these needs into account when supporting them with their day-to-day communication.

Evidence opportunity

1.2 How communication affects relationships in the work setting

Identify three different people with whom you have a work relationship. For each one, explain to your assessor how both poor communication and effective communication affects your work relationships with them. Write down details of your discussion. You could also write an account about how communication affects relationships.

AC 1.3 Identify the skills required to be an effective communicator

Being an effective communicator involves understanding others and being understood by others. If you are not an effective communicator then you will not be able to build good working relationships with the individuals you support and care for, their families, friends, your colleagues and others you work with such as professionals from other services, visitors to the care setting where you work, members of the community and volunteers. This is why effective communication is one of the 6Cs in Health and Social Care. The table below includes some of the important skills that are required to be an effective communicator and examples of how you could apply them in your work practices as a Lead; can you think of any others?

Table 5.2 Skills required to be an effective communicator in adult care

Skills required to be an effective communicator	Examples of how you can apply these skills in the care setting/service where you work
Knowing how to initiate and maintain a conversation	<ul><li>asking an individual questions about their day</li><li>encouraging a colleague to share with you their ideas for improving the service</li><li>introducing yourself to a professional who you haven't met before</li></ul>
Active listening skills	<ul><li>nodding your head while an individual is telling you about their hobbies</li><li>responding to an individual's family member who is upset by listening to what they are saying and asking them how you can support them</li><li>responding to a volunteer who seems to be finding it difficult to communicate with an individual by being open towards them and not crossing your arms</li></ul>
Showing empathy	<ul><li>being kind when an individual tells you they are feeling unwell</li><li>being able to see things from your manager's point of view during supervision</li><li>understanding how a member of the public might feel if they have never met an individual who has dementia before</li></ul>
Using verbal communication skills effectively	<ul><li>speaking clearly to an individual who has hearing loss</li><li>avoiding using jargon when discussing an individual's care with their family</li><li>repeating and rephrasing when discussing health and safety with a visitor to the work setting</li></ul>
Using non-verbal communication skills effectively	<ul><li>responding to an individual who is feeling angry by moving away and giving them some space</li><li>understanding how a colleague may be feeling in their new role at work by observing their body language</li><li>making eye contact and leaning forward when a professional from another service asks to speak with you</li></ul>
Being able to clarify what has been said	<ul><li>summarising with an individual what they have just expressed through their non-verbal communication</li><li>repeating back to a colleague how they have carried out a task</li><li>checking with a member of the community that you have understood what they have told you</li></ul>
Understanding and being able to use a range of communication methods and styles	<ul><li>using signs and pictures with an individual who has a learning disability</li><li>using an interpreter with a volunteer who does not speak English</li><li>checking that the **hearing loop system** is working at the start of a training session for volunteers</li></ul>

> **Reflect on it**
>
> **1.3 Your own communication skills**
>
> Reflect on your communication skills. Which ones are your most effective? Which ones do you think you need to improve? How will these improvements impact on your role as a Lead?

> **Evidence opportunity**
>
> **1.3 Skills for effective communication**
>
> Develop a poster that sets out the skills required to be an effective communicator in care settings/ services.

> **Key term**
>
> **Hearing loop systems** are specialist types of equipment that transmit sounds to individuals who use hearing aids or cochlear implants so that they can communicate with others.

AC 1.4 Describe how communication skills can be used to manage complex, sensitive, abusive and difficult situations in a care setting/service

Managing complex, sensitive, abusive and difficult situations effectively requires you to be a highly skilled communicator.

Different types of situations and behaviours can arise in adult care settings for a range of different reasons, and we will discuss these here.

> **Reflect on it**
>
> **1.4 Difficult situations**
>
> Reflect on a difficult situation that you were involved in. For example, this may be a situation where another person behaved in an angry, threatening or offensive manner towards you or someone else. What happened? How did you communicate with the person? Why? Write a short reflective account about this situation. If you have not experienced such a situation, what might you do?

Complex situations and behaviours

The situations that may arise in the care setting where you work may be complex. For example, as a Lead Adult Care Worker you may be required to manage two care workers who cannot agree on how to work together to provide support to one individual because they have different values, or you may be asked to help resolve a complex situation involving an individual and their family who have different opinions as to how much support the individual requires to live independently.

To manage these complex situations, you will need to have the ability to communicate clearly and in such a way that you can ensure that others listen to what you have to say. You will need to be able to express what you want to say in a non-judgemental and non-biased way so that no one feels that you are being unfair. You will also need to be able to communicate your thoughts calmly and remain patient to try and diffuse any tense or awkward moments and to ensure that the communications remain focused on the individual.

Some individuals may also show complex behaviours because they have complex needs. For example, as a Lead Personal Assistant you may be required to support other personal assistants to provide high quality care to an individual who has a learning disability as well as mental health needs and physical support needs. Complex behaviours can also arise because of individuals' past experiences. For example, if an individual has been denied their rights to make their own choices, then they may find being encouraged to do so very difficult and may as a result develop and show complex behaviours such as becoming distressed and fearful.

To manage individuals' complex behaviours and to support others to do so effectively will require you to be knowledgeable about effective strategies and be able to share this knowledge with others so that they respect what you say and follow your instructions for how to work together as a team. You will also need to be able to answer others' questions in relation to the individual's condition or impairment and how this affects their care or support needs. If you are unable to answer others' questions, then you must show that you are organised and professional by seeking advice and guidance from others, such as from speech and language therapists, and show your commitment when feeding this back to others. You can do this by ensuring your communications are clear, informative and professional.

Sensitive situations and behaviours

Sensitive situations may arise in the care setting where you work as you and others are supporting individuals with their care or support needs and to live their lives as they wish. For example, you may be asked by an individual who you know well whether you would like to go to a barbecue for his thirtieth birthday outside of your working hours. This is a sensitive situation because on the one hand you do not want to disappoint or offend the individual by not going, but on the other hand attending the barbecue may conflict with your duty of care because you will have clear boundaries in place for what you can and cannot do as part of your job role. You are providing a service to the individual; the individual is not your friend.

Other sensitive situations may involve you discussing topics of a personal nature with individuals such as in relation to their personal care needs, their relationships, their emotions and thoughts, or their plans for their future care needs.

Managing sensitive situations requires you to be an empathetic communicator. This means you need to be able to identify with another person's situation and understand their feelings or 'to put yourself in their shoes'. You can communicate this by using sensitive language that is not patronising. For example, you may approach an individual who is feeling anxious about a new relationship by saying to them, 'I can see you're worried about this relationship. Do you want to talk about it?'

In relation to the example of the barbecue perhaps you could explain that part of being a professional means that you have boundaries that you must uphold and so there are certain situations like the barbecue that you are not able to go to because this would fall outside of your work role duties.

Abusive situations and behaviours

Abusive situations can also arise where you work and may involve not only individuals but others too. For example, you may be asked to manage a situation where two individuals have become physically abusive towards each other over a disagreement, or where a visitor to the care setting where you work has become verbally abusive towards you or another care worker when they were refused entry as they were unable to provide any proof of their identity.

Abusive behaviours can also occur when individuals cause harm to themselves such as by cutting their arms, biting their hand, banging their head or refusing to eat or drink. This is known as self-harm.

Managing these abusive situations requires you to use effective verbal and non-verbal communication skills. For example, you can do this by always using respectful language when an individual is abusive and encouraging the individual to talk about how they are feeling. It is important that when speaking, you remain calm and non-confrontational. You can also make use of eye contact but remember that each individual is different, so how this is used will depend on what is effective for the individual. Making eye contact may calm one individual down but may further distress another.

Other non-verbal communication skills involve creating space between you and the abusive person so that the person does not feel threatened and also so that you and others can move to a place of safety where the risk of being injured or harmed will be reduced.

Challenging situations and behaviours

Challenging situations and behaviours in the care setting where you work may arise because of individuals' conditions and differences between individuals' and others' views. They may also occur due to levels of expertise that different professionals have. Other examples include:

- Challenging behaviours presented by individuals who have dementia may include inappropriate touching, restlessness and verbal abuse.
- Challenging situations may arise when care workers disagree with the time that has been planned for their allocated duties or with an individual's family over the care or support the individual requires, for example when eating and drinking, getting dressed, mobilising.

Effective communication is key in overcoming challenging situations. You will need to ensure that you remain calm and professional at all times. It is also important that you use positive language and non-confrontational body language such as holding an open posture and not waving your hands about as this may be misunderstood and lead to further distress. Being understanding and providing reassurance is important but remember to ensure that this is not done in a patronising manner.

To manage challenging, complex, sensitive and abusive situations and behaviours effectively, recap the communication skills you have learned about in this unit and remember to:

- recognise that every individual is unique
- ensure you treat every individual with compassion, dignity and respect
- understand individuals' behaviours
- use non-confrontational approaches
- spend time with the individual.

(This is not an exhaustive list but some useful points for you to remember.)

Research it

1.4 Your setting's guidance on managing challenging situations and behaviours

Research the guidance in place in the care setting where you work for managing challenging situations and behaviours. If you work as a personal assistant in an individual's home, refer to your employer's guidance which may have been provided to you verbally or in the form of a code of conduct that is expected from you.

You could write down your findings or produce a leaflet.

Evidence opportunity

1.4 Communication skills to manage complex, sensitive, abusive or challenging situations and behaviours

Discuss with your assessor the communication skills you used to manage a complex, sensitive, abusive or challenging situation and how you used these.

What communication skills do you share with one of your colleagues? Which skills are different? Explain why. Provide a written account of your discussion. If you do not discuss this with your assessor, provide a written account addressing these questions.

AC 1.5 Explain the importance of maintaining open and honest communication in a care setting/service

Maintaining open and honest communication is essential for building effective working relationships. This means that it is important to be open and honest with each other when communicating because not doing so may lead to:

- misunderstandings that can cause unnecessary distress
- mistrust that can cause a lack of confidence in the relationship
- a reluctance to share opinions and thoughts that can cause a lack of learning from each other.

Being open and honest when communicating with individuals and others means that you will develop relationships based on trust and respect. Open and honest communication is also important for enabling individuals and others to approach you and share with you information that may be quite difficult or sensitive at times. For example, being open and honest with an individual about what actions you will be taking following their disclosure of abuse to you will enable them to feel safe and understand the safeguarding process. Similarly, having an open and honest relationship with the team members you support will encourage them to also be open and honest with you and others, even when doing so may be difficult such as if they witness a colleague following unsafe practices. You will also find it useful to review your previous learning from Unit 303 Understanding duty of care in relation to how maintaining open and honest communication forms part of your duty of care in your job role and relates to duty of candour.

Reflect on it

1.5 The importance of honesty

Reflect on how you would feel if you found out that your manager was not being open and honest with you. Why would you feel this way? Why is it important that your manager is open and honest with you?

> **Evidence opportunity**
>
> **1.5 Maintaining open and honest communication**
>
> Develop a short presentation for a group of volunteers who work in your care setting on the importance of maintaining open and honest communication. Remember to include in your explanation the consequences of not doing so.

LO2 Understand the variety in people's communication needs and preferences

AC 2.1 Describe a range of communication methods and styles available

You will have to demonstrate how to use a range of communication methods and styles. Choosing the most appropriate way of communicating with individuals will depend on what their needs are. As these will vary for different individuals and situations it is important that you are aware of the communication methods and styles that can be used. Remember too that very often individuals use more than one method to communicate with others.

Communication methods

There are many different types of communication methods available and these may include verbal and non-verbal methods, as well as other communication methods:

Verbal methods

- Words – such as spoken words, the level of vocabulary you use, i.e. whether you use simple phrases or long, complex sentences as well as the type of vocabulary you use, i.e. whether it includes regional vocabulary and whether it is jargon free.
- Voice and tone – refers to the tone you use when speaking, for example the volume, mood and feeling.
- Voice and pitch – refers to the quality of sound you hear, for example degree of highness or lowness of tone.
- Spoken communication – also referred to as oral communication and uses spoken words to share ideas, thoughts, emotions and information.

Non-verbal methods

- Eye contact – such as making eye contact, using eye contact intermittently and avoiding eye contact.
- Touch – such as placing your hand on an individual's shoulder to show your empathy or offering a supporting arm to support an individual who has difficulties mobilising.
- Gestures – including face gestures (e.g. smiling, frowning), hand gestures (e.g. pointing, waving) and body gestures (e.g. standing, sitting with legs not crossed).
- Body language – such as leaning towards/away, looking away, crossing your arms.
- Proximity – such as how close or far away you are from the other person.
- Behaviour – such as sitting upright, moving towards/away, turning your back.

Additional methods to support communication

- Written communication – such as written words, phrases, pictures or a combination of two or more of these. **Braille** is another method of written communication using characters that are represented by patterns of raised dots that are felt with the fingertips and used by individuals who have a **visual impairment**.
- Signs – such as British Sign Language. BSL is a system used by individuals who are deaf or have a **hearing impairment**, to communicate and interact with others and involves using hand signs, gestures, facial expressions and body language.
- Symbols – such as those that represent objects, actions, people, places and events. Symbols can be used with or without words, signs and speech.
- Pictures – such as photographs, images and drawings.
- Objects of reference – such as items that are representative to the individual, e.g. a fork to represent lunchtime or a photograph of a place to represent an activity.

> **Key term**
>
> **Braille** is a method of written communication using characters that are represented by patterns of raised dots that are felt with the fingertips and is used by individuals who are blind or partially sighted.
>
> **British Sign Language (BSL)** is a system used by individuals who are deaf or have a hearing impairment, to communicate and interact with others. It involves using hand signs, gestures, facial expressions and body language.
>
> **Visual impairment** refers to loss of vision, either severely (i.e. the individual is blind) or partially (i.e. the individual is able/unable to see to some degree).
>
> **Hearing impairment** refers to hearing loss that main occur in one or both ears. This can be partial or complete loss of hearing.

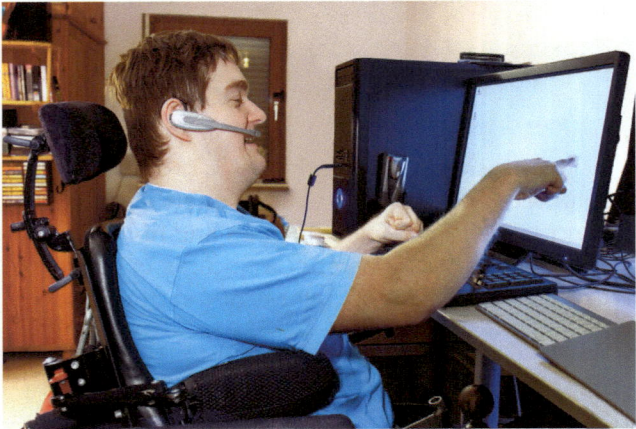

Figure 5.2 Using technology to communicate

Other communication methods

Other communication aids available to support effective communication can include the following:

Picture Exchange Communication System (PECS): these are used by individuals with learning disabilities or autism spectrum conditions to communicate with others using pictures. For example, pictures can be exchanged by individuals for items they would like such as a book or something to eat as well as to answer questions such as 'What do you want to wear today?'. These pictures can also be presented in the form of a communication book or board that is personal to the individual and can be used solely with them. PECS encourages individuals who have difficulties communicating to approach others to initiate communications.

Talking Mats: these are an application used by individuals with dementia who have difficulties with their verbal communication to enable them to communicate using a combination of pictures and symbols with text. For example, the individual could be given options of different activities available and the individual could then choose the ones they would like to participate in as well as those that they wouldn't. Cue cards or picture cards could be used instead where technology equipment, i.e. tablets or PCs, are not available.

Objects of reference: these are used by individuals who may find it difficult to understand spoken words or photographs. Objects of reference are items that represent to the individual an item, a person, an activity and/or a place. So, you may use different objects of reference for the same item for two different individuals; for example a plate can mean lunchtime to one individual while a sandwich may mean lunchtime to another.

Communication passports: these are used by individuals who have difficulties communicating with others to provide information about themselves such as their likes, dislikes or medical condition. These may be used, for example, by the individual when accessing a college course for the first time or during a stay in hospital.

Demonstrating your knowledge and skills of which communication methods are available is an essential part of promoting positive and engaging communications and meeting individuals' needs. It is also important that you are aware of your communication style and how to adapt it so as to ensure that you build respectful and good working relationships with individuals and all others you work with.

When considering a range of communication methods and styles to meet individuals' needs, you will also need to consider the different forms that communication can take. For example, communication does not just take place face-to-face, there are various ways that you use to communicate including over the telephone/mobile phone, through email, through social media such as Facebook and Twitter, through electronic messaging such as texts and WhatsApp, and through video phone calls such as through FaceTime and Skype.

There is more information about this in Unit 301 Safeguarding and protection in adult care settings/services.

Communication styles

In your role as a Lead there are a range of communication styles available that can help you to communicate with individuals and others. Below are some examples of the main communication styles that are available:

- Assertive: this style involves using open and honest communication with individuals and others that involves sharing information with them but without imposing your own beliefs or values. It involves respecting their ideas, opinions and beliefs. Assertive communication also involves communicating clearly to promote a good understanding.
- Enabling: this style involves encouraging individuals and others to take the lead in communications. Enabling communication makes the person the communication is about the focus and empowers the person to take the lead.
- Flexible: this style involves adapting the way you communicate with individuals and others depending on the situation, their needs and your skills. It involves being able to combine two or more different communication methods at the same time, e.g. verbal and non-verbal skills during communications.
- Professional: this style involves being able to communicate with people in appropriate ways depending on the situation, e.g. writing an email to an individual's family and ensuring it contains no spelling or grammatical errors or providing support to an individual who has been recently bereaved without being over friendly. You will learn more about how you can demonstrate professionalism when using a range of communication methods in AC4.4.

Research it

2.1 High and low pitch and tone

Search the internet for clips to understand what high pitch, low pitch, high tone and low tone voices sound like. That way, you will have a better understanding of what these are and what they may mean when communicating with individuals.

Reflect on it

2.1 Communication styles

As you read about communication styles, think about which ones you recognise in yourself the most. Are there any you don't use as much but think you should? What qualities do you think you need to be able to use these? Do you think you need to be kind? Do you need to be empathetic? Do you need to be patient? Are there occasions where a more formal style of communication is needed and some where a less formal one is needed? What are your expectations of others in your interactions? Do you expect certain professionals such as doctors to communicate in a more formal way? What kind of communication style do you think others such as individuals expect of you?

Evidence opportunity

2.1 Communication methods and styles

Design an information handout for staff in your care settings that details a range of communication methods and styles available.

AC 2.2 Describe how people may use or interpret communication methods and styles in different ways

Our family background and the culture we live in affect how we use and/or interpret communication methods and styles. For example, if you have been brought up in a family where you were encouraged to talk and interact with others then you will have developed the confidence and skills to use verbal communication and may prefer this as a method when communicating with others; an assertive communication style would also be appropriate to use. If, by contrast you have been brought up in a family where communications and interactions with others were not encouraged then you may not have the confidence to initiate communications with others and may prefer instead to let others initiate conversations; flexible and enabling communication styles would also be appropriate to use. It is important to be aware of people's different backgrounds as these may affect how individuals communicate with you and how effective your communications are with them.

Different cultures also have different beliefs and behaviours associated with how they use and interpret communication methods and styles. Table 5.3 includes some examples of how verbal communication methods and styles can be used and interpreted in different ways. Table 5.4 includes some examples of how non-verbal communication methods and styles are used and their meanings in different cultures. As you will be working with people from various backgrounds, cultures and religions, it is important that you are aware of these examples and conduct further research into what is acceptable and unacceptable for different cultures.

unintentionally offend individuals and others; this may in turn lead to them not wishing to interact and communicate with you. Misunderstandings can also be avoided by ensuring that the verbal and non-verbal communication methods you use with individuals and others meet their needs.

Research it

2.2 Different cultures, communication methods and styles

Research the different ways that people from two different countries or social groups may use and/or interpret communication methods and styles. Discuss your findings with a colleague and explain the differences that exist. Remember rules around confidentiality.

Reflect on it

2.2 Different backgrounds and communication methods and styles

Reflect on how your background impacts on the way you use and interpret different communication methods and styles. Think about what communication methods and styles you tend to use and the reasons why you prefer them. Are there any communication methods and styles you prefer not to use? Why? Now think about the communication methods and styles others who know you well such as your family and friends tend to use. How do these compare to the communication methods and styles you use?

Evidence opportunity

2.2 How people use and interpret communication methods and styles in different ways

Develop two case studies of two individuals from different backgrounds. For each individual explain how their background influences how they use and interpret communication methods and styles. Make sure you provide a written account.

Individuals with disabilities

You should remember that individuals with disabilities may also use and interpret communication methods and styles in different ways. For example, individuals with hearing loss may use touch to communicate or finger spelling as a means of communication.

As you will learn in LO4, it is important to establish the communication and language needs, wishes and preferences of the people you are going to communicate with so that you can ensure that the message you intend to communicate to others is received in the way you intended it to be and is understood fully. If it is not, then you may

How to check how people from different backgrounds may use and/or interpret communication methods in different ways

For communication and interactions to be effective between you and the individual you provide care and support to, it is important that you find out about their background and how they use or interpret communication methods and styles. You could:

- speak to the individual and find out if there are any particular communication methods or styles they prefer or avoid.
- speak to the individual's family, carer or advocate.
- consult their care plan or notes to find out if there is information about their preferences for communication methods and styles. You could consult the care plans of those from similar backgrounds but with the understanding that people of similar backgrounds are not the same and have their own unique needs and wishes.

Table 5.3 Verbal communication methods and styles, and examples of their uses and meanings in different cultures

Verbal communication methods and styles	Examples of use and meaning in different cultures
Words and a professional style	Individuals in some cultures may prefer to address others using their surnames and to be addressed themselves in this way. In other cultures, this may be interpreted as too formal and inappropriate when addressing an individual who is well known to you. More formal respectful terms may be used to address elders in some cultures and a professional style adopted.
Voice and tone and a flexible style	Speaking loudly when communicating with others may be considered welcoming and clear in some cultures. In other cultures, however, it may be interpreted as being rude or patronising, for example treating an individual as if they have hearing loss when their hearing is fine. Using a flexible style of communication would be appropriate to different situations.
Voice and pitch and an enabling style	Speaking in a high pitch when communicating with an individual can convey your excitement and genuine interest in what they have to say in some cultures. In other cultures, this may be interpreted as patronising, for example treating the individual as you would a child rather than an adult by speaking to them in what is interpreted as a childish, inappropriate way. A more enabling communication style would be more appropriate.

Table 5.4 Non-verbal communication methods and styles and their uses and meaning in different cultures

Non-verbal communication methods and styles	Use and meaning in different cultures
Eye contact and a professional style	Eye contact with an older individual may be deemed appropriate and seen as a way of showing a genuine interest in the individual in some cultures. In other cultures, it may be interpreted as rude or disrespectful particularly if the individual is older than you. A more formal professional communication style may be expected in some cultures.
Touch and a flexible style	Gently placing your hand on an individual's head when they are unwell may be interpreted as a sign of empathy in some cultures. In other cultures, it would be rude and inappropriate as the head is interpreted in some cultures as a part of the body that is sacred. In some cultures, physical contact such as handshakes or hugs between those of opposite genders may be unacceptable or inappropriate, even in a professional capacity. A flexible communication style that can be adapted to different situations and individuals' needs may be more appropriate.
Gestures and an enabling style	Using big physical gestures such as waving your hands when speaking may be interpreted as being warm and friendly in some cultures. In other cultures, big physical gestures may be seen as overwhelming and intimidating. Using an enabling style of communication would mean you could take the lead from the person you're communicating with, and thus ensure your communication is received by them in the way it was intended.
Body language and an assertive style	Using body language such as a nod of the head may indicate that you are listening to the individual and showing your agreement in some cultures. In other cultures, nodding your head during communications may actually mean the opposite, i.e. that you are showing your disagreement. Using an assertive style of communication is useful in these situations.
Behaviour and a flexible style	Your behaviour, such as standing during communications with others, may be interpreted as respectful in some cultures. In other cultures, standing rather than sitting down with the person you are communicating with may be interpreted as rude and inappropriate. Using a flexible communication style can mean you can adapt your behaviour and communications to ensure it remains respectful.

- consult colleagues who have worked with the individual, and other professionals such as the National Autistic Society, who may have a greater understanding of issues around autism for example, including cultural sensitivities.
- do some research into different cultures or backgrounds, including disabilities, to find out about their communication preferences, methods and styles.

AC 2.3 Describe factors that need to be considered for effective communication

When communicating with individuals it is very important to be aware of the many different factors that may have an impact on how effective your communications are. As you will have learned in AC 2.1, individuals' communication and language needs are diverse depending on their conditions and abilities. It is important therefore to be aware of how these and other factors may impact on you being able to communicate effectively with them.

Individuals' conditions

Table 5.5 lists conditions and examples of how they may impact on individuals' abilities to communicate. It is also important to remember that individuals with the same condition may experience it differently and so do not assume that the factors that you will take into account will be the same.

> **Reflect on it**
>
> **2.3 Communication differences**
>
> Think about the differences that exist in people's ability to communicate for various reasons. How do you react to these differences in a way that promotes effective communication? Write a reflective account.

Individuals' abilities

Sensory loss

Individuals who have a **sensory loss** require different levels of support with their communication depending on how much sight or hearing they have. For example, when communicating with an individual who is partially sighted but has no hearing loss you may be able to gain their attention by speaking to them first, such as saying their name, to make them aware that you are speaking to them. By contrast, when communicating with an individual who is blind and deaf you may gain the individual's attention by placing your hand on the top part of their arm (so that you do not startle them) and then using **block alphabet** to spell your name on the palm of their hand (so they know who you are).

Autism spectrum condition (ASC)

An individual with **autism spectrum condition (ASC)** may have difficulty using non-verbal communication and understanding others. ASC can affect individuals' communication in different ways; no two individuals with the same condition are the same and therefore their individual communication and language needs must be taken into account. For example, one individual with ASC may communicate with some people verbally but may find it difficult to initiate conversations and have discussions with others.

Another individual with ASC may have limited speech and find it difficult to understand non-verbal communication such as body language, gestures and facial expressions. It is important to understand these differences to avoid individuals becoming frustrated and not being able to express their ideas, thoughts and feelings.

Table 5.5 Conditions and examples of how they may impact on individuals' communication

Condition	How it impacts on communication
Dementia, e.g. **Alzheimer's disease**	Difficulties in remembering and retaining information, unable to follow thread of conversation, inability to find the right words for objects. An individual with a different type of dementia such as fronto-temporal dementia may, for example, due to their condition appear indifferent or lacking in empathy when communicating and interacting with others.
Stroke	May affect an individual's speech or understanding. May also affect an individual's expression of what they want to say. Individuals who have had a stroke find that it usually causes damage to one side of the brain. For example, if it causes damage to the left side of the individual's brain then it can affect the brain's functions that are responsible for an individual's speech, ability to understand communications as well as their reading and/or writing skills; in other words, an individual's ability to use language. This is a condition known as **aphasia** and sometimes also referred to as **dysphasia**. However, not all individuals who have had a stroke find that it affects their ability to use language; for example, if it causes damage to the right side of an individual's brain then the individual may have difficulties with putting information together such as being able to say what they see or hear. Aphasia can also range from being mild and only affecting one form of communication such as reading, to severe and affecting an individual's speech and understanding when communicating with others (known as mixed or global aphasia). For example, some individuals may not be able to understand what others are saying to them (known as receptive aphasia), others may not have difficulties understanding what is said but may instead find it difficult to express what they want to communicate (known as expressive aphasia).
Arthritis	May cause pain, and the individual may appear distracted or disinterested so this will affect when you approach them.
Mental health conditions	Lack of concentration, anxiety around others in busy environments.

Key terms

Alzheimer's disease is the most common cause of dementia; symptoms can include the gradual loss of memory and communication skills and a decline in the ability to think and reason clearly.

Aphasia is most often caused by stroke. It is a complex language and communication disorder which affects the ability to produce or comprehend speech, and the ability to read or write. It can also be caused by disease, injury or damage to the language centres of the brain. People who suffer from aphasia experience a complete disruption to their communication; they will not understand what others say and will be unable to speak.

Dysphasia is a language disorder that is caused by damage to the brain. People with dysphasia will often have difficulty with verbal communication. It is different to aphasia because here people will experience partial loss of speech. They will still experience difficulty in comprehending and understanding language.

Arthritis is a medical condition that affects joints by causing pain, stiffness, swelling and decreased mobility of the joints.

Sensory loss refers to hearing loss, sight loss or both hearing and sight loss.

Block alphabet is an adapted form of finger spelling taken from British Sign Language (BSL) where you use your finger to trace the outline of capital letters on the palm of the deafblind individual thus enabling communication by touch alone.

Makaton is a method of communication using signs and symbols that can be used by individuals who have learning disabilities.

Learning disabilities

Individuals who have learning disabilities will also require a different approach when communicating depending on the level of their learning disability. Some individuals may communicate using adapted forms of communication such as **Makaton**, others may require you to speak clearly and use short sentences, and others may use photographs and objects of reference to make themselves understood. Knowing how every individual communicates will enable you to adapt your approach, communicate and interact with them positively.

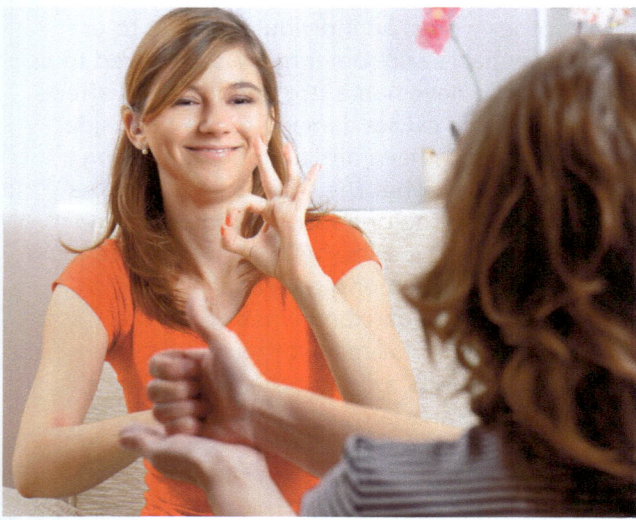

Figure 5.3 How and why do you adapt your communication to meet the needs of individuals?

Research it

2.3, 2.4 Learning disabilities

Research what a learning disability is, then write your own definition. You will find Mencap's factsheet, 'What is a learning disability?' a useful source of information.

Research best practice when communicating with individuals who have different levels of learning disabilities and then produce a 'Top Tips' information guide for how to communicate with individuals with learning disabilities. You will find Mencap's factsheet, 'Communicating with people with a learning disability' a useful source of information.

Individuals who use recreational drugs and alcohol

Recreational drugs are substances that individuals take to make themselves feel better when they do not feel good about themselves or their lives and these can be harmful to the individual's health. These can include both legal and illegal substances such as tobacco, alcohol, cannabis, cocaine, heroin and controlled drugs such as sedatives that can be used to help individuals who have anxiety attacks and difficulties with sleeping. Individuals can, when under the influence of recreational drugs and alcohol, feel disorientated, confused and unable to think logically or respond rationally to situations and interactions with others because their thinking and understanding may be impaired as a result of taking these substances. It is important to be patient and remain calm when interacting with someone who may display behaviour that challenges, and not take anything they say or do personally because it may be the substances that they have taken that are making them act in this way.

It is also important to observe what an individual is trying to express through their behaviour. For example, although an individual may be shouting, their facial expressions and body language may tell you that they're feeling unhappy or frightened. Recognising these signs can help you recognise what may be contributing to their behaviour and address it so that it allows for more effective interactions. If you find that you have tried everything you can and the individual is still behaving inappropriately it may be best to take some time out and leave the individual to calm down before approaching them again later on.

Language used by those who work in care settings

Senior care workers, like individuals, are diverse and may originate from different parts of the UK or other countries. This means that their preferred language and the dialect they use may be different to those of individuals. For example, they may use phrases that are specific to the area or country they originate from but can have different meanings in other areas or countries, such as the term 'darling', which can be received as a term of endearment or be seen as patronising. Similarly, when senior care workers use abbreviations and 'professional speak' individuals may feel uncomfortable if they cannot understand what is being said, for example being referred to as 'customers' or people with 'LDs' (learning disabilities).

> **Evidence opportunity**
>
> **2.3 Factors to consider when promoting effective communication**
>
> Develop a case study of an individual who has care or support needs. You can base this on an individual who you know but you must remember to keep their details confidential when including the case study as part of your portfolio. Describe a range of factors that you and others must take into account when communicating with this individual. For each one, explain the reasons why not doing so may prevent effective communications from taking place. Make sure you provide a written account.

Approaches used by those who work in care settings

The approaches used by senior care workers to communicate and interact are also important. For example, not using an individual's preferred name can mean that the individual will not engage, and rushing your communications can also mean that individuals feel devalued by you and therefore will be less likely to engage with you. Approaches that have the individual's needs at the centre are commonly referred to as person-centred approaches; these are ways of working that are focused on the individual and that enable the individual to be in control of their life; this is covered in great detail in Unit 306 Promoting and implementing person-centred practice.

AC 2.4 Explain how digital and other technologies can be used to promote and enhance effective communication between self and others

Technological aids

- **Voice Output Communication Aids (VOCA)** help individuals to communicate by speaking recorded messages and displaying words and symbols on a screen, e.g. a BIGmack is an electronic device that speaks a recorded message when it is pressed to communicate with others.
- Mobile phones can include features such as words and pictures that can be enlarged and used by individuals with sight loss.
- PCs, tablets, laptops can include software applications with pre-recorded phrases or that enable you to record your message through voice activated software.

You may also find it useful to read through Unit 301 Safeguarding and protection in adult care settings/services, LO7, which includes additional information about how communication can also take place through electronic communication devices, the internet and social networking sites.

> **Key term**
>
> **Voice Output Communication Aids (VOCA)** help individuals to communicate by speaking recorded messages and displaying words and symbols on a screen.

> **Evidence opportunity**
>
> **2.4 Technologies and communication**
>
> Develop a short presentation that explains how you can use technologies to effectively communicate with others.

Table 5.6 Technological aids and how you can use them to meet the needs of individuals

Technological aids	How you can use technological aids to meet individuals' needs
Voice Output Communication Aids (VOCA)	• Technological aids that help individuals to communicate can be used alongside verbal and non-verbal communication methods depending on individuals' needs. Technological devices can range from simple electronic devices to more complex speech output devices and specialist communication software. Knowing how individuals use these can also greatly aid your communication. • For example, an individual with hearing loss may use a hearing aid or cochlear implant to help with making the sounds they hear louder. This can mean that they may find it easier to participate in communications if they can hear when you or others are speaking to them. • For example, an individual with a moderate learning disability may use a Voice Output Communication Aid (VOCA) such as a BIGmack, which is an electronic device that speaks a recorded message when it is pressed to communicate with others. An individual may wish, for example, to say hello to their friends when they arrive at their home. The word 'Hello' can be pre-recorded and the switch on the BIGmack can be pressed by the individual to release the recorded message as each of their friends arrive. • For example, an individual who is blind or partially sighted may use a piece of software such as a screen reader to access a computer, tablet or smartphone. The screen reader reads the information that is displayed on the screen out loud to the individual. This can mean that the individual is able to receive emails and participate with their friends in social networking sites.
Mobile phones	• These can be helpful as some mobile phones include features like 'increased magnification' for an individual with sight loss (the words and pictures on the phones can be enlarged) and hearing aid compatibility so that it is easier to hear for those with hearing difficulties.
PCs, tablets, laptops	• These include software applications designed to enable individuals with a range of needs to communicate more effectively, such as an app that lets you choose a pre-recorded voice or records your own voice saying the words.

Research it

2.4 Technological aids

Research the different types of technological aids available for three individuals with different disabilities or conditions. Remember, each individual is a unique person and therefore how they use the technological aid may vary from another individual who has the same disability or condition.

Develop a visual handout that shows how to use each technological aid with these individuals.

AC 2.5 Describe barriers that may be present when communicating with others

As adult care workers, we should strive for our communications to be effective in order to build strong relationships with those we provide care for, and those we work with. However, for different reasons, sometimes our communications are not effective. Barriers are anything that prevent or stop you or others from communicating and understanding the communication. Barriers can occur not only when communicating with the individuals that you provide care or support to, but also when communicating with others such as their families, your colleagues and other professionals.

It is important that you are aware of the barriers that may prevent effective communications from taking place because being aware means that you can avoid presenting barriers through the ways you use to communicate with others. Being aware of the barriers that exist is also essential for knowing how to overcome them. Below are some examples of different barriers to communication. Can you think of any others?

Barriers present in individuals

Barriers to communication can be present in the individuals you communicate with. Remember though that each individual is unique and therefore the barriers they experience will also be unique.

Speech and hearing impairments

Impairments in relation to speech and hearing may mean that some individuals have difficulties making themselves understood when communicating with others. An individual who has a stutter, for example, may find it difficult to express the words they want to say and may repeat vocal sounds. This may make the individual reluctant to communicate with others, particularly with those they don't know very well as they may feel inadequate or embarrassed about their stutter.

An individual with a hearing loss may find it difficult to participate in conversations with a group of people. Their impairment may mean that the individual finds it difficult to hear what each person is saying, particularly if more than one person is speaking at the same time or the speaker is not facing them when they are speaking.

> **Key term**
>
> **Cerebral palsy** is a neurological condition caused by damage to the brain that affects the body's movements and muscle co-ordination. Symptoms can include jerky uncontrolled movements, and stiff and floppy arms or legs.

Conditions such as cerebral palsy, autism, dementia, and physical disability

Conditions such as **cerebral palsy**, autism and dementia can affect individuals' speech and understanding of both verbal and non-verbal communications. An individual with cerebral palsy may have difficulties using the correct words when speaking, may not be able to speak at all or may have difficulty using gestures when communicating as they may not be able to control their body's movements. This experience can be a frustrating one if not overcome.

An individual with autism may find it difficult to understand and interpret non-verbal communication such as hand gestures and body language when used by others. An individual with autism may also avoid eye contact when communicating with others and find communicating in different social situations difficult. This can mean that the individual is unable to express themselves when communicating with others and can lead to their needs being unmet.

An individual in the early stages of dementia may have difficulty finding the right words when communicating and lose their train of thought during communications. An individual in the middle stages of dementia may have greater difficulty in using verbal communication and may rely more on non-verbal communication to understand what is being said.

Abilities and skills, learning disabilities, self-esteem and past experiences

Other factors that may act as barriers to communication include individuals' abilities and skills, self-esteem and past experiences. For example, an individual may not be able to communicate effectively or have good social skills required to interact with others due to their background, or an impairment or condition such as a learning disability. An individual's language skills may also present a barrier as they may prefer to speak using another language that is familiar to them.

An individual's self-esteem can also affect communications. If, for example, the individual has low self-esteem they may not feel able or confident to interact and communicate with others and may prefer instead to withdraw from communications. An individual's past experiences can also have an impact on how they communicate with others. For example, if an individual has had bad past experiences when communicating, such as others talking over them, not listening to what they have to say or getting impatient, then the individual may be less likely to want to communicate with others as they may believe that all communications are negative. Understanding what barriers an individual may be facing is crucial for being able to recognise them and putting plans in place to overcome them.

Distress
At times, individuals, their families, or colleagues may be so stressed or distressed that it is difficult to communicate with them or understand what they are telling you. At times like this, it is important to allow them time to calm down and communicate what they are experiencing.

Frustration and agitation
This can make it very difficult to communicate with individuals because you will both not feel relaxed or comfortable. This makes it difficult to think, say and express how you feel.

Difficulties when communicating with others who individuals do not know
This can mean that it is difficult for individuals to convey thoughts, feelings and more private or confidential information.

Barriers present in Lead Adult Care Workers and Lead Personal Assistants
Barriers to communication are also present in those who provide care and support to individuals and their families. It is important you are aware of what these are so that you can avoid them in your working practices.

Time
Allowing sufficient time for communications with individuals and their families is essential as not doing so can result in them being rushed and those you are communicating with feeling devalued and not listened to. This can also result in misunderstandings as you, individuals and others are not able to express what you want to say. Of course, you will find that there are many pressures placed on you and your time, but it is important to give time to individuals to express themselves and understand what it is that they would like to communicate in order to better understand their needs and provide the best care possible.

Lack of training and knowledge
Communicating effectively is a skill. A lack of training and knowledge can mean that you have not developed the required skills, qualities and understanding to be able to communicate effectively in line with good practice. For example, you may not know how to communicate effectively with an individual who has a hearing loss or with an individual with a learning disability, including the various aids that are available.

Stress, illness or tiredness
Being fit to work is important because working when you're feeling unwell, stressed or tired can result in you being less patient than you would usually be. It can also affect your concentration and listening skills because you are not feeling relaxed or comfortable. This can impact negatively not only on your communications with others but also on your working relationships, making you less approachable and more likely to misunderstand what is being communicated.

Language and cultural differences
The language you use may vary because of your background, accent or the native language you and others speak. This can mean that misunderstandings can arise, and communications may be ineffective. An individual may not be able to understand you if you speak too quickly or use words that they do not know; for example, vocabulary may be too complex or abbreviated, such as PRN ('pro re nata' in Latin) for medication that is given as and when required. Dialect and different styles of speech can also present barriers to understanding. It could be that the meaning of non-verbal communication methods such as eye contact differs in your culture and theirs – remember, eye contact can be seen as showing a genuine interest in some cultures, but as rude in others. You could revisit Unit 309 Promoting equality, diversity, inclusion and human rights in adult care settings/services.

You will also have to consider revising the way you interact with individuals from different cultures and faiths. For example, a hand shake may be seen as respectful in one culture but not appropriate in another because of the contact made.

Differences in culture or beliefs may also mean that you have certain prejudices and stereotypes, perhaps some that you are not even aware of.

Poor understanding of communication and language needs and preferences
A poor understanding of an individual's communication and language needs and preferences will mean that you cannot tailor the methods you use to communicate to the individual's needs. As a Lead Adult Care Worker, it is your responsibility to find out as much as you can about the individual's communication and language needs and preferences so that you can tailor your methods to suit them.

Barriers present in the environment
Noise and poor light
There are also many environmental barriers that can arise in different care settings and situations when you are communicating with individuals and others. For example, if a room is too noisy others may not be able to hear what you are saying. If a room is too dark, then you and others may not be able to see each other's facial expressions and body language. This may affect the quality of the communications.

> **Reflect on it**
>
> **2.5 Barriers to communication**
>
> What barriers do you think you may present when communicating with individuals and others in your work setting? Now ask someone who knows you well – this may be a colleague you work with – what barriers they think you present when communicating with them, individuals and others. Did anything surprise you? Why? Write a short reflective account.

Lack of privacy and distractions
A lack of privacy when communicating can lead to individuals and others not sharing with you everything they want to say. This may be because there are too many distractions or people walking past, resulting in them feeling anxious that others may be able to overhear. This is particularly true if what they want to say involves a sensitive topic such as their personal care needs or a safeguarding concern. They may also interpret this as you not being a good professional, one that they can trust and confide in.

Room temperature and unwelcoming factors
Other factors that may lead to an uncomfortable environment may include rooms being too hot or too cold, untidy or unwelcoming. Rooms that are too hot or too cold will make individuals and others feel uncomfortable and unable to relax and therefore communicate effectively with you. They may get distracted by trying to open windows to cool the room down, or turn the heating up to make the room feel warmer.

Environments that are untidy and unwelcoming can act as barriers to effective communications. Think about how you might feel if you went to meet a Lead Adult Care Worker in the care setting where your relative was living, and the meeting was in an untidy room with a stained carpet and dirty chairs. What would you think about the professional? The care setting? Similarly, it is important that all environments where communications take place are warm and welcoming – have you ever entered a room or building that felt unwelcoming, perhaps it made the hairs on the back of your neck stand on end?

Cluttered rooms with tall furniture can also prevent reading of facial expressions and make eye contact difficult. It may also mean that people in wheelchairs, for example, may struggle to communicate if they cannot see over tall tables.

> **Research it**
>
> **2.5 Barriers**
>
> Carry out your own research to find out about the potential barriers to communication that may exist in the care setting where you work. For example, think about the individuals where you work and the different barriers that they may present as well as the barriers that you and your colleagues may present. Remember to also think about the physical and social environment where you work and the potential barriers that could exist to communication. Produce a written account with your findings.

> **Evidence opportunity**
>
> **2.5 Barriers to effective communication**
>
> For one individual with care and support needs that you know, make a list of the potential barriers to effective communication. Don't make assumptions about what these may be; find out instead! Provide a written account but make sure that you maintain confidentiality and do not reveal any personal details about the individual.

AC 2.6 Explain how to access support or services to promote effective communication

The care setting where you work will contain a range of sources of extra support or services to enable individuals to communicate effectively.

Internal sources of support

Internal sources of extra support can include:

- people who know the individual well, for example the individual's family, friends, advocate
- experienced colleagues, for example your manager, the individual's key worker
- records, for example the individual's care or support plan, their communication profile.

These sources of additional support are available to you in the care setting where you work and can be accessed in a variety of different ways. For example, perhaps you are unsure about how to use an individual's communication book. You could ask the individual's family or key worker who knows them well and can tell you how they use the communication book with the individual to communicate. You could also read the individual's care or support plan or communication profile that provides more specific information on their communication needs, including guidance on how they communicate and the aids they use. An individual's care or support plan and communication profile will contain personal and **confidential** information – for this reason, you must follow your care setting's procedures for accessing these records.

Key terms

Confidentiality means keeping information private. Confidentiality is important in an adult care setting because it respects individuals' rights to privacy and dignity, instils trust between you and others, promotes individuals' safety and security and shows compliance with legislation such as the Data Protection Act 2018.

Reflect on it

2.6 Accessing support

Reflect on an occasion when you accessed support from someone else in the care setting where you worked. What support did you require? Why? Who did you go to? Why?

External sources of support

Sometimes, you may need to access other communication services from specialist external organisations and professionals to overcome barriers to communication as they can be useful sources of information support and advice. Table 5.7 provides you with details about how these services can enable individuals to communicate effectively and how you can access them.

If your employer is the individual you care for and support, then the individual will provide you with the services and people they prefer to access and make use of to enable them to communicate more effectively. For example, perhaps they prefer to use a family member or a friend to act as a translator or interpreter. The individual may also request your help in accessing a speech and language therapist and/or an advocate; the individual may prefer to use a local service in their area and access other groups available to them such as a support group for people with hearing loss. Some of these services can be accessed directly by the individual; others may require the individual to be referred, for example by their GP or social worker.

Sources of support available to you

See Table 5.10 for more information on sources of support that may be available to you and the importance of also looking after your own health and emotions.

Table 5.7 How services can enable individuals to communicate effectively and how you can access them

Service	How the service enables individuals to communicate effectively	How you can access the service
Translation	Translators are professionals who convert text written in one language to another language so that it can be understood, for example from English to Polish, from Braille into English, from Makaton into English.	To access a professional translation service such as Language Line UK to overcome a language barrier and translate a document, you must first discuss this with your manager or employer as they will have a preferred list of organisations to contact. Your manager or employer will then advise you on the support you need to provide to the individual either by supporting them to access the service directly or by accessing it on their behalf.
Interpreting	Interpreters are professionals who convert spoken language from one language to another so that it can be understood, for example from English to British Sign Language, from Romanian to English, from English to Spanish. Interpreting can take place face-to-face such as in a meeting and/or over the telephone.	To access a professional interpreting service such as UK Interpreting Services to overcome a language barrier and understand what an individual is communicating, you must first discuss this with your manager or employer as they will have a preferred list of organisations to contact. Your manager or employer will then advise you on the support you need to provide to the individual either by supporting them to access the service directly or by accessing it on their behalf.
Speech and language	Speech and language therapists and psychologists carry out assessments and provide care, support and treatment for individuals who have communication difficulties. They work closely with individuals and others such as individuals' families, care workers and GPs to provide an individual plan of support. The Royal College of Speech and Language Therapists (RCSLT) is the professional body for speech and language therapists and is another useful source of information.	To access a speech and language therapist or psychologist you can refer an individual directly to these services or a referral can be made by another professional such as the District Nurse or by the individual themselves contacting their GP. You must first discuss this with your manager or employer who will advise you on the referral process to follow.
Specialist organisations	The Alzheimer's Society, Mencap and the Stroke Association can provide specialist information and practical advice on how to communicate with individuals who have conditions that affect their communication, for those that have dementia, a learning disability and/or a stroke, for example. They not only provide useful factsheets and leaflets but can also provide access to support groups and helplines for further information. You may also need to seek the support of counselling services. You are of course able to speak to the individual, but you should not act as a **counsellor** unless you have been trained in this.	All these organisations can be accessed directly over the telephone and email. You should check with your manager or employer first that they agree that you can do so and if so, agree on the type of information that you will need to access to communicate with individuals more effectively.

Table 5.7 How services can enable individuals to communicate effectively and how you can access them *continued*

Service	How the service enables individuals to communicate effectively	How you can access the service
Advocacy	Advocacy workers support and enable people to express their views, wishes and concerns when they are unable to, for example when the individual has a learning disability, a mental health need or low self-esteem. There are many different types of advocacy services depending on the type of support needed, for example some organisations and charities such as Mencap provide advocacy services for individuals with learning disabilities. There is also statutory advocacy that provides professional advocates, for example Independent Mental Health Advocates (IMHAs) who provide support to people being assessed or receiving treatment under the Mental Health Act 1983. There are also **Independent Mental Capacity Advocates (IMCAs)** who provide support to individuals who lack capacity to make decisions under the Mental Capacity Act 2005, and Care and Support Advocates who provide support to individuals under the Care Act 2014.	**Independent advocates** are appointed by the local authority and so you must first discuss this with your manager or employer who will be able to provide you with further advice and guidance. Some advocates are provided by organisations and charities, but again, to access these you must first discuss this with your manager or employer who will be able to guide you with the type of advocacy needed and how this can be accessed. You will learn more about the purposes and principles of independent advocacy in AC 5.1 and how to access advocacy services in AC 5.3.

> **Key term**
>
> **Counsellors** are trained therapists who listen to you talk through your feelings and emotions and help you find strategies for managing emotional issues.
>
> **Independent advocates** are trained independent people who are appointed to represent/speak on behalf of an individual who may be unable to speak for/represent themselves due to a disability or condition such as dementia.
>
> **Independent Mental Capacity Advocate (IMCA)** refers to a person who provides support and representation for a person who lacks capacity to make specific decisions where the person has no one else to support them.

> **Research it**
>
> **2.6 Local services**
>
> Research two services in your local area that enable individuals to communicate effectively. For each one write down what they do and what services they provide.
>
> Your local authority's website and/or your manager are two useful sources of information.

> **Evidence opportunity**
>
> **2.6 How to access support or services to enable individuals to communicate effectively**
>
> Develop a case scenario of an individual who has communication difficulties. Explain the additional support and services available to support the individual to communicate effectively. Provide a written account of this case scenario.

AC 2.7 Describe the impact that poor or inappropriate communication has on practice

As you will have learned in AC 1.2 of this unit, communication can affect relationships both positively (if it is effective) and negatively (if it is poor). Table 5.8 provides some examples of poor or inappropriate communication and the impact it has on practice.

Evidence opportunity

2.7 The impact of poor communication

Discuss with your assessor or manager the impact that poor or inappropriate communication has on practice.

Table 5.8 Examples of poor communication

Poor communication
Speaking to a care worker who has requested to speak to you in private, but you decide to speak to them in a busy corridor of the day centre where you work: In a situation like this, the care worker will be unlikely to share with you what they wanted to say because it will be difficult for them to feel comfortable if it is busy. Others may overhear and so this will also impact what they decide to tell you in this environment. The care worker will also feel that you are not genuinely interested in hearing what they have to say if you ignored their request to meet privately. This in turn will have a negative impact on your relationship with the care worker.
Supporting an individual to attend their care review but slouching in your chair during the whole meeting: Your body language and behaviour may make the individual feel uncomfortable, embarrassed and undermined by your slouching as it gives the impression that you are not genuinely interested in them or supporting them at their care review. You will also be giving this negative impression to the other people attending the individual's care review such as the individual's family, your manager and other professionals such as the individual's social worker. This in turn will make it difficult to work with these other people as not only will they feel you are disinterested, but it will also reflect badly on you as they may not have any confidence in your abilities and may mistakenly think that you do not have the necessary expertise and knowledge required to provide good quality care and support. This in turn will have a negative impact on your relationship with the individual and others.
Responding to an email sent by an individual's family using an informal style of writing and not proof reading the email for spelling and grammar errors before sending it: The family may worry that you and the organisation you work for are not professional and therefore not providing good quality care to their relative. The individual's family will also be less likely to trust you and respect you if the language used in your written communication is unprofessional. This in turn will have a negative impact on your relationship with the individual's family.

LO3 Be able to communicate effectively with others

Getting started

Think about an occasion when you had to communicate with another person and it worked well. Why was the communication effective? What communication methods and styles did you use and why? How did you ensure that the message you wanted to convey had maximum impact on the person?

AC 3.1 Demonstrate a range of effective communication methods and skills

For assessment criterion AC 3.1 you will be observed and you will need to demonstrate that you can use a range of effective communication methods and skills when communicating with others, e.g. individuals and their carers, loved ones, families, friends, colleagues and peers, managers and supervisors, professionals from other services, visitors to the work setting, members of the community and volunteers. To do so, you need to know about the range of communication methods and skills available.

> **Reflect on it**
>
> **3.1 Communication methods and skills**
>
> Reflect on the communication methods you learned about in AC 2.1 and the communication skills required to be an effective communicator you learned about in AC 1.3. Which ones do you use when communicating with others and why?

Active listening skills including paraphrasing, reflection, summarising, reframing, providing encouragement

Active listening is a communication technique that involves understanding and interpreting what is being expressed through verbal and non-verbal communication so that communications can be fully understood.

SOLER, a theory developed by Gerard Egan, can be used to describe how to practise active listening:

- **S**it squarely: think about how to position yourself in relation to the person you are communicating with to show you have a genuine interest
- **O**pen posture: think about how to maintain an open posture, for example do not cross your arms.
- **L**ean: think about the way you can lean towards the person you are communicating with to show your interest, but take care not to invade their personal space.
- **E**ye contact: think about how and when to maintain eye contact to show you are listening, i.e. not too little, as this may show you are not interested, or too much, as this may make the person feel uncomfortable.
- **R**elax: think about what effect you being relaxed can have on the individual, for example it can show that you have time for them.

Developing active listening skills is important because the person you are communicating with will feel that you are truly listening to them; in this way they are more likely to trust you and tell you confidential and sensitive information that you may need to know to better inform the care or support you provide. Active listening skills include for example the following:

- **Paraphrasing** – this refers to a way of repeating back what has been said or heard using different words to ensure that you have fully understood what has been communicated.
- **Reflection** – this refers to thinking about what has been communicated by taking a step back to examine what has been communicated, including the positives and negatives, to ensure that you have thought about what can be done to improve the communication.
- **Summarising** – this refers to a way of providing a description of the main points and ideas of what has been communicated to ensure that you have fully understood the most important aspects of the communication.
- **Reframing** – this refers to responding to what has been said, or expressed, in an angry or derogatory way without taking it personally to ensure that you can then paraphrase and reflect it back to the person in a constructive way.
- **Providing encouragement** – this refers to using both verbal and non-verbal communication methods during communications to ensure that you are showing respect, understanding and genuineness when communicating.

> **Reflect on it**
>
> **3.1 Active listening skills**
>
> In pairs tell each other about a situation that happened in your work setting. Actively listen to each other and provide encouragement. Then, take it in turns to reflect it back to each other using paraphrasing and summarising. Reflect on your active listening skills. Where could you have made improvements?

AC 3.2 Demonstrate the application of communication skills appropriately in relation to message and audience for maximum impact

For assessment criterion AC 3.2 you will be observed and you will need to demonstrate that you can apply communication skills appropriately in relation to the message you are conveying to others and the needs of those you are communicating with for maximum impact. Maximum impact means that your communications are understood and received in the way they are intended. Ensuring that your message is communicated effectively is important for avoiding misunderstandings.

The following are some top tips for how to use different strategies to clarify misunderstandings. Can you think of any others that you have used that have been effective? You may find that you use different strategies at different times. It is important that you know what you can do when misunderstandings arise because if you don't, not only will your communications with individuals be ineffective but this may also affect the quality of your working relationships and the care or support you provide.

Top tips for use of different strategies to clarify misunderstandings

1 **Be alert:** when you recognise that a misunderstanding has occurred, try and find out the reasons why as soon as you can. For example, perhaps it was because the individual could not hear you because there was a lot of background noise; perhaps it was because the meaning of the sign you used was mistaken by the individual to mean something else. Don't forget there will also be clues in the individual's non-verbal behaviour. For example, perhaps their facial expression will show that they are confused, or their body language shows that they are frustrated. As you will have learned in AC 3.1, this strategy is referred to as **active listening**.

2 **Be clear:** when you think you know the reason why a misunderstanding has occurred, do not assume that you are correct; check your understanding with the individual. For example, you may sign to the individual to go somewhere quieter or ask the individual or their representative 'Did I use the wrong sign?'.

3 **Be responsive:** show the individual concerned that you have noticed that there has been a misunderstanding, that you are sorry that this has happened and that you want to clarify it. For example, you may sign or say to the individual, 'I am really sorry that there has been a misunderstanding. Can you show me what I can do to help?'.

4 **Be resourceful:** if you are still unable to clarify the misunderstanding with the individual then seek advice from your manager or from the individual's representative – this could be their advocate, family member or friend. They will know the individual well and may be able to share with you the strategies that they have used to clarify misunderstandings, including what works well and what doesn't.

For example, you may need to rephrase what you have said, **paraphrase** or use a **closed** rather than an **open question**. If an individual's misunderstanding is due to a language difference, then a translator or interpreter may be required; you may find it useful to review your previous learning in AC 2.6 about these types of specialist services.

5 **Be flexible:** be prepared to adapt your communication with the individual to clarify the misunderstanding. For example, if you are using signing with the individual and this is not working, you could try writing down the message that you are trying to communicate instead. If you are using a sign that an individual does not understand, you could use an object of reference or a photograph instead to convey your message. You will find it useful to review your previous learning in AC 2.1 about the range of communication methods that are available to meet an individual's needs.

Research it

1.4, 3.2, 3.4 Active listening

Research how active listening can be used to clarify misunderstandings. You may find the resource below from Mind Tools, 'Active Listening, Hear What People are Really Saying' including the video clip, a useful source of information for your research: www.mindtools.com/CommSkll/ActiveListening.htm

Show a colleague how you use active listening in communications with two different individuals.

Key terms

Active listening is a communication technique that involves understanding and interpreting what is being expressed through verbal and non-verbal communication.

To **paraphrase** means to restate what has been said or heard in order to clarify.

Closed questions such as Who? Where? encourage short, less complex responses.

Open questions such as What? Why? How? encourage the expression of opinions and feelings.

Case study

2.1, 3.2, 4.3 Clarifying misunderstandings

Yanis is an experienced Personal Care Assistant and provides day-to-day support to Bokamoso, who is a young person with physical disabilities living in her own flat. Yanis and Bokamoso are from different backgrounds in terms of the native languages they speak and the way they were brought up.

This morning Yanis is supporting Bokamoso to search for jobs that may interest her using the internet. There is one job advert that Bokamoso is very interested in and she has asked Yanis to clarify what some of the job's responsibilities are in the attached job description as she does not fully understand what these are.

Yanis reads through the job description carefully but is also unsure what the job's responsibilities involve as he does not understand the meaning of some of the terminology used in the document. Yanis is worried about telling Bokamoso this because she has asked him for his support and so decides it's best to tell Bokamoso that she should look at another job advert while he tries to find out from a colleague what the terminology used means.

Bokamoso misinterprets what Yanis says to her and believes that Yanis doesn't think she is suitable for the job. Bokamoso tells Yanis she is not happy with his attitude towards her and looks very upset.

Discuss:
1. Why has this misunderstanding arisen?
2. How should Yanis respond? Why?

It will be useful to go back and think about the ways in which you can overcome misunderstandings. In the context of what you have learned about language and cultural differences, for example, think about how you can prevent misunderstandings and overcome these barriers. Revisit what you have learned about verbal and non-verbal communication and think about how you can use your knowledge and skills in using these to overcome misunderstandings. Ensure that you use your skills of compassion and care effectively when there are misunderstandings.

AC 3.3 Demonstrate the use of communication skills to build relationships

For assessment criterion AC 3.3 you will be observed and you will need to demonstrate how you use communication skills to build relationships with others. To do so, you will need to understand how the way you communicate in the care setting/service where you work affects your relationships with others.

Evidence opportunity

3.1, 3.2, 3.3 Effective communication

Demonstrate to your assessor how you communicate effectively with others by:

- using a range of communication methods and skills
- applying communication skills appropriately in relation to the message you are conveying and the people you are communicating with
- using your communication skills to build relationships with others.

Your manager could also provide you with a Witness Testimony of your work practices.

AC 3.4 Demonstrate how to overcome barriers to effective communication

For this assessment criterion, your work practices will be observed; you will need to demonstrate that you know how to use different ways to overcome barriers to communication so that effective communication can happen. As individuals' and others' experiences of barriers to communication are different, it is important that you know how to use different methods to overcome these, particularly if the first method you try isn't effective.

Tables 5.9, 5.10 and 5.11 provide you with some suggestions of how to overcome barriers present in individuals, others, lead adult care workers/lead personal assistants and the environment. As you will see, each of the examples below requires you to be able to demonstrate a set of skills, knowledge and qualities for them to effective.

Table 5.9 Barriers that may be present in individuals and ways to overcome them

Barriers present in individuals and others	Ways of overcoming barriers present in individuals and others
Impairments, illness, abilities and skills	For all of the different barriers that are discussed here, it is important to find out from the individual or someone who knows them well, such as a family member or advocate, what their specific communication needs are – do not make any assumptions about what communication methods they prefer to use and how. Professionals such as speech and language therapists can also be useful sources of guidance and information. You will find it useful to review your previous learning around support services in AC 2.6.
Impairments (such as a hearing or visual impairment)	If an individual with a hearing impairment cannot hear what you are saying do not be afraid to repeat what you have said. Speak clearly but not too slowly, otherwise an individual may interpret this as patronising. For individuals with sight loss, effective verbal communication will be key, using the tone of your voice to convey meaning, also non-verbal communication such as touch if/when appropriate and if the individual is comfortable with this.
Conditions such as dementia	If an individual with dementia is not responding to what you have asked them, rephrase the question. Ensure you speak in short sentences so that they can understand and remember the question you are asking them. Remember not to become impatient or look frustrated at having to rephrase and repeat information because doing so may mean that the individual withdraws from the communication.
Communicating with someone who has a learning disability and uses Makaton or sign language	If you do not understand what an individual with a learning disability is communicating in Makaton, then ask the individual to repeat the sign. If you still don't know, then ask a colleague who is familiar with Makaton. You may also decide that you need further training about how to use Makaton. You may also need to use specialist services such translators, interpreters and signers who can support individuals.
Communicating with someone who is not an effective communicator and has had negative past experiences of communication	If you are supporting an individual who isn't an effective communicator and has had negative past experiences of communications, be patient and see if you can find out how they communicate. You may be able to do this by observing them with others and taking note of the methods used to communicate.
Low self-esteem	If an individual with low self-esteem withdraws from their communication with you do not take this personally. Try and put yourself in their 'shoes' and be empathetic. Be patient, stay positive and gently encourage them to communicate with you by perhaps using less verbal communication and more non-verbal communication. A smile and an open posture can go a long way!

Table 5.9 Barriers that may be present in individuals and ways to overcome them *continued*

Barriers present in individuals and others	Ways of overcoming barriers present in individuals and others
Distress/stress	There may be times when your colleagues or others you work with such as volunteers and professionals from other services are going through stressful times or are distressed due to family issues or bereavement, for example, which may affect your communication with them. In such cases it is important to be supportive and offer practical as well as emotional support – you could, for example, ask if they would like to speak to a counsellor or if there is anything you could help with in terms of any arrangements. Ensure that the person knows that you are there if they would like to talk, or that they can speak to a family member or another person in the setting. At the same time make sure you do not pressure them into opening up about what is bothering them. It is important that people do not feel alone and as if no one cares for them, especially at times of distress, which is why you should offer compassionate support as a Lead. However, it may be that they do not want support, and so it is important that you ensure their wishes are at the centre of the support you provide. It may be tempting to try and support the person at times like this as you may feel you are fulfilling your duty of care. However, it is important not to force support on them when they do not want it. We all want our own space at times and it is important to remember that the people you work with may feel the same. Giving unwanted help may make the person feel that you are not respecting their wishes and taking their decision-making powers away from them, or that you are trying to obtain information that they do not want to share, which is not part of providing compassionate support. If a person you work with is particularly distressed, you will need to decide on the best course of action, and it may be that you need to seek the help and advice of your manager or other colleagues or professionals. It may be that the person is showing signs of anger or is becoming increasingly anxious and upset in which case you should seek help immediately to protect the safety of others (this may be help from your manager, colleagues, another professional or the emergency services). You should remember to seek help immediately, but also inform the person that you are seeking help so that you can protect them.
Differences in language	Speaking a different language to those around you or not being able to understand what others are saying can be a lonely and distressing experience for the person. As a compassionate adult care worker, it is your responsibility to ensure that you find out about the people you support and work with, including whether they have any language preferences, and whether you require a translator or interpreter; your manager will be able to advise on this. It may be that you speak the same language as the person, in which case you are able to communicate with them. Or it could be that you can speak a little of the language but still require an interpreter who has a better grasp of the language than you, or it may be that a colleague or a relative of the person has been asked to translate. Remember that speaking a different language to those around you or not being able to understand what others are saying can be a lonely experience for the person and so it is important to be empathetic and make the person feel supported. It may be that the person does not want to discuss private matters in front of family members, so you should take this into account before suggesting that a family member translate or interpret for them. See more on this in Table 5.10. As mentioned, you may also use specialist services such as translators or interpreters; translators can help with translating written communication from one language to another and interpreters with spoken language.

Table 5.10 Barriers that may be present in Lead Adult Care Workers/Lead Personal Assistants and ways to overcome them

Barriers present in Lead Adult Care Workers/ Lead Personal Assistants	Ways of overcoming barriers present in Lead Adult Care Workers/Lead Personal Assistants
Insufficient time	Planning communications with individuals and others at times when you are not busy will ensure that communications are effective and all those involved feel valued. You should allow sufficient time to meet and find out their specific communication and language needs. If it is quite simply impossible to schedule in enough time, you may like to look at your diary and schedule a meeting for a time when you will be able to devote enough time to them.
Lack of training and knowledge	Ensuring that you attend the training planned for you by your employer will help you keep up to date with best practice and new working approaches and techniques used when communicating with individuals and others. Similarly, if there are any areas you are unsure about or want to learn more about it is important to be honest and raise this with your employer so that you can be an effective communicator.
Illness, stress, tiredness	If you are not fit to work because you are physically unwell or emotionally stressed, it is best to not go into work. In this way you will avoid getting frustrated or becoming impatient when you are communicating with others. Similarly, if you are tired this can impact negatively on your communications. Recognise when you are tired and ensure you have the rest that you need; eating healthily will also keep you of sound body and mind. If you are at work and sense that you're getting stressed or tired then take 'time out', compose yourself and return when you feel able to. You can also access further support from your employer in terms of support groups, counselling services or leave from work. It can also be distressing when individuals and others are upset or when they are relating distressing stories to you, after all you will be responsible for people from various backgrounds who may have experienced trauma, and this may pose a barrier to effective communication. In situations such as this it is important to speak to your manager or a colleague and discuss the support that is available to you and think about your own emotions. It may be that a colleague has to take over the support of the person. It may also help to speak to a friend or family as well as your manager and colleagues about what has upset you, although you must remember rules around confidentiality and not relay any personal details about the person or their circumstances. Your manager may also refer you to external sources of support. Remember that it is important that you take care of your own health and feelings as well as those you provide support to.
Language and cultural differences	Be aware of your own and others' language and culture differences. Do not let your own differences affect those of individuals and others. Be open to different languages and cultures and find out as much as you can about what the different meanings that verbal and non-verbal communication methods have; you could even try and learn some words from the person's language which may help you to form a connection. It may be that you use more non-verbal communication in place of verbal communication. Being warm and friendly can help to create positive relationships and rapport. You may need to use sign language and/or picture or flash cards. You may also need to access further support and guidance from interpreters and translators; you will find it useful to review your previous learning in AC 2.6 around accessing support and services to promote effective communication.

Table 5.11 Barriers that may be present in the environment/setting and ways to overcome them

Barriers present in the environment	Ways of overcoming barriers present in the environment
Noise	If the environment you are communicating in is too noisy, if possible try and find a quieter place to speak. If this is not possible, try and reduce the noise levels by finding out first where the noise is coming from, for example is it from the telephone that doesn't stop ringing, from others talking loudly or from a noisy vehicle outside the room? Perhaps you can put the telephone on silent or divert the calls to another room, ask others politely whether they can speak more quietly, close the window or move to the other side of the room away from where the noisy vehicle is parked. If you cannot avoid the noisy environment, you will need to make sure that you still communicate clearly, by perhaps speaking in a slightly louder tone, and use gestures and signing if needed, so that the person can understand you. You may even need to use written communication.
Lack of lighting/ poor lighting	A poorly lit or dark environment can be overcome by finding out the cause of the problem. Perhaps the light bulb needs changing, or you need a brighter light. A blind may need pulling up or a curtain may need to be drawn to let the natural light in. You can also think about where you position yourself in the room – are you in a well-lit area where you are clearly visible and you can see others? This is particularly important when communicating with individuals who use sign language and non-verbal communication methods such as eye contact, facial gestures and body language. If you cannot avoid being in a room where the light is poor, you will need to make sure that the individual is able to understand you. You will need to speak clearly so that they can hear you and also listen to what they communicate. If they cannot see your facial expressions, then it may be that you could change the tone of your voice to express what you are feeling. Likewise, if you cannot see the individual very well, then you should pay attention to the tone of their voice to understand how they may be feeling.
Lack of privacy	A lack of privacy can be overcome by ensuring that windows and doors are closed when communicating so that others cannot overhear. Stopping what you are saying if someone enters the room is another method of maintaining individuals' and others' privacy. If it is not possible to book a private room, you could perhaps delay the meeting slightly and schedule it for another time when the individual may feel comfortable. Also, if the environment is not suited to people with wheelchairs, it may be that you need to adjust the environment accordingly, for example by including ramps that will allow individuals and others to access the building, or counters/tables that wheelchair users can use comfortably.
Temperature – too hot/too cold	Prepare the environment where you are going to communicate by ensuring that it is comfortable and neither too hot nor too cold, for example by switching on the heating, air conditioning or opening/closing windows. If your communication takes place outside or in a public building, then observe how the person you are communicating with is feeling and if they show any signs of being too hot or too cold, then suggest you continue the communication in another area where they feel more comfortable.
Untidiness, unwelcoming	Preparing the environment where you are going to communicate involves making it tidy and welcoming. Ensure it is free from clutter, has been cleaned, any spillages have been wiped up and there are no unpleasant odours. If you come across an untidy environment then suggest you continue the conversation in another area that is more welcoming and where they will feel more comfortable.

6Cs

Compassion

It is important to empathise and understand how those with an impairment may feel when communicating. It may be that they experience feelings of anger and frustration if they are unable to effectively communicate and understand what you are communicating; this may be exacerbated if they cannot hear what you are saying. There may be a significant impact on their wellbeing and quality of life if they are unable to convey their feelings and needs. You should remember that hearing loss does not necessarily mean complete hearing loss but can mean partial loss of hearing, which can also affect individuals' quality of life. Thinking about how you would feel in their situation or when you are not understood or misunderstood will enable you to empathise and be a compassionate adult care worker. Would you feel excluded or left out if you were unable to hear what others were saying?

It is important to understand the various ways in which those who have impairments may be feeling. Make it known that you understand the issues around this and find out how they would like to be supported with their communication needs; you can then enable them to achieve their goals in their own ways. Although it is important to do your research and find out about the ways you can support those with impairments with their communications, remember that not everyone with deafblindness, visual impairments or a learning disability will want to be supported in the same way. It is, therefore, important that you find out how each individual would like to be supported.

It is also important to remain compassionate and calm when there are frustrations around communications. For example, in some cases you may need to repeat information or words so that the individual can understand you, and you will need to remain patient while doing so. Likewise, when working with an individual who has dementia, there may be times when they make statements that do not make sense or are not logical or rational; it is important to find constructive ways to support them and not undermine them. For example, you could observe what their body language is trying to tell you and then check with them the meaning. For example, an individual who is feeling hungry may look at the fridge, place their hand over their stomach or go to the kitchen. You could then confirm this by showing them an object related to food such as a fork or ask them 'Are you hungry?'

Research it

3.4 Understanding how to overcome barriers – communicating with individuals who have a hearing impairment/hearing loss

Research what the Care Act 2014 says about the meaning of safeguarding adults who have care or support needs. Produce a poster with your findings.

You will find it useful to access Skill for Care's resource about the Care Act and its role in safeguarding adults:

www.skillsforcare.org.uk/resources/documents/Developing-your-workforce/Care-Certificate/Care-Certificate-Standards/Standard-10.pdf

Communicating with individuals who are deafblind

You will find the RNID website a useful source of information:

www.rnid.org.uk

Communicating with someone with sight loss

You will find the RNIB website a useful source of information:

www.rnib.org.uk

Macular degeneration

You will find the NICE website a useful source of information:

www.nice.org.uk

Communicating with someone with dementia and sight loss

You will find the RNIB website a useful source of information:

www.rnib.org.uk/professionals/health-social-care-education-professionals/social-care-professionals/dementia-and-sight-loss/

Communicating with someone with a visual impairment

How does it affect an individual's communication if they are unable to see and interpret someone else's verbal and non-verbal communication and are unable to respond accordingly? How does this affect your relationship with the individual? Could this lead to misunderstandings? How have you tried to overcome this barrier? Did you, for example, use more verbal communication? How did you assist them with activities, for example? Did you use Braille to assist them, or suggest an eye sight test? Were there other methods you use? Did you assist them in describing their surroundings? Did you use touch? (You will also find it useful to refer back to ACs 2.3 and 3.1 and the sections on touch.)

Communicating with people with a learning disability

You will find the Mencap website a useful source of information:

www.mencap.org.uk/learning-disability-explained/communicating-people-learning-disability

The degrees to which someone's communication will be affected as a result of a learning disability will vary from communication not being affected at all to severe communication difficulties. Communication needs will also vary depending on what the learning disability is. The communication difficulties they face may also vary in that it may not just be their communication that is affected but other factors that affect their ability to communicate, for example their attention span. You will therefore need to ensure that you work in an empathetic and compassionate way to use your communication skills to enable you to support the individual, to enhance communication, and to not let frustration overcome you if communication difficulties are a hinderance.

Even though a learning disability can mean reduced intellectual ability and difficulty with everyday activities, you will still need to find out what the individual's communication needs are and not assume that individuals will struggle with communication. You can do this by asking the individual or their family, by consulting colleagues who may have worked with the individual or by looking at their care plan.

Communication with someone with a stroke (aphasia and dysphasia)

You will find the Stroke.org website a useful source of information. The following page includes useful links:

www.stroke.org.uk/resources/helping-someone-communication-problems

You will need to think about how to enable more effective communications with someone who is suffering from aphasia or dysphasia. Could you, for example, use gestures and flashcards, or straightforward language that requires simple responses to make it easier for the individual? Also see AC 2.3 for more information on stroke, aphasia and dysphasia.

Communicating with someone with dementia

You will find the NHS and Alzheimer's Society website useful sources of information:

www.nhs.uk/conditions/dementia/communication-and-dementia

www.alzheimers.org.uk/sites/default/files/2019-09/500lp-communicating-190521.pdf

The degree to which someone with dementia has their communication and memory affected will vary. This might be memory loss, which is short or long term, inability to remember things or details, to complete loss of speech. Confusion, seemingly irrational speech and using incorrect or inappropriate words may also be symptoms. Part of being a compassionate care worker is supporting individuals to understand or correcting them in an empathetic manner, one that does not undermine or question them.

Cerebral palsy and motor neurone disease

Do some research into how to address communication issues with those who have cerebral palsy or motor neurone disease and how you can do this effectively. How does their condition affect their verbal and non-verbal communication skills and how can you communicate with them? If non-verbal communication is affected by such illnesses, how can this affect the messages that you receive through their body language or non-verbal communication?

> **Research it**
>
> SOLER is a theory that was developed by Gerard Egan and can be used to describe key techniques that are essential for active listening:
>
> - **S**it squarely: think about how to position yourself in relation to the person you are communicating with to show you have a genuine interest.
> - **O**pen posture: think about how to maintain an open posture, for example do not cross your arms.
> - **L**ean: think about how you can lean towards the person you are communicating with to show you are interested, but not too much or you will invade their personal space.
> - **E**ye contact: think about how and when to maintain eye contact to show you are listening, i.e. not too little as this may show you are uninterested; not too much as this may make the person feel uncomfortable.
> - **R**elax: think about the effects that being relaxed can have on the other person, for example it can show that you have time for them.
>
> Research Gerard Egan's communication model and theory, SOLER, in relation to how a person's posture and body language can have an impact on effective communication.
>
> Demonstrate how you can use SOLER when communicating with others.

Make notes about what you have researched. It is important that you develop your knowledge and skills in communicating with people with different impairments and disabilities as you will encounter and be required to support individuals with these as an adult care worker.

> **Evidence opportunity**
>
> **1.4, 3.4 Ways to overcome barriers to effective communication and using communication skills to manage complex, sensitive, abusive or challenging situations and behaviours**
>
> Read through the short case scenario below and then demonstrate to your assessor different ways of overcoming the barriers to communication being experienced by Ted:
>
> *Ted has mental health needs and experiences high levels of anxiety when in new or different environments. Today is Ted's first day at the day care centre where you work as a Senior Mental Health Worker. You notice that as you walk up to welcome Ted, who is being supported by his sister, he immediately retreats backwards and stares at the floor, his hands are clenched, and he begins to sweat profusely.*
>
> Or you could demonstrate or explain to your assessor how you overcame barriers to effective communication, providing a written account of your actions.

LO4 Be able to meet the communication and language needs, wishes and preferences of individuals

> **Getting started**
>
> Make a list of the key people you communicate with on a day-to-day basis. For each one, write down the ways that you use to communicate with them. Compare the methods you use across all of these. What similarities and differences are there? Why do the methods you use vary? What are the potential consequences if you do not adapt the communication methods you use with different people?

AC 4.1 Demonstrate how to establish the communication and language needs, wishes and preferences of individuals in order to maximise the quality of the interaction

Your work practices will be observed for this assessment criterion; you will have to demonstrate how to establish the communication and language needs, wishes and preferences of individuals in order to maximise the quality of the interaction and get the most from it.

Why is it important to establish communication and language needs, wishes and preferences of individuals?

We are all different and therefore we all communicate in different ways. In order for communication to be effective, you must find out individuals' unique communication and language needs, wishes and preferences that may be based on their beliefs, values and culture. It is important to establish what their communication and language needs, wishes and preferences are because doing so will mean that your interactions will be respectful, person-centred, effective, empathetic, appropriate and sensitive.

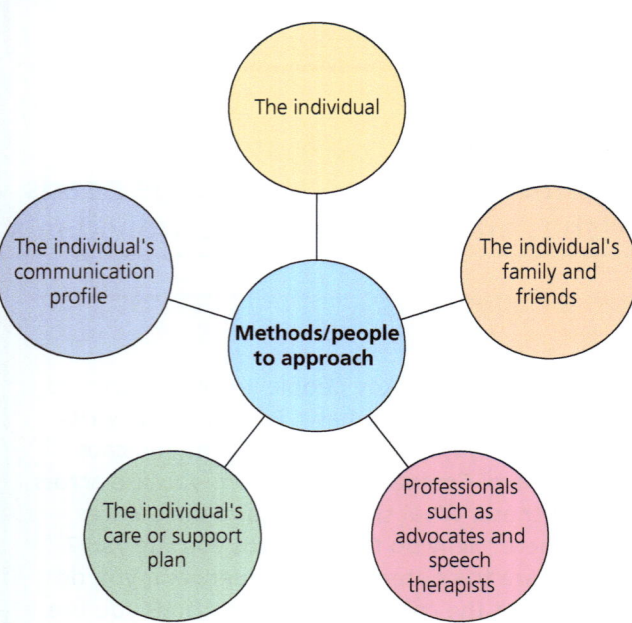

Figure 5.4 Methods/people to approach when establishing communication and language needs, wishes and preferences

How to establish individuals' communication and language needs, wishes and preferences

As you will have learned, individuals' communication and language needs, wishes and preferences will vary. As Figure 5.4 shows, there are a range of methods that you can use to establish what these are and the people you can approach.

The individual themselves can provide you with useful information about their communication and language needs, wishes and preferences. How you establish this with them will vary across individuals but may involve asking them or observing how they communicate with others who know them well, such as their families and friends. Individuals may be able to tell you themselves how they prefer to communicate with others; they may for example prefer to use verbal communication and short sentences or a mixture of words and signs. Individuals can also show you how they prefer to communicate with you by showing you how they use their communication aid to express their thoughts, feelings and ideas with their friends and family when they visit. They may even show you through non-verbal communication what their preferences are by using facial gestures or body language, for example.

The individual's family and friends can be another very useful source of information in relation to establishing the individual's communication and language needs, wishes and preferences because they know the individual well and can therefore provide a valuable insight into the individual. For example, they may use the individual's preferred language when communicating with them such as British Sign Language (BSL) which they may have adapted to reflect the individual's preferences. The individual's family and friends will also be able to tell you the dos and don'ts when communicating with their relative, for example do stand opposite them so that they can see you, do sign clearly, don't rush your communications as this means the individual may misunderstand what you are communicating and can make the individual feel frustrated, don't turn your body away from the individual during communications as they may interpret this as you ending your communication.' Dos and don'ts such as these will apply with most individuals you work with but the advice of those who know them best will be useful to you as you will be able to learn about communication methods specific to the individual.

Advocates and other professionals such as **speech and language therapists** will also know the individual well and will be able to share with you what works best from their perspective during communications. The individual's advocate may provide you with useful tips in relation to establishing the individual's wishes during interactions by suggesting, for example, that you only provide two options at a time when asking the individual to make a choice; for example when asking an individual what they would like to drink you could show them the orange bottle and the blackcurrant bottle. If the individual points to the blackcurrant bottle you could show them both bottles again to check that they are choosing what they prefer to drink. If the individual points to the blackcurrant bottle again then you know that they have chosen to have a drink of blackcurrant.

Speech and language therapists can provide you with guidance on different techniques and approaches that they use when communicating with individuals. For example, they may suggest when communicating with an individual who has had a **stroke** to provide the individual with sufficient time to respond to you during interactions, otherwise the individual may not be able to express what they want to, feel frustrated that they didn't do so and may therefore be reluctant to participate in further communications with you.

An individual's care or support plan can include useful background information about the individual, for example in relation to their culture and beliefs and how these may affect their communication preferences. For example, the care or support plan can help to establish what rules or behaviours must be observed during communications with the individual, such as how to address them (perhaps by using their first name or a nickname) as well as what not to do (perhaps not using a handshake when greeting them as this may be considered inappropriate in their culture).

An individual's care or support plan will also provide up-to-date information about the individual's communication and language needs, wishes and preferences. This information will change over time if the individual's needs change, so it is important to check this document prior to every communication with the individual to ensure that every interaction with them is of a good quality. For example, an individual upon arrival at a care setting may use English as their preferred language but may have developed dementia during their time at the setting. This condition may then cause the individual to revert to using their preferred language when they were a child. It is therefore important that you are aware of any changes that arise so that you can continue to have effective communications with the individuals you support.

Communication profiles provide detailed information about specific communication and language needs individuals may have and usually include specific guidance about how to communicate with individuals effectively. They are used alongside the individual's care or support plan. For example, an individual who is **deafblind** will use more than one method of communicating with others, such as touch to explore the world around them and **objects of reference** to interact with others. Establishing how these are used will be central to the quality of your interaction with the individual.

> **Reflect on it**
>
> **4.1 An individual's care plan**
>
> Reflect on the individuals in the care setting where you work. Think about the information contained in an individual's care or support plan in relation to communication. What details are provided? Why are these important for establishing the individual's communication and language needs, wishes and preferences? Remember that if you provide a written account or have a discussion about this, you must respect confidentiality and not include any details that will give away the individual's identity.

Research it

4.1, 4.2 Communication methods for people who are deafblind

Research different methods of communicating with individuals who are deafblind; remember that every individual is a unique person and so the methods they may choose to communicate with will also vary. Produce an information leaflet with your findings.

You may find the Sense website a useful source of information.

Evidence opportunity

4.1 Establishing communication and language needs, wishes and preferences

Your work practices will be observed for this assessment criterion; you will have to demonstrate how to establish the communication and language needs, wishes and preferences of individuals.

Show your assessor how you establish the communication and language needs, wishes and preferences of two individuals in order to maximise the quality of the interaction. You will need to begin by presenting a brief profile for each individual in terms of their condition or disability and how this affects their communication.

Key terms

Deafblind refers to an individual who has both hearing and sight loss. The combined loss of their hearing and sight means that their ability to communicate and mobilise is severely affected.

Objects of reference are used as a means of communication by individuals and can be any object which is used to represent an item, activity, place or person. For example, a fork can represent lunchtime, and a photograph of a train can represent going to visit a family member.

AC 4.2 Demonstrate a range of communication styles, methods and skills to meet an individual's needs

For this AC, you will need to demonstrate a range of communication styles, methods and skills that support an individual's needs. You will find it useful to review your previous learning in AC 2.1 around different communication styles and methods available as well as your previous learning in AC 1.3 around the skills you require to be an effective communicator.

Communication styles

The range of positive communication styles that can be used to meet individuals' different needs are varied; some examples are included below.

- **Assertive:** You can show an assertive style of communication by using a calm and clear tone of voice when speaking and by using clear and appropriate language and vocabulary (see the section on communication methods for more information). An assertive style of communication creates a respectful, relaxed and warm environment to communicate in. This style of communication can enhance the ways that others view you, as a professional who has the knowledge and skills and is able to convey this through the way that they carry out their role. At the same time, you should ensure that you respect the individual's rights to their opinions and their right to be assertive. This mutual respect can therefore lead to positive communications.

- **Enabling:** this style of communication can show your ability to communicate with individuals in a way that supports individuals to take the lead in communications so that they feel in control of the interaction. You can show an enabling style of communication by always taking the lead from the individual and letting them tell you about their communication preferences; in this way the individual will feel in control and competent to be able to state their needs clearly.
- **Flexible:** this style of communication can show your ability to adapt to different situations and meet individuals' needs. You can show a flexible style of communication by being observant in relation to what the individual is communicating both verbally and non-verbally through tone and pitch, body language and gestures and then responding to this appropriately using the form of communication that the individual is using with you. You will need to be both patient and creative. For example, if an individual with dementia starts using gestures rather than words, then you could interact with them in the same way; this will make the individual feel you are communicating with them at their level. Similarly, you may need to adjust the level of language that you use depending on the person you are speaking to. For example, a person with a learning disability may find it difficult to understand you if you use long, complex sentences or jargon.
- **Professional:** this style of communication can show your ability to communicate with different individuals appropriately in different situations. For example, the verbal and non-verbal communication methods you use to communicate with an individual who is feeling very upset may involve using reassuring words or placing your hand on their shoulder to show your empathy and understanding. The communication methods you use with an individual who is very agitated may involve little or no speech and no touch; instead you may decide that you are going to increase the personal space between you and the individual so that they can have an opportunity to calm down.

There are also a number of things that you should avoid. For example, you should not sit with crossed arms and legs as this suggests you are not open to what the individual has to say. Instead actively show that you are listening by appropriate body language, leaning forward, nodding and showing genuine interest in what the individual has to say. You should not interrupt when the individual is speaking as this suggests that you do not care for what they have to say, nor should you dismiss what they have to say. Instead, value their fears and concerns and be understanding and empathetic towards them. Make sure you focus on the individual and what is best for them rather than giving your own opinions and advice based on your own life experience. Instead focus on giving them the knowledge and information they need to make their own informed choices and decisions, thus ensuring your practice is person-centred.

> **Reflect on it**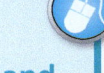
>
> **4.2 Reflecting on communications and interactions**
>
> Reflect on an occasion when you communicated with someone else such as an individual with care or support needs, or a friend or a family member, but it did not work the way you intended it to.
>
> What happened? Why do you think the communication wasn't effective? What communication method and style did you use and why?
>
> What could you have done differently? What might have been the impact if you had done this?

Communication methods

Written communication uses words that are written down to share ideas, thoughts, emotions and information. It can also be adapted to individuals' needs and may take the form of single words, phrases or sentences.

Written communication is also used to communicate information by colleagues, managers and professionals, with individuals and their families such as in the form of letters, reports, and daily records. Written communication can be used both in the form of paper records but also in the form of electronic records and online such as in emails and text messages.

Table 5.12 includes examples of how non-verbal communication methods can be used to meet individuals' needs. Table 5.13 includes examples of how verbal communication methods can be used to meet individuals' needs.

Table 5.12 Non-verbal communication methods and how you can use them to meet the needs of individuals

Non-verbal communication methods	How you can use non-verbal communication methods to meet individuals' needs
Braille	● **Braille** can be used as a method of written communication using characters that are represented by patterns of raised dots that are felt with the fingertips and used by individuals who are blind. Braille is not only available on paper; some smart phones can offer Braille and also keyboards for PCs are available in Braille meaning that individuals with sight loss can access the internet and communicate with others using the internet and social networking sites such as Facebook. ● Being able to read Braille if you are sighted will mean that you will be able to communicate with an individual who uses it and engage in communications with them. ● An individual may use Braille and other similar forms of communication differently depending on their needs. For example, individuals who have sight loss and other communication difficulties may use Moon, which is similar to Braille and based on touch but instead of dots, letters are represented by 14 raised characters at various angles.
Eye contact	● Making eye contact with an individual can be used to gain their trust and engage the individual. Some individuals may prefer to avoid eye contact, and this may be due to their culture so don't maintain eye contact during communications if this is the case, as this may make these individuals feel uncomfortable. ● Eye contact should be used intermittently rather than for longer periods as doing so may create tension and lead to an awkward atmosphere. For example, you may do so when empathising with an individual who is worried about going into hospital for an operation. ● Eye contact can also be a way of an individual expressing their choice, for example, of a drink they wish to have or a person they wish to see. Every individual will use eye contact in different ways; some may prefer to look at the item, others may prefer to blink when the item or person's name is spoken to them. ● Avoiding eye contact is not always a negative sign, and in some cultures it is actually a sign of respect. It is important to be aware that your own cultural traditions may differ from those of the individuals you care for.

Table 5.12 Non-verbal communication methods and how you can use them to meet the needs of individuals *continued*

Non-verbal communication methods	How you can use non-verbal communication methods to meet individuals' needs
Touch	• Touch can be a way of letting an individual know that you want to speak to them. For example, you may place your hand on the top of a deafblind individual's arm when you enter the room to let them know you are there or you may use your finger to fingerspell your name on the palm of a deafblind individual's hand. • Touch can be a method of showing your empathy. For example, an individual may have received some sad news and may be upset. Placing your hand on an individual's shoulder may show that you are empathising with their sad news. • Touch can also be a method of providing reassurance. For example, when an individual has had a fall they may be frightened that they will have another fall and be less likely to want to mobilise again. Offering a supporting arm or placing your hand in theirs can encourage them to mobilise again and gradually increase their confidence. • Touch may also be useful when supporting someone with a visual or hearing impairment, where they are unable to see your facial expressions, so there may be times when you need to place a reassuring hand on the individual's shoulder, for example, but always check with them first, and allow them to guide and direct you. • You should always check whether individuals are happy to have their hand held or have a reassuring hand on their shoulder. You can do this simply by asking the individual if they are happy to receive a hug, or have their hand held. At times, the individual will show if they find touch acceptable through their body language. However, they may not do this if they do not want to cause offence and so it is important to check with them. This will mean that the only interaction that takes place is that which the individual is comfortable with. • Rules around touch also vary according to the culture and beliefs of the individual so it is important that you do some research to find out if a hug or handshake is okay. You could ask them or their family members or relatives. It will be important to think about factors such as the gender, age and religion of the individual. For example, an older woman may find it acceptable to have her hand held by a female adult care worker, but not by a male care worker.
Gestures	• Physical gestures can be used with or without words and can express how you are feeling. For example, this may involve face, hand and/or gestures with other parts of the body. • Facial gestures such as a smile or a nod of the head can show your agreement. Nodding your head can have different meanings to different individuals and can mean the opposite of what you intend, for example a nod may mean a 'No' instead of a 'Yes' as you intended. • An open body posture where your arms and legs are not crossed when sitting down talking to an individual can show the individual that you are interested in what they are saying. Crossed arms and legs suggest a 'closed' posture and could be interpreted as you hiding something.

Table 5.12 Non-verbal communication methods and how you can use them to meet the needs of individuals *continued*

Non-verbal communication methods	How you can use non-verbal communication methods to meet individuals' needs
Body language	- Your body can also show how you are feeling and gives out non-verbal messages with or without you realising, so it's always a good idea to pay attention to what your body language is saying and how it will be interpreted by the individual. - For example, if you lean towards an individual when speaking to them this can mean that you are interested in what they are saying, but too much may make them feel uncomfortable as you are stepping into their personal space and may mean they withdraw from the communication. - Rolling your eyes, looking away or yawning when an individual is talking to you may indicate that you are bored or disinterested in what they are saying because you are too tired to listen. This will make the individual less likely to want to communicate. - Crossing your legs and arms also conveys a 'closed' posture, suggesting that you may not be open to what the individual has to say.
Proximity	- Your proximity when communicating with individuals is also important to take into account, because it can be interpreted in different ways. - For example, if you sit down next to an individual when they are telling you about a shopping trip they have been on, you are showing the individual that you are genuinely interested in what they are telling you. - Sitting too close to an individual, however, may make them feel awkward or embarrassed and this may make the individual less likely to continue their conversation with you. - Maintaining too big a distance from individuals you are communicating with will make it more difficult for them to communicate with you, because they may not hear what you are saying or see the facial gestures you are using. - For example, sitting at one end of the room when explaining to a group of individuals how to participate in a cookery session instead of sitting closer to them may mean that some individuals will not engage with you and may lose interest in the session.
Behaviour	- How you behave when you communicate with individuals is important. Positive behaviour encourages positive communications because it promotes mutual trust and respect. - For example, sitting upright and not slumping in your chair when speaking with an individual will show that you are paying attention to them and that you are taking a genuine interest. - Pacing up and down, leaving the room and re-entering or doing small jobs while talking to someone that involve moving or walking away from the individual, not paying attention to the individual or turning your back on them will give out messages that you are not listening to what they are saying; this may result in the individual withdrawing from the communication.

Table 5.13 Verbal communication methods and how you can use them to meet the needs of individuals

Verbal communication methods	How you can use verbal communication methods to meet individuals' needs
Words	• The spoken words you use can be adapted to meet individuals' specific needs. For example, you may use short, single words to make yourself understood when speaking to an individual with dementia rather than long sentences or phrases that the individual may find confusing and not be able to understand. • The level of vocabulary you use can also be adapted. For example, an individual who has limited understanding because of a disability may understand basic words but not be able to understand complex ones. • The type of vocabulary you use is also important to consider when meeting individuals' needs. Too much jargon may mean that the individual cannot understand what you are saying. Similarly, an individual who speaks a language that is different to your own may misunderstand regional vocabulary such as 'peepers' (meaning eyes) or 'tea' (meaning dinner). • Repeating phrases and what the individual is saying can also show that you are listening and be encouraging for the individual. • Asking a mixture of open and closed questions will allow you to gauge different responses. Open questions starting with 'how', 'what', 'why', 'where' and 'when', such as 'how did you feel when your daughter visited you?' will encourage individuals to speak in more detail and help build your relationship. Closed questions such as 'would you like to go to the shops?' will allow you to receive more straightforward 'yes' or 'no' responses.
Voice and tone	• Your linguistic tone when speaking to others can be adapted in different ways to meet individuals' needs; for example, by speaking in a quieter tone when empathising with an individual who is anxious about moving home. • You can also use your linguistic tone to create a positive mood when communicating with individuals. For example, a positive, pleasant tone of voice can be motivating when encouraging an individual with depression to leave their home and go out to socialise with others. • Your linguistic tone can also create different feelings that individuals can sense when you communicate with them. For example, an abrupt linguistic tone will not encourage communication between you and the individual.
Voice and pitch	• Similarly, the pitch of your voice when speaking to an individual can also create different feelings and moods during communications. It is important to be aware of this so that you can ensure your pitch mirrors your intended message. • For example, when listening to an individual who is excitedly telling you about a new skill they have learned such as cooking or a language, you can show your excitement for their news by congratulating them using a high pitch of voice when saying 'Well done!' • By contrast, a low pitch of voice may be more appropriate for when an individual is confiding in you. For example, they may be sharing with you the concerns they have over their future care needs as their illness progresses or a sad event that they have experienced in their life.
Spoken communication	• Spoken communication may take the form of single words that an individual can understand, e.g. 'park', 'lunch', 'happy', 'sad', or may include words combined in phrases and sentences, e.g. 'Did you enjoy the park?', 'What did you have for lunch today?', 'Are you happy with the outcome of your meeting?', 'Why are you feeling sad?' • Spoken communication may also take the form of informal conversations with individuals and their families or formal presentations such as to colleagues.

Table 5.13 Verbal communication methods and how you can use them to meet the needs of individuals *continued*

Verbal communication methods	How you can use verbal communication methods to meet individuals' needs
Silence	- Silence during communications can also be used to provide the person with the space they need in order to say or express what they want to communicate, without feeling pressurised or rushed. - Silence can also act as a form of support to the person, because it shows that you are genuinely listening to what they have communicated. - For example, you can use silence to provide space when an individual is telling you about a difficult situation they experienced. - Silence in the situation described above will also demonstrate that you've listened carefully to what the person has experienced and are taking it seriously. It provides both reassurance and support to the person.

Table 5.14 Additional methods to support communication

Additional communication methods	How you can use additional communication methods to meet individuals' needs
Signs	- Sign language can be used to communicate with individuals in different ways depending on how they use this. - For example, although two different individuals may use British Sign Language (BSL) they may use the same sign to mean a different word or may express it slightly differently. Knowing the individual and the signs they use is key to avoiding misunderstandings. - Individuals with learning disabilities may use their own adapted form of sign language to communicate with others. They may use signs to mean phrases or signs alongside words and/or gestures. Knowing the meanings of these will help you to be able to understand an individual's needs.
Symbols	- Symbols can be used to communicate with individuals and can represent objects, actions, people, places and events. Communication with symbols can be useful for individuals who have limited speech or who cannot sign or who prefer not to sign. - For example, Makaton combines signs, symbols and speech and can be used with individuals who have learning disabilities and communication needs. A symbol showing a 'thumbs up' can be used to communicate when something is good. A symbol showing a 'happy face' can be used by an individual to express how they are feeling to their support worker. - For example, Blissymbols is another system of symbols used by individuals who are unable to communicate by using speech. The symbols consist of simple shapes that are fast and easy to draw, some look like what they represent such as a circle to represent the sun and others represent ideas such as half a circle to represent the mind. - For example, Picture Communication Symbols (PCS) are symbols that consist of black and white line drawings and can be used to communicate with individuals who have a range of communication and language needs. A high contrast picture communication symbol consists of a simple, brightly coloured symbol with a dark background so it can be clearly seen by an individual with a visual impairment.

Table 5.14 Additional methods to support communication *continued*

Additional communication methods	How you can use additional communication methods to meet individuals' needs
Pictures	• Pictorial information can be used with or without words. When used with words it can often reinforce the meanings of communications. For example, a list of recreational activities for an individual to choose from could be accompanied by pictures or photographs of each activity to ensure the individual understands what each activity involves. • Pictorial information such as photographs can also be used by some individuals without words and as a substitute for words. For example, in response to an individual wanting to know whether they are having any visitors today, you could show them the photographs of the people that will be visiting them. • Pictorial information must be used sensitively, and it is important that it represents the messages you intend to give out. It should include images that are positive and representative. For example, using images of only young female women or individuals from specific cultures may mean that individuals from other genders and cultures will not be able to relate to these and therefore communications may be more difficult. Ensuring pictorial information is representative of individuals' diverse needs is important.

Communication skills

You will find it useful to review your previous learning for AC 1.3 where you explored the different skills required to be an effective communicator. After reading through this section again complete the activity below.

Evidence opportunity

4.2 Range of communication styles, methods and skills to meet an individual's needs

Read through the case scenario below and then demonstrate to your assessor a range of communication styles, methods and skills that you can use to meet the needs of Mr J, who has a hearing loss.

You are Mr J's personal assistant. You see Mr J walking down the corridor towards you. He looks angry, is waving his arms above his head and is shouting at the top of his voice: 'My sister hasn't visited me again this evening and I've been waiting for her all day!'.

Think about why you selected these communication styles, methods and skills. What could be the impact of using these on Mr J? What would the impact be on the communication? What would the impact be on your working relationship with Mr J?

You could also provide a written account detailing your responses to these questions.

Reflect on it

4.2 Meeting an individual's needs

Think about an individual you care for or support. What skills do you use to meet their individual needs? Why do you use each of these skills? How do they impact on the individual?

AC 4.3 Demonstrate how to respond appropriately to an individual's reaction when communicating

Your work practices will be observed for this assessment criterion; you will have to demonstrate how to respond appropriately to an individual's reaction when communicating.

As you have learned, there are a diverse range of communication methods and styles you can use to respond to an individual's reactions during communications that may include, for example, individuals being non-responsive, distracted, happy, angry, upset or anxious.

The following are some top tips for how to respond appropriately to an individual's reactions when communicating with them:

1 **Listen carefully:** active listening is key to understanding an individual's reactions and how they are feeling. Think about what you have learned earlier on in this unit about body language, eye contact and the importance of

not only listening to what an individual is saying verbally but also what they are saying through their body language and gestures. Leaning forward, nodding and maintaining eye contact will show your interest and may help the individual to feel more confident when speaking to you. Appropriate facial expressions and reactions will also display that you are paying close attention to what the individual is saying. For example, a serious expression in a conversation of a serious nature will be more appropriate. Of course, this should come naturally but this is also something you can learn, practise and improve.

2 **Respond accurately:** this involves you responding not only to the words that individuals say but also to the way individuals act and behave. It is important to observe an individual's verbal and non-verbal reactions when communicating with them so that you can respond appropriately. For example, if you ask an individual whether they want to go out on the train and they do not respond, find out what their non-response means. Do not assume they do not want to go out on the train. The individual may not have responded because they have not understood the question, because they have not heard because of background noise or because their hearing aid is not working. Investigate further – perhaps you need to repeat the question clearly or use another form of communication such as a photograph of a train.

3 **Respond promptly:** this involves you taking action immediately; delaying responding to an individual's reactions when communicating is not an option. For example, if you are communicating with an individual with a learning disability and you notice that they become easily distracted when doing so then this could be a sign that the individual is not understanding what you are saying or does understand what you are saying but is finding the communication difficult. It is important to acknowledge to the individual that you've noticed that they appear distracted; not saying anything may make the individual think that you're not interested in what they have to say. It is also a good way of gaining their attention and once you have this you can try and use a different form of communication with them.

You can do this in a positive and supportive way by asking them what support they would like to participate in the communication with you.

Reflect on it

4.2, 4.3 Difficult communications

Reflect on an occasion when you found a communication with someone else difficult. For example, this may have been because you couldn't understand what they were saying, or you were in a rush and didn't have time to communicate with the person or you didn't like the way the person spoke to you.

How did you feel? Why? Did you show the person you were communicating with that you were finding the communication difficult? How did you do this? Was it verbally? Non-verbally? How did the other person respond to you? Why? Was this helpful? If not, why not?

Write a short reflective account addressing the questions above.

4 **Respond appropriately:** this involves you demonstrating your empathy, in other words showing that you can relate to how an individual is feeling. For example, if an individual is sharing with you that they've had a very enjoyable weekend with their family then it would be appropriate for you to respond showing that you are pleased for them. You can do this by paying attention to the tone and pitch of your voice when communicating with the individual, i.e. you could use a higher pitch and an excited tone that creates a happy feeling to the interaction. By contrast, if an individual is upset over experiencing a recent family bereavement you would need to adapt your tone and pitch to reflect that you empathise with the individual, i.e. by using a lower, quieter tone.

5 **Respond professionally:** this involves you recognising that when responding to an individual's reactions when communicating you have a duty of care towards every individual to ensure their safety, health and wellbeing. Duty of care is covered in more detail in Unit 303.

	Dos and don'ts for responding appropriately to an individual's reactions
Do	**Listen actively.** Listen to what the individual has to say to you so that you respond appropriately. Listen to the tone and pitch of their voice as this will convey their emotions and how they are feeling. It may be that they are speaking in an unusually loud voice, or faster or slower than usual.
Do	**Look at the individual's eyes and the contact that they are trying to make.** Check to see whether they make direct eye contact or if they avoid eye contact. It may be that the individual does not feel comfortable or confident in speaking to you.
Do	**Ask questions to check how the individual is feeling.** This might be a simple 'Are you all right?' or 'Is there anything that is upsetting you? Would you like to speak to me about it? If you'd rather not speak to me, is there anyone else you would like to speak to?'
Do	**Look out for overall changes in behaviour and behavioural patterns and moods.** It may be that the individual's reactions in a one-to-one conversation are part of a bigger shift in behaviour. It may be that someone you have cared for and know to be mild-mannered has suddenly become rather violent. Or someone who is normally positive and bubbly looks withdrawn and distressed. Changes in their health may also be indicators of other things. For example, they may be experiencing cardiovascular/heart-related issues due to stressful situations (issues at work, with family or bereavement for example). Having this information and understanding the triggers for any changes in behaviour will allow you to better understand the individual's reactions during your communications and respond to an individual's needs.
Do	**Look out for signs of distress so that you can tailor your communications appropriately.** Sometimes these will be very obvious in the individual's physical reactions. For example, you might notice that they are fidgeting and showing unease. There may be even more concerning health issues visible such as heavy breathing.
Don't	**Forget the things that you have learned about effective communication skills.** For example, remember to retain eye contact in your interactions but not to stare; remember rules around personal space and ensuring the individual is comfortable; show that you are actively listening to the individual by leaning forward and having an open body posture where you are not crossing your arms and legs; remember the rules around touch and only doing this if this is acceptable with the individual. Remember how important it is to understand what is acceptable based on the individual's culture.
Don't	**Ignore body language.** Pay attention to how the individual is seated. Are they sitting upright, and looking relaxed? This might show that they are feeling confident and happy. Are they leaning towards you? This might show that they are interested in what you have to say. However, someone who is slouching in their seat or who has their arms and legs crossed, sitting back in their chair shows signs of low confidence and disinterest.

Case study

2.3, 4.3 Factors to consider when promoting effective communication and how to respond appropriately to an individual's reactions when communicating

Mira's mother lives on her own and has always had a good relationship with her daughter; they usually spend hours talking on the phone and Mira visits every weekend. A few weeks ago, Mira started noticing that her mother didn't always pick up the phone when she rang in the evenings and when she did she appeared distracted and not really interested in what she was saying. In fact, on more than one occasion Mira's mother told Mira she wasn't in the mood to waste her time speaking on the phone and put the phone down mid-way through their conversation.

Mira is really upset by her mother's behaviour towards her and is thinking about not telephoning her as much or visiting her every weekend.

Discuss:
1. What factors could be causing Mira's mother to respond in this way?
2. Discuss how Mira should respond to her mother's reactions during their communications and the reasons why.

> **Evidence opportunity**
>
> **2.1, 4.3** Responding to an individual's reactions, and communication methods and styles
>
> Demonstrate to your assessor how you respond to an individual's reactions when communicating. For example, an individual may be anxious or upset over something that has happened to them (AC 4.3).
>
> Make sure you demonstrate a range of communication methods and styles to meet the individual's needs (AC 2.1).

AC 4.4 Demonstrate professionalism when using a range of different communication methods

Being able to meet the communication and language needs, wishes and preferences of individuals also involves being able to demonstrate professionalism when using different communication methods. Professionalism involves doing your job to the best of your ability so that you can be a good role model and an inspiration to others.

Professionalism when communicating with others means demonstrating for example:

- your expertise and knowledge, e.g. using British Sign Language with an individual who is deaf.
- your competence, e.g. using verbal and non-verbal communication methods when communicating with an individual
- your approach, e.g. being polite and respectful when communicating with an individual.
- your integrity, e.g. being honest when communicating with individuals.
- your ability to adapt, e.g. being able to use different communication methods, skills and styles so the communication is appropriate to the individual and takes into account their unique needs.

> **Reflect on it**
>
> **4.4** What does being a professional mean to you?
>
> Think about what being a professional means to you. How do you demonstrate your professionalism at work? What do you do and how do you do it? Why? Think about other professionals you know in the care setting/service where you work. What makes them professionals?

> **Evidence opportunity**
>
> **4.4** Demonstrating professionalism
>
> You will be observed for this assessment criterion. You will need to demonstrate your professionalism when using a range of different communication methods with individuals. Your manager could also provide a Witness Testimony.

LO5 Understand the role of independent advocacy services in supporting individuals to communicate their needs, wishes and preferences

> **Getting started**
>
> Think about an occasion when you were unable to speak up for yourself. For example, perhaps you were feeling unwell or tired and unable to put forward to others what you wanted to say. How did this make you feel? Did you access any support? If so, who and why?

AC 5.1 Explain the purpose and principles of independent advocacy

As you will have learned in AC 2.6, independent advocacy services support people to speak up for themselves when they are unable to do so because of a condition or a disability, thus ensuring any barriers to communication are overcome and

Table 5.15 Independent advocacy

Independent advocacy is …	Independent advocacy is not …
Speaking up and representing individuals and/or groups who are unable to do so for themselves.	Speaking up for individuals and/or groups when they are able to do so for themselves.
Actively listening to individuals/groups, getting to know and understand them, their views, wishes and concerns.	Telling individuals/groups what you think they should do, putting others' views and interests before those of individuals/groups.
Enabling individuals/groups to understand what options they have and make their own choices by exploring with them the full range of options, their benefits and drawbacks.	Providing individuals/groups with information and advice about the options that you think are suitable for them and making decisions for them.

individuals' views are heard. Independent advocacy services are separate from other organisations that provide services to individuals such as the NHS, housing organisations or providers of care and support such as the care setting where you work. In this way, they can ensure that they truly represent only the views of the individuals they are representing, and have no other vested interest in the service that may make them biased or cause a conflict when providing support and guidance.

Purposes of independent advocacy

The purposes of independent advocacy are:

- to empower individuals or groups to express their views and make them known to others, for example supporting individuals with learning disabilities to express their views in relation to the quality of local health services
- to safeguard individuals who are vulnerable, for example to support an individual in early stages of dementia to be in control of their future care and treatment options
- to speak up for individuals when they are unable to do so, for example they may speak up for an individual who has been detained in hospital for further treatment under the Mental Health Act 1983
- to enable individuals to gain access to information, for example they may enable an individual with a physical disability who is unhappy about the treatment they received from their GP to find out what their rights are and how they can make a complaint.

Principles of independent advocacy

The principles of independent advocacy are:

- the individuals who use independent advocacy are at the centre of the support or service provided; the individual's needs always come first
- the individuals who use independent advocacy are enabled to have more control over their lives; the individual is involved in making decisions, considering the options available to them and the advantages and disadvantages
- independent advocacy is an impartial service provided separately from other services and organisations and with no conflicts of interest
- independent advocacy aims to be accessible to everyone who needs it; referrals can be made directly by the individual and/or through other professionals and organisations.

Table 5.15 provides you with further information about what independent advocacy involves.

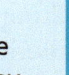

> **Reflect on it**
>
> **5.1 Advocacy**
>
> Reflect on an occasion when you were unable to speak up for yourself. For example, this may have been because you were feeling unwell or did not feel very confident to do so. How did this make you feel? Why?

The different types of independent advocacy

Independent advocacy can be provided in many different situations and for many different reasons. The following are examples of the different types of independent advocacy that can be provided:

One to one advocacy

One to one advocacy is provided on an individual basis for specific issues and can be both short term and long term. One to one advocacy workers can be both paid and unpaid. For example, an individual may require an advocate from the housing charity Shelter to support them at a meeting to discuss their housing options – the advocate could provide information about the options available and explore these with the individual.

Citizen advocacy is another example of one to one advocacy where people are encouraged to support an individual living in their community who may need their support. Citizen advocates are unpaid and usually provide long-term support. For example, an individual may require an advocate to support them to access their local health centre once a week as part of their wish to improve their health and wellbeing. The unpaid advocate may be living close to the individual and share an interest in health and fitness.

Peer advocacy is also one to one advocacy where advocates share their experiences with individuals to support them to develop their confidence and self-esteem. For example, a peer advocate may use their experience of being bullied at work to empathise with an individual who has also been bullied.

Group advocacy

Group advocacy is provided on a group basis to individuals who share experiences, views or interests. For example, a group of people with mental health needs may be finding it difficult to share their experiences of accessing services in their local community with their local authority. Group advocacy can enable the group to find alternative ways of raising their concerns and can enable them to feel more effective and influential as a group. The National Survivor User Network for Mental Health (NSUN) is an organisation made up of individuals and groups all over the UK that share their experiences of mental distress to provide a collective voice for those who have a mental health condition.

> **Research it**
>
> **5.1 Self-advocacy**
>
> Research the benefits of self-advocacy for individuals with disabilities. You may find Disability Rights UK's website a useful source of information: www.disabilityrightsuk.org/self-advocacy
>
> Produce a factsheet with your findings.

Self-advocacy

Self-advocacy is the basis of all types of independent advocacy and empowers individuals to increase their confidence and self-awareness so that they develop the skills to self-advocate, in other words to speak up for themselves. Self-advocacy can be provided by both paid and unpaid advocates to both individuals and groups, on a short-term and long-term basis. An individual with a learning disability may seek to self-advocate so that they can feel more confident when discussing their wishes and preferences with their family.

Statutory advocacy

Statutory advocacy is provided to individuals who are legally entitled to an advocate. There are three types: Independent Mental Health Advocates (IMHAs), Independent Mental Capacity Advocates (IMCAs) and Care and Support Advocates.

Independent Mental Health Advocates are trained advocates who provide support to individuals accessing or receiving treatment under the Mental Health Act 1983. For example, the IMHA may support the individual to understand their rights under the Mental Health Act 1983 and the treatment.

> **Evidence opportunity**
>
> **5.1 Purposes and principles of independent advocacy**
>
> Explain to your assessor the purposes and principles of independent advocacy in relation to two individuals with care or support needs from the care setting where you work. Provide a written account of your explanation or discussion.

Independent Mental Capacity Advocates are also trained advocates who provide support to individuals who lack capacity under the Mental Capacity Act 2005. For example, the IMCA may act on an individual's behalf if the individual lacks capacity to make decisions in relation to plans for their long-term care, for example living in a residential care home as opposed to continuing to live at home.

Care and Support Advocates are trained advocates who provide support and representation to individuals under the Care Act 2014 so that they are involved in exploring the options available and the decisions made in relation to their care and support needs. For example, a Care and Support Advocate may support an individual during a review of their care or support plan to understand what care or support will be provided as well as to express their wishes and feelings about the options available.

AC 5.2 Outline when to offer support to individuals to access advocacy services

As you have learned, independent advocacy can be provided for many different reasons. But how do you know when to offer support to individuals? You don't want to involve an advocate unnecessarily or not involve an advocate when you should. Perhaps there has been a change in an individual's needs that means that they are no longer able to speak up for themselves due, for example, to the onset of a medical condition or being temporarily unwell. Perhaps the individual is finding it difficult to make their views or wishes known and is agreeing with everything you and others are saying. Perhaps you feel that the individual's rights are at risk of being ignored and involving an advocate would safeguard these. Perhaps the individual, an individual's relative and/or a care worker has requested an advocate be involved to provide independent and direct support to the individual, for example when the individual's care or support plan is being reviewed, or during an assessment of the individual's needs to discuss their future care and/or support.

> ### Reflect on it
>
> **5.2 Qualities that an advocate should have**
>
> Imagine that you require an advocate to help plan for your future care needs. What kind of qualities do you think are important for an advocate to have?
>
> For example, you may feel that you need to be able to trust and confide in them. How important is it that they are assertive and patient?

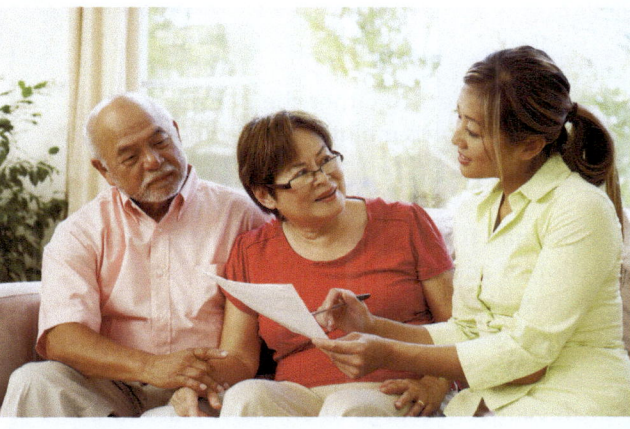

Figure 5.5 Do you know when to involve an advocate?

Other occasions when it may be necessary or desirable to involve an advocate and offer individuals support to do so include finding somewhere to live or moving to a new house, getting a job, making new friends, learning a new skill and/or using health or social care services.

AC 5.3 Explain how to support individuals to access advocacy services

The first action you should take if you think you may need to involve an advocate on behalf of an individual is to make your suggestion to your manager who will be able to advise you. Similarly, if another care worker reports to you that they think an individual requires an advocate then find out from the care worker what their concerns are and the reasons why they think the individual requires an advocate and report these immediately to your manager. It is important to document your suggestion or a care worker's concerns as well as the actions that have been taken by you and your manager so that there is a clear **audit trail** of the actions taken.

If you are a Lead Personal Assistant and the individual you work for is also your employer and you think the individual may require an advocate, discuss this with the individual and/or their representative. Again, it is important to document what actions you have taken and the reasons why, for example that you have been asked to access advocacy services on behalf of the individual or the individual has refused.

If you are asked by an individual or their family directly about supporting them to access advocacy services, it is important though that you first check the process that you are required to follow in the care setting where you work; you can do this by

> **Key terms**
>
> **Audit trail** refers to either the paper-based or electronic records maintained about an activity or situation.
>
> **Community treatment order** enables you to be discharged from hospital when you have been sectioned and treated in hospital as long as you meet certain conditions such as living in a certain place or accessing medical treatment.
>
> **Responsible clinician** refers to the mental health professional in charge of an individual's care and treatment while the individual is sectioned under the Mental Health Act.
>
> **Approved mental health professional** refers to the mental health professional responsible for co-ordinating an individual's assessment and admission to hospital when the individual is sectioned. These professionals can be nurses, adult social care workers, psychologists or occupational therapists.

accessing the care setting's agreed ways of working for involving advocates and accessing advocacy services as well as discussing this with your manager. There are different ways of accessing advocacy services depending on the type of advocacy the individual requires; below are some examples of how you can access different services:

- **One to one advocacy:** You can approach organisations that offer one to one advocacy directly. For example, Shelter, the housing and homelessness charity, accepts referrals directly from individuals and/or their representatives over the telephone via their free, confidential and independent helpline, via email and in person at one of their advice centres. You will be asked to provide the name and address of the individual and your organisation's name and address as well as other information such as details of the difficulties being experienced by the individual, the actions taken to date, and the local authority where the individual currently lives.
A one to one advocate service may also be provided by someone who knows the individual well, perhaps by a friend or a neighbour who shares similar interests with the individual.
In these situations, the person may also be approached directly.

- **Group advocacy:** Organisations that offer group advocacy can also be approached directly. For example, the National Autistic Society (NAS), like most organisations, provides different types of advocacy including group advocacy. NAS can be approached directly via their helpline or indirectly through an adviser at the individual's local Citizens Advice Bureau. NAS can put you and/or the individual in contact with groups in their local area that share the same interests or concerns that they can meet up with.

- **Self-advocacy:** Advocates who support individuals to speak up for themselves can usually be accessed through the organisations they are employed by. For example, Mencap provides access to a number of 'Speaking Up' groups all over the UK where individuals with learning disabilities are supported to meet with other individuals with learning disabilities in their local area, get involved in their communities and learn how to become more confident in speaking up for themselves and making their voices heard. Individuals can make self-referrals to these groups; third party referrals are also accepted.

- **Statutory advocacy:** Under the Mental Health Act 1983 you are entitled to an Independent Mental Health Advocate (IMHA) if you are what is known as a 'qualifying patient'. This means that you have a right to an IMHA if you satisfy certain conditions, for example if you are detained or liable to be detained under the Mental Health Act 1983 or you are subject to a **community treatment order**. The individual can request an IMHA at any point after they have become a 'qualifying patient' by asking a member of staff or their **responsible clinician** or an **approved mental health professional**. If an individual lacks the capacity to request an IMHA then the manager of the hospital must request for an IMHA to visit the individual.

- **Independent Mental Capacity Advocates (IMCAs)** represent individuals who lack the capacity to make decisions. Individuals may access the support of an IMCA when there is no one independent of services available to represent them, such as a family member or friend. Each local area in the

UK will have an IMCA service provided by different organisations. To access this service an individual must be referred by a specific professional such as their doctor because an IMCA can only support an individual as per the conditions set out in the Mental Capacity Act. For example, an individual may lack capacity to make a decision or there may be no one independent of services, such as a family member or friend, who is appropriate to consult and so they may access the services of an IMCA.

- **Care and Support Advocates** who provide support to individuals under the Care Act 2014 can be accessed through the local authority where the individual lives. Care and support advocacy is not provided by the local authority, but it can refer individuals to independent organisations in the local area that provide care and support advocacy. Alternatively, individuals can refer themselves for care and support advocacy or be referred by their representative who may be a family member or advocate, for example. Examples of organisations who provide care and support advocates include both national and local organisations such as: seAp Advocacy, Empower me service through Mencap, Diabetes UK Advocacy service, Age UK, VoiceAbility.

Research it

5.2, 5.3 The Care Act 2014 and advocacy services

Research the impact of the Care Act 2014 on the provision of advocacy services and discuss your findings with your assessor. You may find SCIE's guide, '6 ways to better advocacy under the Care Act' a useful source of information.

Evidence opportunity

5.2, 5.3 When and how to support individuals to access advocacy services

Explain to your assessor when to offer support to individuals to access advocacy services and demonstrate the process to follow for supporting them to access the advocacy service. Provide a written account explaining when you would involve an advocate and how to support individuals to access advocacy services.

LO6 Understand confidentiality in care settings/services

Getting started

Think about a sensitive piece of information that only a few people know about you. For example, this may be in relation to your family background or an experience you had at school or at work. Who would you trust with this personal information? Why? How would you feel if the person you shared this information with told you they would have to share it with someone else you didn't know? Why?

AC 6.1 Explain the meaning of the term confidentiality

AC 6.2 Explain the importance of maintaining confidentiality when communicating with others

Confidentiality is an essential part of providing good quality care and support to individuals who have care and support needs as it aims to protect the personal information of individuals and their families from being shared or made known to others who have no right to access it or use it.

As a Lead Adult Care Worker or a Lead Personal Assistant your job will involve accessing individuals' personal information and therefore it is essential that you uphold individuals' rights to privacy when doing this. This may be in relation to their family background, their date of birth, their medical treatment, or their care or support needs. As all these items of information are personal to individuals, it is important that they are kept private and that their details are restricted to only those who have authorisation to access them; this may include you, your colleagues, or other members of the team. As an adult care worker, you will need to ensure that you do not disclose any personal information without the consent of the individual.

Your role will also involve you accessing the personal information of others. For example, as a Lead Adult Care Worker you will be responsible for monitoring and supporting other care workers in the team. This may involve accessing information that is personal to them, for example in relation to their training needs, their sickness records, or their next of kin details. All this information is confidential and must therefore be treated with care so that it remains private.

Individuals should be supported to understand how policies around confidentiality affect them, and what their rights are. They should also be supported in contributing to records about them. You would have to take into account the best way to involve individuals – this means finding out about their communication preferences, including those in relation to culture and disabilities, and taking these factors into account.

'Need to know'

Individuals have the right to have all personal information obtained from them and held about them kept private. Sometimes there may be occasions when it may be necessary to share their personal information with others in confidence. This process of sharing confidential information with others is referred to as doing so on a 'need to know basis' only. This means that only relevant information is shared with only those who require it.

Respecting confidentiality and how this can impact positively on working relationships

Protecting the confidentiality of those you care for and work with is key to maintaining strong working relationships as it means that others will consider you as a professional who can be trusted not to share their private details, and that you will not breach their trust. It will also mean that individuals feel that both they and the information they share is protected. This can impact positively not just on the relationships in the work setting but also in terms of the individual's wellbeing where they feel valued and respected.

Data Protection Act 2018

In your role, you will make and keep records for various reasons, whether it is to document an individual's care, health or the activities they have taken part in – whatever the reason, this information will be shared and used in various ways.

The Data Protection Act 2018 places strong emphasis on confidentiality and a duty for organisations to report certain types of breaches when it comes to personal data. You can find more information on this here: https://ico.org.uk/for-organisations-2/guide-to-data-protection/guide-to-the-general-data-protection-regulation-gdpr/personal-data-breaches/ and here: www.gov.uk/data-protection

It would also be useful for you to read about the DPA and discuss how this will affect you as a Lead Adult Care Worker or Personal Assistant. If you work in a care setting, you could also find out how your setting's agreed ways of working reflect the DPA with regard to keeping records and information as well as the types of information you are able to retain and the information you must discard.

Reflect on it

6.1, 6.2 Meaning and importance of confidentiality where you work

Reflect on your job role and the meaning of confidentiality in the care setting where you work. Why is it important? Reflect on the individuals, their families and others you work with. What does confidentiality mean to them? Compare your understanding of this term to their understanding of it – are there any similarities, differences? Write a reflective account addressing the points here.

Evidence opportunity

6.1, 6.2 Meaning and importance of the term 'confidentiality'

Discuss with your assessor the meaning of confidentiality in relation to the care setting where you work. Why is this important? You could also provide a written account detailing what confidentiality means and why it is important.

AC 6.3 Explain why and when confidentiality may need to be breached

Obtaining consent from the individual and examples of when you may need to break confidentiality and pass on information without consent

It is important to remember that you cannot pass on information without the consent of the individual. You should not assume that the individual already understands this or will agree. However, there may be times when you will need to pass on information without the consent of the individual. For example, this may be when a young individual shares with you that a friend of theirs stole some goods from the local shop. In this instance, you would need to inform the person that it is your duty to pass this information on to your manager in the first instance. Your manager may then need to inform the police; if so, the individual will be informed of all actions taken and why they are required.

The role of a personal assistant

A personal assistant is employed directly by the individual with care or support needs or by a family member when the individual does not have the capacity to be the employer. If you are a personal assistant, you will have a contract of employment that will set out your rights and responsibilities as an employee including who you can share information with, such as doctors, and when this may be required, such as during hospital appointments. Sometimes, however, it may be necessary for you to share confidential information without your employer's consent. For example, if you identify that your employer is being abused you have a duty to report this to the council's safeguarding board.

In AC 6.4 we discuss the tension that may arise between your duty of care to protect the individual's confidentiality and the need to disclose concerns.

> **Evidence opportunity**
>
> **6.3 Necessary confidentiality breaches**
>
> Discuss with your assessor or manager why and when confidentiality may need to be breached.

6Cs

Courage

Courage may be required when you need to break confidentiality and pass on information if you believe that this is in the best interests of the individual. Not doing so may put the individual and others at risk. For example, if you do not disclose that an individual is being abused or harmed, then the abuse may get worse, and the individual's health and wellbeing may deteriorate.

Competence

Competence refers to effectively putting your knowledge and skills into practice. Doing so will show that you are able to provide high quality care and support to individuals. In this section, you can show that you are competent by demonstrating confidentiality in your day-to-day communications with individuals and others that you work with. This will include being competent and effectively putting into practice the knowledge and skills you have when recording and storing personal information and maintaining and promoting confidentiality in your daily communications with individuals, their families and colleagues, for example. Think about what you have learned in this AC. How can you show your competence in the different aspects we have discussed?

AC 6.4 Describe the potential tension between maintaining an individual's confidentiality and disclosing concerns

There are times when an individual's right to have their personal information kept confidential cannot be upheld and you need to disclose the concerns you have. When personal information is shared, it is done so in confidence and only with those who require it. Situations in which it is important to disclose information include those where:

- **there is a risk of abuse or neglect:** for example, if an individual tells you that they are going to harm themselves and they do not want you to tell anyone, you will not be able to keep this information confidential. Your **duty of care** towards the individual is to keep them safe and free from harm and therefore you will need to pass this information on to your manager in the first instance or if your employer is your manager then onto the Adult Social Care team. In this way you can show that you have taken action to prevent the individual from harming themselves.
- **someone is in danger:** for example, if a visitor to your care setting tells you that they overheard two individuals talking about another individual who lives in the home and how they are planning to challenge them in their room later that evening but that it was probably a joke and they therefore want you to keep it to yourself, you will not be able to keep this information confidential. Your duty of care towards the individual is to keep them free from danger but you also have a duty of care towards the two individuals who are planning this action to ensure that they do not become involved in something serious which could ultimately result in a crime being committed. You will need to pass this information on to your manager or to the Adult Social Care team. In this way you can show that you've taken action to prevent the individuals from coming to harm and becoming involved in a serious crime.
- **a crime has taken place or there is a potential risk that a crime may take place:** for example, if an individual's family tells you that they witnessed another individual who lives in the care setting stealing from the local shop and they ask you not to report it but to have a word with the individual instead because they have learning disabilities and probably did not fully understand what they were doing, you will not be able to keep this information confidential because a crime has been committed. You will need to pass this information on to your manager or to the Adult Social Care team. In this way you can show that you've taken action to report that a crime has taken place. The police will also need to be made aware if a serious crime has taken place.

Although it is easy to see why in some situations confidential information may need to be shared to protect individuals and others from danger, harm, abuse and neglect it is not so easy to disclose the information because very often the person making the disclosure will not want you to share this information with others. In addition, you may feel that disclosing the information will damage the relationship and trust you have with the person and may mean that they do not approach you in the future with their concerns.

> ### Reflect on it
>
> **6.4 'In confidence'**
>
> Reflect on how you would feel if you told a friend something about yourself in confidence, but they told you they would have to report it to someone else. How would you feel about your friendship? Why?

Managing the relationship with the individual

It is important to remember that as an adult care worker your duty to promote individuals' safety and wellbeing is of paramount importance. The tensions that arise between maintaining an individual's confidentiality and disclosing concerns can be managed by explaining to the person making the disclosure that although you will be sharing their personal information it will be kept confidential and will only be shared with a named person; this may be your manager, the safeguarding officer in the care setting where you work, or the social worker, for example. You can also explain that you have a legal duty of care as part of your job role to maintain their and others' safety and wellbeing and therefore you are following your responsibilities as part of your job role. Finally, you could show the person the policies and procedures of the care setting where you work to reassure the person that you are following an agreed way of working.

Remember:

- You must gain consent from the individual before disclosing any information unless the individual's safety is at risk, or if the safety of others is at risk. You must only disclose information if it is in the best interests of the individual and others 'need to know' in order to provide the best possible care for the individual.
- If you need to pass on information and the individual has not consented to the information being shared, you must still inform the individual that you will be sharing the information. This also applies if they have consented to information being shared. Make sure that they know what information will be shared exactly, and with whom.
- You must speak to your manager or a senior colleague before sharing any information with others.
- Refer to Unit 305 Handling information in adult care settings/services for information on the things you need to be aware of when sharing information.
- If you are a personal assistant, you may need to disclose your concerns to the police, medical or social services. Remember to inform the individual that you are doing so.

Research it

6.4 The Care Act 2014 and duty of care

Research what the Care Act 2014 says about the duty of care of care workers. How does this concept relate to the need to disclose confidential information? Develop a leaflet to present your findings.

As a personal assistant, the individual who you provide care and support to may also be your employer. This may make you feel awkward about disclosing any concerns you have about the individual, in the event of it affecting your employment with them. When you started your role as a personal assistant you should have received information and/or training about how to maintain confidentiality in your work. In terms of sharing information about the individual, they and/or their representative would have told you what information they would want passed on and what information they would not want passed on, with whom it can be shared and under what circumstances. There may be circumstances where you have to share information about the individual without their consent, such as in a medical emergency or if they have disclosed to you they have been abused or committed a criminal offence.

The reflective exemplar guides you in reflecting on the potential tension between maintaining an individual's confidentiality and disclosing concerns and the skills required to manage these situations effectively.

	Reflective exemplar
Introduction	I work as a Lead Personal Assistant with Si who has autism. My duties involve leading a team of personal assistants to enable Si, who lives at home with his parents, to maintain his independence.
What happened?	This morning at the end of my shift, Si's parents asked me whether they could speak to me in private. I agreed, and they proceeded to tell me how they overheard one of the personal assistants (PAs), who happens to be Si's favourite PA, tell Si that if he didn't get up in the next five minutes he wouldn't be eating for the rest of the day. Si's parents explained to me that although they didn't agree with what the PA said they thought that he probably didn't mean it as they know that he is very fond of Si and also because it was probably due to him being a little stressed; he had already been trying to encourage Si to get up for at least 30 minutes.
	I thanked Si's parents for telling me and explained that I would be reporting this to the office in the first instance. Si's parents stated immediately that they didn't want the PA getting into trouble or losing his job because he had developed such a good working relationship with Si. They asked whether I could just have a private word with the PA informally.
	As I was rushing off to carry out an assessment for another individual, I agreed with what they said and when I returned to the office reported what was disclosed to me in confidence as per the procedure. I also recorded what was said to me in private in the office on the allocated disclosure form and then handed this personally to the Office Manager.
What worked well?	I listened attentively to Si's parents and knew the process to follow when information needs to be disclosed. I was not persuaded by Si's parents to not follow the agreed ways of working.
What did not go as well?	I agreed with Si's parents without being honest with them or taking the time to explain in full what would happen next; this may mean that they do not approach me again with their concerns. I could have phoned the office and requested another Lead carry out the other individual's assessment or if this was not possible I could have rescheduled it for a time when I was available. In this way, I could have spent more time with Si's parents.
What could I do to improve?	I will need to revisit my previous training in how to manage situations such as this one where there are potential tensions between maintaining confidentiality and disclosing concerns. Perhaps I also need to work on my confidence level in managing situations such as this one.
Links to assessment criteria in this unit	ACs: 6.1, 6.2, 6.4

Evidence opportunity

6.4 Potential tension between maintaining an individual's confidentiality and disclosing concerns

Develop a case study of an individual who trusts you and wants you to keep something they have told you a secret. Describe the potential tensions between maintaining confidentiality and disclosing what the individual has asked you to keep a secret. You could develop a presentation or provide a written account. Make sure you follow rules around maintaining confidentiality when it comes to including details about the individual in your write-up.

Legislation	
Act/Regulation	Key points
Care Act 2014	Health and social care workers have a legal duty of care to maintain individuals' and others' safety and wellbeing.
	Individuals with care and support needs can access care and support advocates to enable them to be fully involved in all aspects of their care and support.
Equality Act 2010	Employers and providers of services for individuals with disabilities have to make reasonable adjustments when these are required, such as by making information available in large print for individuals with sight loss and installing a hearing loop system in a meeting room.
Mental Capacity Act 2005	Individuals are entitled to an Independent Mental Capacity Advocate (IMCA) when an individual lacks the capacity to make decisions and where there is no one independent of services, such as a family member or friend, who is able to represent the individual.
Data Protection Act 2018	Information and data must be processed fairly, lawfully, used only for the purpose it was intended to be used for, be adequate, relevant, accurate and up to date, held for no longer than is necessary, used in line with the rights of individuals, kept secure and not transferred to other countries without the individual's permission.
	The arrangements in place protect the security of individuals' personal information. In May 2018 the Data Protection Act came into force. It provides detailed guidance to organisations on how to govern and manage people's personal information. This will need to be included in care settings' policies, procedures, guidelines and agreed ways of working.
The Freedom of Information Act 2000	Individuals have rights to apply for access to information held by a wide range of public bodies, such as local authorities and hospitals.
Human Rights Act 1998	Individuals are entitled to have their human rights respected such as their right to privacy in relation to their personal information being shared.
Mental Health Act 1983	Individuals are entitled to an Independent Mental Health Advocate (IMHA) if they are what's known as a 'qualifying patient'.

305 Handling information in adult care settings/services

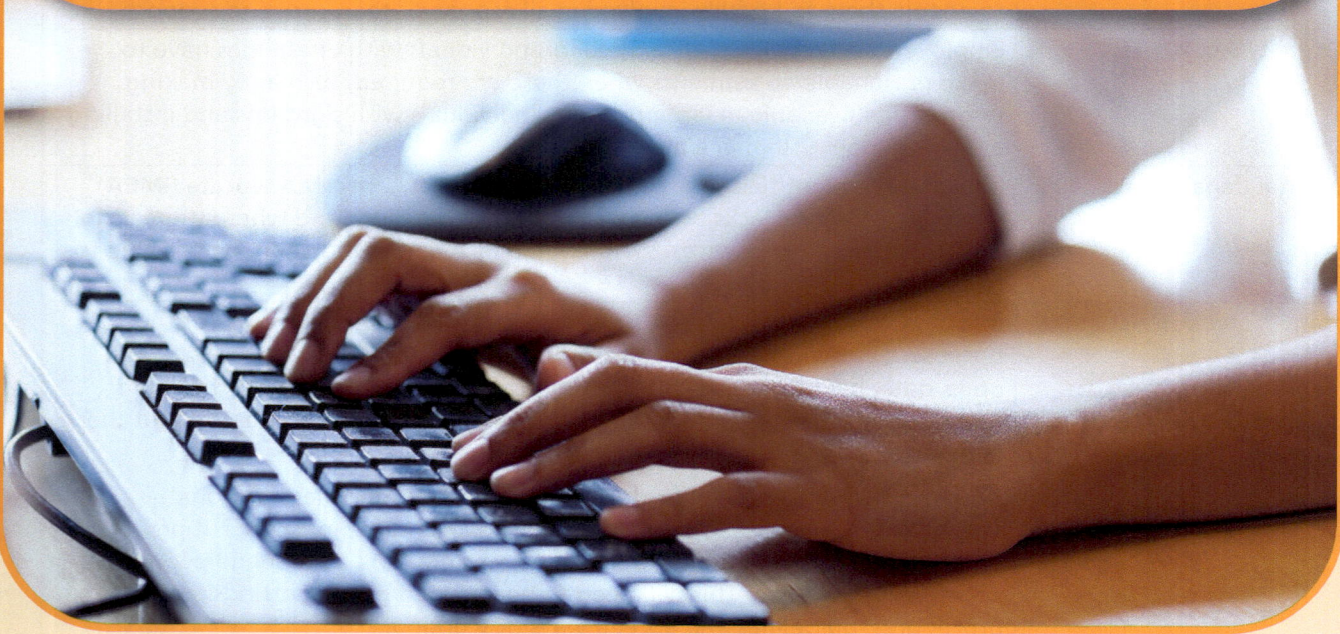

About this unit

Credit value: 2
Guided learning hours: 15

Understanding the requirements of legislation and codes of practice for handling information in care settings is essential for the delivery of safe and effective care. In this unit you will learn about the relevant key pieces of legislation and the working codes of practice.

Being able to implement good practice in handling information requires you to know about and use different manual and electronic information systems so that the information they contain can be kept secure. You will also learn more about your agreed ways of working for maintaining records and ensuring that they are up to date, complete, accurate and legible, ensuring data security when storing and accessing information, including how to support audit processes in line with your role and responsibilities.

Finally, as a Lead Adult Care Worker or Lead Personal Assistant you must also be able to support others to handle information effectively, including ensuring they understand the importance of keeping information secure, and be able to respond to data breaches that may occur in the setting/service where you work.

Learning outcomes

By the end of this unit, you will:

LO1: Understand requirements for handling information in care settings/services

LO2: Be able to implement good practice in the handling of information

LO1 Understand requirements for handling information in care settings/services

> **Getting started**
>
> Think about the care setting where you work and the information you handle on a day-to-day basis. This may, for example, be written information that you record manually and/or electronically, files or reports that you store and verbal information you discuss and share.
>
> Why is it important that you and your colleagues handle all information professionally and in line with legislative requirements? What would be the consequences if you didn't? If you work in an individual's home, how do you make sure that you follow legislative requirements? How does this protect the individual's confidentiality?

Handling information

Handling information in care settings is a big responsibility. There is lot of information that is recorded about individuals in care settings and this is held in different records and reports. The information we record about individuals is personal and private to that individual and so it is very important that these documents are handled with care. These are legal documents and need to be completed, stored and shared by following agreed ways of working and legal requirements.

Your role in handling information

As an adult care worker, it is important that you know about the legal requirements and codes of practice that relate to the recording, storage and sharing of information in care settings. These set out the **rights** individuals and others have in relation to their personal information. Legislation and codes of practice also set out your responsibilities and the working practices you must follow to ensure you maintain the confidentiality and security of all the information you handle at work.

As a Lead Adult Care Worker or a Lead Personal Assistant, your job role will involve you competently handling different people's information, and recording and reporting information about them. For example, you may need to:

- handle and record the information obtained from an individual and their family while developing the individual's care plan with them in relation to their family background, their support needs and/or interests. You may also need to record and report any changes in these
- supervise the work of other care workers and this may involve writing reports about care workers' performance at work, such as their strengths and areas for further training and development
- get involved in recruiting and supporting new care workers, meaning you will need to read job application forms containing information about the applicants' previous work experience and current qualifications
- record information about an individual's health, for example any changes you may have noticed or signs and symptoms of injury or illness
- record any actions you have taken with regard to an individual's care, any discussions you have had and any decisions you or the individual have made
- document any areas of concern with regard, for example, to an individual or a colleague
- provide an audit trail for actions (this would be particularly important in any investigation about abuse or an incident).

6Cs

Competence

As an adult care worker, you will be responsible for handling various pieces of information and recording and reporting in a complete and accurate way. You will be recording and reporting information so that you can make decisions and plan the care and support for individuals; you will be sharing information with those inside and outside the care settings to inform individuals' care; you will be providing information about individuals to your colleagues to ensure consistent care and support.

It is therefore important that you equip yourself with the knowledge and skills that are required to be capable and competent in this area of your job. This will apply whether you work in a large care home, or as a personal assistant in an individual's home. For example, you will need to ensure you are able to handle confidential information in an appropriate way and follow and abide by the various laws around recording, storing and sharing of information; you will need to ensure that you are able to maintain records that are up to date, complete, accurate and legible. You will need to show that you can write accurate reports about individuals, keep individuals' reports safe where you work and share information about individuals only when you have permission to do so.

Think about your own practice. How do you show your competence when handling individuals' and others, information in the care setting where you work? What records do you complete as part of your work role? What type of information do these records contain? Who does this information belong to? How do you ensure that you handle this information safely? Is there any information that is sensitive? How do you maintain its confidentiality? Do you always return any files or records? Have you ever, accidentally or otherwise, not returned files to their correct place? What could the consequences of this be when you are working in a nursing home or day centre? What could the consequences be if you are working in someone's home? If you work in someone's home, how do you ensure information is safely stored?

AC 1.1 Outline the main points of legal requirements, policies and codes of practice for handling information in care services

Legislation that relates to handling information

Table 6.1 outlines detailed points for each of the main pieces of legislation with regard to handling information. However, below is some information to introduce you to each piece of legislation and how it relates to handling information and the rights of people in relation to the handling of their personal information.

Data Protection Act 2018

The Data Protection Act 2018 is the UK's implementation of the EU's General Data Protection Regulation (GDPR) 2018. The GDPR enhances people's rights by placing more emphasis on how organisations share people's personal information as well as the records that they are required to keep, to show that they are handling people's information in accordance with the Regulation.

The Data Protection Act 2018 sets out the rights people have in relation to how information about them can be legally used, recorded, stored and shared. Its aim is to protect people from having information about them misused or abused, by ensuring that organisations follow a set of agreed standards or principles when handling people's personal information. In certain circumstances it allows people to see the information that has been recorded and is held about them.

The Care Act 2014

The Care Act sets out the rights people have in relation to being able to access information and advice about their care and support from local authorities. It also sets out the rights people have in relation to information being shared when there are safeguarding concerns.

The Health and Social Care Act 2008 (Regulated Activities) Regulations 2014

These Regulations established the Fundamental Standards which the care you provide must never fall below. It also established the duty of candour that requires providers to be open and transparent with individuals and their representatives, such as their advocates or families, regarding their care and treatment and providing them with truthful information when care goes wrong.

Freedom of Information Act 2000

The Freedom of Information Act sets out the rights people have in relation to accessing **general information** held by public authorities such as local authorities, the NHS, and the police. The Data Protection Act 2018 by contrast protect people's rights to access personal information held about them, such as their health records.

Access to Personal Files Act 1982

This Act sets out the rights a person has to access personal information that is held about them by public authorities and organisations. For example, a person may want access to their housing or social services records; these may be paper-based or held electronically.

Human Rights Act 1998

The Human Rights Act sets out the rights and freedoms that everyone who lives in the UK is entitled to. It asserts that everyone has the right to be treated with respect, dignity and to be treated fairly by public organisations such as the government and the police. It incorporates the rights set out in the European Convention on Human Rights (ECHR) into British law.

The Caldicott Principles

The Caldicott Principles are a set of eight principles that were developed in the 1990s following a review into the use of patient information across the NHS. Organisations should adhere to these principles to ensure that patient identifiable information is protected and only used when necessary. Although these guidelines are not the law as such, it is important that you are aware of them. For more information, take a look at: www.gov.uk/government/publications/the-caldicott-principles

> **Reflect on it**
>
> **1.1 Legislation**
>
> Reflect on the reasons why there is legislation in place for the handling of information. What are the consequences of there being no legislation for the handling of information in care settings? What impact could this have on individuals? What impact could this have on you and other care workers?
>
> Write a piece addressing these points here.

Policies that relate to handling information

Every adult care setting/service is required to have in place policies for handling information that describe how to follow safe working practices in ways that comply with the legislation you've learned about in this AC. Policies set out what practices for handling information must be followed and the reasons why. Policies for the handling of information in care settings/services may also include other agreed ways of working as well as formal policies, for example how to access electronic information.

The following are some examples of the policies that are in place for the handling of information in care settings/services:

- Data Protection – this policy sets out how all the personal data in the care setting/service will be handled. It also includes the data protection principles, as set out in the Data Protection Act 2018 legislation you learned about and how they will be complied with.
- Access to records and files – this policy sets out how manual and electronic records and files can be accessed, when and by whom including different levels of authorisation depending on the sensitivity of the information contained within these.
- Record keeping – this policy sets out how manual and electronic records will be maintained and the period information will be held for.
- Confidentiality – this policy sets out the meaning of confidentiality and how confidentiality must be respected when handling information at work.
- Cyber security – this policy sets out the meaning of cyber security, how it applies and includes the steps to take when a data breach occurs.

> **Key terms**
>
> **General information** that is recorded and held by a public authority may include information in relation to complaints received, accidents that have taken place, and correspondence exchanged between organisations. For example, an individual may request access to find out about the number of infections there have been in a hospital or the number of accidents there have been in a residential care home so that they can decide which setting is best for their relative to access.
>
> **Information Governance Alliance** includes the Department of Health, NHS England, NHS Digital and Public Health England. Its aim is to improve how people's information is handled by health and care services.
>
> **Health and Social Care Information Centre** (now called NHS Digital) is responsible for providing information and systems for handling individuals' information.

- Internet, email and mobile phone – this policy sets out the requirements that must be followed when using the internet, sending/receiving emails and using mobile phones in the care setting/service.

> **Research it**
>
> **1.1 Handling information policies**
>
> Identify the policies for handling information that you have in the care setting/service where you work and discuss their purpose.

Codes of practice that relate to handling information

A code of practice is usually voluntary and provides guidance on how to follow best practice. It is not mandatory like legislation but rather a set of standards that are recommended to be followed for best working practice. The care setting where you work will have a code of practice in relation to handling information setting out the standards you and your colleagues are expected to follow while you carry out your day-to-day work responsibilities. There are also some general codes of practice that relate to handling information in care settings. You will learn more details about these in this AC.

> **Research it**
>
> **1.1 Codes of practice in your setting**
>
> Research the code or codes of practice you have in place for handling information in the care setting where you work. Where did you find it? How did you access it? Why is it important? What is its relevance in relation to handling information? Whose information is it relevant for? If you are a personal assistant working in an individuals' home, what standards are expected from you in terms of handling information?

Records Management Code of Practice for Health and Social Care 2016

This code of practice was published by the **Information Governance Alliance** and sets out the rights people have when their records are handled by those working in or with NHS organisations. It includes the handling of both digital and paper records such as health records, x-ray reports and GP records.

HSCIC Code of Practice on Confidential Information 2014

This code of practice was published by the **Health and Social Care Information Centre (HSCIC)*** and sets out the rights people have when confidential health and care information is collected, analysed, published or shared by organisations. It also refers to the Caldicott Principles. This is similar to the HSCIC Guide to Confidentiality 2013 below. However, the code was updated and renamed to make it clearer.

HSCIC Guide to Confidentiality 2013

This code of practice was also published by the Health and Social Care Information Centre (HSCIC)* and sets out the rights people have to ensure that their personal information is respected and shared safely and confidentially by health and care workers.

In 2016 the HSCIC changed its name to NHS Digital.

In Table 6.1, you can learn more about how you and your setting can comply with these codes of practice.

The main points of legal requirements, policies and codes of practice for handling information in care services

Now that you have learned about the importance of having legislation, polices and codes of practice in place for the handling of information in care settings it is important that you understand these so that you can comply with them. By following the legislation, policies and codes of practice outlines, you will be helping to:

- uphold individuals' right to have all their information handled safely
- protect individuals from having their information misused or abused
- respect individuals' right to confidentiality when handling their information
- maintain the security of all information you handle.

Table 6.1 details some of the main points of key legislation and includes examples of how you can ensure that you comply with these when handling information in the care setting where you work.

Table 6.1 Legislation for the handling of information in care settings

Legislation	Main points covered and examples of how you can comply with the legislation
Data Protection Act 2018	In May 2018, the UK implemented the EU's General Data Protection Regulation (GDPR) 2018 into the Data Protection Act 2018. Although the new DPA shares many of the principles of the Data Protection Act 1998, the new DPA enhances individuals' rights and the arrangements organisations must have in place for handling information. The DPA 2018 gives individuals greater rights over their personal information: - Organisations will have to demonstrate how they have obtained individuals' consent when handling information. - Individuals will have the right to give and to withdraw their consent for processing information. - Individuals' rights and interests must be safeguarded when information is being processed, i.e. to rectify inaccurate personal data. - All public authorities must have a named data protection officer who is responsible for ensuring the organisation is complying with the DPA 2018 and is the main point of contact. You will find it useful to visit the ICO website for more information on the DPA 2018. You will also find it useful to research (online) the DPA 2018 and the accountability principle, privacy notices, individual's rights, requests for information, processing personal data, consent, breaches of data, Data Protection Officers, assessments and how the DPA 2018 affects children's data/consent. You/your setting must comply with this legislation and your manager/setting will be able to further advise you on this. There may even be training that you are required to attend.

Table 6.1 Legislation for the handling of information in care settings *continued*

Legislation	Main points covered and examples of how you can comply with the legislation
Data Protection Act (DPA) 1998	The Act has a set of principles as its basis for the handling of all information and they state that all personal information or data must be: Principle 1 – processed fairly and lawfully Principle 2 – processed for specific purposes Principle 3 – adequate, relevant and not excessive Principle 4 – accurate and up to date Principle 5 – not kept for longer than is necessary Principle 6 – processed in accordance with the rights of the data's subjects Principle 7 – kept secure Principle 8 – not transferred to other countries without adequate protection. You can comply with these main points in the following ways: ● Principle 1: You must ensure that the information you include in reports about the care and support provided to individuals is written respectfully and must only include information that you have had permission to collate. You must seek permission from the individual or the individual's representative. ● Principle 2: You must be clear about the information you wish to obtain about an individual or team member by explaining to them why you are collating the information and what you intend to do with it. This might, for example, be in relation to their health needs or in the case of a colleague, training needs. ● Principle 3: You must ensure that all the information you hold about an individual, for example in relation to the support they require, is sufficient, relevant to that individual and that you do not hold more information than you need, as this could be irrelevant information about the individual's background. ● Principle 4: You must ensure that all the information you record about an individual is true, factual and up to date, such as all information relating to their care and support needs. The information you record must be in line with any changes in the individual's care and support needs so that the care and support provided can meet these. ● Principle 5: You must ensure that all information you hold about an individual is not retained for longer than necessary. For example, the information you hold about individuals that no longer live in the care setting must be archived or deleted securely in line with your care setting's agreed ways of working. ● Principle 6: You must ensure that all information you record about an individual or colleague, for example, is in line with their rights. You must, for example, respect and uphold their right to access a copy of the information you have recorded about them and you must respect their right to have any inaccurate information recorded about them corrected. ● Principle 7: You must ensure that all the information you record and hold about an individual is kept safe and secure. For example, you must ensure that you only write reports in a private office, that the individual's electronic files held on the computer are password-protected, you must ensure that you do not leave files or correspondence about the individual in a public area and that information is only accessed by those who have permission to do so.

Table 6.1 Legislation for the handling of information in care settings *continued*

Legislation	Main points covered and examples of how you can comply with the legislation
	• Principle 8: You must ensure that all the information you obtain about an individual is protected when transferred to another country overseas. For example, you may need to do this when an individual's information needs to be sent abroad, or you will need to inform an individual when supporting them with booking a holiday abroad that the information they are providing online will be accessed by an overseas company, and seek the individual's permission for their information to be transferred in this way. You should always ensure an individual's information is not transferred to other countries without adequate protection or without the individual's permission as these countries may not have legislation in place in relation to how personal information about individuals is used and stored.
The Care Act 2014	The underpinning principle of this Act is achieving 'wellbeing' for individuals and their carers in terms of their physical, mental and emotional wellbeing.
	It established new duties for local authorities to make available information, advice and advocacy on care and support, for example in relation to the different types of care and support available, how to access services, and costs of services.
	It is important that you are aware of the new duties the Care Act placed on local authorities in relation to ensuring information is made available when individuals need it.
The Health and Social Care Act 2008 (Regulated Activities) Regulations 2014	The 2014 Regulations established the Fundamental Standards of care that providers are expected to meet at all times. According to the Standards, care providers are expected to ensure care is person-centred, individuals are treated with dignity and respect, their consent is sought and gained, that individuals' safety is ensured, that they are safeguarded from abuse, that their needs with regard to food and drink are met, that the premises and equipment used in relation to their care is maintained, complaints are handled and addressed appropriately, that there is good governance in the setting, issues around staffing are addressed, that fit and proper staff provide care, duty of candour is upheld, and that the CQC rating is displayed.
	The duty of candour requires providers of care to be open and transparent with individuals and their representatives such as their advocates or families, regarding their care and treatment including when it goes wrong.
	You can meet the standards of care in relation to handling information by, for example:
	• treating all information about individuals with respect
	• obtaining individuals' or their representatives' consent in relation to obtaining and sharing information about their care or support needs
	• informing individuals and their carers of their rights to complain if they are not satisfied with their care or support
	• informing individuals if a mistake has been made in relation to handling their information by being honest about what happened, apologising and providing support
	• promoting openness by supporting individuals and others to raise any concerns and complaints they may have
	• promoting transparency by allowing information about the organisation's services and their outcomes to be shared, for example with individuals and their families.

Table 6.1 Legislation for the handling of information in care settings *continued*

Legislation	Main points covered and examples of how you can comply with the legislation
Freedom of Information Act 2000	This Act promotes people's rights to access general information held about them by public authorities such as the NHS and local authorities. This right is referred to as the 'right to know'.
	It is important that you are aware of people's rights to access general information held about them. In this way you can provide individuals with information about their rights to request and access information held about them, unless there are reasons for them not to do so, for example it may put them at risk if they do so, and unless doing so may, for example, impact negatively on an individual's mental health.
	Examples of information they may want to access are care files, medical reports, documents, letters, test results, or minutes of a meeting held about their care needs.
	Each public authority will have their own procedure for how to request access to general information. You can support individuals by ensuring they understand the process to follow.
	You should remember this when you are recording information about individuals as they may access the files and will be able to read what you have said. You should remember that this Act does not allow people to access the personal data of other people, only themselves.
Human Rights Act 1998	This Act sets out the rights and freedoms that everyone who lives in the UK is entitled to in a series of articles. Article 8 under this Act states that people are entitled to the following right in relation to the handling of information: the right to respect for their private and family life, home and correspondence such as letters, telephone calls and emails.
	You can comply with Article 8 by ensuring that when you handle an individual's personal information you keep it secure by writing your reports in private, ensuring that files are safely stored and protected, ensuring you only discuss their personal information with those with whom you have permission to do so, and only sharing without their permission in exceptional circumstances, in the case of a medical emergency, for example.

Research it

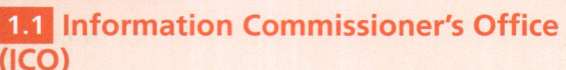

1.1 Information Commissioner's Office (ICO)

Research the ICO's guide to the Data Protection Act 2018. You can access this from the ICO website:

https://ico.org.uk/for-organisations/guide-to-the-general-data-protection-regulation-gdpr

Or go to https://ico.org.uk/ and search for 'Data Protection' or 'GDPR'.

Produce an information handout about how you can comply with these requirements in your day-to-day role.

Complying with legislation when you work in an individual's home

If you work in an individual's home you are not exempt from complying with these pieces of legislation. In fact, it is even more important that you are aware of the individual's rights and your responsibilities to ensure their information is kept safe and handled securely at all times. Not doing so may mean that you are in breach of your employment contract and not providing the individual with the protection and confidentiality of their information that they are entitled to.

Consequences of not complying with legislation

If a setting does not comply with legislation then the setting will be breaking the law, which means that the setting will be fined. The setting's working practices will also be reviewed and its reputation will be damaged as a result.

The policies in care settings that you learned about earlier on in this unit are also important for detailing how information must be handled.

Table 6.2 Policies for handling information

Policies	Main points covered and examples of how you can comply with the policy
Data protection	This policy sets out the types of personal data that the care setting/service will be handling and processing, the personal data protection principles, the rights of how data subjects' information is handled, including their rights to consent and complain, the responsibilities of the care setting/service and those of others in the work setting.
	You can comply with the data protection policy by ensuring you follow the eight personal data protection principles when handling information in your care setting/service. It is also important that you understand the rights of data subjects and ensure that you promote them in your day-to-day communication such as treating all information that you handle in confidence, fairly and keeping it secure.
Access to records and files	This policy sets out how and when data subjects can access their manual/electronic records and files and the processes to follow.
	You can comply with the access to records and files policy by ensuring you are aware of the records and files you have authorisation to access in your Lead role and complying with this. You can also ensure that you know how to respond to for example an individual's family if they ask to access their relative's records, including who you could seek advice from if you are unsure.
Record keeping	This policy sets out the records that will be maintained in the care setting/service as well as the purpose and use of the information held on these and how the information on these must be completed to ensure it is complete, accurate and legible.
	You can comply with the record keeping policy by ensuring you know what records you are expected to keep as part of your job role, and how, when and where, so that you can ensure you are completing them fully, accurately and in confidence.
Confidentiality	This policy sets out how confidentiality will be maintained in the care setting/service.
	You can comply with the confidentiality policy by ensuring that your practices promote confidentiality when handling all types of information, i.e. spoken, written, electronic. You will learn more about how you can maintain and promote confidentiality in AC2.2.
Cyber security	This policy sets out how to maintain cyber security when accessing information on websites, sending and receiving emails, and how to report a data breach in the care setting/service.
	You can comply with the cyber security policy by being aware of the processes to follow when sending and receiving information over the internet to/from others outside of the care setting such as by only using secure sites, protecting confidential information with passwords and only opening emails from recognised sources/addresses.
Internet, email and mobile phone	This policy sets out internet, email and mobile phone usage, including when these can be used, where and by whom.
	You can comply with your care setting's/service's internet, email and mobile phone usage by familiarising yourself with, for example, the internet sites you must and must not access at work, the requirements that must be followed when sending and receiving emails and when mobile phones can and can't be used while at work.

In addition to policies, there are also codes of practice in place that provide health and social care workers with specific guidance on how to handle information effectively. Table 6.3 provides you with more information about what these include.

Table 6.3 Codes of practice for the handling of information

Codes of practice	Main points and examples of how you can comply
Records Management Code of Practice for Health and Social Care 2016	The Code provides guidance on how to manage records effectively for people working with or in NHS organisations in England. You can comply with the Code, for example, by ensuring that your records are: ● **authentic:** by ensuring you provide a true record of what has happened and you sign and date your entry. ● **reliable:** by ensuring you include the facts only rather than personal opinions about what has happened and that you complete the record as soon as possible after the activity/event happened. ● **honest:** by ensuring you write records that are complete and if you make an error you put a line through it and add your initials next to it to show clearly that it was an error and who it was that made the error. ● **usable:** by ensuring that you follow the agreed ways of recording and handling information in the care setting where you work so that your written records can be understood and retrieved when required.
HSCIC Code of Practice on Confidential Information 2014 *The HSCIC has changed its name to NHS Digital.*	This Code of Practice outlines how health and social care workers can follow best practice when handling confidential information. The Code is also based on the Caldicott Principles that outline other principles that all health and social care staff are expected to follow in addition to the data protection principles. These are: 1 Justify the purpose. 2 Only use personal confidential data if it is absolutely necessary. 3 Only use the minimum necessary personal confidential data. 4 Access to personal confidential data should be on a need-to-know basis only. 5 Ensure that everyone with access to personal confidential data is aware of their responsibilities. 6 Comply with the law. 7 The duty to share information can be as important as the duty to protect patient confidentiality. 8 Inform patients and service users about how their confidential information is used. You can comply with the Code of Practice by ensuring you always: ● explain to the person you are collecting information from why you need it ● respect a person's right to not have confidential information about them used ● use secure systems for recording and sharing confidential information.

Table 6.3 Codes of practice for the handling of information *continued*

Codes of practice	Main points and examples of how you can comply
HSCIC Guide to Confidentiality 2013 *The HSCIC has changed its name to NHS Digital.*	This Guide provides health and social care workers with information about how to share information safely and confidentially and is based on the following key principles: 1 All confidential information about individuals must be respected. 2 Individuals' rights to not have confidential information shared about them should be respected. 3 Confidential information should be shared within a team when it is needed for providing safe and effective care to an individual. 4 Organisations must have in place effective systems, policies and procedures for maintaining confidentiality. You can ensure that you comply with the Guide by, for example, ensuring you: • only discuss confidential information about individuals in the care setting where you work, not outside • know what process to follow if an individual asks you to not share their confidential information with a member of the team • know the rules for when you can share confidential information with other team members • read and understand what the procedures say in the care setting where you work about how to handle confidential information about individuals.

6Cs

Competence

Applying your knowledge and skills in relation to handling information effectively in the care setting where you work is essential for the provision of high quality care and support. This is because you need information that is accurate and up to date to be able to plan and meet individuals' care or support needs. Here, you can show your competence by ensuring that you respect individuals' rights to confidentiality when recording, storing, accessing and sharing their personal information.

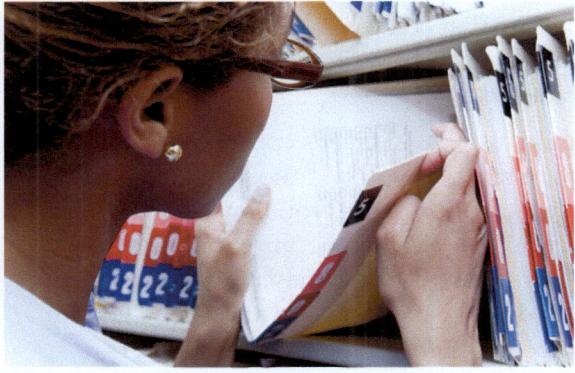

Figure 6.1 Do you know how to handle information effectively and securely?

Evidence opportunity

1.1 Main points of legal requirements, policies and codes of practice

List three key pieces of legislation, three policies and three codes of practice that relate to handling information in care settings.

For each one, write down details of their main requirements, why they are important and how you comply with them when handling personal information in the care setting where you work. How could you improve your practice?

AC 1.2 Describe how to ensure data and cyber security is maintained in care services when using a) electronic information systems, b) manual systems

Importance of effective storage systems

Before we discuss how to ensure security when using electronic information systems and manual systems in care services, it is important to understand the importance of effective information systems. As you will have learned in AC 1.1 it is important that you comply with legislative and organisational requirements so that all the information that you record can be read and understood by those who require it and request access to it. It is also very important that all the information you document can be retrieved quickly and easily when it is required, otherwise it cannot be accessed or used.

Importance of effectively recording and storing

Recording and storing individuals' personal information securely will mean that you will be able to support individuals to be in control of their care and support needs to live the lives they want safely and independently. If individuals trust you and your abilities, they will be able to trust that all information held about them is recorded accurately and kept safe.

Not ensuring the provision of safe care and support to individuals when recording and storing information can have serious consequences for the continuity of their care and support and will in turn impact negatively on their lives. For example, if information is not recorded accurately and stored safely, your colleagues will not be able to provide care that continues to meet individuals' needs in a consistent way and so their needs may remain unmet.

This could also have serious consequences for the care or support you and the team provide to individuals. For example, you may need to update an individual's care plan because their dietary needs have changed; they may now require a soft food diet because they are at risk of choking. If you document this but other care workers cannot retrieve or find the individual's care plan because you filed it incorrectly then the team will not know about the change in the individual's dietary needs and may not provide the individual with a soft food diet; this in turn may result in the individual choking and requiring emergency medical treatment. Similarly, if you document that you have observed a member of your team use unsafe practice when supporting an individual to move from one position to another, and this record is left lying around and not stored securely on the computer or in the moving and handling folder, you risk other members of the team being able to access and read it. This may result in the member of your team who used unsafe practices being victimised. Knowing how to use both manual and electronic information storage systems to help keep personal information safe and confidential is therefore essential.

The importance of clear, accurate and legible records

Whatever the information you record, it is important that you record it accurately, that the information is dated so it is clear when the record was made and that it contains factual information. You will need to ensure that it is legible and easy to read, and that it is clear to understand and makes the point in a straightforward way. This is because, in a care setting, information is shared on a day-to-day basis, so others will need to access the information you have recorded. Even if you work in an individual's home, the individual or family members who have permission may also want to access and read their records. The individuals that you care for need to be confident that the information that they give to you will be recorded and secured safely. If they do not trust that this will happen, it could stop them from giving you information or affect the things that they decide to tell you.

There is more information on maintaining up-to-date, complete, accurate and legible records in AC 2.3.

Monitoring storage systems for their effectiveness

It is important that you monitor systems for their effectiveness. This means that you and your colleagues should review feedback on how well the systems in place are working. What is working well when it comes to recording and storing information? What is not working well? This includes being open and honest about when things go wrong. Regular monitoring of information storage systems will ensure that if some things are working particularly well in terms of keeping information safe and secure this can be maintained; if not they can be improved.

Protecting the privacy of individuals and building trust

Protecting the privacy of individuals' personal information and safely storing it will mean that you will be supporting individuals' rights to have their personal information kept private at all times. This will help you to form a relationship with the individual based on trust.

Not protecting the privacy of individuals' personal information can have serious consequences as individuals may lose their trust in you because you are not keeping their information safe. It may stop them from sharing further information with you.

Individuals' personal information could also be accessed by those who do not have permission to do so, which places individuals in danger and/or at risk of harm and abuse.

What do we mean by data and cyber security?

Ensuring data and cyber security when using systems means ensuring that the information that these systems contain can only be accessed by those who have permission to do so. For example, a manual system may be a filing cabinet full of individuals' paper records that contain information about individuals' background, health, care or support needs, or an electronic system could be a folder on a PC that contains files full of individuals' risk assessments. The filing cabinet will be accessed with a key that only those with permission can use and the PC or electronic files will be accessed with a password that only those with permission will know.

Data and cyber security means using systems securely where the information contained is kept safe from damage in the event of, for example, a fire. Fire is not the only way that paper records can be damaged; electronic systems need to be backed up in the event of PC failure or virus attack that may cause information to be deleted or be prevented from being accessed.

Security and privacy of records

Records that need to be left in individuals' rooms will usually be kept safe in a drawer or cupboard, out of sight. Other records will be held in the file. In residential settings, some records such as the care worker's daily report may be left in the individual's room in a place of their choosing; this might be in their drawer or cabinet. The individual can read the report and their family may also access it with their permission. If a record contains sensitive information, for example about an allegation towards a staff or family member, then a separate confidential report would be made about this.

Manual or electronic?

Below, we discuss the various manual and electronic systems that are used to store information. Let's consider how you decide whether something needs to be recorded manually or electronically in the first place? In other words, how do you know when you can just write something down, and when you will need to input information into a computer? In order to answer this question, it would be useful to consider the reason or purpose you are documenting the information. For example, you may need to add information about a change in an individual's diet on the daily menu that you give to the cook. The menu may be the best place to record it if this is the record that your colleague is most likely to access. However, there may be further information that you need to include about the individual's health needs. This may include changes to their weight or their condition that need to be taken into account when supporting the individuals with their care needs. In this case, you may decide that updating the individual's main electronic record on the PC is the best way to record these changes because in this way everyone who has access to this will be made aware of the changes and adapt their work practice accordingly. Whatever way you choose to record the information, you must do so securely.

> **Research it**
>
> **1.2 The policy in your setting**
>
> Research what the records policy in the care setting where you work says about what information must be documented and how. For example, what does it say about the records that you must hand write and the records that you must complete electronically? Why must you complete these records in this way?
>
> Discuss your findings with a member of your team and write notes to document your discussion.

Familiarising yourself with filing systems

Whether files are stored manually or electronically, the setting where you work will have a filing system in place which you will need to familiarise yourself with and learn how to use. Being able to use the system efficiently will only help you in your role if you are able to find and access the information you need quickly and if you have a sound understanding of how files are to be returned and stored. It will also help your colleagues to work efficiently if you are all able to keep an ordered and organised filing system. You might use an alphabetical system to organise your files, or one that uses numbers, or one that is organised by the topic or type of care you offer. Whatever system you use, you are far more likely to be able to find what you are looking for if you and your setting has an easy to follow and organised system in place. It is also important that those who use the system understand how this is to be used, for example where, how and when files must be returned, the importance of returning files and what may happen if files are not returned or are misplaced, and who is responsible for handling files – whether anyone in the setting can access the files or if there is a designated person in the setting that is responsible for the filing system. Whether or not there is a designated person will depend on the setting; the designated person may be an administrator in a care home, or they could be a manager or team leader.

Electronic information systems that help ensure cyber security

Many care settings and perhaps your own care setting will use electronic systems for some or all of the information they hold about individuals, staff and the organisation. Keeping records and information on a computer means that they can be updated easily and accessed quickly when required. They often have the potential to store a lot more information than manual systems and in much smaller spaces as files on a computer take up much less space than files located in a filing cabinet. You are also unlikely to leave electronic files lying around, or misplace them either inside or outside of the setting.

Each care setting will have procedures in place for accessing and using their electronic information system – you should find out if you have an electronic information system in the care setting where you work and whether there are any rules for using it that you need to be aware of. It may be that you and others are not used to using the types of computerised systems that your setting has implemented, in which case it is important that you receive guidance and appropriate training in how to develop your knowledge and skills in this area. If you work in an individual's home, you will need to find out what electronic information system, if any, they use and how they use it, including what types of information and records are held on it and whether there are any rules you need to be aware of when using it.

Just as we discussed with manual electronic systems, files on computers may also be indexed and organised alphabetically, numerically or by topics/areas and job roles. There may be levels of sub-folders that you need to familiarise yourself with so that you can find what you are looking for efficiently and know where to store files.

Like manual systems, electronic systems can also be kept secure in a variety of ways; here are some examples of how:

- **Passwords:** secure passwords to enter computer-based systems can ensure that only those with authorised access do so. For example, different passwords and security levels can be set for different types of records such as those that contain information about individuals or care records; these may include records about staff members such as supervision records or they may be records that relate to the organisation, for example organisational risk assessments. These records will only be accessed by those who have authorisation to do so – a care worker, for example, will not require access to another staff member's personal information file but may require access to an individual's care plan. Remember, do not write passwords down.

- **File protection:** files on computers can be protected as a permanent record by ensuring that the information contained in them cannot be deleted or altered in any way. They may be 'read only' files that you cannot edit or change. There may be some records, such as manual handling risk guidelines or health and safety assessments, that can only be read when accessed by the team and can only be updated by a nominated person such as you or another senior colleague.

- **Firewall protected:** computers that store personal details, data and information should be protected by a 'firewall.' This is a piece of software that protects the computer and the information stored on it from people outside who do not have permission to access the network or the stored information. It can also stop people 'hacking' into the computer and stealing information. Hacking occurs when people access a computer without permission, and possibly misuse the information. Firewalls can also stop other internet viruses from infecting the computer. They can be installed as part of anti-virus software which will stop any harmful virus from entering your computer.

- **Anti-virus software and virus scans:** it is important for organisations to protect their electronic systems from viruses that can interrupt, interfere with and even delete personal information held. Computers in your setting (and in the home of the individual you support) should have anti-virus software installed which will stop any harmful virus entering your computer. You may know from personal experience of having a virus on your computer that viruses can harm documents or files that you have stored! You may even have had your computer or laptop repaired and lost files. Some security alerts can be viruses themselves, so seek advice from a senior colleague or an IT expert if a security alert pops up on the screen while you are using the computer. You should also familiarise yourself with the rules relating to opening emails in your care setting, for example you should understand the rules around ensuring that they are from who you think they are. If you receive an email from someone you don't know, carefully check the sender's address is valid, and do not click any hyperlinks in the email, in case the sender is trying to gain access to the electronic system where you work. Check your agreed ways of working to find out what they say about this. How serious might it be if a virus infected a computer in your setting? While anti-virus software may not stop all viruses, it is something that should definitely be installed on computers in your setting as this can stop important information and files from being lost or accessed by potentially harmful sources.

- **Screen savers:** computers that have screen savers are useful for maintaining the security of the information stored. For example, if you access electronic records containing individuals' personal information and someone distracts you from what you are reading by asking your advice or sharing a concern, the screen saver can automatically switch on and prevent anyone else seeing or accessing the information on the screen. Screen savers can be set for different time periods, so you can ensure it switches on automatically when the computer is not in use or after a minute of you not using it. A password will very often then need to be entered to be able to access the electronic system again.
- **Information back-ups:** it is important for organisations to back up the electronic information being collated so that it is not lost and can be retrieved when required. Most organisations will back up their electronic systems once a day, usually at the end of the day; some electronic systems back up information on an automatic basis throughout the day – you should find out which system the organisation you work for uses. Most organisations will have a procedure in place for who is responsible for backing up information and how often this will take place. It may be someone at your setting or may be done outside your setting (this will depend on the size of the setting you work in, for example a larger setting or organisation may need to back up and store information externally). You can, for example, backup and store electronic information externally on a hard drive, on a server or in the cloud. Sometimes there may be systems in place where information is backed up with paper copies in case the electronic copies are lost. These should also be stored safely.

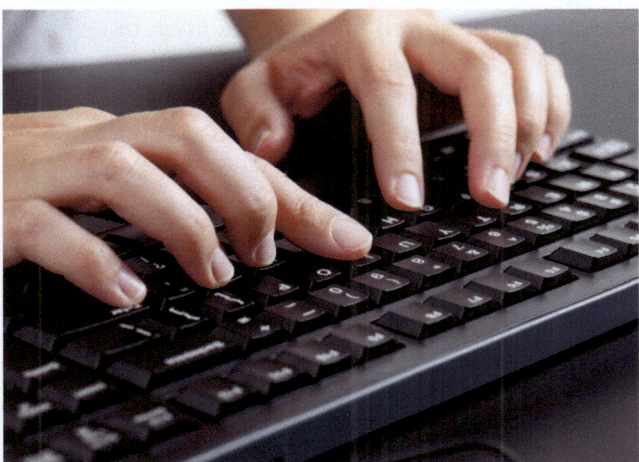

Figure 6.2 How do you keep electronic information secure? How do you promote best practice and encourage others to keep electronic information secure?

- **Safe use of email:** emails are used to send and receive information. Some information may be personal and confidential and so it is important to ensure that all information remains secure and free from hacking and viruses. The safe use of email involves changing the passwords you use frequently as well as keeping them in a safe place and not giving them out to others to prevent unauthorised others from getting access to personal and confidential information. It is also important that you don't open email attachments from people you don't know as doing so may result in a virus infecting your computer and gaining access to confidential information.

- Other practices that can help ensure data and cyber security include: not sharing sensitive information such as in relation to a person's medical condition or a person's finances over email, having anti-virus software installed kept up to date, and being able to recognise unsolicited emails that claim to have come from a recognised source but are in fact fraudulent, i.e. by looking closely at the email address and reporting spam emails to the email provider.

Manual systems that help ensure data security

Records that contain handwritten information are stored in a manual filing system. These might include reports about individuals' daily tasks, menus, medication records and activity records. Each care setting will have in place their own arrangements for filing records. For example, records may be stored in a filing cabinet, in lever-arch files in a cupboard or in box files on a shelf. It is important that you know how these are stored in these various different storage systems so that you and others can retrieve them easily when you need them, use them and keep the information they hold safe and secure.

Box files on a shelf may be colour coded to indicate what records they hold, for example blue for general information on activities, yellow for leaflets on community services, or green for useful telephone numbers about care or support services in the local area. Do you know the system used in the care setting where you work?

Records about individuals that are stored in a filing cabinet may be filed in various ways. They may be stored:

alphabetically: under individuals' surnames. This may be more effective in smaller settings where you are unlikely to have many people with the same surname. Records about members of the team that are stored in files in a cupboard, for example, may be filed alphabetically under team members' surnames.

numerically: you may have noticed in some settings such as hospitals, individuals have a number alongside their surname. Or their information could be filed under their room numbers.

by topic/area of work or job role: files may be organised or categorised, especially in large organisations, under job roles of care workers, or services or areas where they work, for example there may be files allocated to individuals with specific needs such as learning disabilities and mental health needs. They may have sub-folders where files are then organised alphabetically or numerically.

Ensuring the security of data when using manual systems

Every manual information storage system must be secure, otherwise the personal information it holds may be at risk of being accessed by those who are not authorised to do so. If you think about all the personal information that is held in the manual systems used in your care setting you can begin to see the consequences of this type of information falling into the 'wrong hands' as it could be misused, abused and/or lost. Failure to comply with legal requirements for handling information and records correctly can also mean that the organisation you work for may be fined and that you may also lose your job.

It is also important that you do not take personal information about individuals anywhere with you as you could accidentally misplace or lose this, meaning other people have access to the information. For example, if you are supporting an individual to learn how to travel independently on public transport it is important that you do not complete your daily records while travelling; you can do this safely when you return to the care setting. The consequences of losing information could be serious. 'Identity theft' is a crime and has become a bigger issue in recent years. This is when people steal other people's personal details to commit fraud. They may pretend to be that person in order to buy goods or get loans in that person's name. This has increased with the sharing of information on the internet which means that the protection of all personal data has become a very important issue.

Manual systems can be kept secure in a variety of different ways. Here are some examples:

- **Filing cabinets:** the security of records and the information they contain can be maintained by ensuring all filing cabinets are lockable and are locked at all times when not in use. Keys to filing cabinets can be kept safe if they are held by nominated people only and are kept with them at all times while at work. For example, in the care setting where you work this may be you or a senior colleague. The filing cabinet can also be located in a private area such as in an office rather than in a communal area such as an entrance hall.

- **Drawers and cupboards:** when storing records that contain personal information in drawers and cupboards these also should be lockable. For example, in an individual's home it may be that their bedside drawer is lockable and therefore they may decide that this is where they would like their daily notes kept. Cupboards that hold information and records in files and/or books such as accident forms and health and safety risk assessments can also be kept secure by ensuring that they are locked when they are not in use. In some care settings it may be a requirement for you to document when and why you accessed a record, including who you sought authorisation from to do this. Is this a requirement in your care setting?
- **Storage areas:** some records such as those relating to individuals who no longer live at the care setting or staff who no longer work at the setting may need to be filed away or archived for a limited period of time when no longer in use. It is important that these are also stored securely so that they can only be accessed by those who have authorisation to do so as they may contain personal confidential and/or sensitive information.
- **Other systems:** other personal information may also be contained in different types of records. For example, a visitors book for documenting who enters and exits the care setting, an accident or incident book for recording accidents and/or incidents that may arise, a communication book for recording telephone messages that are received by the care setting and for recording messages exchanged between team members. It is important that these systems for recording information are also kept secure. You can do this by, for example, ensuring the visitors book is not left wide open on the desk in the entrance to the building for everyone to see, and that the accident, incident and communication books are returned to their allocated areas when no longer in use, for example to the private office, the locked drawer or cupboard.

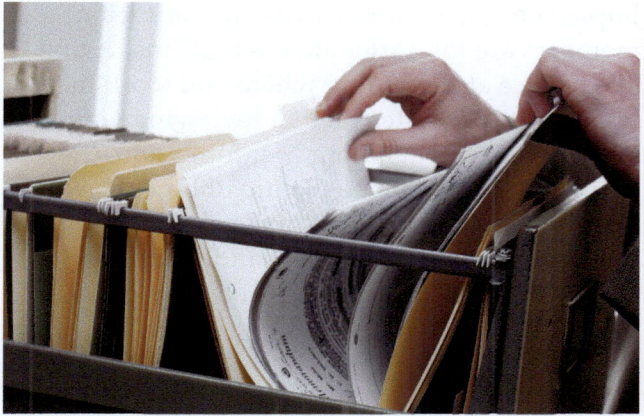

Figure 6.3 What manual information systems do you know how to use? Which systems do you use in your setting?

Reflect on it

1.2 Manual systems in your setting

Reflect on the security practices you follow when accessing records and personal information from manual systems in the care setting where you work. Are you using your care setting's systems for storing manual records correctly? How do you know you are? Write some short notes to document your thoughts.

Evidence opportunity

1.2 Data and cyber security when using manual and electronic information

Produce a PowerPoint presentation aimed at the team you lead, that describes and details the most important security features of both manual and electronic information systems in the care setting where you work and how to ensure data and cyber security is maintained.

AC 1.3 Describe how to support others to keep information secure

As you have already learned, you have an important role to play in the handling of information. As a Lead Adult Care Worker or Lead Personal Assistant you will also be responsible for supporting others to handle information effectively in the care setting where you work. This will ensure that not only are you implementing good practices but your team members are too. After all, if a CQC inspection takes place at the setting where you work they will not only be interested in reviewing your practices for the handling of information, they will want to gain a true picture of how the whole team, including visitors to the care setting and the individuals themselves, handle information and are complying with the procedures and systems in place.

Support team members and colleagues

Your team members and colleagues may not have full understanding of the need for keeping information secure. You may find that they do not understand the reasons why security is very important. You can support them by explaining to them the reasons why they must comply with, and the consequences of not complying with, the systems in place in the setting, and this explanation should include the legal and organisational requirements. You could provide this information to your team members and colleagues in a variety of ways; this could be formally through training sessions, team meetings and one-to-one support meetings. You could also hold discussions with your team members and colleagues to reinforce the need for the secure handling of information and provide them with information updates and examples of good practice you have read about or heard about locally or in other care services. You can also reinforce the need for keeping information secure by carrying out your role and responsibilities to the best of your ability.

> **Reflect on it**
>
> **1.3 Supporting your team**
>
> Reflect on an occasion when you provided support to a team member or colleague in relation to keeping information secure. What happened? What support did you provide? How effective was your support? Why?

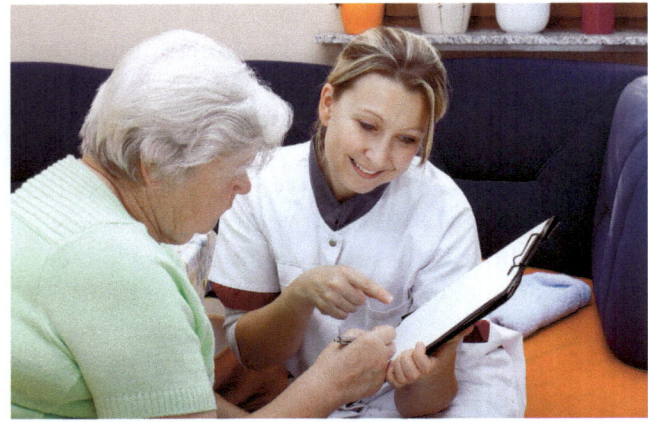

Figure 6.4 What type of support do you provide to individuals when handling information?

Support individuals

The individuals you care for and support may not be fully aware of their and your responsibilities in relation to the need for the secure handling of information. For example, they may think this only applies to you and your team members and not to them. They may also not fully understand the reasons why securely handling information is so important and what type of information needs to be handled securely. You can support individuals by making this information available to them. This might include informing them of the ways in which they can protect information about themselves and the importance of doing so; it might include telling them about what information is held about them, where it is kept and how it is kept secure. Remember that the way that you inform them will depend on their needs. For example, an individual who has sight loss may prefer for you to talk to them about this. An individual who has hearing loss may prefer you to write the information down or use sign language when you explain this to them. An individual with a learning disability may require their advocate to be present when you are explaining this to them using a combination of words, pictures and signs. Remember that all information can be easily forgotten and so it is useful to ensure that you reinforce the need for the secure handling of information at different times and in different ways; for example you could do this regularly, on a one-to-one basis, at group meetings or at social occasions.

Working in a compassionate way

The individuals that you care for also need to be confident that the information that they give to you will be recorded and safely secured. This involves showing compassion when handling their personal information – in other words, thinking about how you would feel if it were your personal and private information and how safely and securely you would want it to be handled. If individuals do not trust that this will happen, it could stop them from giving you information or affect the things that they decide to tell you.

It is important that individuals in your care setting understand that you will only share the information they have given you if you have their permission to do so. Any information that you do share about them, with your colleagues or other professionals, will only be shared in private to ensure its confidentiality and that it is on a 'need to know' basis.

When deciding what information can be shared and not shared on a 'need to know' basis, the individual's personal situation must always be taken into account as well as their best interests. You can only do this if you know the individual. When making a decision to share or not to share information on a 'need to know' basis, the pros and cons must be fully explored, and a decision made in the individual's best interests only.

You will also need to keep in mind any capacity issues – does the individual have capacity to make the decision to share or not share details? The issue of capacity is covered in Unit 306, Promoting and implementing person-centred practice, AC 1.8.

It is important the individual understands that sometimes you have to share information about them without their permission – a process referred to as 'breaching confidentiality'. This might be, for example, when an individual tells you that they are going to harm themselves or someone else. You would need to share this kind of information without their permission, probably with your manager, because not doing so may mean that they will put themselves and others in danger, something that you cannot allow to happen.

Compassion is central to keeping individuals' personal information secure as doing so involves showing your kindness towards individuals and upholding their rights to dignity, respect and being taken seriously.

Research it

1.3 Communicating the need for security

Research how maintaining the security of information in your care setting is communicated to the individuals with care or support needs. Write down all the different methods used. Which ones are most effective? Why?

Support families, carers or advocates

Individuals' families, carers and advocates may also require support from you to understand the need for the secure handling of information in the care setting where you work. For example, a family member may want to know how best to access their relative's file, who to approach or when it is best to discuss their relative's care or support with you. They may also have questions about recent legislation changes such as the Data Protection Act 2018 and what it means to them and for their relative. They may want to ask you about what happens to their relative's records if their relative moves or passes away.

You will also need to decide how to communicate this information to them. You may decide that this is best done through a written communication such as an email or a letter – remember if you select this as a method, you should ensure the information you provide is up to date, complete, accurate and legible. Other families, carers or advocates may prefer to speak to you face-to-face about this, so you could make arrangements to speak to them as a group or individually, if you think this will be more appropriate. Be prepared to be able to answer any questions they may have, and if you can't answer their questions be prepared to find out the answers. You could also signpost them to other useful sites for more information such as CQC or the Information Commissioner's Office's (ICO) website and even to the person responsible for data protection in the care setting where you work.

Support others to understand and contribute to records

Supporting others, such as your team members, colleagues, the individuals, their families, carers or advocates to understand and contribute to records can mean that you are able to promote effective handling of information in the care setting where

6Cs

Communication

Supporting others to understand the need for keeping information secure involves you being able to communicate effectively both verbally and in writing with different people; doing so is central to working effectively and in partnership with others. Communicating effectively with others and being able to show that you have the relevant knowledge about handling information will mean that they feel they can approach you when they do not understand an aspect of a record, for example, and ask you for advice. It can also mean that others will be more likely to want you to support them with contributing to their records. In this way you can show them good practices when understanding and contributing to records.

Reflect on it

1.3 Supporting others

Others include team members, colleagues, individuals accessing or commissioning care or support, families, carers or advocates. You will need to ensure that you can support these different people to understand and contribute to records. Look back over AC 1.3 on supporting others to understand the need for secure handling of information.

you work. Knowing that others will also be accessing and using the information that you record will mean that you are more likely to include only relevant information as well as ensure that the records you are keeping are up to date and accurate. If others are able to understand and contribute to records in a consistent way, the team will be gathering more authentic information and will therefore be able to use this to provide more effective care that meets individuals' care or support needs because fewer misunderstandings will arise. You will also be able to form good working relationships as you will be seeking others' involvement.

How to support others to understand records

It is important for others to be able to understand records being completed, particularly if they are about them. In this way you can ensure that you are promoting their rights to understand the information contained within their records or those that they represent. You can support others to understand by ensuring you:

- **make information available in a format they can understand:** you may, for example, need to adapt how you provide information; once you have got to know the person, you will have a better understanding of what format to make this available in

- **explain the purpose of the record:** ensure you fully explain what the record is, and what it is used for
- **explain what will happen to the information obtained:** ensure you fully explain what the information you obtain will be used for and seek their consent to do so
- **show others the records you have to complete:** make sure that you involve others and show them the information you are required to complete, so they can begin to understand the reasons why the record is important and how it is used
- **provide information, advice and guidance:** ensure you provide any additional information others may want to know about the record, including answering any questions they may have, such as: how often does the record have to be completed?, who sees it?, how long is the information kept for?, and any concerns they may have regarding its security or who the information is shared with.

How to support others to contribute to records

It is also important for others to be able to contribute to records or at least to be given the opportunity to contribute to them. In this way you can ensure that you are promoting their rights to be consulted and involved in records about them or those that they represent. You can support others to contribute to records by ensuring you:

- **make records accessible:** ensure they are available and presented in a way that they can use and understand
- **explain the benefits of contributing:** for example, reinforcing how contributing to records will mean that they are in control of the information collated and documented and of ensuring that it is accurate and up to date

- **explain their rights to contribute to records:** for example, promote their rights to be treated with dignity and respect regarding the handling of information contained within their records
- **show others how they can contribute to records:** for example, include comments about individuals' care and support (in the daily report or in individuals' care or support plans, for example), complete the records with them, and review the records with them
- **provide information, advice and guidance:** for example, discuss the options available for them to contribute to records (as mentioned above). You could also look at and read through the records you make, ask them for their comments and you could record these. You could also include their feedback on aspects of the records that worked well and those that didn't work as well.

The benefits of others understanding and contributing to records

By understanding and contributing to records, those involved in the individual's care and support will feel involved and consulted. This can lead to improvements in the accuracy of the information being collated and documented because others will be able to raise any issues or suggestions they have. This collaborative way of working will more likely lead to them asking you questions, discussing their ideas and suggestions with you and therefore will help to improve working relationships.

> **Reflect on it**
>
> **1.3 Skills and qualities for supporting others**
>
> Supporting others to understand and contribute to records requires specific skills and qualities. How many of the skills and qualities shown in Figure 6.5 do you have, and which ones do you think you need to improve on to be able to support others to understand and contribute to records more effectively?

> **6Cs**
>
> **Compassion**
>
> Compassion, in this AC, refers to being able to support others to understand and contribute to records with kindness. In order to do this effectively you will need to be able to empathise so that you can understand how it feels to have others share your personal information and the expectations you have for how you would like to be treated. You can show individuals and others that you understand the importance of supporting them to understand and contribute to their records; you could even explain this to them. You can also work in a compassionate way by involving them and explaining the benefits of them being involved and contributing to records. For example, you could explain that by contributing, they will feel more in control of how their information is dealt with. All of this will also allow you to build a good working relationship with them.
>
> **Care**
>
> Care, in this AC, involves you showing that you have a genuine interest in ensuring that you provide high quality care and support and that everything you do in your job role is focused on enabling the best possible outcomes for individuals. You can do this by supporting others to handle information using positive and respectful ways that are in line with your employer's agreed ways of working.

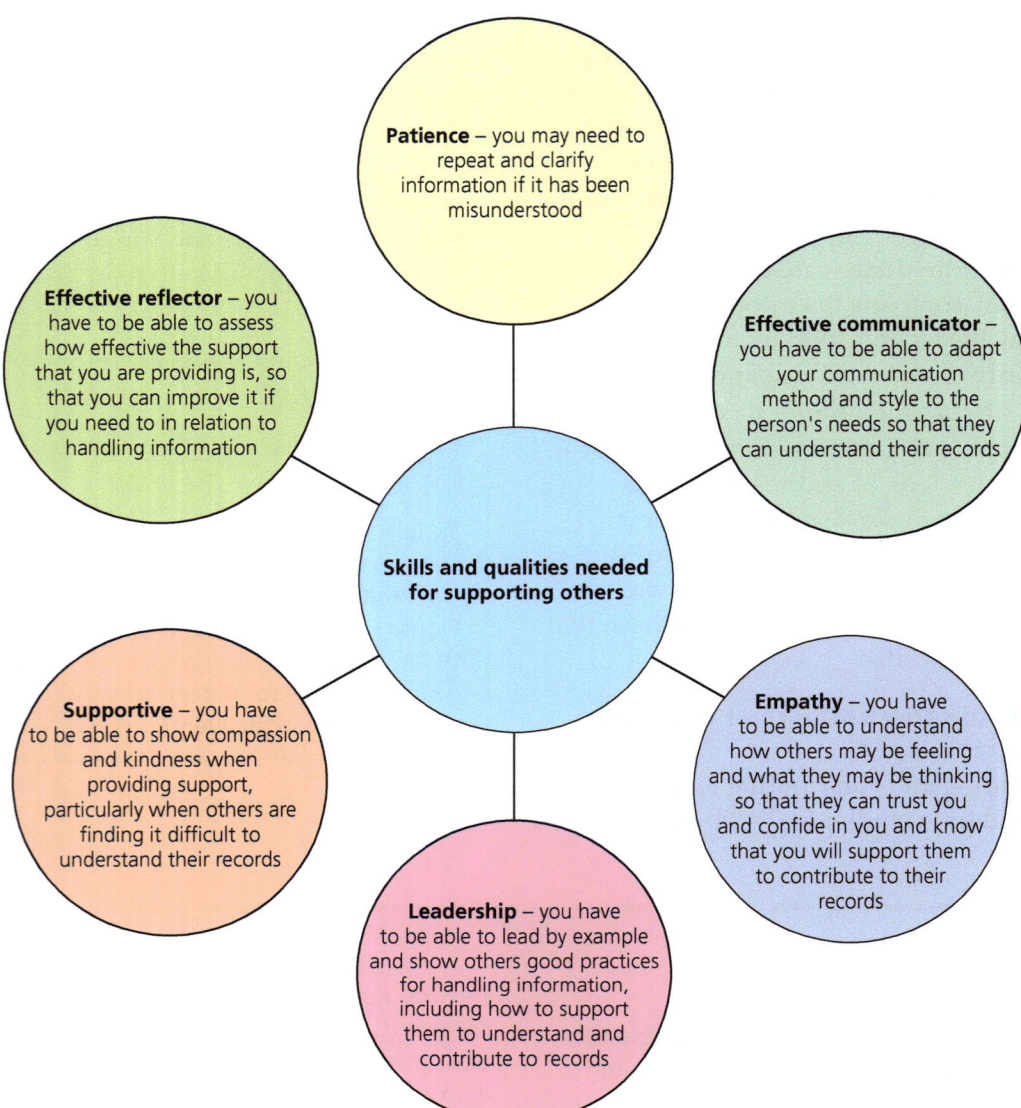

Figure 6.5 Essential skills and qualities for supporting others

The reflective exemplar provides you with an opportunity to further reflect on the impact that supporting others to understand and contribute to their records can have.

Reflective exemplar	
Introduction	I work as a personal assistant providing one-to-one support to Dylan, a young man who has autism.
What happened?	Dylan asked me whether he could get more involved in the review meeting that has been arranged to discuss his support needs. The meeting will be attended by Dylan's parents and social worker.
	Prior to the meeting I showed Dylan a copy of his care plan that will be discussed and reviewed at the meeting. We went through each section of his care plan and discussed why the information contained on it was important. After reading through each section I gave Dylan the opportunity to ask any questions and confirm whether he agreed with the information contained.

Reflective exemplar	
What happened? *Continued*	The section of Dylan's care plan that contained information about the support he requires with day-to-day activities required updating. Dylan explained what areas were out of date and what additional needs he had, such as the support he would like with booking a taxi so that he can access his local gym twice a week. At the end of our discussion Dylan looked happy and he told me that he was really looking forward to the review meeting next week and that he didn't feel scared about it any longer.
What worked well?	It was pleasing to see Dylan take an interest in his care plan and want to actively contribute to the record. Providing Dylan with the opportunity to contribute to his care plan, ask questions and take the lead in deciding the information that was no longer current meant that I was promoting his rights to be an active participant in his care and support.
What did not go as well?	I hadn't fully appreciated how Dylan was feeling about his review meeting, i.e. that he was scared. I should have taken the opportunity when he mentioned this to me to explore why he was feeling that way and how this compared to how he was feeling after he discussed his care plan with me prior to his review meeting.
What could I do to improve?	I think I will need to reflect on how I could have empathised with Dylan over how he was feeling about his review meeting. After his review meeting has taken place I will have a post-review meeting discussion with Dylan and find out how he thought the process went, what worked well and what could have been improved. I plan to reflect on his feedback and use this to improve how I support Dylan to understand and contribute to his records.
Links to unit's assessment criteria	AC: 1.3

> ### Evidence opportunity
>
> **1.3 Support others to keep information secure**
>
> Show your assessor how you support others to keep information secure. You could work with an individual and their family and show how you support them to understand the need for keeping information secure. Think about the methods you are going to use – why will you use them? Think about any questions they may have – how you are going to respond to them?

AC 1.4 Explain what is considered a 'data breach' in the handling of information

What is a data breach?

A data breach is the accidental or unlawful destruction, loss, alteration, unauthorised disclosure of, or access to, personal or secure data. A data breach is not only about loss or theft of personal data; it is also when the confidentiality or availability of personal data has been compromised.

The Information Commissioner's Office (ICO) states that examples of personal data breaches can include:

- deliberately or accidentally losing, destroying, corrupting or disclosing personal data
- accessing personal data without authorisation
- sending personal data to an incorrect person
- devices such as laptops or tablets containing personal data being lost or stolen
- making amendments to personal data without authorisation
- loss of availability of personal data that impacts negatively.

Source: ICO, Personal data breaches, What is a personal data breach?

AC 1.5 Describe how to respond appropriately to a 'data breach' within own work setting/service

How to respond to a data breach

Under the Data Protection Act 2018, the legislation that you learned about earlier on in this unit in AC 1.1, all organisations in the UK are required to report certain personal data breaches within 72 hours to the ICO. Those that are a risk to people's rights and freedoms must be reported; those that aren't, don't have to be reported. If an organisation does not report a notifiable data breach, then the ICO could fine them.

All personal data breaches must be documented, irrespective of whether they have been notified to the ICO. When organisations report data breaches to the ICO the UK's Data Protection Act requires them to provide the following information:

- Details of the personal data breach to include the number of people affected and the number of records involved
- The name and contact details of the data protection officer in the organisation; or if there isn't one the name and contact details of the person from whom more details about the personal breach can be obtained
- Details of the likely consequences of the personal data breach
- Details of the measures taken or planned to be taken as a result of the personal data breach
- Details of the measures that will be taken to reduce any potential negative effects of the personal data breach.

The organisation you work for will have a procedure in place for responding to data breaches. Do you know where it is? Do you know what it says about responding to a data breach, including who you have to report it to? Have you attended any training about responding to data breaches in your organisation?

The NHS hacking scandal 2016/17

Recently, the NHS became victim of hacking (where files and records were accessed illegally). This affected over 100 countries and had serious consequences for the NHS and its hospitals across the UK. Doctors were unable to access electronic information held on IT systems unless a ransom was paid. This meant many operations were cancelled as patients' personal information about allergies and health conditions, for example, could not be accessed. Results of patients' blood tests and x-rays could not be obtained and patients could not be admitted or discharged from hospital without access to their information that was held electronically.

While such a story is rare, with organisations like the NHS having robust or strong systems in place to prevent the likelihood of a cyber-attack or 'hack', this highlights how no organisation is completely safe, and moreover how important it is to ensure you and your setting do the utmost to protect the information you hold. This may be through systems such as locking files away in cabinets, or having firewalls, anti-virus software and password protection policies in place. You will learn more about this in AC 2.1.

> **Research it**
>
> **1.4 NHS Hacking scandal 2016/17**
>
> Look back at the NHS 2016/17 hacking scandal that we discussed about fraudsters gaining access to NHS patients' records and preventing NHS staff from accessing patients' personal information, including medical records and x-rays. Research what happened by looking at articles available on the internet and think about how such an incident might affect where you work.
>
> Write down findings from your research.

Research it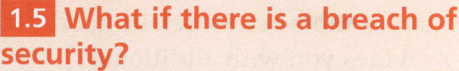

1.5 What if there is a breach of security?

Research what the records policy in the care setting where you work says about what you should do if there is a data breach when handling information. For example, you may identify that a member of the team has not followed the required processes for maintaining and keeping an individual's personal information safe, or has tried to access an electronic information system without authorisation.

Discuss your findings with a colleague and make some notes to document your discussion.

Evidence opportunity

1.4, 1.5 What is a data breach and how do you respond?

Discuss with your manager what is a 'data breach' in relation to the handling of information and how to respond appropriately to a data breach in your work setting/service.

LO2 Be able to implement good practice in the handling of information

Getting started

Think about the care setting where you work and the records you are required to complete as part of your job role. For example, you may have to update individuals' care or support plans, pass a message on to a colleague about an individual's GP appointment or complete a training request for a member of the team. If you work in an individual's home, you may need to update the individual's daily record or their risk assessment. You will also need to update this if you work in residential care settings.

How do you record these different types of information? Do you use paper or electronic records, or both? Where do you store these records? Why? How do you access these records? Why?

AC 2.1 Demonstrate how to ensure data security when storing and accessing information

For this AC you will be observed on how you ensure data security when storing and accessing information in the care setting where you work. You must therefore familiarise yourself with your care setting's procedures for storing and accessing both manual and electronic information. It is important that you know not only the procedures to follow but also the reasons why. In this way, if you are asked for information or advice by a member of your team you can explain and show them good practices to follow when storing and accessing information that are in line with your care setting's agreed ways of working and that comply with legislative requirements and codes of practice.

One of your responsibilities will be to read and understand what your employer's agreed ways of working are in relation to recording and storing information.

- Complying with or following your employer's agreed ways of working correctly will mean that you are following best practice.
- Not following your employer's agreed ways of working can have serious consequences for you, your colleagues at work and the individuals you provide care and support to. For example, you may lose your job, you will prevent your colleagues from providing the care the individual needs, and the individual may not have their unique needs met.

Reflect on it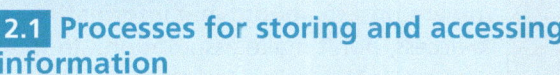

2.1 Processes for storing and accessing information

Reflect on the reasons why you have different processes in the care setting where you work for storing and accessing different types of information. For example, you may want to think about the different types of information you access compared to others in your team. How might this affect what information you can access and how you store information? Write a short reflective account detailing your thoughts.

The information in LO1 will be useful to you here as it will provide you with an understanding of how to use manual and electronic information systems effectively so that they help to ensure information remains secure. You should be able to demonstrate this knowledge and understanding in your skills and behaviours as part of your role.

The 'dos and don'ts' table below details good practice and provides you with additional information about ensuring data security when storing and accessing information.

	Dos and don'ts for ensuring security when storing and accessing information
Do	Store information correctly, using the system agreed. For example, if an individual's communication profile is always documented, reviewed and then stored electronically then ensure that you follow this process too. Doing so will mean that others will be able to access the most up-to-date record in relation to the individual's communication needs.
Do	Store information securely. For example, if you are reading through a team member's training record in preparation for a meeting with them, then ensure you return their training record to where you retrieved it from and ensure that it is kept secure by locking the filing cabinet afterwards. When you retrieve information, make sure you make it clear that you have borrowed the file by leaving a note to say who has borrowed it and when it will be returned by.
Do	Seek permission to access information about an individual in the care setting where you work, irrespective of whether this information is held manually or electronically. Ensure you familiarise yourself with the process to follow. This may be different for different individuals, for example depending on the individual's capacity, and the information you are seeking.
Do	Return files after you have accessed them and return them as soon as possible, to exactly where you got them from.
Do	Access information respectfully. Show consideration towards accessing individuals' and or staff's personal records as they may contain sensitive information; you should ensure you only access information you are allowed to access, whether this is stored manually or electronically. Treat people's personal information with respect and be empathetic towards how they may be feeling knowing that you are accessing it.
Don't	Use poor practices when storing manual and electronic information. Not filing records correctly, not keeping your password secure, or not logging out after you have used the computer may mean that records cannot be found and that others who do not have permission may gain access to confidential information.
Don't	Rush and forget to store information securely. Not returning records to their secure locations can mean that others who do not have permission to read them may do so. Not ensuring the safe keeping of records can also increase the likelihood of them getting lost.
Don't	Access information without following your care setting's agreed ways of working. For example, if you are unsure about what information you can access and what information you are not authorised to access, don't make assumptions. In this way you will be showing your professional duty to handle personal information correctly.
Don't	Access information that you do not require. For example, if you require information about an individual's interests so that you can support them in actively participating in different activities do not access additional information about their family history or their health. Only access the information you require and for the purpose you intend to use it for.
Don't	Make copies of documents, whether these are paper-based or electronic copies. You may not be able to keep track of where the other copies go and who handles them. Make sure that information is not duplicated unless absolutely necessary. If copies are needed, allocate version numbers to them and then once they are no longer required you can delete/destroy the previous version.
Don't	Edit and make changes to any file unless you are allowed to. This includes moving pages around, removing information or moving folders and files around in an electronic system. This may mean that others cannot find what they are looking for.

6Cs

Competence

In the context of this assessment criterion, competence means that you are able to ensure data security when storing and accessing personal information and promote individuals' rights to have all their information treated with dignity, respect and privacy. You could show this by effectively and efficiently following your care setting's processes for storing manual and electronic records and by seeking permission to access information about individuals and other team members who you support.

Now read Case study 1.1, 1.2, 2.1, 2.2. It will help you to think about how secure practices apply in different care settings and with different individuals. You may also want to think about the similarities and differences there are between Stefan, the individual in the Case study, and the individuals who you support.

Case study

1.1, 1.2, 2.1, 2.2 Ensuring safe storage of individuals' records

Giorgio is a Lead Personal Assistant and is visiting Stefan for the first time to assess his current situation. Stefan is an older adult who has been recently diagnosed with dementia; Stefan lives on his own and requires support with his personal care tasks. During the assessment, Stefan shows Giorgio round his home. Giorgio asks Stefan whether there is anywhere secure that can be used to store his records and any other personal information such as the copy of his risk assessment. Stefan tells Giorgio that he does have a lockable cupboard in his living room but that he lost the key several months ago and has not been able to find it. He suggests to Giorgio that his personal information could be left out on his coffee table, the only table he has in his living area.

Discuss:

1. How do you think Giorgio should respond to Stefan? Why?
2. How can Giorgio protect Stefan's personal information?
3. What legislative requirements apply to Stefan's situation?
4. What codes of practice apply to Stefan's situation?

Reflect on it

2.1 Communication: how do you receive and pass on information?

Think about the different ways in which you receive and pass on information before you are in a position to record and store the information. Is this verbally by telephone or face-to-face? Is this electronically via email, fax, text or instant messaging? Is it through the post? Do you also use these methods to share information?

What are the advantages and disadvantages for each method? What communication issues are there for different methods? For example, emails may be a quick way to share and pass on information, but they do not allow you to observe the person's reactions and facial expressions; meanings may be misinterpreted as a result, and files could accidentally be shared or forwarded to people you did not intend to send to.

Think about the things you need to consider with regard to the different methods you use for receiving and sharing information. What are the advantages and disadvantages of each method? What are the rules you have to follow with regard to confidentiality?

Research it

2.1 Policies and procedures

Research the policies and procedures (agreed ways of working) for receiving and sharing information.

What does your setting say about handling post? What post are you allowed to open, for example? How about any confidential information you receive via email? What are the rules regarding this?

What if you receive an email by mistake? How are you expected to deal with this?

Write down your thoughts and findings.

> **Evidence opportunity**
>
> **2.1 Storing and accessing information securely**
>
> Using secure practices, demonstrate to your assessor how you store and access:
>
> - two pieces of information about an individual with care and support needs
> - two pieces of information about a team member.
>
> You will need to show that you can store information both manually and electronically.

AC 2.2 Demonstrate how to maintain and promote confidentiality in day-to-day communication

For this assessment criterion you will be observed demonstrating different ways you use to maintain and promote confidentiality in day-to-day communication. Your working practices in relation to confidentiality must be in line with your employer's agreed ways of working; these include policies and procedures in relation to data protection and confidentiality. Your employer's agreed ways of working are based on the requirements set out by relevant **legislation**.

Maintaining and promoting confidentiality in day-to-day communication

Maintaining and promoting confidentiality in day-to-day communication is not only relevant to written information and paper-based records but also when speaking to individuals and others and when using technological aids in communications. Below are some top tips that you can use for maintaining and promoting confidentiality in day-to-day communication with individuals, their families, your colleagues and other professionals.

- **Sharing personal information (and obtaining consent):** only share personal information when you have the person's permission to do so and when you have the authorisation from your employer to do so. Ensure that you do not share personal information about a person when you do not need to do so; only share information that is necessary and required for the intended purpose. For example, an optician may only

> **Research it**
>
> **2.2 Confidentiality legislation and policies**
>
> It is important that you know and understand the pieces of legislation, policies and codes of practice around handling and processing personal information.
>
> - Research what the Data Protection Act 2018 say about confidentiality and handling and processing personal information and data.
> - You will also find it useful to research the Care Act 2014, Human Rights Act 1998, and Freedom of Information Act 2000 which also include points relating to confidentiality.
> - Research what the Care Quality Commission (CQC) says about confidentiality and how you must comply with rules around handling and processing personal information.
> - Research what various inspection agencies in adult care settings say about the rules around handling and processing personal information and data.
>
> You may find the following websites useful sources of information:
>
> - Data Protection Act 2018: https://www.gov.uk/data-protection
> - Data Protection Act 1998: www.legislation.gov.uk/ukpga/1998/29/contents
> - CQC Code of Practice on confidential personal information: www.cqc.org.uk/sites/default/files/20180419%20Code%20of%20practice%20on%20CPI%20with%20GDPR%20and%20IRMER%20updates.pdf

need to know about health conditions relevant to the individual's vision but not their whole life history or health profile. Another example may be when a colleague shares with you the reasons why they have been off sick; do not mention the reasons they have disclosed to you to another colleague if they have not given you permission to do so. Even if you have not discussed permission, you should under no circumstances pass this on; the new Data Protection Act 2018 stresses the importance of not passing on private information. An individual's family may ask you about their relative's care or support needs; do not share this personal information about the individual unless you have been authorised to do so by the individual or your employer. If the individual is unable to consent, then you must have permission from their representative. Working in this way is essential for building trust and promoting professionalism.

- **Discussing personal information:** all personal information that is related to those who live, work and visit the care setting where you work must be kept confidential. This means that when you discuss personal information about individuals or others in the care setting you must ensure that you do so in a private place. For example, choose a private room when communicating using BSL with an individual about their care plan; doing so will mean that others will not be able to see what you are both communicating. A colleague may approach you to tell you that they wish to raise a concern with you about an individual. Ensure you do this in a quiet and private location in the care setting so that others will not overhear what you are both discussing and to ensure that the concern raised can be kept confidential.

It is also good practice to not discuss personal information outside of the care setting where you work. In fact, this will be part of the rules in your setting. All personal information about individuals, their families and your colleagues with whom you work should be discussed only within the care setting and not outside in a public place such as on a train or in the high street. In this way, the risk of others overhearing what you are saying can be minimised. Working in this way is essential for building good working relationships.

However, it may be that a situation has been upsetting and you feel you need to share this. It is of course okay to discuss your feelings around the issue, and your actions, but you should not divulge information about the person's name, age, gender, ethnicity, family circumstances or any personal data that might give away who the individual is, i.e. their identity. You should also not discuss individuals in a negative way. The way you describe and discuss the individuals you care for and the people you work with is important, and through this you can show your professionalism and commitment to protecting the confidentiality and trust of those you work with. For example, when writing about the care and support you have provided to an individual ensure you do this by using a respectful and professional tone. This will not only mean that you are following confidentiality rules and guidelines, but it will also mean that individuals, as well as colleagues and those outside the workplace, know that you can be trusted and relied upon.

You should also remember not to discuss individuals with other individuals that you care for. Think about how you would feel if people you knew discussed you with others. Again, creating and maintaining trust between yourself and the individual you care for is key to your relationship and the care that you offer them.

If you have to share personal information, remember not to give confidential details over the phone if possible. If you do need to give details over the phone, then check the identity of the person who has called you. You may need to take their number and call them back so that you are able to take some time to check the identity of the person requesting information.

- **Recording personal information:** all written information such as that contained in records, documents, emails and letters must be kept confidential. Ensure when you are documenting personal information that this takes place in a private area in the care setting where you work, such as in an office that can only be accessed by those who have authorisation to do so. When you are writing information electronically, for example when emailing a professional, ensure that you do so in private and that others cannot access your computer screen when you are doing so if they do not have access to this personal information. Also ensure that you state in the email whether this information can be forwarded on and to whom it can be disclosed. Working in this way is essential for keeping all documented personal information private. You will also need to ensure that the information that is recorded is done so in an accessible, accurate, legible and clear fashion, so that others who access the document are able to read and understand what has been recorded. The information should also be up to date.

- **Storing personal information:** you must uphold the confidentiality of all personal information by storing it securely. Ensure that after you have used a record or document containing personal information you return it to its secure location, for example to a locked filing cabinet or locked drawer and in the case of electronic records, to a secure (password-protected) electronic folder on the computer with a security system in place to prevent hacking. Ensure that you do not leave records or other confidential documents out, even for a few minutes, as others may be able to access personal information that they did not have authorisation to see, such as a colleague's home address or a letter from an individual's GP. Working in this way is essential for storing personal information in line with your employer's agreed ways of working and relevant legislation. The same principles apply if you are a personal assistant working in the individual's home; you will need to ensure that information is safeguarded whether these are hard-copy paper documents, or electronic files. However, the individual may not have a lockable cabinet where files can be stored, so you will need to discuss the best ways to safely store records in the individual's home.

6Cs

Commitment

Commitment means to be dedicated. In an adult care setting this means commitment to improving the experience of people who need care and support, ensuring it is person-centred. In this section in particular, you will need to show commitment to maintaining the confidentiality of individuals' and others' personal information at all times. This is important for building good, honest and open relationships with individuals and others.

Evidence opportunity

2.2 Demonstrating ways to maintain and promote confidentiality in day-to-day communication

Select three aspects of confidentiality that are relevant to your day-to-day communication in the care setting where you work. For each one, demonstrate to your assessor how you put these into practice in your current job role. Make sure you show how you promote confidentiality in your day-to-day communication.

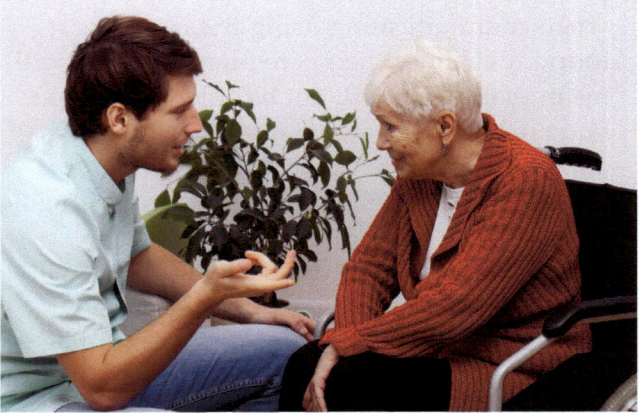

Figure 6.6 How committed are you to confidentiality?

Reflect on it

2.2 Confidentiality where you work

Reflect on how you maintain confidentiality in the care setting where you work. What guidance have you been provided with about following the rules of confidentiality? Perhaps there is a code of practice in place for you and your team members to follow, perhaps you have attended a training update on confidentiality or perhaps someone explained this to you?

Why is it important to receive and understand information and guidance about how to maintain confidentiality in your day-to-day work responsibilities?

What if you work in an individual's home? How can you ensure that you respect their privacy and confidentiality?

Case study

1.1, 1.2, 2.2 Requirements for handling information

Sally is a senior support worker and leads a small team who support three young adults with learning disabilities to live independently. Sally will be providing the team with an information update about handling information in relation to the Data Protection Act 2018, focusing on how, through their working practices, they can ensure they uphold individuals' rights to confidentiality and to having all their personal information treated with respect.

Discuss:

1. Where can Sally access up-to-date information about the Data Protection Act 2018?
2. What legislation is relevant to handling confidential information in care settings?
3. What policies are relevant for maintaining confidentiality in care settings?
4. What codes of practice are relevant to handling individuals' personal information in care settings?

AC 2.3 Demonstrate how to maintain records that are up to date, complete, accurate and legible

For this assessment criterion you will be observed on how you maintain records in the care setting where you work to ensure that they are up-to-date, complete, accurate and legible. All the records you complete as part of your job role are legal documents and a permanent record of what has happened. It is therefore important that when you complete records you do so correctly and effectively, however the information has been communicated to you (whether this is verbally in person or over the phone, electronically via email, fax or text message, or in paper format via a letter, for example). Doing so will mean that you will be able to show that you are:

- **complying with legal requirements:** for example, the requirements of the Data Protection Act 2018 and other legislation you learned about in LO1
- **complying with organisational requirements:** for example, the agreed ways of working, the policies and procedures for maintaining records effectively in the care setting where you work
- **complying with your duty of care:** in relation to handling information; this includes promoting people's rights to privacy, confidentiality, safety and wellbeing
- **complying with your responsibilities:** for example, by providing accurate, reliable and clear information about individuals or team members to others such as GPs or your manager who may need to access it promptly.

Maintaining up-to-date records

Always add date and time to records

You can keep records that contain up-to-date information by ensuring you always date the written or computerised records you make, and include the time, so that if you or someone else needs to refer to them at a later date you can check when the record was made and therefore whether the information you recorded at the time is still current or needs to be added to. For example, you may have recorded in an individual's care plan that the individual has recently returned from hospital after sustaining a fall and is now using a walking frame indoors. This information may no longer be up to date in two weeks' time; the individual may, for example, have recovered well from their previous fall and may no longer be using a walking frame indoors. By updating your first entry and dating both entries you will be able to communicate clearly to others in your team the individual's care needs and the support they require at that particular time and ensure that the individual receives safe and effective care that meets their needs.

Record information as soon as possible

You can do this by making an entry into an activity record as soon as you have completed an activity such as cooking a meal with an individual and any relevant information. This means that you are unlikely to forget important information or 'mix up' information, especially if you are providing support for more than one individual. In addition, recording information as soon as possible after something has happened will ensure the records are current and you will be less likely to forget to include important details. In safeguarding or emergency situations the timing of the records is important.

Record information regularly and consistently

You could, for example, make an entry into the daily report at the end of every shift. This will also help to ensure that your records are up to date as they will log or document the individuals' progress and the care they have received. You should also ensure that you document information consistently, for example by documenting information about an individual in all the records that you use for that individual.

Update records with changing needs and preferences of team members and individuals

Maintaining records that are up to date is also important for establishing the current needs of the individuals you care for and the team you lead. For example, ensuring that you update a team member's training record will mean that you will be able to plan how to meet their training needs effectively and ensure that they have received all the training that they require to carry out their role safely and effectively.

Not updating an individual's record can mean that individuals' information becomes out of date and does not provide a true picture of the support they require, the care needs they have, and their preferences for how they want to live. This may then mean that the care and support you provide does not meet an individual's needs and can result in it being unsafe.

Update records to help families understand the care that individuals receive

Keeping records that are up to date will instil confidence and show you and your team's professionalism when providing care to individuals. For example, individuals' families may request an update of an individual's condition or progress with a task they are learning such as cooking – imagine how it may feel to not receive up-to-date information about their relative and how the team member may feel to not be able to provide it?

Maintaining complete records

Include sufficient and relevant detail

You can keep records that are complete by ensuring that when you document information it contains all the necessary details. Include too many details and it may be difficult for others to understand what you are trying to say; include insufficient details and you may not have included all the relevant details that the next person who accesses the record may need. For example, when completing a risk assessment in full before supporting an individual to go shopping, you may like to clearly record the hazards you identified, potential risks and the ways you and the individual agreed to use to manage these.

Keeping records that are complete is important because not doing so can mean that important information about, for example, a change in an individual's health condition may not be recorded. This can mean that the individual is not provided with the correct care and their health condition may worsen as a result. Not writing records completely can therefore have serious consequences for individuals but can also mean that you risk putting your own job and career at risk.

> **Reflect on it**
>
> **2.3 Up-to-date information**
>
> Reflect on an occasion when you were asked for information about an individual's care or support needs. Were you able to provide this information? Was it up to date? How do you know it was up to date? Did you carry out any checks? Why?

Sign and date documents

Ensuring that records are complete also involves including your signature and the time and date at the end of what you have written – not only does this show that you have written everything you wanted to but it also means that no one else can add anything else to your entry at the end. Records that are signed and dated will also reflect their authenticity and will make it easy to refer back to the person who completed them if, for example, more information is required or something needs to be clarified.

23/01/2023	Provided J with the usual support this morning. All is fine. J's sister requested the time of J's hospital appointment next week.
24/01/2023	J feeling unwell this morning and stayed in bed. Discussed with J the reasons why she was feeling unwell; she explained that she had a headache. I asked J whether she would like to book an appointment with her GP. J refused but requested that I inform her sister. I informed her sister immediately over the telephone. J's sister will be visiting J this afternoon at 2pm to see how she is; I informed J of this. Please can you ensure that you check how J is when you provide her with care this evening and inform the office before you leave.

Figure 6.7 Examples of entries in a communication book

Reflect on it

2.3 Complete records

Read through the two entries in Figure 6.7. These are examples made by a Lead Personal Assistant in a communication book about the support provided to an individual. Reflect on how complete they were and, more importantly, how effective you think they were and the reasons why. You could think about what the main message being conveyed is and whether there is sufficient information provided.

Research it

2.3 Maintaining complete records

Research two records that you have completed as part of your daily responsibilities in the care setting where you work. For example, these may be contained in a document or in a book. Read them through and check whether they are complete. Explain to a colleague why they are complete. If they're not complete, what information is missing and what could you do to improve your record-keeping in the future?

Record details as soon as possible

Recording details as soon as possible after, for example, a task or an accident will mean it is less likely that you will forget details and will ensure that you include all the important information to provide a true picture of what happened.

Maintaining accurate records

Writing accurately into records is very important for ensuring that all information included provides a true picture of what really happened. Not doing so can mean that important decisions about individuals are made and based on inaccurate information. For example, if an individual has a fall it is important that you record what happened accurately, including the date, the time, how the fall happened, what injuries were sustained, what actions you took and whether there were any witnesses. In this way, the record will provide a true picture of how the accident happened and how the individual was supported. This will help to ensure your records are accurate. The Data Protection Act allows people to view any information/records held about them and so it is important to ensure the information you include is accurate, as well as complete and legible.

Differentiate between facts and opinions

You can keep records that are accurate by ensuring that you document the facts. It is fine to include opinions, but you must identify them as such, and they must be based on evidence – you should be able to justify (provide clear reasons for) what you have written. Accurate records mean that to the best of your knowledge they contain information that is true and based on fact or evidence. Basically, the record must clearly state what you have seen and/or heard, and if you include any opinions, you must support them with evidence and clearly state that this is an opinion.

Relate to the individual only

You should also ensure that you only write about the individual and not anyone else in their notes, so it is clear that the information relates to that individual only. This is true in most circumstances and you should follow your agreed ways of working and organisational procedure where another person is involved in the situation you need to record. For example, if there has been a disagreement between two individuals, the names of the individuals need to be recorded on both sets of daily logs.

Record details soon as possible

Updating records as soon as possible after, for example, a task has been completed will mean that you will be more likely to include only the most relevant and important information.

Include all relevant details

Accurate records will have a positive impact on individuals' safety and wellbeing. They should reflect the current state of the individual, what they have told you about how they are feeling, whether they have disclosed any information and exactly what they have told you. If this information is not recorded accurately, this may lead to individuals not being safeguarded, and they may be at risk of danger, harm or abuse or not having their needs met and their wellbeing promoted. For example, recording that an individual has lost 3 kg in weight in one week will lead to a concern being raised about the individual's wellbeing and a request for the individual to receive medical attention quickly so that the reason for the weight loss can be established and their dietary needs can be reviewed; it may be that the individual requires additional food supplements or additional support with their eating. Including the relevant information on an individual's support plan will mean that the key areas of support are clear and understood by your colleagues so that they can provide consistent care.

By contrast, if you record that 'it appears' or 'you think' an individual may have lost some weight but do not provide specific information in your record about how much weight the individual has lost and over what period, then your record may not be perceived as urgent or requiring any action and hence be overlooked. In addition, using vague language such as 'it appears' or 'I think' implies that this is your personal opinion rather than the facts.

Including inaccurate information in your records could therefore have disastrous consequences for the individual – their condition and health may continue to worsen and could even lead to death and you will have failed in your duty of care. This will in turn put your own job and career at risk. The individual's family may decide to complain about this serious failure in care, which may in turn put the organisation you work for at risk of being unable to continue to provide care to individuals with care needs. These are, of course, worst-case scenarios, but they all illustrate the importance of recording information accurately to ensure that individuals receive the most effective care and support possible.

Maintaining legible records

Keeping records also means that you must ensure that all information you include is legible. This means that individuals, your colleagues and others accessing your records must be able to read your handwriting and understand what you have written. Not doing so may mean that important information about individuals is not understood, that misunderstandings arise and that the required care and support are not provided when individuals need this. It also means that colleagues may spend more time trying to work out what you have written. How would you feel if you accessed a record and could not read what was written? Would this make you worried that you may miss important information simply because the writing was not clear and legible?

Write clearly

You can keep records that are legible by ensuring that they are written in a way that they can be read easily by others. This means that if you are hand writing records or using the computer to do so, your handwriting and the typeface must be clear so that it can be read easily and quickly by others. If not, then again you risk not being able to share important information about either an individual or a team member with others, which can in turn mean that their needs remain unmet.

Write concisely

Try not to write too many paragraphs. Bullet points are often a good way to convey information and will save time for the next person who needs to read the records. You should cover all important and correct information, and be clear, but if you can be concise, even better!

Clearly delete errors

If you make an error when you are hand writing a record, ensure it is crossed out clearly with a single line struck through it so that it is evident that you have made an error and also so that your original entry can still be read; this is important in case of the information being referred to at a later date.

Use permanent ink

Some records such as an individual's daily report must be written in permanent ink so that they can be read but also so that they cannot be altered or deleted.

Ensure records are grammatically correct

Keeping legible records ensures that they can be understood by others easily. This means that records must be free from spelling and grammar errors. Writing in complete sentences and having good punctuation will also help the information contained within records to be understood. Not doing so can lead to misunderstandings and inaccurate information being passed on. If you are writing records on a computer, then you can make effective use of the spelling and grammar check tools that are available. If you are hand writing records, then it is a good idea to proof read them carefully when you have completed them, or ask a colleague to do so for you.

Evidence opportunity

2.3 Maintaining records that are up to date, complete, accurate and legible

Demonstrate to your assessor the techniques you use in the care setting where you work to ensure the records you keep are up to date, complete, accurate and legible.

Discuss how effective the techniques are that you use. How do they compare to the techniques others use in the care setting where you work? Are there any improvements that you can make to the way you maintain records? You might like to write notes to document your discussion.

AC 2.4 Demonstrate how to support audit processes in line with own role and responsibilities

For this assessment criterion, you will be observed on how you support **audit processes** as part of your agreed job role and responsibilities in the care setting where you work. The organisation that you work for will have in place specific practices that you are expected to follow for handling information. These will be set out in the organisation's policies and procedures and will be reviewed to ensure that they remain up to date and reflect current legislation and codes of practice for the safe and effective handling of information. Your organisation will monitor that you and other members of the team are complying with these. They will also monitor how effective the practices for handling information in the setting are.

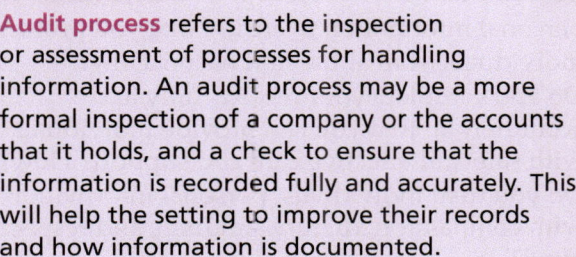

Key term

Audit process refers to the inspection or assessment of processes for handling information. An audit process may be a more formal inspection of a company or the accounts that it holds, and a check to ensure that the information is recorded fully and accurately. This will help the setting to improve their records and how information is documented.

Care Quality Commission (CQC) inspections

In addition to the requirements of the organisation you work for, all registered providers of care are also inspected by the Care Quality Commission (CQC) to check that they meet the minimum standards of quality and safety; this includes the safe and effective handling of information. The CQC inspectors visit providers of care services so that they can observe the care being provided to individuals but also so that they can read and review the organisation's policies, procedures, records and documents that hold personal information in relation to, for example, individuals' needs, including how they are documented and met. Inspectors will also take the opportunity during their visits to speak to and listen to the experiences of individuals and others who work and/or visit the care setting. In this way they can build up a picture of how effective the systems in place are; this could, for example, be those in relation to handling information as well as other systems that support the care being provided to individuals.

CQC inspections are based on five questions that they ask of all providers of care; these are then further broken down and referred to as the key lines of enquiry:

1 Are they safe?
2 Are they effective?
3 Are they caring?
4 Are they responsive to people's needs?
5 Are they well-led?

In terms of relating the five questions to handling information you could, for example, ask yourself the following:

1 Do you maintain the security of individuals' personal information to ensure that you protect individuals from abuse and harm? How?
2 Do you complete your records fully and accurately so that you can provide individuals with safe and effective care and support? How?
3 Do you treat individuals' personal information with compassion, dignity, kindness and respect? How?
4 Do you handle all information effectively so that it meets individuals' needs? How?
5 Do the procedures and systems in place for handling information enable you to deliver high quality care and support to individuals? How?

How many of these questions did you answer 'yes' to? It is also important to be able to provide evidence of how you are handling information effectively in your work setting. This may be gathered by the CQC inspectors observing you while you work or speaking to the individual you provide care to and/or their relatives, or they may review records that you have completed. It is important therefore to ensure that your practices for handling information are consistent and apply good practice at all times.

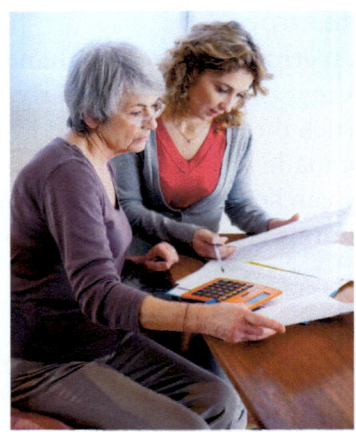

Figure 6.8 How do you comply with inspections?

If you work in the individual's home

If you work for a care setting that is not registered as a provider of care and therefore not inspected by CQC, for example if you are a carer for an individual in their own home, then you are still bound by the requirements of relevant legislation and codes of practice. The individual you provide care to may have additional requirements that they wish you to comply with and so you must also familiarise yourself with these.

6Cs

Commitment

Commitment means to be dedicated. In this AC it would involve you being dedicated to ensuring that you and the team you lead handle information in effective and efficient ways and are able to support the audit processes. You can show your commitment by working with your employer's agreed ways of working for recording, storing, accessing and sharing information as discussed in this section.

Courage

Courage in this AC would involve you making sure that you speak up for individuals if you are aware that they or their personal information is at risk of being placed in danger, harmed or abused. It is your duty of care to ensure their safety and wellbeing, including when it comes to information that is about them, or personal or confidential to them. You can show your courage by always reporting immediately any concerns you have about individuals' personal information being recorded, stored, accessed and/or shared. In this way you can ensure that you are safeguarding them and their information and not placing them in any further danger.

Table 6.4 is a useful checklist that you can use to assess how effective you are in supporting audit processes for the effective handling of information where you work. It will help you to raise your awareness of your role in the audit process and think about your responsibilities for handling information, including what to do if you have any questions or concerns about handling information.

Table 6.4 Checklist for supporting audit processes for handling information

	Checklist for supporting audit processes for handling information
Recording information	• Do you know what records you are responsible for completing? • Do you know how to access the records you are responsible for? • Do you know when to complete these records? • Do you know how and why you must complete these records? • Do you know who you must report to if you have any concerns about the recording of information? • Do you know about issues such as confidentiality when recording information? Do you know how to comply with data protection legislation and the Data Protection Act 2018 when it comes to recording information?
Storing information	• Do you know how to store manual records you are responsible for? • Do you know how to store electronic records you are responsible for? • Do you know the reasons why manual and electronic records are stored in this way? • Do you know how to keep secure all the records you are responsible for? • Do you know who you must report to if you have any concerns about the security of stored records? • Do you know about issues such as confidentiality when storing information? Do you know how to comply with data protection legislation and the Data Protection Act 2018 when it comes to storing information?
Accessing information	• Do you know how to access manual records you are responsible for? • Do you know how to access electronic records you are responsible for? • Do you know the reasons why manual and electronic records are accessed in this way? • Do you know how to seek an individual's consent to access their records? • Do you know who you must report to if you have any concerns about accessing information or security around accessing information? • Do you know about issues such as confidentiality when accessing information? Do you know how to comply with data protection legislation and the Data Protection Act 2018 when it comes to accessing information?
Sharing information	• Do you know what information about individuals you can share with others and the reasons why? • Do you know what information about individuals you cannot share with others and the reasons why? • Do you know when information can be shared with others? • Do you know the checks you must make before sharing information with others and the reasons why? • Do you know who you must report to if you have any concerns about sharing information? • Do you know about issues such as confidentiality when sharing information? Do you know how to comply with data protection legislation and the Data Protection Act 2018 when it comes to sharing information?

Reflect on it

2.4 Your strengths and weaknesses

Reflect on how effective your working practices are in terms of the requirements that your organisation has in place for the handling of information as part of your day-to-day role and responsibilities. What are your strengths? What are your weaknesses? How can you develop your strengths and improve your weaknesses? Present your findings as a SWOT (strengths, weaknesses, opportunities, threats) analysis.

Evidence opportunity

2.4 Supporting audit processes

Show your assessor how you follow good practices in line with your current job role and responsibilities for handling information. Show them how you support audit processes in line with your own roles and responsibilities.

Legislation	
Act/Regulation	Key points
Data Protection Act 2018	Personal information must be recorded, used, stored and shared according to a set of principles or rules, i.e. information and data must be processed fairly, lawfully, used only for the purpose it was intended to be used for, be adequate, relevant, accurate and up to date, held for no longer than is necessary, used in line with the rights of individuals, kept secure and not transferred to other countries without the individual's permission. People's rights are more enhanced than they were under the Data Protection Act 1998. Organisations have greater responsibility for ensuring that they have effective arrangements in place for handling information and that those who work for them are complying with their procedures and systems.
The Freedom of Information Act 2000	Individuals have the right to request information held about them by a wide range of public bodies, such as local authorities and hospitals.
The Care Act 2014	Local authorities must provide comprehensive information and advice about care and support services in their local area so that individuals can make informed decisions about their care and support. The information provided must be able to be understood by individuals.
The Health and Social Care Act 2008 (Regulated Activities) Regulations 2014	Personal information about individuals in care settings must be used in line with organisations' agreed ways of working. It promotes transparency by supporting the sharing of information with individuals and their families.
The Human Rights Act 1998	Everyone in the UK is entitled to the same rights and freedoms. In relation to the handling of information, Article 8 established the right to respect for your private and family life, home and correspondence.

306 Promoting and implementing person-centred practice

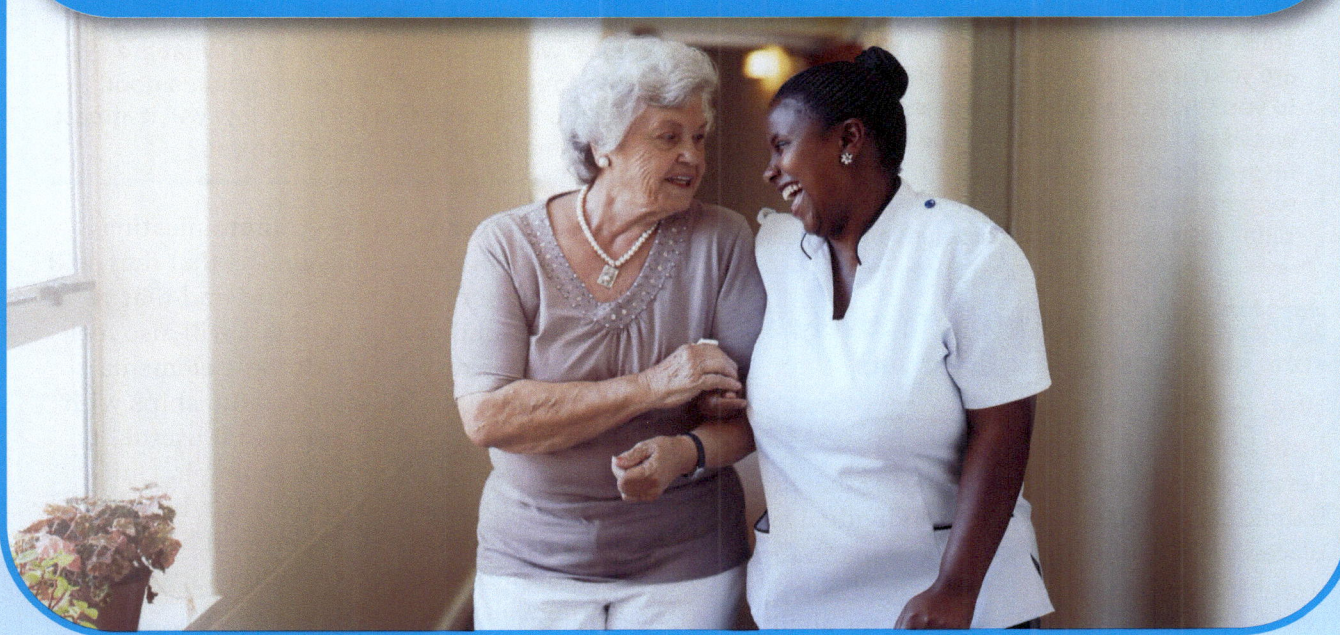

About this unit

Credit value: 3
Guided learning hours: 22

Person-centred care involves individuals with care or support needs being actively involved in the planning and provision of their care. Working in a way that embeds person-centred values is crucial for ensuring individuals are in control of their care or support.

Other person-centred approaches that you will learn about include positive risk taking, using an individual's care plan and finding out about individuals' unique histories, preferences, wishes and needs.

You will also learn about how to establish consent when providing care or support to an individual and what to do when you cannot. Encouraging active participation and reducing the barriers that may arise, as well as supporting individuals' rights to make informed choices and considering how this can be done in line with best practice and risk assessment processes, are also aspects of person-centred working that you will be able to use your skills to practise.

Promoting individuals' wellbeing and showing how you can do so effectively are some additional areas of expertise that you will have an opportunity to develop and explain the importance of.

Learning outcomes

By the end of this unit you will:

LO1: Understand the application of person-centred practices in care settings/services

LO2: Understand the importance of individuals' relationships

LO3: Be able to work in a person-centred way

LO1 Understand the application of person-centred practices in care settings/services

Getting started

Think about what makes you who you are. What are your likes and your dislikes? What is important to you? What do you believe in and why? How would you feel if your family and friends didn't respect these? Now think about the people you support; how do you think they would feel if you didn't respect their personal values and beliefs?

AC 1.1 Explain how to effectively build relationships with individuals

Why is building relationships with individuals important?

Person-centred care involves ensuring that the individual is valued as a unique individual and placed in the centre of any decisions made about their care and support. Central to applying person-centred practices is therefore having the ability to build relationships with the individuals that live in care settings and access care services. Without good relationships with individuals, you and others will not be able to meet individuals' unique needs and preferences because you will not be able to create an environment where individuals feel that they can approach you and tell you about themselves. It will also make it difficult for you to get to know individuals, provide them with quality care to meet their current needs and support them to plan for their futures if you have not built a relationship with them. You may find it useful to refer back to Unit 300 Responsibilities and ways of working in adult care settings/services and review your previous learning in LO1 around working relationships with individuals and why it's important to work in partnership with individuals.

How to effectively build relationships with individuals

Building relationships with individuals is a two-way process that involves both you and the individual working together to build that relationship as you interact with each other as part of your day-to-day work tasks. Below are some of the ways how you can effectively build relationships with individuals; can you think of any other ways?

Reflect on it

1.1 Importance of relationships with individuals

Reflect on a person you have a working relationship with. Why is the relationship you have with this person important? What are the consequences of not having built a good relationship with this person? How will it impact on them? How will it impact on you?

- **Good communication** – Communicating clearly with individuals means that they will feel that they have been heard and that you understand them. Individuals will also feel valued and respected. All these elements are essential for building relationships with individuals. You will also find it useful to review your previous learning in Unit 304 Effective communication in adult care settings/services, AC 1.2 around how communication affects relationships in a care setting/service.

- **Good care and support** – Providing good quality care and support that is designed in partnership with the individual and takes into account their individuality, their rights, choice, privacy, independence, dignity and respect will promote a warm and genuine environment that is perfect for building relationships with individuals. Without good care and support individuals will not engage with you in a meaningful way as they will not feel valued and will not trust you; two elements that are essential for building effective relationships.

- **Being open and honest** – Being open and honest with individuals that you work with on a day-to-day basis means that individuals will begin to trust you and engage with you because they will feel that you value them and place them at the centre of their care and support. Being honest involves being truthful with individuals even when you know that they are not going to like what you tell them. Without openness and honesty, it is very difficult to build relationships with individuals because they will not feel that they can trust you and therefore they will not be themselves. As a result you will not get to know them or who they really are.

- **Being respectful** – Being respectful towards individuals involves treating them kindly and politely; in other words how you like to be treated in relationships. Respecting individuals including their culture, beliefs, lifestyle, views and preferences that may be different from yours is essential as this shows that you are accepting of them and who they are, which in turn makes them feel valued and listened to. Without respect, it is very difficult to build relationships with individuals because they will not trust you.
- **Being empathetic** – Being empathetic towards individuals involves being understanding and sensitive towards them. It involves not only understanding how an individual feels but also feeling how individuals must feel in particular difficult situations, for example in situations where individuals experience sadness, such as in a bereavement of a close family member, or where individuals experience anger, such as in being refused access to a café because of their disability. Without empathy, it is very difficult to build relationships with individuals because they will be less likely to interact with you if they think that you do not understand how they feel.
- **Making time** – Making time is essential for building relationships with individuals as relationships do not just happen after meeting someone on one occasion or after providing support to an individual over a week; they take time to build and how long they take will vary from individual to individual. Some individuals may have had a bad experience with a relationship and may therefore take a little more time to trust you, others may be more open to building a relationship with you quite quickly. Every individual will be unique and what's important is that you spend time with them and get to know them, which will be difficult to do at times if you are very busy. Without time spent together, it is very difficult to build relationships with individuals because you will not be able to get to know them.
- **Being committed** – Being committed is essential for building relationships with individuals because doing so may be challenging at times. For example, you may be very busy and have very little time to sit down with individuals and spend some meaningful time together getting to know them, or an individual may have acted disrespectfully towards you and not been very honest with you. Being committed to working around these challenges so that you do not let these negatively influence the relationships you have with individuals is a good personal asset to have and a quality that can't be taught. Without commitment, it is very difficult to build relationships with individuals because you will not be able to maintain the quality of the relationship and continue to convey to the individual that you have a genuine interest in getting to know them and work with them.

As mentioned earlier building relationships is a two-way process and therefore good relationships can only be built if individuals also commit to good communication, being open and honest, respectful and empathetic with you and others who they work with. When individuals are not able to engage with you in this way due to a disability or condition that prevents them from doing so, it is important to involve others who know the individual well such as their family, friends and/or representative such as an advocate who can help to maintain and build the relationship between you and the individual.

> **Research it**
>
> **1.1 Effective relationship building**
>
> Research the psychologist Carl Rogers. The features of good relationships that were described by Rogers provide a good basis for thinking about how to effectively build relationships with individuals.
>
> You will find the link below useful:
> www.simplypsychology.org/carl-rogers.html
>
> Take it in turns to discuss with a partner the three most important qualities you think are needed for building effective relationships with individuals. Explain to your partner your reasons for your choices. How did your choices differ from those of your partner's?

> **Evidence opportunity**
>
> **1.1 Building effective relationships with individuals**
>
> For one individual you know about describe who they are including any care or support needs they have.
>
> Then, explain why it is important to have an effective working relationship with them, including the consequences of not doing so.
>
> Explain how you and others have built an effective relationship with them. What skills did you use and why? What qualities were essential and why?

AC 1.2 Describe how person-centred values can be applied in a range of situations

What are person-centred values?

Your values are unique to you; they make you who you are and influence what you do and how you do it. Values represent what we believe to be important to us; they also guide us with how we live our lives and the decisions we make.

The care and support that you provide and support others to provide as a Lead Adult Care Worker or Lead Personal Assistant is also underpinned by a set of values. These are commonly referred to as **person-centred values**. Practising person-centred values means placing the individual or person you care for at the heart of everything you do and ensuring that you support others to do the same; it is about ensuring care suits individuals and fits around them and that they don't have to adjust to rigid care systems; it is about enabling individuals to control how the care they receive is planned and delivered.

By making sure these values underpin and influence all aspects of your work, the care you and others provide will be:

- focused on the individual and represent their unique needs, wishes and preferences
- focused on enabling the individual to be in control of their life including how they want to live it
- focused on enabling the individual to plan for the care and support they would like (including changes that may arise in the future).

The person-centred values that underpin high-quality care and support are set out below.

You will need to show that you can apply these to the way that you practise in your **care setting**.

Applying person-centred values

As you will have learned in previous units, individuals communicate and interact with others in many different ways. When individuals are in **complex or sensitive situations** this may influence how they feel and interact with others because they may feel upset, frightened, angry or frustrated.

Putting person-centred values into practice is important because doing so can:

- reduce individuals' distress, anger or frustration
- improve individuals' quality of life
- improve individuals' wellbeing
- support individuals' needs, preferences, history, wishes and strengths
- encourage positive relationships between individuals and others
- create an environment that is positive and safe for everyone
- ensure individuals feel safe
- ensure individuals are treated with compassion, dignity and respect
- empower individuals to be in control of their lives.

> **Key terms**
>
> **Complex or sensitive situations** may include those that are distressing or traumatic, threatening or frightening, likely to have serious implications or consequences, of a personal nature, or involving complex communication or cognitive needs.

> **Reflect on it**
>
> **1.2 Complex and sensitive situations**
>
> Reflect on an occasion when you or someone you know dealt with a complex or sensitive situation. What happened? Why was the situation complex or sensitive? How did you or the other person feel about the situation? Why? Write a reflective account.

Putting person-centred values into practice in a complex or sensitive situation is very important because you will require an enormous amount of skill and knowledge to be able to handle these types of situations effectively.

How to put person-centred values into practice

You can put person-centred values into practice when handling a complex or sensitive situation by using a variety of person-centred approaches to ensure the individual remains at the centre. Table 7.1 provides you with some examples of the different ways you can do this.

Table 7.1 Examples of ways to put person-centred values into practice in complex or sensitive situations

Examples of complex or sensitive situations	Ways to put person-centred values into practice
Distressing – an individual is bereaved of their parent	<ul><li>Individuals may experience distress if they have been bereaved.</li><li>Reassure the individual that it is OK to feel the way they do. This will show your understanding and care.</li><li>Listen to what the individual tells you; do not pressurise the individual to speak with you if they do not want to. You could ask them whether they would like to be left alone, speak with you later or whether they would prefer to speak with someone else. This will show your compassion, and that you are promoting their rights to respect and choice in allowing them to retain control of the situation.</li><li>Offer the individual support. This can be from you, others who know the individual well within your setting or even the use of outside support services, such as bereavement helplines or counselling services.</li><li>Reassure the individual that you will maintain their privacy and confidentiality when you record and report what has happened. Continue to monitor the individual.</li></ul>
Traumatic – an individual receives the bad news that they have been made redundant	<ul><li>Individuals may experience trauma when they have been given bad news.</li><li>The individual will be feeling shocked, overwhelmed, upset and even angry about what has happened.</li><li>Show your care and compassion towards the individual by asking them if they are OK.</li><li>Listen to what the individual tells you; don't interrupt them or ask questions. Let the individual tell you about the bad news they've received at their own pace. This will show your compassion and understanding that you are giving them time to adjust to the bad news they've received.</li><li>Offer the individual support. This can be from you, others who know the individual well within your setting or even the use of outside support services to help with finding work, training, finding and applying for benefits, debt, budgeting and money advice such as from organisations that can offer emotional support such as Mind and Mental Health UK.</li></ul>
Threatening or frightening – an individual witnesses another individual get physically assaulted	<ul><li>Try and calm the individual down as they are likely to be very upset by what they have witnessed. The individual may also not be able to sleep at night because of what they have witnessed and/or feel frightened for their own safety. You will need to reassure the individual that they are safe and free from harm.</li><li>Discuss what has happened with the individual; if they want to repeatedly go over the incident, do not become impatient or prevent them from doing so. Let them tell you what happened and how they are feeling as this is likely to be their way of making sense of it all.</li></ul>

Table 7.1 Examples of ways to put person-centred values into practice in complex or sensitive situations *continued*

Examples of complex or sensitive situations	Ways to put person-centred values into practice
	• Respect the individual's choice in relation to what they would like to do next. Perhaps they do not want to provide a witness statement, perhaps they do. It is important to be honest with the individual and explain to them that the police may want to interview them; this is likely to make them feel anxious, but you can reassure them by telling them that they will only be interviewed by someone who is experienced and has been trained to do so. • Offer the individual support to overcome the incident they have witnessed; ask the individual if there is anyone they would like you to contact. Continue to monitor the individual.
Likely to have serious implications or consequences – an individual self-harms	• The individual will be feeling very low in mood and anxious. • Show your consideration towards the individual by not ignoring any signs you see that they have self-harmed, for example perhaps you notice bruises or cuts or that the individual's behaviour has changed. • Be sensitive towards the individual by choosing the words you say to them and taking account of your body language; do not scold them, appear angry or show that you are shocked by what they have done. • Ask the individual how they feel and give them the choice as to whether they want to share anything with you about how they are feeling. Offer them any support you can, for example by showing you genuinely care about maintaining their safety and/or by giving them the contact details of other people they can talk to in confidence, such as a helpline or support group. • Reassure the individual that you will maintain their privacy and confidentiality when you record and report what has happened. Continue to monitor the individual.
Involving personal care – an individual is supported with their personal care for the first time	• The individual will be feeling anxious, embarrassed and even upset about being supported with their personal care. • Show your care and compassion towards the individual by asking them how they want to be supported with their personal care. • Reassure the individual by explaining that you are there to support them and make them feel comfortable. • Be sensitive towards the individual by not giving them eye contact when supporting them with their personal care as doing so may make them feel embarrassed. • Be respectful towards the individual by respecting their privacy, i.e. by placing a towel around them and closing the door, and their independence, i.e. enabling them to do as much for themselves as they are able to. • Reassure the individual that you will maintain their privacy and confidentiality when you record and report how you supported them with their personal care. Continue to monitor the individual.
Involving complex communication or cognitive needs – an individual with dementia accuses you of stealing their personal possessions	• The individual will be feeling very upset and anxious and maybe even angry. • Do not contradict what the individual is saying or take their accusations personally because although you know it is not true, for the individual who has this condition they truly believe it is. Respecting what they are saying will mean that they will feel listened to and valued. • You can reduce the individual's distress by distracting them once they have told you about why they are distressed; perhaps the individual can go for a walk or perhaps you can suggest they try an activity.

Table 7.1 Examples of ways to put person-centred values into practice in complex or sensitive situations *continued*

Examples of complex or sensitive situations	Ways to put person-centred values into practice
	• You may also be able to reduce the individual's distress by helping them to look for their personal possessions. If you do find them, tell the individual that you are pleased and reinforce this with them rather than tell them that they accused you wrongly; this will more likely lead to positive feelings. • Reassure the individual that you will maintain their privacy and confidentiality when you record and report what has happened. Continue to monitor the individual.

> **Research it**
>
> **1.2 Types of complex and sensitive situations**
>
> Research different types of complex and sensitive situations that have arisen in your work setting. What person-centred values were put into practice? Why? Discuss with your assessor or a colleague.

> **Evidence opportunity**
>
> **1.2 Person-centred values in practice in different situations**
>
> Discuss with your assessor the different person-centred values you have put into practice in three situations.

AC 1.3 Describe how to use care plans and other resources to apply person-centred values and strength-based approaches

What are strength-based approaches?

Strength-based approaches are ways of working that are also referred to as asset-based approaches and place the focus on the individual's strengths, resources and what they can do themselves to keep well and maintain independence. They focus on:

- what the individual can do rather than on what they can't, i.e. their abilities, strengths, skills, knowledge, potential
- developing a good working relationship between the individual and those who support them so that the individual can work with those supporting them to live their life how they want
- the individual's support network, i.e. the relationships the individual has with others in their life such as loved ones, their family, friends, neighbours, professionals, and how they can support the individual to achieve what they want.

What are care plans?

A care plan is the document where day-to-day requirements and preferences for care and support are detailed. Care plans can be developed and updated by the individual receiving the care, with the help of others who know the individual well, such as family and friends. You or the manager will then look at the care plan, assess and agree to it. As well as looking at the overall plan, it may be that the manager needs to approve any budget with regard to the plan.

As you have learned, a key part of person-centred care is to encourage the individual to do as much as possible themselves, so a key part of the care plan will be to identify the areas that the individual is able to manage without assistance, then work out where the individual requires some help. By being focused on the individual, the care can be based on what they want and tailored to match their needs. This is why the care plan is so important when it comes to delivering person-centred care. Essentially, the care plan should be informed by what the individual wants from their care. This can then be used as the basis to determine how you can provide that care and support.

Sophie's care plan
All about me My name is Sophie Donning. I am 26 years young and up until a year ago I lived with my mum, dad, younger brother and two dogs. My family and friends are very important to me and I enjoy spending time with them and enjoy visiting them at weekends and going away on holiday. My family and friends know me very well and are the people who are the closest to me. They say that I am fun to be around and admire my patience and kindness, especially towards my younger brother who, like me, also has a physical disability. I enjoy helping people and always try to keep busy. **How to support me** When I need support, I will let you know; I am very good at asking for help when I need it. Some things I can do for myself. These include getting washed, dressed, doing the laundry and cleaning my flat. There are other things that I need you to support me with. This is because I use a wheelchair and sometimes I may feel a bit low in myself and might feel unable or not confident enough to do these things on my own. These things usually involve going out shopping, attending appointments – especially those at the hospital – and going to new areas or places I've never been to before. Please remember not to assume I will always need your support when I go out. Sometimes if I'm having a good day I won't need your help. Always ask me, just to make sure.

Figure 7.1 Example of a care plan

Figure 7.1 is an extract from an individual's care plan to give you an example of what one might look like. It is important to remember that as care plans are personal and unique to the individual, no two care plans will be the same. This is why writing plans in the first person is good practice.

Other resources

When applying person-centred values and strength-based approaches other resources as well as care plans can also be useful and may include, for example, one-page profiles, advanced care plans, assessments from other organisations, and information from other people important to the individual.

- **One-page profiles** – as the name suggests this resource commonly consists of a single page and summarises what is important to the individual and how they want to be supported. **One page-profiles** provide useful information about the individual such as their likes, including what others like about them, their interests, strengths, who they like being with and how they would like others to support them. Their inclusion of concise information means that they can be quickly referenced to provide a clear overview of the individual.
- **Advanced care plans** – are care plans that record details about the care and support an individual would like to receive in the event that they are unable to speak up for themselves, i.e. if they become unconscious due to an accident or if they have the onset of a condition such as dementia or a mental health need. **Advanced care plans** involve individuals planning for their futures by sharing their preferences, wishes, personal values and beliefs about their future care with those that are important to them such as their loved ones, family, friends and carers. For example, this may relate to their:
  - *living arrangements* – e.g. the area they wish to live in, where they want to live such as in their own home as opposed to a residential care home, who they want to live with such as with their sibling as opposed to on their own.
  - *health and wellbeing* – e.g. their physical health and wellbeing, their mental health and wellbeing, what they value as important regarding their wellbeing such as maintaining a healthy lifestyle or a lifestyle where they can spend time outdoors, practising their beliefs.
  - *relationships* – e.g. the relationships that are important to them, the relationships they value such as loved ones, partners, family, friends, neighbours, how they wish to maintain these relationships.
  - *education or employment* – e.g. skills they would like to develop further, areas of interest, opportunities they would like to explore, career and/or studying ambitions.
  - *end of life care* – e.g. preferences for how the care is provided such as at home or by accessing hospice care, preferences for who is involved, how to take into account any beliefs such as in relation to who provides the end of life care and in relation to medication and treatment options.

- **Assessments from other organisations – assessments** involve the gathering and recording of information about an individual and are aimed at finding out how best to support the individual. For example, individuals who wish to access a mental health service must complete a mental health assessment. The mental health assessment involves speaking with mental health professionals such as a nurse, psychologist or psychiatrist about an individual's needs such as their mental health symptoms, their wellbeing, their physical health, their culture, their relationships, their strengths and skills, and their wishes, hopes and aspirations for the future.
- **Information from other people important to the individual** – family, friends, loved ones, carers, advocates and others who are important to the individual are another excellent resource for information as they may be able to share insights and information about the individual in relation to what they enjoy doing and how they do it that is not recorded anywhere else. For example, an individual's partner will be able to share a valuable insight into the individual's past experiences, social and family relationships.

> ### Key terms
>
> **One-page profiles** are resources that typically consist of a single page and provide an outline of what is important to the individual and how the individual would like to be supported.
>
> **Advanced care plans** are resources that document the care and support an individual would like to receive in the future in the event they are no longer able to speak up for themselves.
>
> **Assessments** are resources that involve obtaining and recording information about an individual with the aim of supporting them and meeting their unique needs.

Using care plans and other resources for applying person-centred values and strength-based approaches

Using care plans and other resources such as one-page profiles, advanced care plans, assessments and information from other people important to the individual contributes to applying person-centred values and strength-based approaches because:

- it promotes the individual's rights: the individuals you care for are fully involved or lead how their care and support needs are met. They may not only write the plan or profile but they may also have a copy of what has been agreed. They can also maintain control over their personal information by discussing only what they want to as part of their assessment or agreeing with others who are important to them what they would like to include in their plan
- it supports individuality: the care and support you provide meet an individual's unique needs, preferences, culture, beliefs and personal values. It is drawn up in a format that the individual understands and may even use photographs or video
- it enables the individual to live independently: by focusing on their strengths, abilities and wishes, it enables the individual to achieve as much as they can for themselves to keep well and maintain independence. By focusing on and recognising their strengths, abilities, wishes and needs, care plans and other resources can enable an individual to have the quality of life they desire and enable them to gain confidence to self-care and achieve as much as they can for themselves to keep well and maintain independence.

> ### Reflect on it
>
> **1.3 Person-centred values and care plans**
>
> Reflect on your learning at the beginning of this unit around how and why person-centred values must influence your working practices.
>
> What person-centred values are you promoting when using an individual's care plan for the provision of their care and support?
>
> - Reflect on person-centred values and strength-based approaches.
> - Reflect on your learning about how to use care plans and other resources to apply person-centred values and strength-based approaches.
> - What resources do you use? What person-centred values and strength-based approaches are you promoting when supporting individuals with their care and support?

Evaluating the use of care plans

The use of care plans, one-page profiles, advanced care plans, and information from other people in applying person-centred values and strength-based approaches will only be effective if:

- the care plan and other resources are developed with the individual, otherwise it will not reflect the individual's strengths and wishes, promote their rights or make use of the resources they have
- the care plan and other resources are updated – otherwise it will not reflect the individual's wishes, promote their rights or make use of the resources they have
- the care plan and other resources are used and referenced before and during the provision of care and support – otherwise you will not be able to use them to inform your working practices.

Below is an example of an assessment that uses strength-based approaches:

Table 7.2 Example of an assessment that uses strength-based approaches

Assessment areas	Questions to ask and information to find out
Individual's strengths	- What does the individual enjoy doing? - What is the individual good at? - What does the individual think they can do better? - What does the individual think they can do to improve themselves?
Individual's support network	- Who is important to the individual? - Who supports the individual? - Who does the individual communicate with? - What if anything does the individual want to change about their support network?
Individual's personal challenges	- What personal challenges does the individual have? - What is preventing the individual from doing what they want? - What does the individual think they can do themselves to overcome these? - What support does the individual think they need to overcome these?

> **Evidence opportunity**
>
> **1.3 Using care plans and other resources**
>
> Identify an individual's care plan and other resources that you have used in your day-to-day work practice – you may find it useful to refer to this while completing this activity.
>
> Remember that the care plan contains personal information that does not belong to you, so make sure that you have the individual's and your manager/employer's permission to access it and that you do so in private. You must pay strict attention to confidentiality.
>
> With your manager, discuss the reasons why you used these resources in your working practice and how they helped you deliver person-centred care according to the needs and strengths of the individual. Then provide two examples of how you used the resources. Include in your discussion how doing so impacted on the individual and the quality of care and support you provided. How effective were the care plan and other resources in applying person-centred values? What aspects of the individual's life have improved as a result? Are there any areas where further improvements are required?
>
> Write up notes to evidence your discussion.

AC 1.4 Explain why person-centred values and strength-based approaches must influence all aspects of adult care work

Embedding person-centred values in your everyday work practice is central to providing person-centred care. As you know, person-centred care is about providing support that keeps the individual as the focus. This involves supporting the individual to be in control of their life and the decisions they make both in relation to now and in the future. These person-centred values will underpin everything that you do, from mealtimes to personal routine tasks, and activities that they participate in will need to have the individual and their **preferences** at the centre. It is important to ensure that these underpin all aspects of your work because in your lead role you will be expected to set a good example to others.

Working in a way that embeds person-centred values in all aspects of health and adult care work is important and benefits individuals because:

- By involving individuals in the care they receive and supporting them to make their own choices and decisions, you will allow individuals to live as independently as possible, helping them to feel in control of their lives and to feel more confident. It is worth thinking about how you would feel if someone made decisions about your life for you. What if someone else made the decisions about where you lived, what you ate and what medicine you could or could not take? Everyone is allowed the right to make their own choices, including those in care settings, and taking away this control denies people their right to make choices and live the way they want to.
- It can make a positive difference to individuals' lives as the care and support you provide will reflect individuals' needs, views and preferences. It will be in line with what the individual prefers, enabling them to live how they want to.
- You will be able to find out more about individuals' unique likes, dislikes, abilities and preferences and can tailor your care to meet their requirements. This will show individuals that you respect and value them. It will show you have a genuine interest in them and that you care.

Working in a way that embeds person-centred values in all aspects of health and adult care work is important and benefits you and other adult care workers because:

- **It ensures you are meeting the expected standards:** embedding person-centred values into your work practices means that the way you provide care and support to individuals will meet the standards that are expected of you as a Lead Adult Care Worker and Lead Personal Assistant, and demonstrates that you have the right values and behaviours.
- **It ensures you provide high quality care and support:** you will be following best practice which will in turn impact on the quality of the care and support you provide. For example, showing you are able to support individuals to be in control of their lives, including their own care and support, will lead to the provision of safe and effective care and support.
- **It ensures you promote partnership working:** you will be getting to know how to work alongside individuals and others who are involved in their lives, such as their families, other professionals and services, thus showing you are able to work as part of a team for the best interests of individuals.

Not working in a way that embeds person-centred values in adult care settings is unthinkable and must be avoided. Below we explore some of the consequences of not ensuring that person-centred values influence all aspects of your work.

Consequences of not embedding person-centred values

- **Ignoring individuals' rights:** individuals will not feel valued or respected and may become frustrated and anxious.
- **Disempowering individuals:** individuals will not feel in control of their care or support and may stop interacting with you.
- **Influencing individuals' lives negatively:** individuals who have not participated in their care and support will experience a poor quality of life because they will feel disappointed that their views were not taken into account.
- **Providing poor-quality care and support:** the care and support will not meet individuals' needs, views and preferences.
- **Not working in partnership:** a lack of trust between individuals, others and you means not being able to work together effectively when providing care and support.
- **Not meeting the required standards:** not working competently can result in you working in unsafe ways and not being able to continue with your career.

AC 1.5 Describe how person-centred values and strength-based approaches must influence all aspects of adult care work

Person-centred values

Individuality
This means treating people as individuals and supporting and encouraging an individual to be their own person, for example assisting an individual to dress in the way they want to. It means understanding that everyone is different and unique. The people you care for may have similar impairments or conditions, but they will all have different needs and preferences. For example, not all individuals will want assistance with eating and drinking – some individuals with physical disabilities may be able to eat and drink independently while others may require support to eat and drink or use adapted cutlery to do so.

Think about your own personal morning routine. What do you like to do as soon as you get up in the morning – do you like to get up straightaway when your alarm goes off or do you like to switch the snooze button on for five minutes? Perhaps you like to have a cup of tea in the morning before you have a shower, or perhaps after you have a shower. Perhaps you like to have time to have breakfast in the morning, as long as it's not too early. If you didn't follow your morning routine, how would you feel? Not your usual self? Disorganised and not ready for the day ahead? This is what makes you, and what makes individuals who they are. It's thinking about these small touches that are important to delivering good quality care.

Rights
This means helping individuals to understand and access their rights and supporting and encouraging an individual to understand what they are entitled to, for example ensuring individuals' rights are met and that there are no barriers to stop them from accessing their rights. Having a disability or being in a wheelchair should not be a barrier to joining in activities, and fear of upsetting a care worker should not be a barrier to making a complaint. Not being able to read or read English should not be a barrier to signing a form. Instead, you and others should support individuals to access their rights and ensure activities allow everyone to participate. You must make sure that individuals are aware of the process for making complaints and are supported to make a complaint should they need to. You will make sure that you support anyone who cannot read to understand what they are signing before they do so.

Choice
This means supporting, encouraging, empowering and enabling an individual to make their own choices and decisions. Everyone is entitled to make their own choices in a care setting. Individuals should choose how they would like to be supported and be given information about what options are available in order to make informed decisions. For example, you should tell individuals about the different care and support services that are available in their local area so that they can decide which one is best for them.

Privacy
This means showing respect for an individual's personal space and personal information and allowing them their privacy. For example, this could include something as simple as knocking on the door of an individual's room before entering, making sure that individuals can spend some time alone if they want to, giving individuals privacy should they request it when family members visit, and ensuring that they are able to privately carry out personal care should they want to.

Independence
This means supporting an individual to be independent and in control of their life by doing as much for themselves as they are able, for example encouraging an individual to find out about the range of services that are available to them to enable them to remain living in their own home. Supporting individuals to be independent also means assessing the risks that they face but ensuring that they understand these and are able to live as independently as possible.

Dignity and respect
This means treating people well and showing respect for their views, opinions and rights. Respect for individuals involves taking into account their differences and valuing them as individuals with their own needs and preferences. It also means promoting an individual's sense of self-

respect by ensuring they do not feel humiliated or embarrassed in any way. Although you are there to support them, individuals should still feel that they are in control of their lives and treating them with dignity and respect is a big part of this.

Care – one of the 6Cs

Providing care is of course perhaps the key person-centred value that underpins your and others' roles. But more specifically, it means providing care in a way that is consistent, sufficient and meets the needs of the individual. For example, one of your responsibilities may be to support an individual with their mealtimes. However, in order to make sure that you provide good quality care and fulfil this duty adequately, you will need to ensure that the meal is prepared in a way that meets their dietary and nutritional requirements and is enjoyable, and you may also need to support them in eating and drinking should they need it.

Compassion – one of the 6Cs

This means providing care to an individual in a way that shows kindness, consideration, empathy, dignity and respect. For example, this might mean taking time out from a busy shift to sit with an individual who has received some sad news.

Courage – one of the 6Cs

This means providing care in a way that is morally acceptable, to do the right thing for the individuals we care about, and to constantly develop and change our ways of working if this will lead to improved, more efficient practice. It also includes speaking up if you have concerns about practice at work or about an individual. This could include speaking up for an individual who is being abused and is too scared to report it.

Communication – one of the 6Cs

Good communication is key to providing high quality care and support and to effective team working. It includes actively listening to what the individuals have to say and is necessary for building strong relationships with them and colleagues. You may like to refer to Unit 304 Effective communication in adult care settings/services for more information.

Competence – one of the 6Cs

Being competent in your job role means having the knowledge, skills and expertise to provide high-quality care and support, and working effectively and efficiently with individuals. It means understanding the needs of the individuals you care for and providing effective care to meet their needs. For example, this could include applying the knowledge and skills you have learned in relation to moving and handling to assist an individual to move safely from one position to another.

Commitment – one of the 6Cs

As an adult care worker, you will need to be committed to upholding person-centred values and ensure that they inform your practice. Being committed to the people we care for is a key part of our role. This also means being committed or dedicated to continuously improving the quality of care that we offer individuals so that their experience is a positive one.

It means dedication to providing care that has the person at the centre and is underpinned by person-centred values. It also means striving to improve your practice to ensure it is person-centred. How can you show you are committed to providing person-centred care and support in your current job role? How have you contributed to an individual's positive experience of accessing care and support? Look at the areas we discussed above and think about how you apply person-centred values in your role.

Partnership

This means working together, alongside the individuals for whom you provide care and support, to ensure that they are at the centre of the care you provide and are in control of the care they receive. It also includes working with others, their families, your colleagues and those outside the organisation. Working in partnership is essential for the provision of high quality person-centred care. You might want to look at Unit 300 Responsibilities and ways of working in adult care settings/services, AC 1.4, 1.5 and 1.6, which cover partnership working.

Strength-based approaches

Individuals' personal strengths and abilities

Working together with individuals by building on their personal strengths and abilities forms part of all strength-based approaches and is essential for promoting individuals' wellbeing. Recognising an individual's strengths and abilities involves taking into account what the individual considers to be important to them. It can only be achieved by getting to know the individual and what they are good at rather than what they're not good at, and what they can do rather than what they can't. In this way, the care and support accessed by the individual can be centred on their strengths and abilities rather than on what's wrong or any difficulties they are having, i.e. in relation to a disability or condition or their age. For example, you can recognise and show respect for an individual's strengths and abilities by asking them what they are strong at rather than what's wrong with them. In this way, the individual may then share with you that they are a patient person, have a good sense of humour, have a keen interest in the environment, can cook for themselves and their friends and have learned how to use public transport to travel independently to places that they like to go to. Recognising an individual's strengths will therefore promote the individual's wellbeing by improving their self-confidence in their ability to self-care.

Individuals' support network

Working together with individuals by using the support they have around them is essential for ensuring that you build on their current support with those people that are important to them and that know them. Recognising an individual's support network involves finding out who and what support they have around them from either the individual and/or their representative who is involved in their lives. For example, an individual may have their sister visit them at home once a week for a chat, a neighbour phone them to ask them if they need anything from the local shops, or a carer support them twice a week with completing their housework. It is important that this support network for the individual is recognised by involving both the individual and others who are not just meeting the individual's needs but rather form part of the individual's life. In this way you can find out a lot more about the person rather than about their condition, in other words what makes the individual unique. You will learn more about how you can treat an individual as a whole person by meeting their holistic needs in AC 1.7.

Individuals' wider community

Working together with individuals by recognising the community they are part of is essential for ensuring that the individual can live their life how they want to in line with their desired outcomes. Recognising an individual's community involves having a discussion with the individual and others involved in their lives to find out about how the individual is involved or would like to be involved in their local area and/or other communities. For example, an individual may have enjoyed going swimming at their local leisure centre, or they may like to be part of their local neighbourhood watch team or volunteer at the community centre in the town near them or attend a sports club that they have an interest in. It is important that individuals' wider community is recognised so that individuals continue to feel that they belong and so that their wellbeing is promoted.

Strength-based approaches do not ignore individuals' needs but rather build on individuals' strengths and use these to meet their needs and the outcomes that individuals would personally desire for themselves to ensure that they lead content and fulfilled lives and achieve their full potential. As well as having discussions with individuals and others to identify their strengths, strength-based approaches can also include using the **recovery model** and **motivational interviewing techniques** to build an individual's confidence, express empathy with the individual and show the individual that they are being listened to and are understood.

> **Key terms**
>
> **Recovery model** is a model often used with individuals who experience mental illness. It takes a holistic view of a person's life and is lead by the person themselves and takes into account the benefits of having supportive networks and relationships for aiding mental health recovery.
>
> **Motivational interviewing techniques** are positive ways of promoting an individual's strengths by, for example, using open-ended questions, i.e. those beginning with 'what' and 'how', affirmations, i.e. confirming back to the individuals their strengths and abilities, reflection and summaries.

> **Research it**
>
> **1.4, 1.5 Legislation, embedding person-centred values and strength-based approaches and the consequences of not doing so**
>
> Research how key pieces of legislation such as the Human Rights Act 1998 and the Care Act 2014 can help with embedding person-centred values and strength-based approaches when providing care and support to individuals. Explain to a colleague the reasons for embedding person-centred values in your working practices, then explain the consequences of not doing so.
>
> Produce a written account of your research findings.

> **Evidence opportunity**
>
> **1.4, 1.5 How and why person-centred values and strength-based approaches must influence all aspects of your work**
>
> As a Lead Adult Care Worker or Lead Personal Assistant, imagine that you have been asked by your manager to write some guidance for a new member of staff, outlining the reasons why it is important to work in a way that embeds person-centred values and strength-based approaches.
>
> Write down how you would explain to the new staff member what person-centred values are. Which values would you say are the most important? Why?
>
> What examples could you use to explain how to work in ways that embed person-centred values? Ensure you explain all of this in your written work.

AC 1.6 Describe how to seek feedback to support the delivery of person-centred care in line with own role and responsibilities

Seeking feedback from others is an essential part of delivering person-centred care. It is important to seek feedback from as many sources as possible so that you can build a true picture of how effective the care you and others are delivering is and what improvements, if any, need to be made to ensure that the individual and their needs remain at the centre of the care you provide.

Sources of feedback

To deliver person-centred care you need to find out how effective the care being provided is in terms of whether it is having a positive impact on the individual and whether it is of a high quality. You can obtain feedback from individuals, carers, loved ones, family and friends of individuals. Colleagues, peers, managers, supervisors, professionals from other services, visitors to the work setting, members of the community and volunteers can also provide feedback.

> **Reflect on it**
>
> **1.6 Seeking feedback**
>
> Reflect on the people you can seek feedback from in the setting where you work. Now think about an occasion when you obtained feedback from someone at work. Why did you approach this person and not someone else? What was the feedback for? Was it useful? Why?

Remember to observe how an individual responds to you by observing their body language, for example, as this can give you and others a lot of useful feedback.

Feedback methods

There are many different ways you can seek feedback from individuals and others. Once you have obtained feedback from various different sources, you need to organise it in a meaningful way so that you can make sense of it. This is important in order to understand which aspects of the care you provide are working well and which areas require improvement. You will also be involving the individual throughout the whole process, which is part of person-centred care.

There are different methods you can use to seek feedback:

- **Face-to-face:** if you decide to meet with people individually or in small groups you can obtain their feedback directly. You may devise a set of questions that you would like everyone to answer and record people's answers by making notes or by recording what they say. It is always a good idea to clarify the answers you have received by checking your understanding of them with the person.

  If you are working with a small group of people you may have a discussion around a set of key topics and then ask one person from the group to record people's views and provide feedback to you at the end of the discussion. If you have a discussion with a person on a one-to-one basis you may decide to ask a colleague to make notes of the key points discussed. You will need to ensure that you meet in a private room where you will not be disturbed.

  When collating the feedback you have received, either directly from a person or group of people or indirectly through a representative, you will need to develop a way of recording this. For example, you could create a form where you can record the questions you ask and the answers you receive, or a record sheet where you can summarise the key points and perspectives shared during discussions.

- **Telephone:** you may decide to telephone individuals' relatives or friends to obtain their feedback, particularly if, for example, they live too far away to meet with you or are too busy to arrange a meeting. You will need to think about how to ensure that you get the person's full attention over the telephone. For example, you may decide to telephone the person first to introduce yourself and explain why you want to obtain their feedback and what you are going to do with the information. Once you have obtained their permission to be interviewed for feedback you could then agree a mutually convenient time when they can speak with you over the telephone; you will need to provide them with an indication of how long it is going to take and what it is going to involve – will it be a series of questions for them to answer or more of a discussion? It might be useful to provide the person with an outline of the questions you are going to ask or the topics you are going to discuss beforehand.

  You must decide how you are going to record the feedback you receive over the telephone. If you are going to make notes, then ensure that you have a format for recording these. If you record the phone call, then you will need the person's permission to do so.

- **Email:** you may decide to email questionnaires to people. If you do so, then you will need to think carefully about your wording and how you are going to explain to the person why you are contacting them, the purpose of obtaining their feedback and how you are going to use it. Remember when emailing invitations to people requesting that they respond to questionnaires you should ensure that these are written clearly and professionally and that you include your name, role and contact details, so that if the person has any questions or wants to clarify who you are, they can do so.

  You must also then think about how you are going to collate the questionnaires you receive over the email. Are you going to store these electronically or print them out and store them in a file? How will you ensure their confidentiality? Will you use a password with a dedicated folder that only you have access to, or a lockable filing cabinet that you can store them in securely? Remember confidentiality – you may need to look at the rules around Data Protection Act 2018 (see Unit 305 for more information).

Analysing feedback sought

To ensure the feedback you have collated is valid and that you will be able to make sense of it you will need to know the following information – perhaps you can use key points, like a checklist,

Feedback checklist

Sources
- Who did I ask for feedback? Why?
- How many people did I ask for feedback?
- How many people responded?
- How many people did not respond or take part? Why?

Methods
- Which methods did I use to obtain feedback? Why?
- Did I agree the methods used with those involved?
- Which methods were most effective? Why?
- Were any methods used ineffective? Why?

Timescales
- What timescales were agreed to obtain feedback?
- What timescales were agreed to collate feedback?
- Who did I agree these timescales with? Why?
- How am I going to communicate these agreed timescales?

Factors
- How am I going to maintain confidentiality?
- Are there any arrangements I need to make to obtain people's feeback?
- How am I going to handle negative feedback?
- How am I going to share the feedback received?

Figure 7.2 Example of a checklist to help you determine the quality of feedback you have obtained

to help you determine the quality of the feedback you have obtained. Figure 7.2 is an example of a checklist you could use.

Understanding sources of your feedback

Understanding the sources of your feedback is essential for determining the purpose of your feedback so that when making a judgement as to its effectiveness you can measure it against your original aims. This is referred to as analysing your feedback, i.e. deciding whether the feedback you obtained provides you with answers to the questions you were asking. You also need to ensure that the feedback you obtain is representative. For example, two out of six responses obtained from a team of care workers is not representative of the team's views compared to five out of six responses. The latter number of responses will mean that you have obtained feedback from more people within the team and therefore this is likely to be more representative of what the team thinks.

Justify the methods you use

It is important that you are able to justify the methods you use including those that worked well and those that didn't. This will help you show that the methods you used for obtaining feedback were open and transparent and that they generated valid and accurate information. For example, you may decide to interview an individual who has a hearing impairment in person and with a sign language interpreter present so as to ensure that they are able to understand you, express what they think and make themselves understood. You can refer to Unit 304 Effective communication in adult care settings/services.

Seek feedback in a timely manner

All feedback needs to be obtained in a timely manner, and those you have requested feedback from should not be rushed. Not giving enough time for people to provide feedback can result in some people not being able or willing to participate. Feedback obtained also needs to be analysed in a timely manner so that your analysis reflects people's current views and perspectives. Not doing so can result in people involved forgetting why they provided feedback in the first instance as well as delay your findings and therefore their relevance to the impact they had on the person. For example, if you obtained people's feedback during the months of March and April but did not analyse it until September and then fed back your findings to all those involved in December, then it is likely people may have forgotten what they said.

Other factors

Your analysis must take into consideration a number of important factors. Again, not doing so may compromise your findings because they may not be considered valid. For example, it is important that confidentiality is respected throughout the process so that all those involved can be confident that their feedback will be kept secure; this means that people will be more likely to say what they think.

It is also important that people are supported when required to give feedback; for example an advocate may need to be present or an individual require more time, or a team member may only be able to meet you at the end of their shift.

Your analysis must give a balanced view of all feedback you have received; this means both positive and negative feedback must be recognised and recorded. Not doing so may mean that people involved decide to not provide their feedback in future, feeling it has not been taken seriously.

Finally, it is important that your findings are communicated to all those involved. You can do this using a variety of methods. Doing so will mean that all those involved will know what has happened with the feedback you have obtained from them and that you will have this as something to refer to in the future.

> ### Evidence opportunity
>
> **1.6 How to seek feedback to support the delivery of person-centred care**
>
> Identify an individual you provide care or support to. Identify three sources of feedback you can use to determine the quality of the care or support provided to this individual. For example, you may want to speak to the individual or to a colleague or their advocate who knows them. Collate and analyse each person's feedback received. Ask a work colleague, team member, your manager or employer to observe you doing so; obtain their feedback on the process you followed.
>
> Provide a written account describing how to seek feedback to support the delivery of person-centred care in line with your role and responsibilities.

AC 1.7 Describe how the active participation of individuals and others in care planning promotes person-centred values and strength-based approaches, to meet the holistic needs of an individual: a) for the present and b) planning for their futures

Active participation

Active participation of individuals and others in care planning is a way of working that promotes person-centred values and strength-based approaches because it recognises:

- individuals' and others' rights to participate in their care and support for both the present and when planning for their futures
- individuals' rights to maintain relationships with others that are important to them both for the present and when planning for their futures
- individuals' abilities to be active partners rather than passive recipients in making decisions about their care and support for the present and when planning for their futures
- individuals' potential to be in control of their care and support and influence how their present and future needs are met.

You may also find it useful to refer back to the role of advanced care plans in AC 1.3 to help individuals with planning for their futures.

Benefits of active participation

Active participation is a person-centred way of working that can lead to person-centred care and support. This is because it recognises:

- **an individual's rights:** to participate in activities fully and to maintain relationships in everyday life as independently as possible
- **an individual's abilities:** to be an active partner who is involved in their own care or support rather than a passive recipient who is not involved and on the receiving end of care or support
- **an individual's potential:** to be in control over their care or support and influence how their care or support needs are met.

The active participation of individuals and others in care planning involves supporting and enabling individuals to live their lives as independently as possible.

This does not mean doing things for them but instead helping them to do things for themselves as much as possible. This might mean enabling them to go out shopping on their own or take part in a social group.

There are many benefits of active participation for individuals who have care or support needs. Some of the main ones are included in Figure 7.3. Can you think of any others?

> ### Reflect on it
>
> **1.7 The benefits of active participation**
>
> Reflect on the benefits of active participation in care planning identified in Figure 7.3. Now think about the difference each of these benefits would make to your life.
>
> - What impact could it have if you feel good about making your own decisions?
> - How can an increase in confidence benefit you?
> - Why is being in control of your life important?
> - Why is it important that your unique strengths, abilities, preferences and needs are taken into account and understood?

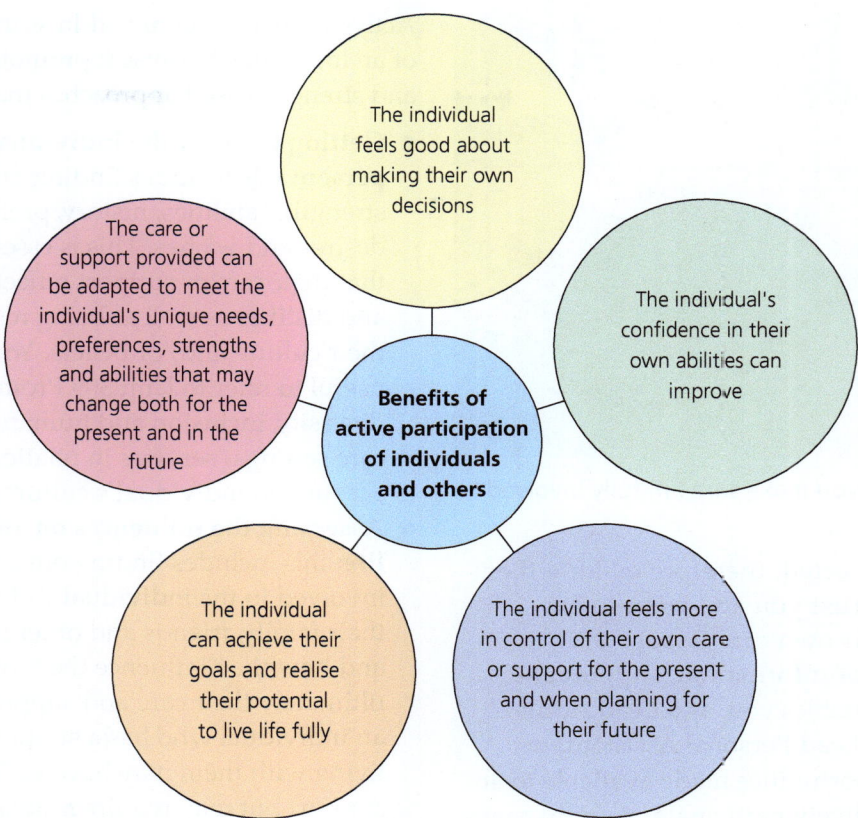

Figure 7.3 The benefits of active participation of individuals and others in care planning

Barriers to active participation

There may be occasions when it is difficult to encourage active participation, for example a new adult care worker may lack the knowledge or skills, have not received training or does not feel they have sufficient time; or perhaps individuals and others don't understand the benefits of active participation in care planning.

Promoting person-centred values and strength-based approaches to meet the holistic needs of an individual

You have already taken the first step towards understanding how active participation promotes person-centred values and strength-based approaches by learning about the different barriers that can exist for individuals who have care and support needs, and by raising your awareness of what these are and how they can vary for different individuals and care settings. You are now therefore ready to take the next step towards finding out about the different approaches that can be used to reduce these barriers:

- **Keep your knowledge and skills about best practice up to date:** this enables you, as a Lead Adult Care Worker or Lead Personal Assistant, to ensure that your working practices and approaches are effective. Maintaining your knowledge and skills through continuous professional development activities, such as training, reading articles and working with experienced colleagues, can be crucial for developing positive ways to encourage individuals' active participation.
- **Spend time getting to know the individual:** this enables you, as a Lead Adult Care Worker or Lead Personal Assistant, to build up a good working relationship with the individual that can be crucial for applying active participation. You will get to know their strengths, abilities, preferences and needs which means that you can take these into account when encouraging them to become more involved. For example, if you know that an individual does not like noisy environments then you could make arrangements to discuss their care or support in a quiet area where the individual will feel relaxed and you will not be disturbed. At the same time, the individual will get to know you, which means that they will feel valued

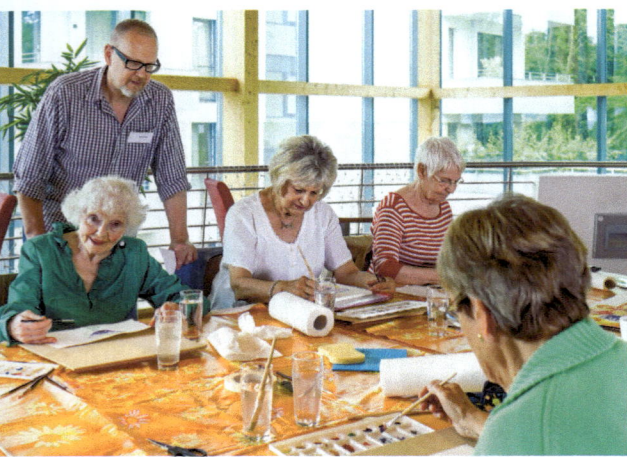

Figure 7.4 How can you make sure I'm fully involved?

by you and respected, therefore making them more likely to trust you and want to get involved in their own care or support.

- **Access sources of information, support and guidance:** this enables you, as a Lead Adult Care Worker or Lead Personal Assistant, to increase the opportunities made available to an individual to actively participate. Your manager can be one such source of information and guidance; for example, they can ensure that you are aware of different ways of supporting individuals' choices about their care or support as well as your responsibilities for doing so. The individual's representative, such as their advocate or a family member, can also act as a good support for ensuring the individual understands the information you are providing, including their options. In addition, involving others can ensure that the individual's strengths, abilities, preferences and needs are being supported and continue to be the main focus of all care or support provided.

One of the most important benefits of active participation involves focusing on the individual as a unique and whole person; it involves recognising that an individual's needs will involve looking at all aspects of their personhood and their life, in other words their '**holistic** needs'.

> **Key term**
>
> **Holistic** in this context refers to treating individuals as a whole person, i.e. considering all of their needs, such as physical, emotional, spiritual, etc.

Active participation can address the holistic needs of an individual because it promotes person-centred and strength-based approaches that involve:

- **Getting to know the individual as a whole person:** this includes finding out about their strengths, abilities, history, preferences, needs, desires and wishes. This is essential for ensuring that their care or support reflects their likes and dislikes as well as being respectful of their culture and/or beliefs. You will find it useful to refer to Unit 309 Promoting equality, diversity, inclusion and human rights in adult care settings/services in relation to taking into account an individual's culture and beliefs.
- **Assessing the influences on an individual's life:** this includes finding out about all those involved in the individual's life such as their family, friends and other professionals and how they influence the individual and ultimately their care and support. For example, an individual who has a supportive partner living with them may have sufficient emotional support but may require more practical help with household tasks to reduce their dependency on their partner and enable them to improve their emotional wellbeing (a concept you will learn more about in LO2 and also in Unit 314 Understanding personal wellbeing). On the other hand, an individual who lives on their own may have developed effective ways of managing household tasks by themselves but requires emotional support as they do not have anyone they can confide in or talk things through with. In both these examples individuals' physical and emotional wellbeing influence different aspects of their lives and impact on their holistic needs.
- **Working closely with the individual:** As you have learned in this AC, active participation is not something that is done in isolation; it is achieved by working closely not only with the individual but also with others involved in their lives and with their care or support. This is essential for ensuring that the individual remains in control of their care or support and that they are treated respectfully and as a whole person with their holistic needs taken into consideration. You will find it useful to review your learning in ACs 1.1 and 1.2 in Unit 300 Responsibilities and ways of working in adult care settings/services in relation to working in partnership with others.

> ### Research it
>
> **1.7 Best practice for applying active participation in care planning**
>
> Research examples of best practice when applying active participation in care planning to meet individual holistic needs. Useful sources of information for carrying out your research could include the care setting where you work, care settings you know about in your local area, newspapers, television and the internet.
>
> Produce an information handout with your findings.

> ### Evidence opportunity
>
> **1.7 Applying active participation in care planning**
>
> Develop a case study of an individual who has care or support needs that includes details of their individual holistic needs and the barriers that may affect this individual in actively participating in their own care or support.
>
> Describe different ways of applying active participation of the individual and others in care planning and how this promotes person-centred values and strength-based approaches. Remember to include anything that may help or hinder this individual's active participation in their own care or support. For example, this may be in relation to the care setting or to those who work with the individual. How is this a help or hindrance? You may want to think about the role other health professionals can play too.
>
> Remember that you cannot include the care plan or individuals' personal details in your portfolio.

AC 1.8 Describe how to support an individual to question or challenge decisions concerning them that are made by others

Making your own choices in everyday life will occasionally involve coming into conflict with others who disagree with the decisions you make or who you may want to question or challenge. Examples might include conflicts relating to starting a new career, going to university or learning to drive. Dealing with these conflicts requires effective support from others who you trust and who know you well, such as family and friends.

> ### Reflect on it
>
> **1.8 Questioning or challenging decisions**
>
> Reflect on an occasion when you questioned or challenged a decision made by someone else about you. What happened? How did you feel? Would you do anything differently next time?

Similarly, individuals who have care or support needs may disagree with decisions made about them by others, such as by their GP, social worker or a family member, and it is their right to be able to question or challenge any decisions made about them. Individuals may find this difficult to do because of:

- **their needs:** a learning difficulty may mean that the individual finds it difficult to communicate their views to others
- **their relationships:** an individual may feel they are being unkind if they disagree with a decision made by their parent or anxious if they disagree with a decision made by the Lead Adult Care Worker or Lead Personal Assistant providing them with care or support in case they withdraw the care or support they are providing
- **their support network:** an individual may feel isolated or not have anyone that they feel they can turn to when they want to question or challenge decisions about them made by others; they also may hold the view that others, such as adult care professionals, know best.

It is important that you are aware of the barriers that may prevent or deter individuals from questioning or challenging decisions made about them so that you can support them effectively. Here are some ideas for how you can do so:

- **Encourage good communication:** for example, you should enable the individual to feel relaxed and trust you so that they feel free to share their concerns. You can also encourage the individual to ask questions and share their views with you. You will need to be patient and prepared to listen carefully, giving individuals the time they need to communicate their concerns. You should ensure that they have all the information they need so they are aware of how they can challenge

any decisions made about them, for example information about the complaints procedure.
- **Seek guidance:** speaking to your manager or supervisor can be useful as they can provide additional support to both you and the individual.
- **Support the individual to ask for a second opinion:** either themselves or by you asking for a second opinion and speaking on the individual's behalf.
- **Support the individual to access support:** from other people who have been in similar situations so that they can support each other.
- **Support the individual to make a complaint:** support the individual to access the complaints procedure, understand and use it. It may be that the individual has made a complaint or challenged a decision in the past and this has not been dealt with well. This could deter the individual from challenging decisions and so it is important to reassure them that support is available and that their complaint will be dealt with respectfully.

6Cs

Communication

How can you build a positive working relationship with the individuals you provide care or support to? Communicating effectively with individuals is crucial for ensuring that they feel relaxed, can trust you and share with you how they are feeling. This is important when you are supporting individuals to challenge any decisions made about them, especially if they feel reluctant to do so.

Research it

1.8 Support groups

Research the support groups that are available in your local area for supporting individuals with mental health needs to speak up for themselves. Your own knowledge of the local area may come in handy here, and the internet is a good source of information. Discuss your findings with your assessor.

Evidence opportunity

1.8 Supporting individuals to question or challenge decisions

Find the complaints procedure for the care setting where you work.

Describe how you can use this to support an individual with care or support needs to question or challenge a decision made about them. Write this down, or write a general account of how you support individuals to question or challenge decisions.

LO2 Understand the importance of individuals' relationships

Getting started

Think about the relationships that are important to you. How many different relationships do you have? Which ones are most important to you and why? Now, think about an individual you provide care or support to. How many relationships do they have? Which ones are the most important to them and why? What do you notice between the relationships you have and the relationships this individual has?

AC 2.1 Describe the different relationships that are important to individuals, including intimate or sexual relationships

Your wellbeing

Your wellbeing refers to your health and whether you feel in good health and happy overall in yourself. Your health not only refers to how you are physically, for example being pain-free, but also to other aspects of your health, such as your mental health (your attitude to life), emotional health (how you feel about life), social health (the relationships you have), cultural health (your sense of belonging to a group that shares your beliefs), spiritual health (your human spirit), intellectual health (your thought processes) and economic health (your finances or housing situation).

As you will have learned in Unit 300 Responsibilities and ways of working in adult care settings/services, the relationships we have are important because they can:

- enable us to get to know ourselves and those around us
- provide us with practical and emotional support
- provide us with love and affection
- provide us with intimacy in a loving and/or sexual way
- provide us with a sense of belonging.

The different relationships that are important to individuals will vary from person to person. You will find it useful to refer back to ACs 1.1 and 1.2 in Unit 300 Responsibilities and ways of working in adult care settings/services for more information about different types of personal and working relationships. The following table provides details of some of the different types of relationships that exist and the reasons why they may be important to individuals:

> **Reflect on it**
>
> **2.1 The importance of relationships**
>
> Reflect on three different relationships you have in your life and why they are important to you. How would you feel if you lost these relationships? Why?

Table 7.3 Relationships and why they are important

Type of relationship	Reasons why it's important to individuals
Family – a personal type of relationship with the people you feel most comfortable with, i.e. relatives such as your siblings that can be related to you through birth or by adoption	- Having a relationship with a sibling who an individual has grown up with can make the individual feel that they have someone in their life who not only knows them but who they can also rely on. - Having a relationship with a sibling can mean that the individual has someone they feel is part of them and part of a family that they belong to. - Having a relationship with a sibling can mean that the individual has someone with whom they can share memories of growing up together and experiences of family occasions such as birthdays.
Partners – a personal type of relationship with a person that you know intimately in a romantic and/or sexual way	- Having an intimate or sexual relationship with a partner will enable an individual to experience and share love, affection, intimacy, and emotional and physical closeness with another person. - Having an intimate or sexual relationship with a partner will enable an individual to express themselves sexually, explore their sexuality and have their sexual needs met. - Having an intimate or sexual relationship with a partner will provide opportunities for an individual to be in a long-term partnership, get married, have or adopt children.
Friends – a personal type of relationship with the people that you have a close connection or bond with; people you have things in common with and have shared or similar experiences with	- Having friendships will mean that an individual has people in their life who they can have fun with and socialise with. - Having friendships will mean that an individual will have the opportunity to be part of a friendship group that they belong to and can pursue their interests with. - Having friendships will mean that an individual can share things that are important to them and can also experience their friends sharing things that are important to them.

Table 7.3 Relationships and why they are important *continued*

Type of relationship	Reasons why it's important to individuals
Acquaintances – a personal type of relationship that may vary in frequency and may not develop into anything more than an acknowledgement, e.g. a next door neighbour, someone from the community	• Having relationships with acquaintances will mean that an individual will feel that they belong to their local community, i.e. saying good morning to their neighbour, having a chat with a person who they see from time to time in the local shop. • Having relationships with acquaintances will mean that an individual will have other sources of support including practical and emotional support, e.g. a chat with a neighbour while travelling on the bus. • Having relationships with acquaintances will mean that an individual will have the opportunity for these acquaintances to develop into other types of personal relationships such as friendships and partnerships.
Care workers – a working type of relationship that provides care and support to individuals accessing adult care settings/services	• Having working relationships with care workers will mean that individuals will have their care and support needs met. • Having working relationships with care workers will mean that individuals can experience building mutual trust and respect and have someone they can confide in. • Having working relationships with care workers will mean that individuals will feel that they have people who are working with them and in partnership to lead their lives the way they want to.
Professionals from other services – a working type of relationship with people that individuals may not see on a day-to-day basis like carers but that can provide access to specialist services, e.g. a hospital consultant, an optician, a dietician	• Having working relationships with professionals from other services will mean that individuals' holistic needs are met. • Having working relationships with professionals from other services will mean that individuals will be able to have access to specialist care and services when required such as access to a bereavement counsellor or a physiotherapist after an accident. • Having working relationships with professionals from other services will mean that individuals will benefit from their expertise, knowledge and skills.
Visitors, including volunteers – a working type of relationship with people that individuals may see from time to time but that can provide individuals with practical support	• Having working relationships with visitors will mean that individuals will feel safe and in control of their living arrangements. • Having working relationships with volunteers will mean that individuals may have opportunities to interact and participate in group and one-to-one activities with others. • Having working relationships with visitors and volunteers will mean that individuals will have opportunities to share their views and ideas with others who do not know them too well and to learn about others' views and ideas that may be different to their own.

Evidence opportunity

2.1 Different types of relationships

Think about a fictional character you know about, such as on a TV programme or in the media. Write a written account that describes the different types of relationships the individual has, including intimate and sexual relationships and why they are important.

AC 2.2 Explain the impact of maintaining and building relationships on an individual's wellbeing

> **Research it**
>
> **2.2 Care Act 2014**
>
> Research what the Care Act 2014 says about what is understood by 'wellbeing' in relation to adult social care. You may find the link below useful:
>
> www.scie.org.uk/care-act-2014/assessment-and-eligibility/eligibility/how-is-wellbeing-understood.asp
>
> Now write down your own definition of wellbeing.

Your wellbeing and your relationships

All the different types of relationships you have in your life impact on your wellbeing. This is no different for individuals who access care and support services. Often individuals who access adult care settings/services have a larger number of working relationships than personal relationships. You have already learned in AC 2.1 how important both types of relationships are and now we are going to explore the impact of maintaining and building relationships on an individual's wellbeing. Table 7.4 provides information about the impact that maintaining and building relationships can have on an individual's wellbeing.

Table 7.4 Factors and how they contribute to the wellbeing of individuals

Wellbeing aspect	How maintaining and building relationships can impact on an individual's wellbeing
Physical health	Relationships can support individuals to maintain their physical health by encouraging them to socialise with others. By taking part in activities with others, individuals are encouraged to mobilise and they can learn from others that they meet about how to live a healthy lifestyle and the benefits of doing so.
Mental health and emotional health	Relationships can support individuals to maintain their mental health by having people that they can trust, confide in and talk to about any anxieties or worries they have. Relationships with professionals from other services can support them to seek additional help when they feel unable to manage; this may include counselling services or their GP.
Social health	Relationships can support individuals to maintain their social health by providing them with opportunities and different experiences of activities where they can meet other people as well as maintain any current positive interactions they have with, for example, their families, friends and others.
Cultural health	Relationships can support individuals to maintain their cultural health because they can encourage individuals to share with others who provide them with care and support information about who they are, their background, history, beliefs and preferences. It is important that you and others take relationships into account through the provision of care and support to individuals.
Spiritual health	Relationships can support individuals to maintain their spiritual health because they can encourage individuals to reflect on who they are, what makes them unique and what they like about themselves as well as what their motivations and goals are in life. Being aware of and respecting individuals' religious beliefs is also important for good spiritual health because their religious beliefs will influence how they live their lives and what they value as important to them.
Intellectual health	Relationships can support individuals to maintain their intellectual health because they encourage individuals to do things for themselves. Relationships can provide them with opportunities to ensure that they are mentally stimulated with activities that will enable them to exercise their intellectual health.
Economic health	Relationships can support individuals to maintain their economic health because they can provide individuals with information and support to access additional support through housing services or the benefits agency, for example. Relationships can also encourage individuals to think about the ways they can improve their own situation.

> **Evidence opportunity**
>
> **2.2 Impact of maintaining and building relationships on an individual's wellbeing**
>
> Explain to your assessor the impact of maintaining and building relationships on an individual's wellbeing. How can different relationships contribute to the wellbeing of an individual? Write an explanation or have a discussion with your assessor.

AC 2.3 Outline how own role supports individuals to maintain and build relationships

You are an integral part of an individual's wellbeing because the way you think, behave and practise in your work role when providing care or support will affect an individual's identity, self-image, self-esteem and overall health.

Your working relationship with individuals must be positive, i.e. your thoughts and behaviours must be positive and promote an individual's wellbeing because doing so will mean that the individual will:

- feel valued
- feel respected
- build a good working relationship with you
- trust you.

Positive attitudes include being kind, caring, considerate and respectful.

You can support individuals to maintain and build relationships by demonstrating good working approaches that promote an individual's wellbeing. You may want to review your learning from Table 7.4 in AC 2.2.

You can support individuals to maintain and build relationships by:

- **spending time getting to know who they are as a person:** for example, their needs, values and preferences and who's important to them. This will show the individual that you are taking a genuine interest in them. You could also support individuals to maintain their relationships with others through arranging visits, telephone calls, emails or contacts through social media.

- **supporting the individual to share their history:** for example, their culture, background, those people involved in their lives, beliefs and any practices relating to these, for example nutrition, religion and dress. Doing so means that you will be reflecting back to the individual who they are and why they should feel proud of who they are. By taking the time to find out and record this information, it also shows that you respect who they are and are interested in finding out about them so as to provide the best possible care.

- **interacting with the individual positively:** for example, using positive language when speaking, using open body language when interacting, reinforcing good ideas, giving praise, supporting the individual to take risks, make mistakes and learn from them, and promoting the individual's rights, for example to dignity, privacy and independence. This will also mean that the individual will feel they can approach you and talk to you about how they are feeling including any relationships they are having or thinking of having, i.e. intimate or sexual relationships. Creating an open and empowering culture is essential for individuals building and maintaining relationships.

- **providing individuals with privacy and space:** for example, ensuring there is a private area or room where individuals can discuss the relationships they are having or have the opportunities to talk about any sensitive topics such as sex, helpful and unhelpful relationships etc.

- **providing individuals with a warm, comfortable and welcoming atmosphere:** where individuals can feel relaxed and be more likely to invite friends and family over.

- **promoting person-centred values:** for example, listening to the relationships individuals want even if they are not what you would choose, respecting individuals' rights to maintain relationships including intimate or sexual ones.

- **being aware of your own prejudices:** for example, being aware of how your values for relationships may be different to individuals' and how your beliefs and values may impact on the choices individuals make about their relationships, i.e. in relation to gender preferences, sexual expression.

> **Case study**
>
> **2.1, 2.2, 2.3 The importance of individuals' relationships**
>
> Charles is a Lead Adult Worker and supports young men who have learning difficulties and mental health needs to live independently in the community. Josh, one of the young men he has been supporting, has disclosed to Charles in confidence that he is feeling lonely and has been thinking about having someone he has recently met but does not know very well stay overnight in his room. He is unsure whether this is a good idea as he has never done this before. Josh also tells Charles that he would like to meet up with some of his friends from college more often but doesn't know how to go about this and asks Charles whether he could help him. Finally, Josh tells Charles to keep his idea about his overnight stay to himself as he doesn't want his mum finding out as she would not approve because his friend is a married gay man.
>
> **Discuss**
>
> 1. Which relationships do you think are important to Josh? Why?
> 2. How could these relationships impact on Josh's wellbeing. Why?
> 3. How can Charles support Josh to maintain and build these relationships?
> 4. How would you feel if one of the individuals you support disclosed this to you? Be honest about how you think you would feel.

- **supporting individuals' choices:** for example, by providing information so that individuals can make their own informed choices or, if they lack the capacity, to following the process to support them. You will find it useful to review your learning from Unit 302.
- **using the care and support planning process:** ensuring that individuals' rights and needs to build and maintain relationships form part of individuals' care and support plans; their needs for relationships should be supported and met just like other care and support needs they have.
- **keeping up to date with how to support individuals with relationships:** ensuring you attend training provided by your employer about how to support relationships, increasing your knowledge and awareness about topics that you may not know about, and developing your skills around how to discuss relationships with individuals as well as any questions they may have.

> **Research it**
>
> **2.3 Approaches that promote the wellbeing of individuals**
>
> Research the approaches that are used in the care setting where you work to promote individuals' wellbeing.
>
> Produce a staff handout with your findings.

> **Evidence opportunity**
>
> **2.3 Promoting identity, self-image and self-esteem**
>
> Write an account that outlines how you provide support with one aspect of an individual's life to help them maintain and build relationships.
>
> Ensure that you include details of how you promote the individual's sense of identity, self-image and self-esteem.

LO3 Be able to work in a person-centred way

> **Getting started**
>
> Discuss with a partner what working in a person-centred way in your work setting involves. What person-centred values do you apply in your day-to-day working practices and why? How does working in a person-centred way improve individuals' lives?

AC 3.1 Demonstrate working with an individual and others to establish and understand an individual's history, preferences, wishes, strengths and needs

As we have discussed, the needs of the individuals that you care for should be at the centre of all the care and support you and your colleagues provide. To make sure this happens, first you will need to find out as much as you can about individuals for whom you will be caring. You must not only understand what they would like from their care, but also find out as much as possible about their history to enable you to understand them as a person, which will in turn allow you to meet their needs and allow them to live their life as they want. In order to do this, you will need to work with the individual and others, who may include team members and colleagues, other professionals, as well as families, friends, advocates or others who are important to the individual.

There are different ways you can build up a picture of who an individual is and what makes them the person they are. In order to find out more about the individuals you care for, you will need to explore different ways to discover this information by working with both individuals and others. The best way is to ask the individual. You will learn more from speaking to them than you will from any other sources and it may be that, depending on your role, you carry out an assessment and complete a form with set information you need to find out. You can also speak to their family, carers or advocates who will be able to help you build up a picture of who the individual is. Team members and colleagues as well as other professionals, such as GPs, will be able to help you understand particular aspects about the individual such as their medical history – this is important of course but will not necessarily help you understand the person as a whole.

Finding out about an individual's history

By speaking to individuals about their history, you will be able to understand more about the experiences that have informed the person they are. You can do this by asking them about their childhood and family background. This is very important, especially when you work with older people. All individuals have a history and they may even be eager to share it with you. You could ask if they would like to show you any photographs or tell you any memories. By doing this, you are valuing the person you care for as an individual, one for whom you should have a genuine interest. Other people involved in their lives who know the individual well, such as their family, friends and advocates, may also be useful sources of information.

Think how you feel when someone asks you for your opinion, or asks you how you are feeling, what your likes and dislikes are or talks to you about your own history. Do you feel that the person asking cares about you and your opinion? Do you feel that they are interested in who you are as an individual? Similarly, asking people about their history will not only allow you to provide better care but will also allow the individuals to feel respected and valued and not just another person that requires care.

The individual's preferences

These may be based on the individual's beliefs, values and culture. You can find out about an individual's beliefs by asking the individual what they view as important. For example, these may be religious values and will impact the support needs that they have, such as nutrition and personal care. You can find out about an individual's values by discussing them with the individual. These may include not eating meat, washing with running water or only being assisted with their personal hygiene by a person of the same gender. You can find out more about an individual's culture by asking them (and others who know them well) questions about their culture and the associated practices they follow. This might affect how they communicate with others, what they eat and what they wear.

The individual's wishes

You can find out about an individual's wishes by asking the individual what their hopes and dreams are for the present and the future. Others who know the individual well may also be helpful when drawing up a picture of what the individual's wishes are.

The individual's strengths

You can find out about an individual's unique personal strengths by getting to know them and finding out more about them and their life; this may be through the individual themselves or through others who know them well. For example, you could ask an individual what do you like about yourself? What do you enjoy doing? What are your interests? What have you done in your life that you're proud of? What achievements have you had? What personal challenges have you had in your life and how did you overcome them? Their answers to these questions will provide you with ideas on what skills, knowledge and abilities they have.

The individual's needs

You can find out about an individual's needs by asking the individual what care and support needs they have and what they require to meet these. This might include asking them what their needs are with regards to nutrition and what activities they would like to participate in so that they can live as actively as possible. You will need to identify the gaps between where they are independent and able and where support is required. Others who know the individual well may also be a useful source of information about the needs they have. It is only by finding out about the individuals that you can truly provide person-centred care.

Remember to discuss all aspects of their life that make up the person they are, such as their health, social interactions, cultural and religious background and educational and employment background so that you build up a holistic and more rounded impression of the person they are.

Collating all this information takes time and may have to be built up over days, weeks and even months. It may involve not only discussions with the individual and others who are involved in their lives but also reviewing previous care plans the individual may have had (letters about the care and support they have received, reports, other records, such as communication records and risk assessments, photographs and images of different activities they have participated in and goals they have achieved). Some of this information may have already been collated by your manager upon the arrival of the individual at the care setting where you work or by other staff who have worked closely with the individual – do not forget to ask them and involve them too.

Case study

3.1 Working with an individual to identify their strengths

Levi is 26 years old and has experienced some mental health problems including depression. As part of Levi's mental health recovery, his mental health worker, Siobhan, is supporting Levi to identify his own personal strengths for use in his care plan by using a tool called the Adult Needs and Strengths Assessment (ANSA). Together, Levi and Siobhan have gone through the following strength areas and identified where Levi's strengths lie:

Strength area	Levi's strengths
Family	Significant strength – Levi is supported and respected by his partner, parents and siblings.
Social	Mild strength – Levi has numerous friends and maintains a good relationship with his partner. Sometimes, Levi's social interaction with others can decrease if he is feeling low in mood, anxious or not confident.
Interests	Significant strength – Levi enjoys water sports and outdoor activities and has good orienteering and hiking skills.
Education	Significant strength – Levi has developed good literacy skills.
Volunteering	Strength is not present – Levi has found it difficult to take up volunteering opportunities he has been offered due to his lack of confidence when meeting new people.
Resilience	Significant strength – Levi has managed some recent challenges he has been presented with well, i.e. moving to a new area and being bereaved of a close friend.
Personality	Significant strength – Levi has many positive personality traits including honesty, kindness and determination.

Discuss

1 What are the benefits of Siobhan supporting Levi to identify his strengths?
2 Which strengths does Levi have already?
3 Which strengths can Levi develop further?

> **Evidence opportunity**
>
> **3.1 Finding out about the individual**
>
> You will be observed working with an individual and others to establish and understand the individual's history, preferences, wishes, strengths and needs. You could also obtain a witness testimony showing that you are able to work with others, so you will need to arrange for your assessor to do this.
>
> Once you have agreed these with your manager or employer, put them into practice. Did you find out anything you didn't know about the individual? How did you find the process? If you did this again would you use the same methods? Explain why. Discuss your responses with your assessor. Remember that you will be observed working with an individual and others to find out the individual's history, preferences, wishes and needs. Remember that you cannot include the care plan or personal details about individuals in your portfolio.

AC 3.2 Demonstrate working with individual(s) to identify how they want to actively participate in their care and support, taking into account their history, preferences, wishes, strengths and needs

As you have learned, in order for you to apply active participation successfully you must be able to work closely with individuals and others; you will be observed doing so for this AC.

Working with individuals

Working with individuals is more than just working alongside them. It involves being committed to:

- **sharing a common set of values:** for example, to take into account an individual's strengths, to respect an individual's wishes, to support an individual's independence, to take into account an individual's unique needs and to safeguard individuals from harm.
- **agreeing goals:** for example, to enable positive outcomes for individuals, goals may be agreed both over short and long periods of time
- **communicating effectively:** for example, communications must be open and honest, timely and regular with individuals, this includes verbal and written communications. You may find it useful to refer to Unit 304 Effective communication in adult care settings/services.

Working with individuals brings many benefits for them, you, and others including:

- improving and developing your understanding of different ways of working and best practice
- encouraging a strong team
- pooling resources
- providing person-centred care.

Agreeing how an individual wants to actively participate

Working closely with individuals to identify how they want to actively participate in their care and support involves making decisions together. This is important if you are to ensure that your care and support is of a high quality and takes into account their history, preferences, wishes, strengths and needs. In this way the individual will feel good about themselves and experience a sense of achievement.

Working with individuals to identify how they want to actively participate in their care and support involves taking a step back to think about who the individual is and what makes them unique, i.e. their background, history, preferences, wishes, hopes, strengths and needs. It is also important to ensure that the individual's independence is promoted so that they are encouraged to do as much for themselves as possible.

You will also need to show your respect for others' opinions even when you don't agree with them, be able to communicate clearly and listen attentively. It also involves providing individuals with active support, in other words, a step-by-step guide of how they can actively participate in their care and support by ensuring they do what they can themselves and are supported in the areas that they need support with.

An example of how you can work closely with an individual and others to enable the individual to retain their independence as much as possible might be:

You accompany an individual with a learning disability to go food shopping. You could ask them what support they think they may need to do their food shopping. For example, this may be with:

- *identifying what foods they enjoy or desire and may include food that reflects their beliefs and/or culture*

- *locating the food items in the shop and accessing them, i.e. they may be on a high or very low shelf*
- *reading the labels on the food items, including their ingredients and identifying that they are in line with their preferences and lifestyle*
- *identifying the food items' cost and that they are within their budget*
- *paying for the food items at the till or using the self-scan facility.*

In this way, the individual will recognise and further build on their strengths and skills in these areas and will gain confidence as well as feel a sense of achievement that they have done this for themselves. Working together in this way will mean that the individual can take the lead on how they actively participate in the support that they need and this will provide both of you with an opportunity to get to know each other better and develop a good working relationship.

Reflect on it

3.2 Skills for working with individuals

Reflect on the skills you require to be able to work with an individual and others to agree how active participation will be implemented. Perhaps you could think about the communication skills you require and how you could show your empathy and understanding.

What are your strengths? What skills could you further develop or improve? How? You will find it useful to refer to Unit 304 Effective communication in adult care settings/services.

Evidence opportunity

3.2 Work with individuals to identify how they want to actively participate

You will be observed working with individuals to identify how they want to actively participate, so ensure that you arrange for your assessor to do this, or that your manager can provide a witness testimony.

With your assessor, discuss an occasion when you worked with an individual from your care setting to identify how they want to actively participate. What skills did you show when working with the individual and others? Why were these skills important? You may find it useful to review your previous learning in Unit 300 Responsibilities and ways of working in adult care settings/services.

AC 3.3 Demonstrate being responsive to an individual's changing needs or preferences and adapting actions and approaches

Working in a person-centred way is not only about finding out about an individual's history, preferences, wishes and needs, and knowing how to handle complex and sensitive situations. It also involves being responsive to individuals' changing needs or preferences and adapting actions and approaches taken so that the individual remains at the centre of all care and support provided. Adapting your ways of working involves putting into practice the person-centred values you learned about earlier on in this unit. This is a good time for you to recap the knowledge you gained about person-centred values for care and support in LO1. Before doing so, how many do you know already? Can you name them? Do you know why they must influence all aspects of your work? Then look back at LO1 and think of all the considerations we discussed, such as an individual's health, family background and religious needs.

Changing needs or preferences

The needs or preferences of individuals may change for many different reasons. For example, it may be due to a change in an individual's condition or health. Perhaps the individual's condition or health has worsened or perhaps it has improved. Perhaps you and others will focus more on building the individual's self-esteem and confidence to improve their mental and emotional wellbeing; you may also decide to find out about additional support that the individual can access to help them to overcome their fears of falling. Perhaps you and others will focus more on enabling the individual to increase their independence and find out about different mobility aids and equipment that they may be able to access to make mobilising around their home easier, such as a walking aid or hand rails.

Changes in individuals' needs and preferences may also occur because of a change in circumstances. For example, an individual may have recently been bereaved of their partner. This may mean that they no longer have the emotional, practical or financial support that they have been used to having when at home. However the individual responds to their situation, you and others will need to ensure that you are able to adapt your actions and approaches to support the individual's choices and preferences.

Table 7.5 provides some examples of how you can adapt your actions and approaches in response to individuals' changing needs or preferences.

Being responsive to individuals' changing needs or preferences and adapting your actions and approaches is a key part of being able to provide high quality care and support. It requires a great deal of expertise and commitment. It means that you need to work in ways that are flexible, maintain the individual as the focus and be prepared to try different ways of working. Working in this way can also have a significant impact on the quality of individuals' lives and can make a positive difference, as Case study 3.3 shows.

Table 7.5 Examples of how to adapt actions and approaches

Changing needs or preferences	Examples of how to adapt your actions and approaches
An individual with dementia begins to require support with their personal hygiene as they are no longer able to do this themselves	• Explain to the individual that you would like to support them with their personal hygiene; you may need to adapt the way you do this by speaking in short and clear sentences and by giving the individual time to understand what you have said to them. • Provide the individual with the opportunity to choose whether they would like a bath or shower and whether they would like a hair wash. Instead of asking them (which they may find difficult to understand because of their condition), you may need to walk round the bathroom first so that they can point and choose what they would like. • Show respect for an individual's culture and beliefs by asking them if there is a personal hygiene routine they prefer to follow, such as using running water when washing, or only having a person of the same gender assist them. Your questions will need to be short and clear. If the individual appears confused or does not understand what you have asked them you may need to show them through your actions, for example by using running water, by going to their preferred bathroom or asking them to place their personal materials in the bathroom of their choice.
An individual wants to try a new activity but is anxious that they will not enjoy it	• Ask the individual whether there are any activities they would like to do but haven't tried yet, such as bowling, or learning a new skill like sewing or painting. If the individual does not know what new activity they would like you could research the local area with them to find out what activities are on offer. • Promote an individual's independence and self-confidence by encouraging them to lead the activity – give only as much support as required and ensure that you do this by going at the individual's own pace. • After the activity, encourage the individual to reflect on their participation in the activity and discuss what they thought worked well. Ask them what they enjoyed, what they didn't like or what they think could be improved. Ask them how anxious they felt before, during and after the activity; you will need to monitor this closely as part of your support to the individual to ensure it is effective and reflective of the changes in their needs.

Case study

3.3 Person-centred working in practice

Kian is a **Shared Lives carer** and is married with two children. Stacey has learning disabilities and lives on her own. She is joining Kian and his family this weekend as they are planning a camping trip to take place the following week to which Stacey has also been invited. As Stacey has never been camping before she is keen to find out more about what Kian and his family are planning and she agrees to discuss the trip with Kian and his family over afternoon tea.

Kian begins by showing Stacey photographs of previous camping trips the family has been on. Kian asks Stacey to take her time to look through these and as she does so he asks one of the children to tell Stacey where the photo was taken and what is happening in it.

Kian is observing Stacey closely and he can see that she is looking a little upset. Once they have finished looking through the photographs, Kian asks Stacey if she can help him with the washing up. Stacey agrees and while the two of them are in the kitchen, Kian asks Stacey what she thinks about camping. Stacey explains that she's feeling very anxious because she has never spent time away from home before.

Kian asks Stacey if she would prefer not to go away at first for a whole weekend and instead to try a day trip to see how she feels. Stacey says that she would really enjoy that. Kian asks Stacey to have a think about where she would like to go, then perhaps she could visit again one afternoon next week and they could discuss this again as a family over tea. Stacey agrees and says that she will also try and bring some information with her about different places where they could all go together.

Discuss:

1 The person-centred values applied by Kian.
2 Examples of how Kian takes into account Stacey's history, preferences, wishes and needs.
3 How Kian adapted his working approaches and why.
4 The impact of Kian's person-centred way of working on Stacey.

Key term

Shared Lives carer are people who open up their homes and family lives to include an adult with support needs so that they can participate and experience community and family life. The individual may stay with them for the weekend and they may even go on holiday together.

Research it

3.3 Shared Lives Plus

Shared Lives Plus is an organisation for Shared Lives carers and schemes. Find out about who they are and what they do.

Produce a leaflet with your findings. You will find the link below useful: https://sharedlivesplus.org.uk/

Research it

3.3 Helen Sanderson Associates

Helen Sanderson Associates have developed a range of person-centred thinking tools. Research the tools they have developed and think about how they might help you in your care setting. You will find their website useful: www.helensandersonassociates.co.uk

> **Evidence opportunity**
>
> **3.3 Being responsive to individuals' changing needs or preferences**
>
> Keep a diary for a week, recording the different occasions you were responsive to individuals' changing needs and/or preferences and you adapted your actions and approaches. Reflect on the person-centred values you have applied and how you have done so.
>
> At an appropriate time, show your diary to your assessor and discuss what you have learned about the importance of person-centred working when supporting individuals. Ensure you reflect on your performance and the benefits that your person-centred values had for individuals.
>
> Remember that for AC 3.3 you will need to show your assessor how you are responsive to individuals' changing needs or preferences and can adapt your actions and approaches.

AC 3.4 Demonstrate respect for individuals' lifestyle, choices and relationships

As you will have learned, showing respect for individuals involves taking into account their differences, needs and preferences. Every individual will have their own view about how they want to live their life. Some individuals may feel that a healthy lifestyle is important to them, others may not value this as much. Individuals are also entitled to make their own everyday choices and decisions about the relationships they have. Irrespective of the lifestyle individuals choose, the choices they make or the relationships they have, you must respect individuals' decisions and support them to live their lives in the way they want. Showing respect for individuals' lifestyle, choices and relationships is crucial to working in a person-centred way because it involves supporting individuals to make choices that they:

- understand
- have been fully involved in
- are in control of.

In other words, person-centred practice involves supporting individuals' rights to make informed choices.

Consent and demonstrating respect
What is consent?

You will already know that person-centred care involves respecting individuals' choices and decisions. Demonstrating respect for individuals' lifestyles, choices and relationships also requires you to provide the individual with sufficient information to be able to understand the lifestyle, choices and relationships they want. Similarly, before providing individuals with any form of care and support, you must ensure that you have their agreement to do so and that you have provided them with sufficient information about their options, the benefits, and the risks and consequences of not doing so to ensure their understanding – this is referred to as 'informed consent'. You will need to answer their questions as best you can and, if you don't know the answer, to check with someone who does or refer them to someone who does. Make sure the person who needs this information receives it, so they can make an informed decision/consent, whether this is the individual or their family, for example.

> **Reflect on it**
>
> **3.4 Consent**
>
> Reflect on an occasion when you gave your consent to something, for example when you were asked where you wanted to go on a night out or what you wanted to eat. How did this make you feel?
>
> Now imagine how you would feel if you were not asked for your consent.

Why is obtaining consent important?

Obtaining an individual's consent when providing care or support is important because:

- **it is a legal requirement:** to comply with legislation, such as the Mental Capacity Act 2005, the individual must give their consent for the provision of care or support. When an individual is unable to give their consent because they lack the capacity due to having a condition such as dementia, then a representative may decide on their behalf, but only if they act in the individual's best interests

> **Research it**
>
> **3.4 Mental Capacity Act 2005**
>
> Research what the Mental Capacity Act 2005 says about the importance of establishing consent when providing care or support and promoting individuals' rights. Find out more about the five principles:
>
> 1. A person must be assumed to have capacity unless it is established that they lack capacity.
> 2. A person is not to be treated as unable to make a decision unless all practical steps to help them do so have been taken without success.
> 3. A person is not to be treated as unable to make a decision merely because they make an unwise decision.
> 4. An act done, or decision made, under this Act for or on behalf of a person who lacks capacity must be done, or made, in their best interests.
> 5. Before the act is done, or the decision is made, regard must be had to whether the purpose for which it is needed can be as effectively achieved in a way that is less restrictive of the person's rights and freedom of action.
>
> Source: *Mental Capacity Act 2005, Part 1, Section 1 The principles* (www.legislation.gov.uk/ukpga/2005/9/section/1)
>
> There is a useful link below: www.mind.org.uk/information-support/legal-rights/mental-capacity-act-2005/overview/

at all times. The 'best interests' principle in the Mental Capacity Act 2005 means that all decisions made on behalf of an individual who lacks capacity must benefit the individual – this may be in relation to the individual's health, care or support. Obtaining consent also means that the individuals you care for have given their agreement for their care and as a result you and your setting are protected legally.

- **it is necessary for working in a person-centred way:** obtaining an individual's consent when providing care or support means that you are respecting the individual's right to agree or refuse, and promoting their dignity by not assuming that you know what care or support, lifestyle or choices the individual wants, needs or prefers. Remember it is the individual who knows best. It is the individual or their representative who decides what care or support is needed and/or preferred. The care and medical professions are able to advise on care and medical treatment but individuals and their representatives must be able to decide what happens to them.

Factors that influence consent

As you will have learned, obtaining an individual's consent is important but sometimes you may come across an individual that may not be able to express their consent. This may be because:

- **the individual lacks capacity** and is therefore unable to make a decision for themselves. This may be due to a learning disability, a condition such as dementia, a mental health need, because they are confused, drowsy or unconscious or because they have misused a substance such as an illegal drug or alcohol.

An individual who lacks capacity will be unable to express their consent. In other words, they will not be able to do one or more of the following: understand or retain the information they have been given, evaluate the information they have received to make a decision or make a decision and express their decision to someone else.

It is also important to take into consideration that an individual's lack of capacity may vary and/or may be temporary. An individual with dementia may lack capacity on some days but not others; similarly some individuals with a learning disability may lack capacity to make some major decisions such as about their future care but not minor decisions such as what to eat or wear. It is important to be aware of all these factors that can influence the capacity of an individual to express consent.

Remember that when an individual does not have capacity for one decision this does not mean that they lack capacity for every decision.

- **the individual is undecided over whether to give their consent** and is therefore unable to express their wishes. This may be because the individual requires more time to make a decision. This may be the case particularly if the decision they have to make is an important one such as changing the type of support they receive or moving house, or because they are anxious about it. For example, in relation to having some medical treatment they may be concerned about going into hospital or the side effects of the medications they will be taking.

- **it is unclear whether an individual has given their consent** and therefore it cannot be assumed that the individual has expressed their consent. This may be because the individual has specific communication needs and it is difficult to understand what the individual is trying to express, or because an individual is feeling anxious or becomes withdrawn and therefore makes it unclear whether they are expressing their consent.

- **it is unclear whether an individual has understood the information provided to them** and therefore again, it cannot be assumed that the individual has expressed their consent. This may be because the information provided to the individual is not in a suitable format that meets their needs; the language used may be too complex or the photographs used may not be easily recognisable by the individual. It could also be due to poor working practices that mean that the information provided is done in a rush or in a way that does not meet the individual's specific communication and language needs and preferences or causes offence to the individual, for example if it is not respectful of their culture and beliefs. You can refer to Unit 304 Effective communication in adult care settings/services for more information about effective working approaches for meeting specific communication needs and preferences.

When consent cannot be readily established

As you will have learned, sometimes it may not be possible to establish consent with an individual for various reasons.

If consent cannot be readily established take the following steps:

- Try explaining the information to them again. This is so that they understand what the procedure entails, the benefits, risks and consequences.

- Seek advice from, for example, your manager. It is your duty to not ignore the concerns you have but to report that the individual has not given consent, seek further guidance and discuss your concerns. Settings will have their own policies and procedures in place in case of such situations. Doing so reflects your competence for providing good care and support and ensuring that the best outcome for the individual can be reached.

- Consult with the individual's representative. In some cases you may be able to seek further clarification from a person who knows the individual well, for example the individual's advocate. Discussing this with someone else may help. You must always check with your manager before doing so as this information is personal to the individual and is therefore protected data.

- Record your findings in relation to the actions you took to establish consent with an individual and the actions you took when you were unable to establish consent with the individual. Include what happened, what the individual said/expressed, the guidance you were given, by whom and when.

If, after trying all these options, consent can still not be established with an individual then it may be that you are unable to do anything. However, this will depend on a number of things, such as the individual's capacity and whether refusal means their health will be in danger. Advice may need to be sought by your manager from external agencies, such as the Courts, who can provide legal clarification, and Professional Councils, who can provide additional support.

> **Reflect on it**
>
> **3.4 Capacity to make informed decisions**
>
> Imagine you had an accident, were experiencing temporary confusion and needed support to make informed choices in relation to day-to-day living. How would you feel if your choices were not respected? What impact might this have on how you live your life?

> **Evidence opportunity**
>
> **3.4 Respecting individuals' lifestyle, choices and relationships**
>
> Identify an activity with which you can support an individual who has care or support needs. For example, putting their shoes on, brushing their teeth, making a shopping list or deciding how to spend the evening.
>
> Think about how you would support the individual with this activity. Ensure you demonstrate how you show your respect for the individual to make their own informed choices. Your assessor could observe you supporting the individual directly, or you could get a witness testimony from your manager.

AC 3.5 Promote understanding and application of active participation amongst others

Active participation, although beneficial and an essential part of high quality care and support, can be difficult for individuals and others to understand and use because everyone views active participation differently:

- **Individuals:** some individuals may have only experienced dependency on others and may not be used to doing things for themselves, so active participation may be something they find frightening or don't believe is right for them. For example, an individual with a physical disability may have lived at home with their parents all their life and will therefore not have experienced living on their own. They may also have had everything done for them by well-meaning parents – this may have even included arranging their day-to-day activities. An individual in this situation will not be used to making their own choices but may instead depend on others to do so.
- **Individuals' families:** some individuals' families may be very protective over the individual, particularly if they have care or support needs because they are aware of their vulnerability and do not want any harm to come to them. For example, an individual with a learning disability may have a very supportive family, but who only allow the individual to socialise with them and not with their friends because they feel that in this way they can safeguard the individual from the risk of being harmed or abused by others. An individual's family in this situation will find it difficult to promote the use of active participation because they believe that their relative does not have the capacity to do so and may come to significant harm.
- **Your colleagues:** some of your colleagues may be new to working in the adult care sector, others may be experienced but have become used to working in ways that are not in line with current best practice, others may not have had in-depth training around dementia care, for example. Perhaps an individual with dementia may have started to become restless at night and your colleagues think that rather than find out what this change in the individual's behaviour means, it is better to prevent the individual from leaving their room at night or to accompany the individual back to their room every time they leave. Your colleagues in this situation may not understand why it is important to find out the meaning behind the individual's behaviour and they may not understand how the use of active participation can be relevant and beneficial to an individual with dementia.
- **Other team members:** some of your team members, such as other professionals who may come from different backgrounds and have different areas of expertise, may not think that they need to understand and use active participation because they perceive this as being your responsibility and that of your colleagues rather than theirs. For example, an older individual may want to learn a new skill such as painting at college. The tutor may believe that their role is to teach the individual to paint and that if they require additional support that you and your colleagues will provide this rather than them. Your role would be to encourage the individual to do as much for themselves when taking part in the painting activity. Team members in this situation may not understand why it is important for them to use active participation and how this can address the individual's holistic needs (you learned about how active participation can address the holistic needs of an individual in AC 1.7).

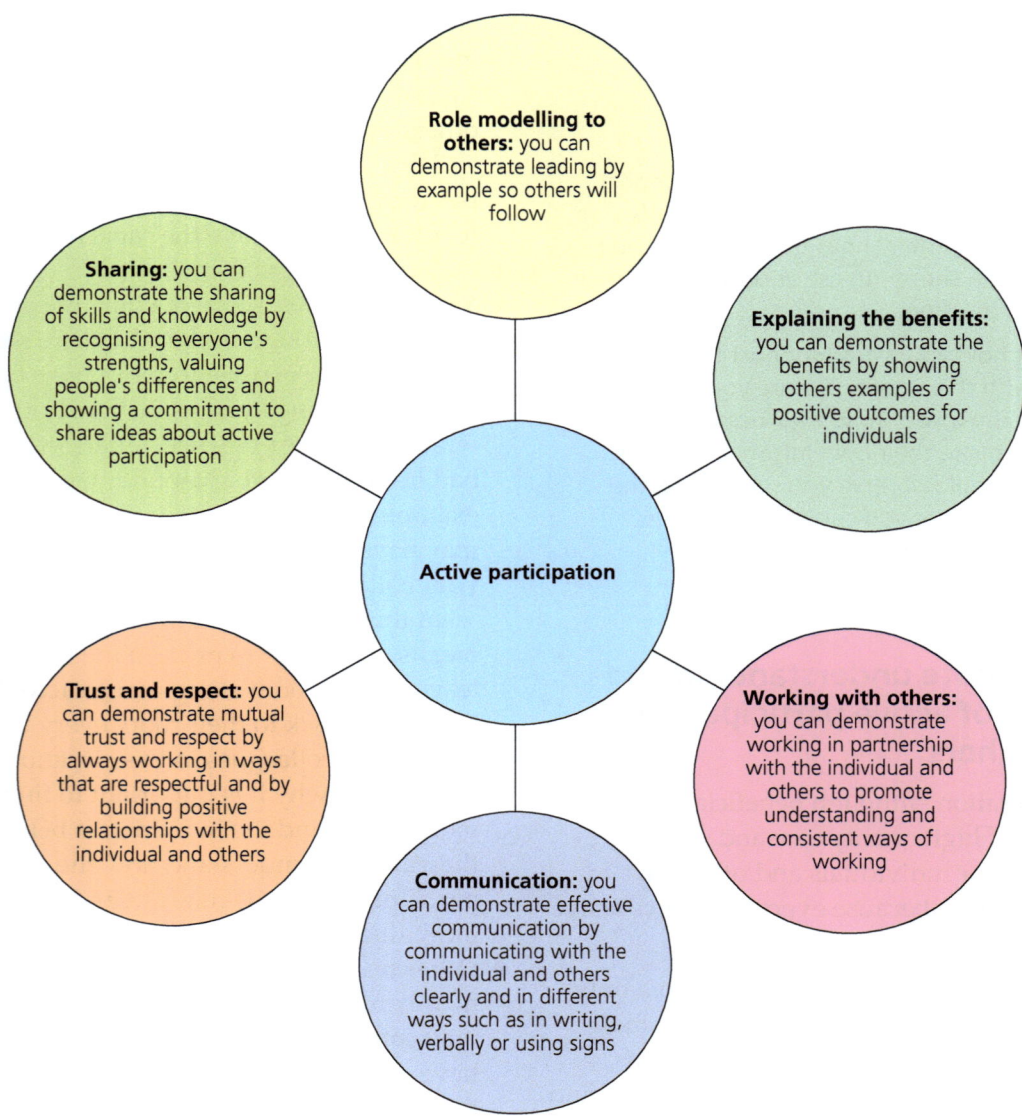

Figure 7.5 Ways to promote understanding and use of active participation amongst others

Ways to promote understanding and use of active participation amongst others

There are many different ways to promote understanding and use of active participation when working with individuals and others and Figure 7.5 provides examples of some of the main ones. Can you think of any others? You may also find it useful to review AC 3.2. You will be observed for this AC.

Reflect on it

3.5 Active participation and others

Reflect on each of the examples you've just read about how individuals, individuals' families, your colleagues and other team members may not understand active participation and its use. How do you think this will impact on the individual, the quality of the care or support provided, and those you work with?

> **Evidence opportunity**
>
> **3.5 Ways to promote understanding and use of active participation amongst others**
>
> Work with an individual and a colleague to promote understanding and use of active participation. What skills and knowledge can you demonstrate that you have? How? Why are these essential for providing high quality care and support? Make sure your assessor observes you or obtain a witness testimony from your manager.

Legislation	
Act/Regulation	**Key points**
Data Protection Act 2018	Personal information must be recorded, used, stored and shared according to a set of principles or rules to ensure the individuals' rights are protected and the security of their personal information is maintained.
	The Data Protection Act 2018 is the UK's implementation of the EU's General Data Protection Regulation (GDPR) 2018. In order to ensure care is person-centred, you will need to ensure information is handled with the utmost care. You can find more information on the Data Protection Act 2018 in Unit 304.
The Human Rights Act 1998	Everyone in the UK is entitled to the same rights and freedoms. This includes individuals who have care and support needs. The Act supports individuals to have the right to take risks and to have their choices and decisions respected.
The Management of Health and Safety at Work Regulations 1999	It is a legal requirement for risks in work settings including care settings to be managed safely and that risk assessments are carried out, documented, reviewed and updated.
The Mental Capacity Act 2005	This Act supports person-centred working by supporting individuals' rights to make their own decisions, including being provided with the necessary support to do so. It also protects the rights of individuals who lack capacity by providing guidance on who can make decisions about them and how to plan ahead for this in case it arises in the future.
The Care Act 2014	This Act supports individuals' rights to make informed decisions about their care and support and promotes a person-centred approach to care planning where adult care workers can support individuals to develop their care plans.
	It also defines the concept of wellbeing and outlines how adult care workers can promote individuals' wellbeing. Also see the government publications:
	● *Personalised Health and Care 2020*, which sets out how technology and data can be used to improve health and the way health and social care services are delivered.
	● *The Adult Social Care Outcomes Framework Handbook of Definitions*, which measures how well care and support services achieve the outcomes that are the most important to people.
The Health and Social Care Act 2008 (Regulated Activities) Regulations 2014	This Act supports the rights of individuals and their representatives to be involved in the planning, provision and review of their care and support. It would be useful for you to research the various Regulations, including 11 which covers consent.

307 Promoting choice and independence in adult care settings/services

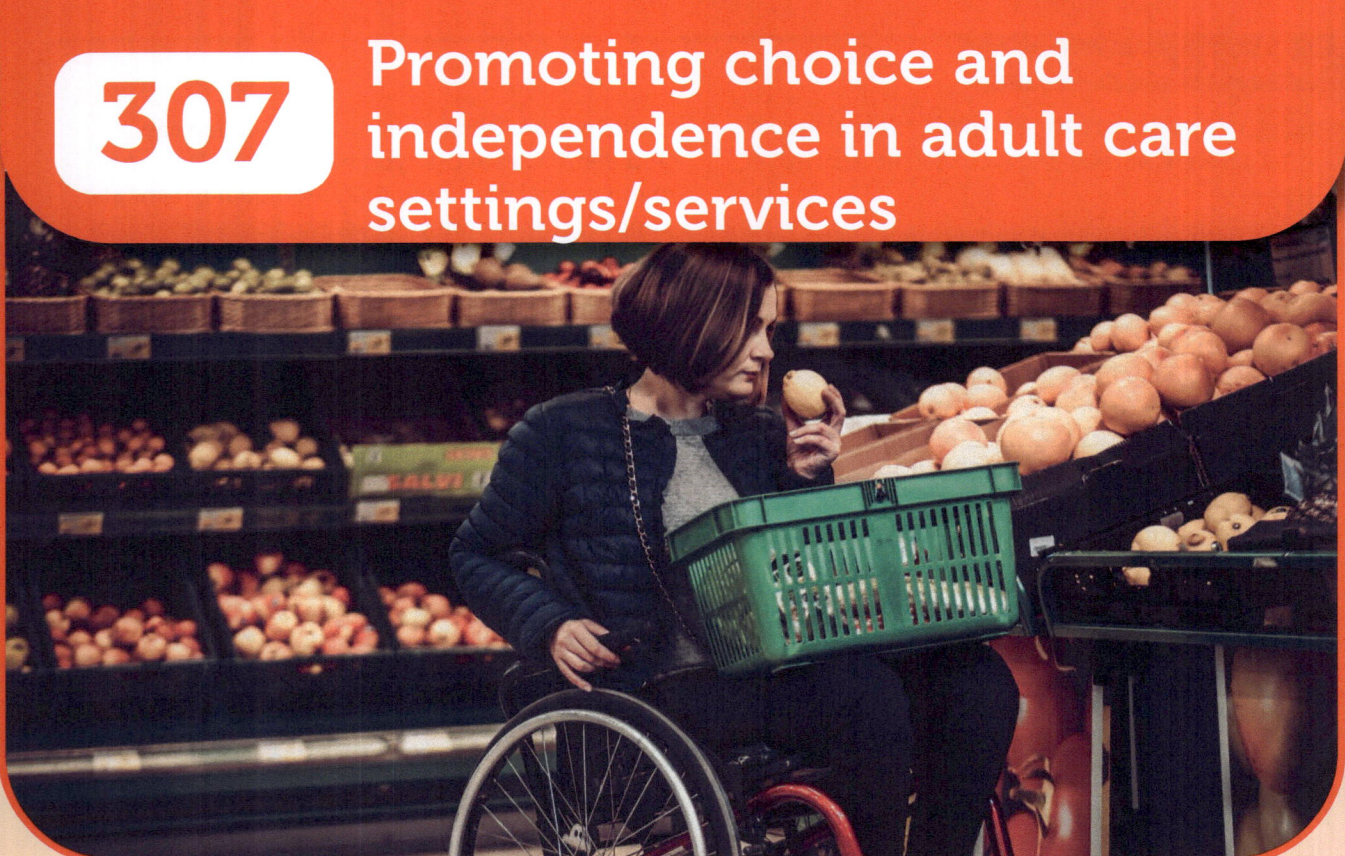

About this unit

Credit value: 3
Guided learning hours: 22

Person-centred care involves working with individuals with care or support needs in a way that embeds person-centred values such as promoting choice and independence, ensuring that individuals are in control of their care or support.

In this unit you will learn about how risk assessments can be used to promote individuals' choices, independence and their right to take risks, including why and when individuals' risk assessments are reviewed and updated.

You will also learn about how to promote individuals' rights to make informed choices and decisions and consider how to do this with support, guidance and risk assessment processes. How to establish individuals' informed consent when providing care and support is another aspect of person-centred working that you will be able to use your skills to practise.

Promoting individuals' independence in their care and support and showing how you can do so effectively is an additional area of expertise that you will have an opportunity to develop.

Learning outcomes

By the end of this unit you will:

LO1: Understand the role of risk assessments in promoting person-centred approaches

LO2: Be able to promote individuals' rights to make choices

LO3: Be able to promote individuals' independence

LO1 Understand the role of risk assessments in promoting person-centred approaches, choice and independence

Getting started

Think about an occasion when you supported an individual to take risks. How did you support the individual to assess the risks involved?

AC 1.1 Explain how risk assessments can be used to promote and enable individuals' choice, independence and right to take risks

Taking risks and using risk assessment to do so is a key aspect of providing person-centred care because taking risks is part of everyday life and an essential part of supporting individuals' rights to make choices, be independent and be in control of their lives, care and support. Robust risk assessments allow individuals to take risks. This approach is also known as positive risk taking and involves weighing up the benefits and harms of different choices and decisions. It is linked to promoting and enabling individuals' choice, independence and right to take risks because it involves:

- enabling individuals to grow in confidence and make their own decisions based on information available on a range of options
- promoting individuals' strengths and abilities
- supporting individuals to take opportunities
- supporting individuals to understand their responsibilities and those of others
- supporting individuals to understand the benefits of taking risks
- supporting individuals to understand the consequences of taking risks
- supporting individuals to learn from their mistakes
- developing good working relationships with individuals and others
- being positive about taking risks.

Reflect on it

1.1 Positive risk taking

Reflect on three aspects identified above of what positive risk taking involves and explain how you do this in the care setting where you work.

Evidence opportunity

1.1 Risk assessments – choice, independence and right to take risks

Provide a written account explaining how risk assessments can be used to promote person-centred approaches. How do you promote and enable individuals' choice, independence and right to take risks in the care setting where you work through positive risk taking?

AC 1.2 Outline risk assessment methods used to promote choice and independence used in different situations

Promoting choice and independence involves doing everything you can to support individuals to make their own choices and decisions and be independent without compromising their or others' safety. The risk assessment process, which you will learn more about in Unit 310, involves supporting individuals to take risks by assessing what the potential dangers are and by considering what can be put in place to reduce those risks and protect individuals from danger, harm, abuse and neglect. The risk assessment process does not prevent individuals from doing what they want but rather helps individuals and you to manage these risks effectively by considering what can be done to reduce them. In this way, you will be exercising your duty of care by supporting individuals' rights to be independent, live in the way that they want to and make their own choices and decisions after giving careful consideration to the associated benefits, risks and consequences.

Reflect on it

1.2 Consequences

Reflect on the consequences of using risk assessment to prevent or restrict an individual's right to make choices and be independent. What would the consequences be for the individual, you and the organisation?

Risk assessment methods

As you will have learned in AC 1.1, risk assessments to promote choice and independence are not form filling exercises or procedures that are carried out quickly; they are instead part of a process that enables individuals to make decisions about their lives and then learn from the outcomes of those decisions. All risk assessment methods used in care settings must be in line with organisational policies, procedures and agreed practices or ways of working. Although risk assessment methods used may vary from one care setting to another, they will all form part of a way of working called risk enablement. Risk enablement includes the following principles:

- The individual's safety, wellbeing and happiness will be the main focus.
- Consultation with the individual to find out what is important to them will take place.
- Consultation with others involved in the individual's life and who know them well may also take place to ensure that everyone is working together to produce the best outcome for the individual.
- All discussions, choices and decisions made, including those agreed, will be documented to provide a clear audit trail that can be referred to and used to provide continuity of care and support.

Below are some examples of different risk assessment methods that can be used to promote choice and independence:

- Consultation with the individual to find out what they would like to do so that they are placed at the centre of their care and support and are empowered to make their own decisions. This may take the form of a discussion with the individual or with their advocate. Alternative and augmentative communication tools and/or digital technology could also be used with the individual depending on their preferred communication needs and abilities. You will learn more about different technologies that can be used to support an individual's independence in AC 3.3 of this unit.
- Consultation with the individual's family and friends to find out more about the individual such as their strengths and abilities so that they can also be involved in the risk assessment process. The individual's family and friends may be able to provide more information on what the individual would like to do and/or what they have enjoyed doing in the past. This may take the form of a discussion with them and/or with the individual.
- Consultation with others who are involved in the individual's care and support, such as colleagues, managers, professionals from other agencies, who will be able to share their ideas based on what they know about the individual.

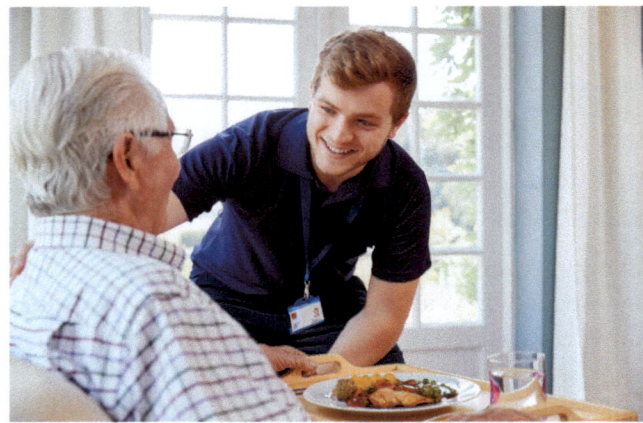

Figure 8.1 How do you promote choice and independence?

AC 1.3 Describe own role when undertaking risk assessments to promote choice and independence

When undertaking risk assessments to promote individuals' choice and independence your role involves:

- following your care setting's policies, procedures and agreed ways of working/practices so you work within the responsibilities of your job role
- spending time with the individual so that they feel valued and can trust you with considering what they want to do
- involving the individual to consider the risks themselves and how to address them by providing them with information about the options available and ensuring they understand the implications of different choices they make. You must ensure that you do not influence an individual's choices and decisions, even if you do not agree with them, as it is your role to support the risk assessment process and enable the individual to achieve what they want to
- involving others in the individual's care and support in line with the individual's wishes so that the individual feels that they are supported

- involving other agencies involved in the individual's care and support so that you have an accurate picture of the risks involved and can share ideas with others of how best to address them
- recording all discussions/decisions made as part of the individual's risk assessment and communicating these to those who work with the individual, including the severity of the risks identified, their likelihood of happening, the strengths and abilities of the individual and the outcome for the individual if they take the risks identified
- seeking additional support and guidance if you are unsure of any aspect of the risk assessment process and/or you have any questions.

You will also find it useful to review your previous learning in Unit 303 Understanding duty of care, LO2 around how to address conflicts or dilemmas that may arise between an individual's rights and the duty of care.

> **Evidence opportunity**
>
> **1.2, 1.3 Risk assessments**
>
> Identify two individuals with care and support needs that you know. For each individual:
> - outline the risk assessment methods you use to promote their choice and independence.
> - describe your role in undertaking risk assessments.

AC 1.4 Explain why it is important to review and update individuals' risk assessments

Risk assessments are only effective if they contain accurate and up-to-date information. This means that when there are changes, either to the individual or to the environment, these must be reflected in the risk assessment to ensure that it is accurate and details a true picture. For example, a moving and handling risk assessment will require updating if the individual begins using a new or different piece of equipment to move from one position to another or, for example, when an individual's health changes as a result of illness.

Regularly revising risk assessments is essential for ensuring that individuals can continue to take risks positively and safely and for minimising any harm or injuries to individuals and those who support them.

AC 1.5 Describe when individuals' risk assessments should be reviewed and updated

Risk assessments usually include a review date once they are completed so that their accuracy and currency can be checked at regular intervals. At the time of completion, the review date may be in one month's time, but should things change before this, such as in a week or two weeks' time, then they must be revised and updated. All changes to a risk assessment must be documented clearly so that it can be used and accessed whenever it is needed by those who have permission to do so.

AC 1.6 Explain who should be involved in the review and update of individuals' risk assessments

When reviewing and updating individuals' risk assessments the individual should be involved as well as all those others that form part of the individual's agreed care and support. In this way everyone will be aware of why and when the individual's risk assessment has been reviewed and updated and so can work together in providing the individual with support to achieve their outcomes in a positive way.

> **6Cs**
>
> **Care**
>
> Reviewing and updating individuals' risk assessments is an effective way to show that care is at the very heart of the support you provide to individuals. For example, think about what would happen if an individual's risk assessment didn't contain accurate and up-to-date information. Consider what would happen if you didn't regularly review an individual's risk assessment and what could go wrong. Care is an ongoing process and something that you should always be striving to improve.
>
> **Communication**
>
> Without effective communication with individuals, and others you work with, supporting individuals' risk assessments would be very difficult. Reviewing and updating risk assessments requires you, individuals and others to work together to support individuals to achieve positive outcomes in a safe way.

Reflect on it

1.4, 1.5 Up-to-date records

Reflect on your learning in Unit 305 Handling information in adult care settings/services in relation to why it's important to ensure records are up-to-date. How does this learning relate to reviewing and updating individuals' risk assessments?

Evidence opportunity

1.4, 1.5, 1.6 Reviewing and updating individuals' risk assessments

Provide a written account explaining why it is important that individuals' risk assessments in the care setting where you work are reviewed and updated, when they should be reviewed and updated and who should be involved.

LO2 Be able to promote individuals' rights to make choices

Getting started

Reflect on an occasion when you supported an individual in the care setting where you work to make their own choice over an aspect of their care or support. What guidance did you follow and why? Did you access any support? If so, why and how did this help you and the individual?

AC 2.1 Demonstrate how to support individuals to make informed choices and decisions

Supporting individuals' rights is crucial to working in a person-centred way because it involves supporting individuals to make choices that they:

- understand
- have been fully involved in
- are in control of.

In other words, person-centred practice involves supporting individuals' rights to make informed choices and decisions.

6Cs

Competence

Supporting individuals to make informed choices and decisions requires you to show your competence. This is because, to do so effectively, you need to show that you know the individuals you are working with, including understanding their needs, strengths, abilities and preferences. In this way you can be sure that you are providing individuals with the support that they need to make their own choices.

Research it

2.1 Making informed choices and decisions

Research best practice when supporting individuals to make informed choices and decisions. You can conduct your research either in the care setting where you work or in another care setting that you know about.

You could also speak to other team members and ask them about the practices they follow when supporting individuals to make informed choices and decisions. You could ask them questions such as: 'What type of care setting do you work in?'; 'What care or support needs do the individuals you work with have?'; 'What ways do you find work best when supporting individuals to make informed choices and decisions? Why?'

Evidence opportunity

2.1 Supporting individuals to make informed choices and decisions

You will be observed for this AC: supporting individuals to make informed choices and decisions. Show your assessor how you support different individuals to make informed choices and decisions.

	Dos and don'ts for supporting individuals to make informed choices and decisions
Do	Find out how an individual makes their own choices and decisions – to ensure that you are providing support to individuals in ways that have been agreed and that match their strengths, abilities and preferences.
Do	Ensure all information presented to individuals is understood – to ensure that individuals can then use this information to consider and choose from different options that are available to them and understand the barriers and risks.
Do	Ensure individuals and/or their representatives or advocates are involved – to ensure that individuals and their representatives put forward the individual's views, ideas and preferences.
Do	Keep records of all options available and agreed upon – to ensure that these can be shared with everyone involved and referred to when required.
Don't	Make decisions for individuals – this does not support an individual's rights to make their own choices.
Don't	Present information in a misleading way – this does not enable individuals to make informed choices.
Don't	Ignore individuals and others who know them well – this does not enable you to take into account their personal views, ideas and preferences.
Don't	Only agree options verbally – if clear written records are not kept, this does not enable information to be shared accurately and reviewed with all those involved.

AC 2.2 Establish informed consent when providing care and support

Before providing individuals with care and support, you must ensure that you have their agreement to do so and that you have provided them with sufficient information about their options, the benefits, and the risks and consequences of not doing so to ensure their understanding – this is referred to as 'informed consent'.

Establishing consent with an individual for an activity or action can only be successful if you:

- work together with the individual. This ensures their rights are respected and their preferences supported
- are flexible in the methods you use. Some individuals may be able to consent verbally, others in writing.

When establishing consent with an individual for an activity or action in any adult care setting it is important to comply with the following best practice guidance.

Top tips for demonstrating respect:

- Respect the individual's views about their lifestyle, choices and relationships; for example you should discuss when the activity or action is to be carried out.
- Listen to the individual and find out about their preferences about the activity or action.
- Discuss or explain what carrying out the activity or action will involve; for example you should tell them about the number of staff required to support the activity and the process to be followed.
- Provide the individual with relevant and accurate information; this may be in response to any questions or concerns the individual may have.
- Don't impose your views or preferences on the individual or make derogatory comments about individuals' lifestyle, choices and relationships even if they are different to yours or you disagree with them.
- Support the individual to make their own decisions and respect these. For example, discuss with the individual the related benefits, drawbacks and consequences and respect their decisions even if you disagree with them.

- If the individual lacks capacity, then you should speak to their advocate but make sure that in the first instance, you consult the individual. Also make sure that you support those with language and communication difficulties to communicate their consent and seek the assistance of translators and communication aids. Remember that if you are unsure about anything or do not have the knowledge about any of this, then you should refer the individual to someone who does (for example, a medical professional). This means the individual has access to the most correct and accurate information available. Also remember the things you have learned about confidentiality when communicating information, especially to those other than the individual. You may be dealing with sensitive and private information, so it is important that you are sure the individual is happy for the information to be communicated to others.

Demonstrating respect for individuals' lifestyles, choices and relationships is not a process that is completed by adult care workers at the beginning of their shift or once a day; it is an ongoing process that takes place for every activity or action they complete with an individual. This is because an individual's preferences, like yours, may change from one day to another and respecting individuals' preferences and right to change their mind is a must. For example, just because an individual chose to have a shower yesterday morning does not mean they want to have a shower every morning; the individual may prefer to have a bath instead, or to have a wash at night before going to bed. You will only know if you seek the individual's consent – not doing so will result in you not providing good care and support.

How is consent communicated?

We have already discussed informed consent, where individuals are asked for their consent or agreement based on the information they have received about the benefits, risks and consequences. However, how do individuals give or communicate their consent? You will find that this will vary depending on the types of things for which you are requesting consent. For example, it might be done verbally (verbal consent) when you ask an individual whether they are happy to have lunch, or would like to take part in a group activity, and they tell you that it is OK. You may need written consent, for example, when individuals are agreeing to serious medical procedures, when an individual agrees for someone to be their advocate or when consent is required around financial matters.

You will find that consent is not always communicated explicitly, but it may be implied. For example, if you ask an individual who is in bed whether they would like to get up and get dressed, and they sit up in bed and look at their wardrobe, then they are implying that they are ready to do so. It is important that you are aware of these different ways of establishing consent, as well as the situations in which it is important to gain more formal written consent.

> **Research it**
>
> **2.2 Health and Social Care Act 2008 (Regulated Activities) Regulations 2014**
>
> Research the Health and Social Care Act 2008 (Regulated Activities) Regulations 2014: Regulation 1. What does it state about how consent must be established when providing care or support to an individual?
>
> There is a useful link below:
>
> www.cqc.org.uk/guidance-providers/regulations-enforcement/regulation-11-need-consent
>
> Discuss your findings with a colleague in the care setting where you work. Make notes based on your discussion.

> **Evidence opportunity**
>
> **2.2 Obtaining consent**
>
> Show your assessor how you establish consent in your work.
>
> Identify an individual you provide care or support to in the care setting where you work and who you know well. Using the individual's care plan and your knowledge of the individual's background, needs and preferences, discuss which methods you can use to obtain their consent when providing care or support.
>
> Do you use these methods already? If not, why not? What are the benefits of doing so? What could be the consequences of not doing so? Ensure you cover all of this in your discussion.
>
> Remember that you cannot include the care plan or individuals' personal details in your portfolio if you write up details of your discussion.

AC 2.3 Demonstrate the use of support mechanisms and guidance to promote an individual's right to make choices

Your role in demonstrating respect

You have a very important part to play in showing respect for individuals' lifestyles, choices and relationships. In your role as Lead Adult Care Worker or Lead Personal Assistant you will be able to do this by:

- **role modelling:** this involves you supporting the individual's right to make choices as part of your day-to-day activities, for example in relation to what to wear, what to eat, where to go out, who they would like to meet up with. In this way, the individual will experience how this benefits them and will be more likely to work with you to be an active participant. Others, such as your colleagues and individuals' families and friends, will observe you applying active participation and therefore be more likely to do this themselves too.

- **providing information:** this involves you informing the individual and others about your duty of care to support the individual's right to make choices, the lifestyle they wish to lead and/or the relationships they have. This may involve you guiding your colleagues on a day-to-day basis or providing them with training. Your role may also involve providing individuals with information in a format they can understand by, for example, meeting with them on a one-to-one basis or arranging a group discussion. This will provide individuals with the information they need to make their own choices and the reasons why this is important.

- **providing support:** this involves you supporting individuals both directly and indirectly to exercise their rights to make their own choices and have the lifestyle and relationships they want. For example, you may be involved in actively supporting an individual to choose what activities they would like to participate in or the type of support they would like, and when and how often they want to receive it. You may be involved in speaking up for an individual who is unable to speak up for themselves when making their own choices because the individual lacks capacity.

> ### 6Cs
>
> #### Compassion
> You will need to ensure that you use your own role and authority in a compassionate way to support the individual's right to make their own choices. For example, you can show your compassion by putting the individual first, before your own views and needs.
>
> When an individual makes a choice that you disagree with, how can you show that you have encouraged them to make an informed choice? How can you show you have taken their views seriously? How can you demonstrate that you have not let your views influence their choice?
>
> #### Commitment
> Being committed to providing high-quality care and support to individuals means that you do everything you can to encourage individuals to make their own informed choices and support them to do so even when others around them may question the choices they have made or may have concerns. In these situations you can show your commitment by ensuring the individuals' views and needs come first.
>
> #### Courage
> Courage is speaking up for an individual if they are at risk – this is an important responsibility that all Lead Adult Care Workers and Lead Personal Assistants have.

> ### Reflect on it
>
> #### 2.3 Skills for supporting individuals to make informed choices
>
> Reflect on the skills and qualities you have as a leader that help you in supporting individuals to make informed choices. Why are these important? How do they influence the care and support you provide?

Support mechanisms and guidance

There are a range of support mechanisms and guidance that you can also use to promote an individual's right to make choices:

- Care/Support plans – these will include how to promote an individual's right to make choices. For example, an individual's care plan may include guidance about how to promote an

individual's choices when eating, such as only being given two options to choose from at a time rather than three or four, or using photographs of meal options and placing them in front of the individual so that they can choose one.
- Risk assessments – these will include agreed ways of how to promote an individual's right to make choices while promoting their safety and wellbeing. For example, an individual's risk assessment may set out agreed ways of how to promote an individual's choice to go on a walking tour, such as by being supported with two members of staff and ensuring the individual uses the walking equipment required.
- Use of advocates – advocates can be a valuable source of support as they will ensure that they put forward the individual's views and that their right to make choices is at the centre of their care and support. For example, an advocate may put forward an individual's ideas for how they want to be supported when choosing activities.
- Alternative communication strategies – individuals' communication needs and preferences will be set out in individuals' care/support plans and/or communication profiles. For example, sometimes individuals prefer to use alternative communication strategies that may include signs, gestures, pictures or photographs. It is important to be aware of how individuals communicate so that they can understand you and vice versa when promoting their choices. You will find it useful to review your previous learning in Unit 304 Effective communication in adult care settings/services around alternative communication strategies.
- Assistive technology – assistive technology is another tool for promoting individuals' right to make choices. This includes devices, equipment and software that enable individuals who have difficulties, for example communicating or carrying out daily tasks, to be more independent and gain the confidence to self-care. For example, an electric wheelchair that has been adapted for an individual with a disability can enable an individual to gain confidence in mobilising the wheelchair themselves and move where and when they want to rather than depend on someone else supporting them. Again, you will find it useful to review your previous learning in Unit 304 Effective communication in adult care settings/services around assistive technology.
- Family/informal carers – family/informal carers have a good insight into the individual because they know them well and very often because they are related to the individual or are friends with them can be valuable sources of information and guidance about how they promote an individual's right to make choices. For example, an individual's mother may share with you that to promote their son's choice over how to spend the day she makes him a cup of tea first and then asks him.

> **Evidence opportunity**
>
> **2.3 Using support mechanisms and guidance to promote an individual's right to make choices**
>
> You will be observed for this assessment criterion demonstrating how to use support mechanisms and guidance to promote an individual's right to make choices. From the range of support mechanisms you have learned about in this AC, ensure that you show how you use some of these when promoting individuals' right to make choices. Which methods will you use? Will these vary with different individuals? Why?

AC 2.4 Work with individuals to manage risk in a way that maintains and promotes an individual's right to make choices

Being in a lead role means not only that you can encourage individuals to be the lead participants in their care and support but that you can also lead the way for others to follow you in providing high quality care and support.

Managing risk while demonstrating respect

Taking **risks** is part of making choices in everyday life for all of us; not doing so would act as a barrier to us achieving what we want to do. Similarly, when Lead Adult Care Workers and Lead Personal Assistants support the right of individuals to lead lifestyles, make choices and have relationships they want, this too may involve individuals taking risks. This doesn't mean that individuals will be placed in danger, be harmed or abused or be persuaded to not take risks – but rather that they will be supported to understand what the **hazards** and risks are and how these can be managed.

Assessing what the risks are and their impact is crucial when supporting individuals' right to make choices because it involves a careful balance between supporting the rights of individuals to make their own choices and maintaining their safety and thinking about protective factors that can be put in place to ensure safety. A thorough risk assessment is not only a useful tool to use for this, it is also a legal requirement for maintaining individuals' safety while they do the activities that they enjoy.

Go to Unit 310 Promoting health and safety in adult care settings/services, LO3, for information on the risk assessment process.

Positive risk taking

Positive risk taking in relation to person-centred care involves weighing up the benefits and drawbacks to the individual of taking the risk. The greater the potential benefits to the individual, the more important it is to try and find a way of managing the risk safely while being able to support the individual to take the risk.

The reflective exemplar provides you with an opportunity to explore in more detail how Lead Personal Assistants use risk assessments as part of working in a person-centred way.

Reflective exemplar	
Introduction	I work as a Lead Personal Assistant providing support to Sean who is 36 years old and uses a wheelchair to mobilise. Sean has panic attacks when he leaves his house and so my role is to support him to manage his panic attacks so that he can visit his local shops independently. I visit him on a weekly basis.
What happened?	This morning I supported Sean to prepare a route that he could use to go to his local shops that are approximately ten minutes away from his house. While looking together on the internet, on Google maps, at the roads we could walk down together Sean began to get very concerned that he may get into difficulties and not be able to return home safely.
	We discussed Sean's concerns together over a cup of tea. Sean began by saying that he may fall out of his wheelchair when travelling over the uneven pavements; we agreed that with me by his side supporting him and with his lap belt done up this was a low risk. Sean then added that he was afraid that he may have his money stolen again like the last time he went out on his own. I explained to Sean that I would be with him and so this again was a low risk. Finally, Sean had concerns over whether he was able enough to do his own shopping; again, I explained that he had already prepared a shopping list and that with my support he would manage fine.
	After much discussion, Sean apologised to me but said that he wasn't ready to leave the house yet and said that he might try again next week when I visited him.
What worked well?	I think identifying the potential hazards that Sean had concerns over was a good first step towards carrying out a risk assessment and reassuring Sean that he could overcome his fears of leaving the house.
What did not go as well?	Having identified the hazards and partly evaluated the level of risk, I think we should have discussed together what could be put in place to control or reduce the level of risk identified.
	This is part of the risk assessment process but I think it would also have reassured Sean more fully over the concerns he had and he would have felt safer. He may have refused to go out because he may have thought I didn't take his concerns seriously.
What could I do to improve?	I think I'm going to review my learning around the five key steps involved in the risk assessment process* and see if I can arrange to attend an update on using risk assessment.
Links to unit assessment criteria	ACs: 1.1, 1.2, 1.3, 2.4

* You can find out about the five key steps of the risk assessment process in Unit 310.

> **Evidence opportunity**
>
> **2.4 Risk assessment and choices**
>
> For this AC you will be observed by your assessor working with individuals to manage risk in a way that maintains and promotes an individual's right to make choices.
>
> Be prepared to discuss with your assessor how you maintained and promoted every individual's right to make choices.

LO3 Be able to promote individuals' independence

> **Getting started activity**
>
> Reflect on what being independent means to you. What do you do independently in your life? Why is this important? How would you feel if you lost your independence temporarily due to an accident or illness? How would this impact on your daily activities?

AC 3.1 Involve an individual in their care and support

Part of your role as an adult care worker is to support individuals to live their lives in the way they want to; not do things for them or make decisions for them but instead work with them and support them to make their own choices and decisions and do as much as they can for themselves. Involving an individual in their care and support has many benefits including encouraging them to take control and maintain their skills, abilities and self-esteem. You will learn more about how to support individuals to recognise their strengths and abilities to gain confidence in AC 3.2 of this unit.

You can involve an individual in their care and support by:

- getting to know the individual – this is an ongoing process that involves spending time with the individual and building a working relationship with them so that you can get to know them as a person and you can both learn to trust and respect each other. This means that you will then understand how to best involve them in their care and support because you will know the type and level of support they will require from you to be involved and to live their life as they choose. As every individual is a unique person, this is a process you will have to go through over and over again when involving individuals in their care and support.
- communicating with the individual – being able to communicate with the individual is an essential skill to have and will help you to involve the individual in their care and support. Communicating with the individual in their preferred way and using methods and techniques they understand will mean that you will be able to find out from them directly how they want to be involved in their care and support. Effective communication with the individual is also important for resolving any difficulties that may arise, such as if the individual lacks the confidence to be involved in their care and support or if the individual disagrees with the type and level of support they require. You may find it useful to review your previous learning in Unit 304 Effective communication in adult care settings/services in relation to communicating effectively using different methods and styles.

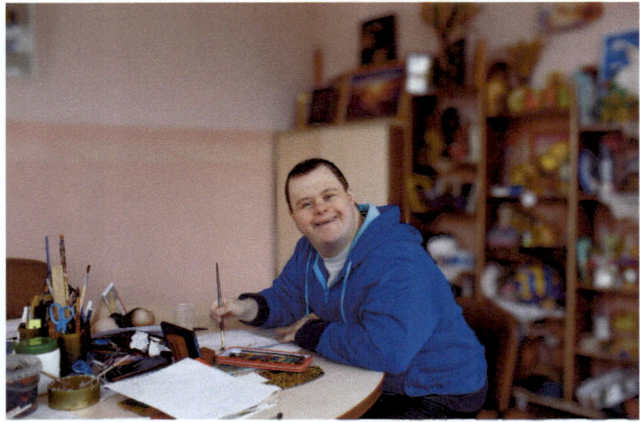

Figure 8.2 Benefits of involving individuals in their care and support

- communicating with others involved in the individual's care and support – being able to communicate with others such as individuals' family, friends, informal carers, or advocates is important because they too are involved in meeting individuals' care and support needs and know the individual well. Asking others for their views and ideas will benefit both them and the individual because it means that others feel that their contributions are listened to and valued and that the care and support provided to the individual is consistent and effective.

> **Reflect on it**
>
> **3.1 Involving individuals in their own care and support**
>
> Reflect on an occasion when you or a colleague involved an individual in the care and support in the care setting where you work. How was the individual involved? What benefits did this bring and to whom? Did any difficulties arise when encouraging the individual to be involved in their care and support?

AC 3.2 Support individuals to recognise their strengths and abilities to gain confidence to self-care

You have explored in AC 3.1 the different ways that you can encourage and support individuals to be involved in their care and support so that they can be more independent.

Sometimes, however, individuals are unsure about being more independent or may not recognise the strengths and abilities they have due to profound disabilities/end of life/circumstances. In these situations, it is your role to work with them to recognise these so that they gain the confidence to self-care. To do this you must know and understand the individual and the agreed ways of working with them. For example, depending on the them situation you can support them to recognise their strengths and abilities to gain confidence to self-care by:

- exploring different activities with the individual that promotes their independence by getting them to use the skills and abilities they have. Doing so will enable them to feel more confident in using the skills and abilities they have
- reinforcing the individual's strengths and abilities by, for example, identifying what these are and communicating these to them, praising the individual when they have used or demonstrated a skill and/or ability, and asking them how they feel afterwards
- enabling the individual to take risks and learn from their mistakes so that they no longer feel anxious or nervous about being able to self-care and can see that they do have the ability to self-care
- reassuring the individual that gaining confidence to self-care is an ongoing process and will vary for every person. It is also important to reassure them that being able to self-care does not mean that they will be on their own or no longer have any care or support. Instead, it means others working with them to help them do as much for themselves as possible
- promoting person-centred values and strength-based approaches when working with individuals to promote their independence and confidence to self-care. You will find it useful to review your previous learning about person-centred values and strength-based approaches in Unit 306 Promoting and implementing person-centred practice
- communicating with others involved in the individual's care and support to find out how they promote the individual's independence and confidence to self-care so that everyone is working consistently together.

Case study

3.1, 3.2 Gaining confidence to self-care

Amandeep works as a community carer providing support to individuals at home. This morning Amandeep visited Therese who is 60 years of age and has recently had a stroke which has left her with reduced mobility and swallowing difficulties when eating and drinking. It has been agreed that Amandeep will support Therese with her personal care by helping her with getting out of bed, getting washed and dressed and then with having some breakfast.

When Amandeep arrived at Therese's house, her sister who lives with Therese explained to Amandeep that she has already washed and dressed her sister and is just making her breakfast now, because otherwise Therese will take too long in getting ready and it's quicker if she just does it for her. Amandeep notices that Therese looks sad, her hair has not been brushed and she is not wearing her favourite bracelet. Amandeep also notices that Therese's sister looks tired and stressed.

Discuss:

1. How could Amandeep involve Therese in her care and support?
2. What would be the benefits of involving Therese in her care and support?
3. How could Amandeep involve Therese's sister in Therese's care and support? Why is this important?
4. How could Amandeep support Therese to recognise her strengths and abilities and gain confidence to self-care? Why is this important?

Evidence opportunity

3.1, 3.2 Support individuals to recognise their strengths and abilities to gain confidence to self-care

You will be observed for both assessment criteria so you will need to show how you involve an individual in their care and support as well as how you support individuals to recognise their strengths and abilities to gain confidence to self-care.

If the individuals you work with are not able to be involved in their care and support or to recognise their strengths and abilities due to profound disabilities/end of life/circumstances then you can instead write a reflection on how ways of working with individuals could support them to be involved in their care and support and recognise their strengths and abilities to gain confidence to self-care.

AC 3.3 Identify a range of technologies that can support or maintain an individual's independence

Technologies that can support or maintain an individual's independence and help them to reach their full potential can include **alternative and augmentative**, communication tools and/or digital technology. The table below includes some examples of these including how they can be used to support or maintain an individual's independence; do you know of any others?

Table 8.1 Examples of technologies that can support or maintain an individual's independence

Technologies	How technologies can support or maintain an individual's independence
Alternative and augmentative	• A BIGmack communicator is a speaking and recording communication device that enables an individual to record messages that can then be activated and played when communicating with others by tapping the top of the device. The top of the device comes in a variety of bright colours that are suitable for individuals who are visually impaired and also has a large surface area that can be used by individuals who have low physical control, i.e. due to a condition such as cerebral palsy. • An Eye-talk communicator is a communication board that enables individuals who have limited mobility to communicate with others. For example, words such as yes/no, phrases and happy/sad faces can be attached to the board and individuals look at these while the person communicating with them tracks their eye movement to find out what the individual is communicating.

Table 8.1 Examples of technologies that can support or maintain an individual's independence *continued*

Technologies	How technologies can support or maintain an individual's independence
	• A ProxTalker is a picture communication system that also talks. It doesn't require software or a PC because it uses **radio frequency identification technology** to retrieve vocabulary stored on sound tags. Individuals can choose from pre-recorded tags or record their own tags that are placed on a button and then are pressed to speak. This alternative and augmentative device enables individuals who have communication, cognitive, and/or physical needs to communicate and develop their speech.
Communication tools	• Social stories can enable individuals to understand how to carry out an activity or task. For example, an individual who wants to be more independent and learn how to bake a cake may find it helpful to first watch a short video or film of someone else baking a cake. In this way they can understand the different steps the activity involves and how to do it. • Photographs and pictures of people and places can enable individuals who have difficulties interacting with others, due to for example being on the autistic spectrum, to identify people they want to get in touch with and places they want to go to. These photographs and pictures can also be stored on an individual's phone and so can be used by the individual when out. • Smart watches can enable individuals to use their voice to carry out tasks independently. For example, individuals can make hands free phone calls, make spoken instead of written notes, i.e. when making a shopping list, surf the internet by using speech rather than the written word to ask questions and find out information.
Digital technology	• Telehealth equipment can enable individuals who live at home to be more independent in managing their health conditions. For example, if an individual has high blood pressure they can use a monitor that checks their blood pressure at home and then sends the results automatically to their GP who can then check these. • Telecare devices can enable individuals to stay living at home independently and safely; they detect when there is a problem and then send alerts so assistance can be arranged. For example, a fall detector is built into a pendant worn around the neck or wrist and can detect when an individual has had a fall and will automatically call the response team. • E-books can enable individuals to access a wide range of reading materials from a portable device such as their tablet without having to depend on others. The font size and style can also be amended on e-books to suit individuals' specific needs.

Key terms

Alternative and augmentative technologies (AAC) refer to technologies, systems and devices that individuals can use to substitute or supplement everyday speech so that they can express themselves and communicate with others.

Radio frequency identification technology (RFID) uses radio waves to identify and track tags or labels that are attached to objects.

Reflect on it

3.3 Technology that supports independence

Reflect on the case study you explored for ACs 3.1 and 3.2 in relation to Amandeep the community carer providing support to Therese. What range of technologies are there that can support or maintain Therese's independence with her mobility?

> **Evidence opportunity**
>
> **3.3 Technology that supports independence**
>
> Research a range of technologies that can support or maintain an individual's independence. Produce a poster with your findings.

Legislation	
Relevant Act	**Key points**
Data Protection Act 2018	Personal information must be recorded, used, stored and shared according to a set of principles or rules to ensure the individuals' rights are protected and the security of their personal information is maintained.
The Human Rights Act 1998	Everyone in the UK is entitled to the same rights and freedoms. This includes individuals who have care and support needs. The Act supports individuals to have the right to take risks and to have their choices and decisions respected.
The Management of Health and Safety at Work Regulations 1999	It is a legal requirement for risks in work settings including care settings to be managed safely and that risk assessments are carried out, documented, reviewed and updated.
The Mental Capacity Act 2005	This Act supports person-centred working by supporting individuals' rights to make their own decisions, including being provided with the necessary support to do so. It also protects the rights of individuals who lack capacity by providing guidance on who can make decisions about them and how to plan ahead for this in case it arises in the future.
The Care Act 2014	This Act supports individuals' rights to make informed decisions about their care and support and promotes a person-centred approach to care planning where adult care workers can support individuals to develop their care plans. It also defines the concept of wellbeing and outlines how adult care workers can promote individuals' wellbeing. Also see the Government publications: ● *Personalised Health and Care 2020*, which sets out how technology and data can be used to improve health and the way health and social care services are delivered. ● *The Adult Social Care Outcomes Framework Handbook of Definitions*, which measures how well care and support services achieve the outcomes that are the most important to people.
The Health and Social Care Act 2008 (Regulated Activities) Regulations 2014	This Act supports the rights of individuals and their representatives to be involved in the planning, provision and review of their care and support. It would be useful for you to research the various Regulations, including 11 which covers consent.

308 Supporting individuals with their health and wellbeing

About this unit

Credit value: 3
Guided learning hours: 22

Supporting individuals with their health and wellbeing involves considering their health, happiness and comfort and is very important as this will have a direct impact on the quality of their lives.

In this unit you will learn about the importance of an individual's wellbeing, the factors that can impact their wellbeing as well as the range of services and resources available to support an individual. You will also learn how to monitor, assess and respond to any changes in individuals' physical and mental health as well as involve individuals in monitoring their own health and wellbeing.

Finally, you will learn about different person-centred ways of working with individuals and others to promote and improve individuals' health and wellbeing.

Learning outcomes

By the end of this unit you will:

LO1: Understand the importance of an individual's wellbeing

LO2: Know how to monitor individuals' health

LO3: Be able to assess and respond to changes in an individual's health and wellbeing

LO4: Be able to promote individuals' health and wellbeing

LO1 Understand the importance of an individual's wellbeing

> **Getting started**
>
> How would you describe yourself? What are your 'positives'? For example, your personality, kind nature or sense of humour? How would others describe you? What do they say are your positives? Do you agree with what others say about you? Why? How can what others say about you impact on how good you feel about yourself? Can you think of an example when this happened?
>
> As well as what others say about you, what other things affect how you feel about yourself? For example, how can your physical health affect how you feel emotionally? How can your emotional health affect your physical health? For example, if you feel unwell does this make you feel more positive or negative? Why?

AC 1.1 Evaluate how identity, self-image and self-esteem can impact on an individual's wellbeing

There are three aspects that make up who you are: your identity, self-image and self-esteem.

Identity

Your individual identity is personal to you and includes the different aspects that make you unique – your background, your values, your personality, your qualities, your wishes, your views. We build up our own personal identity through our experiences in life, through both childhood and adulthood. The types of experiences we have will affect what we think about ourselves. For example, if an individual as a child experienced making friends at school as something enjoyable, this will in turn mean that they will feel good about themselves when meeting new people and making new friends. Making new friends will mean that an individual will have others to share their lives and experiences with; this will make them feel more confident about themselves and means they will have a positive view about themselves and therefore experience wellbeing: that they are liked by others, that they are needed by others and are part of others' lives. Friends, relatives and partners reflect back to us who we are and it is through others that we develop high self-esteem and wellbeing.

Self-image

Your self-image is how you see yourself. This will depend on how you value yourself – whether you see yourself positively or negatively. For example, if an individual has experienced abuse and harm then they may see themselves negatively because this may have made them feel worthless and they may even feel that they are to blame for what happened to them. If an individual has a negative self-image of themselves then this can impact on their wellbeing because they may feel, for example, depressed, and their mental ill health can in turn result in the individual becoming withdrawn and not engaging with others.

If, however, an individual has a supportive network of friends, family and carers around them then they may see themselves positively because this may have made them feel supported and encouraged to be independent and make their own choices and decisions. If an individual has a positive self-image then this can impact on their wellbeing because they will feel empowered to live their life how they want to and therefore experience a good quality of life.

> **Research it**
>
> **1.1 Care Act 2014**
>
> Research what the Care Act 2014 says about what is understood by 'wellbeing' in relation to adult social care. You may find the link below useful:
>
> www.scie.org.uk/care-act-2014/assessment-and-eligibility/determination-eligibility
>
> Now write down your own definition of wellbeing.

Self-esteem

Your self-esteem is what you think and feel about yourself. This will very much depend on how you value yourself as well as how others close to you think and feel about you. When others hold individuals in high regard and praise them, it is likely that they will feel the same about themselves too. When others devalue individuals, however, they are not likely to feel very positive about themselves or their abilities.

Your identity, self-image and self-esteem are all interrelated and one can affect the others:

- A strong sense of identity (who you are) can promote a high self-esteem (how you feel about yourself) and a high self-esteem can make you value yourself and feel good about who you are and therefore enhance a positive view of yourself (self-image).
- Not knowing or being unsure about your own identity (who you are) can lead to low self-esteem (how you feel about yourself) which can in turn make you feel unworthy and have a negative view of yourself (self-image).

It is important therefore when supporting individuals with their health and wellbeing that you remember how identity, self-image and self-esteem can impact on an individual's health, happiness and comfort.

Reflect on it

1.1 Self-esteem

Reflect on an occasion when someone praised you for something you had done well. How did this make you feel about yourself? How did this make you feel towards this person? Now reflect on an occasion when someone devalued you. How did this make you feel about yourself? How did this make you feel towards others?

Evidence opportunity

1.1 Identity, self-image and self-esteem

Think about an individual that you support in the care setting/service where you work. Think about their background, culture and beliefs, what they look like, what their personality is, and their likes and dislikes.

Then discuss with your assessor how this individual's identity, self-image and self-esteem impact on their wellbeing.

AC 1.2 Identify the factors that positively and negatively influence an individual's wellbeing

Wellbeing refers to a person's quality of life and considers health, happiness and comfort. It is important to remember that the factors affecting wellbeing will be different for different people.

Table 9.2 provides information about the different factors that can positively and negatively influence an individual's wellbeing.

Table 9.2 How factors can positively and negatively influence the wellbeing of individuals

Wellbeing aspect	Factors that can positively and negatively influence individuals' wellbeing
Physical health	Good physical health means that individuals can live their lives comfortably and free from pain and distress, which will contribute to their wellbeing. Poor physical health will impact negatively on an individual because they may not be able to do the activities they want to do as they may be in pain or distress.
Mental health	Good mental health means that individuals will feel positively towards themselves and others thus enhancing positive feelings of self-worth and therefore of wellbeing. Mental ill health can result in individuals not being able to manage with daily activities and feeling unworthy and helpless. Relationships can support individuals to maintain their mental health by having people that they can trust, confide in and talk to about any anxieties or worries they have.
Emotional health	Good emotional health means that individuals will have a positive outlook on life and will feel good about their life, themselves and others. Poor emotional health can result in individuals feeling that the world around them is a frightening place, somewhere where they are not welcomed and will not be able to live in. This might be because of psychological illness or issues that have affected them in everyday life that have caused them stress.

Table 9.2 How factors can positively and negatively influence the wellbeing of individuals *continued*

Wellbeing aspect	Factors that can positively and negatively influence individuals' wellbeing
Social health	Good social health means that individuals have positive relationships with others which means that others will reflect back to them positive feelings and images of themselves. Poor social health may result in individuals having destructive or unhelpful relationships with others that may in turn lead to their isolation and withdrawal from daily activities.
Cultural health	Good cultural health means that individuals have a sense of belonging to a group of people who share the same or similar beliefs and values to them, which in turn creates a sense of contentment and happiness. Poor cultural health may mean that individuals feel excluded from society, that no one understands them; this may make them feel isolated and unworthy.
Spiritual health	Good spiritual health means that individuals have a sense of a human spirit that makes them feel that they have a purpose and a reason to live. Poor spiritual health may mean that individuals are frightened of the world around them or may not be able to understand themselves and others. You can support individuals to maintain good spiritual health by supporting them to reflect on who they are and supporting spiritual or religious practices they may follow (or may like to follow) such as prayer or meditation.
Intellectual health	Good intellectual health means that individuals have rational, logical and clear thought processes that enhance their wellbeing. Poor intellectual health may mean that an individual's thought processes become disrupted and they may become more dependent on others, thus losing their own resilience and sense of fulfilment.
Economic health	Good economic health results when individuals' finances, including their housing situation, are satisfactory for them to be content. Poor economic health may result in individuals not being able to meet their day-to-day needs because they have insufficient income or poor housing that is, for example, damp or not heated.

> **Evidence opportunity**
>
> **1.2 Factors that influence an individual's wellbeing**
>
> Using the same individual from Evidence opportunity activity AC 1.1, make a list of the factors that influenced their wellbeing both positively and negatively.

AC 1.3 Describe the range of services and resources available to support an individual's wellbeing

There are a wide range of services and resources available from both within the care setting/service where you work and externally through other organisations that can support an individual's wellbeing, strengths and needs. Individuals' strengths and needs vary and therefore it is not uncommon for individuals to access different types of services and resources which may be provided through more than one type of provision or combination, i.e. internal and external to the care setting/service you work in. To ensure individuals' strengths and needs are responded to fully and quickly the range of professionals that work within these services work together as one team to provide the best possible outcomes for individuals.

Services and resources available in the care setting/service where you work:

- **You and the team you work within** – you, your colleagues and manager/supervisor are equipped with the necessary knowledge and skills to support the individuals you care for and their health and wellbeing. As well as monitoring individuals' health and wellbeing and responding to any changes that may occur (an area you will explore in more detail in LOs 2, 3 and 4 of this Unit) you and the team will also be empowering individuals to make their own choices and decisions about their own health and wellbeing.

- **Individuals' family, friends and others involved** – an individual's family, friends and others involved in their lives will know them well and are a good source of support, understanding and encouragement for individuals when they are monitoring their own health and wellbeing and are more likely to recognise the early indicators of physical and/or mental health deterioration (a topic you will explore in more detail in LO2 of this unit).
- **Peer support** – other individuals who live in/access the care setting/service where the individual lives can also be a source of support for individuals when promoting their health and wellbeing by sharing ideas and discussing difficulties and how to overcome them. This may take place informally on a one-to-one basis or formally in pairs or groups.
- **Information and guidance** – information and guidance on the promotion of health and wellbeing for individuals may also come in the form of leaflets, information handouts, blogs or videos available within the care setting/service, and this can also be made available to individuals in a format that they understand and that meets their communication needs and preferences. (You will find Unit 304 Effective communication in adult care settings/services a useful source of information).

> **Reflect on it**
>
> **1.3 Support for wellbeing**
>
> Imagine a new team member has been recruited and they ask you about what support is in place in the care setting/service where you work to support individuals' wellbeing. What would you say to them? Do you know what's available? If not, how could you find out?

Services and resources available externally

Statutory sector services and resources consist of organisations and services that are managed and led by the government. The following are some examples of these:

- **The National Health Service (NHS).** The NHS provides healthcare services and support to individuals in a variety of settings based in hospitals and in the community. For example, GP-led health centres, pharmacists and dentists can provide treatment to individuals when they are unwell. Individuals may also need to access further treatment and may be referred to other services such as mental health services or may need to access specialised healthcare and treatment from for example physiotherapy departments, occupational therapy services, pain management and rehabilitation clinics.
- **Social services** are provided by local authorities or councils and are funded through the government. For example, individuals may access support from domiciliary care services that provide care and practical support to individuals at home, or through community-based services such as day care centres where individuals can access information, meet with others and participate in activities.
- **Mental health services** are provided by mental health trusts that provide specialist health, treatment, care and support to individuals with mental health needs. This can include one-to-one or group counselling for individuals experiencing mental ill-health, information and training on how individuals can manage their mental health when they've experienced anxiety, anger or bereavement, or psychological therapy for individuals who are experiencing serious mental illness.

Private sector services and resources consist of organisations and services that are not managed by the government and are run to make a profit. Below are some examples of these:

- **Private residential/nursing care** provides different types of care and support to individuals depending on their needs. For example, sheltered housing is aimed at individuals who would like to live independently but with some support; support is usually provided through a 24-hour emergency alarm system by a warden or housing manager. Care homes offer specialist care to individuals who require extra care and support such as individuals who have dementia; support is provided through staff trained in dementia care and qualified nurses.
- **Private hospitals** provide healthcare to individuals, and services are funded by individuals themselves or through medical insurance policies. For example, the private healthcare company BUPA (British United Provident Association) has its own private hospitals and provides residential, nursing and specialist care to individuals who have dementia.

Third sector services and resources consist of organisations and services that are not for profit and are independent of the government and can include charities, community groups and self-help groups.

Table 9.3 gives some examples of third-sector organisations that are registered charities and offer a range of support and resources to individuals.

Table 9.3 Examples of third sector organisations that are registered charities and offer a range of support and resources to individuals

Third sector organisation	How it supports individuals' wellbeing
Mind	• Provides information, advice and support to individuals who are experiencing mental health problems. • Offers information and support through Infoline, a telephone helpline where you can discuss and find out about mental health problems, treatment options, advocacy services. • Offers an online community, Side by Side, where individuals can give and receive support to/from others who are also experiencing or have experienced mental health problems.
The Advocacy People	• Provides information, advice and support to empower individuals to speak up, put their views across, be heard and taken seriously. • Offers different types of advocacy: e.g. mental health advocacy, to support individuals who have been sectioned and are in hospital; care and support; advocacy, to support individuals to be involved and have a say in how they are cared for and supported; advocacy for individuals who lack capacity, to support individuals who have been assessed as lacking capacity to make decisions. • Offers self-advocacy groups where individuals can speak up for themselves and what's important to them, meet with others, make friends and keep up to date with local and national issues that may affect them and their rights.
Beat	• Provides information, advice and support to individuals with eating disorders such as **bulimia nervosa, binge eating disorder, avoidant/restrictive food intake disorder (ARFID)** and **anorexia nervosa**. • Provides a national helpline that people can contact directly either online or by phone to help individuals to understand their illness and take steps towards recovery including getting the help they need. • Provides support and advice to individuals' family and friends so that they develop the skills and knowledge to support their relatives towards recovery while at the same time look after their own health and wellbeing.

> **Key terms**
>
> **Bulimia nervosa** refers to an eating disorder that involved singeing then 'compensation' behaviours for that bingeing.
>
> **Binge eating disorder** refers to an eating disorder where people consume large quantities of food over a short time (referred to as binge eating) but unlike bulimia nervosa they do not try and get rid of it.
>
> **Avoidant/restrictive food intake disorder (ARFID)** refers to an eating disorder where people avoid certain foods or types of foods, restrict the overall amount of food they eat, or both.
>
> **Anorexia nervosa** refers to an eating disorder where people are of a low weight because they limit how much they eat and drink.

> **Evidence opportunity**
>
> **1.3 Services and resources**
>
> Conduct some research into the services and resources available in the care setting/service where you work and in the local area. Develop an information handout about three services/resources that are available to individuals in your care setting/service and three services/resources that are available in the local area. Provide details of the support that they provide including how they can support individuals' wellbeing.

AC 1.4 Describe how to access a range of services and resources

Now that you have learned about the many different services and resources that are available to support individuals' wellbeing, you will also need to know about how these services and resources can be accessed so that you can support individuals to access them.

- Individuals can refer themselves, a process more commonly referred to as self-referral. For example, an individual who lives in a care home and has recently experienced the loss of a close relative may refer themselves to the bereavement support group that is held every Friday at the care home. How they do this will depend on the service they access, i.e. they may have to complete a self-referral online form that asks them for some details about themselves or they may be able to go in person and visit the group. Services that accept self-referrals will have in place a process to follow that is usually available directly from the service either through their website or by telephoning them directly.
- Individuals may require a referral from a professional to access a service. Professionals can also make referrals on individuals' behalf to other services or professionals that they think the individual can benefit from. For example, an individual who has lost their job may visit their GP because they are feeling depressed about their situation and anxious about how they are going to manage financially. The individual's GP may refer them to a mental health professional for emotional support and give them some leaflets on charities/groups available in the local area that can offer information, advice and practical help with managing finances, including finding out about benefits and/or grants that could be claimed and other resources such as using a **local foodbank** or a **community fridge**.
- Individuals may be referred to a service by someone else who knows them but is not a professional, such as a close relative or friend, when the individual is unable to do so themselves; a process more commonly known as a third-party referral. For example, an individual who is caring for their parent who has dementia at home may refer their parent to a specialist Admiral Nurse for further support and advice on managing their **continence care** and **incontinence products** that are available.

>
>
> **Key terms**
>
> **Local foodbanks** provide essential items free of charge to people who are struggling financially to afford these. Items can include food items as well as cleaning materials and toiletries. Items provided are usually donated by members of the public and local businesses.
>
> **Community fridges** are run by community groups in schools, community centres and shops and their main aim is to save fresh food from going to waste. Individuals who live and work locally can access these to meet others and eat together while learning new skills. Food includes surplus from supermarkets, local food businesses, producers, households and gardens.
>
> **Continence care** refers to caring for an individual who unintentionally passes urine (urinary continence) or faeces (faecal incontinence) or both. This may be due to a physical health condition or to an illness such as dementia.
>
> **Incontinence products** refer to products that help people manage incontinence such as incontinence pads, waterproof sheets for beds or absorbent mats for chairs.

>
>
> **Reflect on it**
>
> **1.4 Local services and resources**
>
> Reflect on a local service or resource available in your local area that you've accessed. How did you find out about it? How did you access it?

> **Evidence opportunity**
>
> **1.4 Access to services and resources**
>
> Think about the services and resources that may support different individuals' wellbeing that are available both within and outside of the care setting where you work. Develop a leaflet for the individuals you work with in your care setting about how to access a range of different services and resources. Ensure the information you provide is clear and can be easily understood.

AC 1.5 Identify possible barriers to accessing services and resources available to support an individual's wellbeing

AC 1.6 Evaluate how potential barriers for an individual to access services and resources could be overcome

There are a range of possible barriers that can prevent individuals from accessing the services and resources available to support their wellbeing. It is important to know what these barriers are so that you can provide individuals with the necessary support and information to overcome them. You may find that individuals face one or more of these barriers; providing them with timely and sensitive support and advice will mean that you are doing everything you can to support their wellbeing. Table 9.4 describes some of the barriers that individuals may encounter, and gives some suggestions for how they could be overcome.

Table 9.4 Barriers to accessing services and resources to support an individual's wellbeing and how they could be overcome

Potential barriers to accessing services and resources	Suggestions for how to overcome these barriers
Financial costs of services and resources may exclude individuals who are not able to afford them.	• Support individuals to look for alternative services and resources that may be available locally and free of charge, such as those from charities and local community groups. • Support individuals to review their finances to see if there are better ways of budgeting, or benefits/grants that they may be entitled to.
The geographical location of services and resources may exclude individuals who cannot afford the costs of travelling there or cannot arrange support from a relative who may have other work or family commitments.	• Support individuals to review their finances to see if there are benefits/grants available to help them travel to services and resources. • Support individuals to access advocacy services and find an advocate who may be able to support them to access these services or resources.
The times when services and resources are available may prevent some individuals from accessing them, e.g. some may only be provided during hours of business (9–5) and on weekdays, others on specific days and evenings, others at weekends.	• Support individuals to consider being more flexible and open to accessing services/resources at different times. This might also involve rescheduling other arrangements they have. • Support individuals to put forward their ideas for how their care and support could be provided more flexibly, i.e. on different days/times.
The physical access to services and resources, such as a lack of lifts, wide doorways or adapted facilities, can exclude individuals who have difficulties mobilising or use a wheelchair.	• Support individuals to raise these access issues with the person/organisation providing the service. This can be done through you or someone else who knows the individual well, or through an advocate. • Support the individual to put forward their suggestions for how the access issues could be improved, e.g. could the service be provided in another part of the building? Could a temporary ramp be used? Could an accessible pop-up kitchen be installed?

Table 9.4 Barriers to accessing services and resources to support an individual's wellbeing and how they could be overcome *continued*

Potential barriers to accessing services and resources	Suggestions for how to overcome these barriers
Cultural barriers may prevent individuals from accessing services and resources, e.g. lack of awareness of cultural beliefs with respect to how care or treatments are to be provided can prevent individuals from accessing services and resources.	• Ensure you know what individuals' cultural beliefs and/or preferences are and that you support individuals to communicate these to those providing the services they accessing, e.g. for a female carer to provide personal care to an elderly Muslim woman, or for a hospital consultant to liaise with an individual's family when discussing treatment options for an illness. • Support individuals to provide/get involved in education, training and information about raising awareness of cultural beliefs/preferences. This could be directly to organisations or through local self-advocacy groups.
Communication barriers may prevent individuals from accessing services and resources, e.g. lack of information available in a format the individual understands, or a lack of professionals who can communicate with the individual.	• Ensure individuals have access to information about services and resources in a format that they understand, e.g. in their language, in Braille (for individuals who have visual impairments), in jargon-free language, in a room with a hearing loop system (for individuals who have hearing impairments). • Ensure professionals know how to access interpreting and translation services and how to work with interpreters and translators.
Psychological barriers may also make it more difficult for individuals to access services and resources, e.g. an individual with a mental illness may not recognise that they are unwell, or an individual who lives at home on their own may fear having to go into a care home if they tell a professional that they require more support to live at home.	• Reassure individuals that you are there to support them and promote their wellbeing and that they can trust you; this includes explaining clearly to them, in a way that they understand, why they would benefit from the service/resource and how you can support them to access it. • Ensure you make individuals aware of their rights to access the support/service they require, as well as to change their minds and stop doing so if this is what they want.

Evidence opportunity

1.5, 1.6 Barriers to services and resources

Reflect on the different barriers that may prevent an individual from accessing a range of services and resources as well as the different ways that these could be overcome. Develop a case study of an individual who has care and support needs, and include details of the services and resources they want to access and the potential barriers they may face in doing so. Describe how the individual could overcome these barriers.

AC 1.7 Explain how an individual's wellbeing may affect their behaviours and relationships

Earlier on in this unit, in AC1.2, you considered the different factors that can positively and negatively influence an individual's wellbeing; you may find it useful to review your previous learning for AC1.2. Similarly, an individual's wellbeing can also influence or impact on their behaviours and relationships. When we refer to an individual's behaviours, we mean the way that they act or behave, including towards others, and when we refer to an individual's relationships, this includes both personal and working relationships that the individual has with other people.

Reflect on it

1.7 An individual's wellbeing

Reflect on an individual you provide care and support to. From your experience and knowledge of the individual, make a list of the aspects of their wellbeing that are poor and those that are good. Now ask a colleague who also works with this same individual to do the same. Compare and discuss your lists. What were the similarities and differences? Why?

Let's consider how different aspects of wellbeing may affect an individual's behaviours and relationships. It's important to remember that each of these aspects do not occur in isolation from the others; individuals may experience one or more of these at the same time.

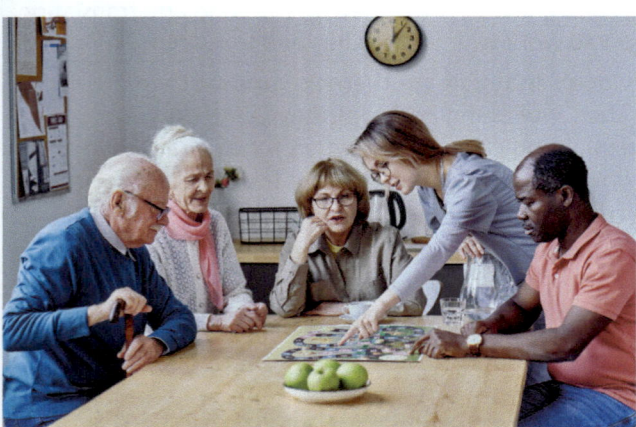

Figure 9.1 Do you know how to improve an individual's social wellbeing?

- **Social wellbeing**: an individual's social wellbeing might be poor if they are isolated from others who they care about and who know them well, such as their family and friends. In this case, the individual will be more likely to withdraw from opportunities to meet with others and maintain the relationships they have in their lives – they may not have the self-confidence to do so, or may not believe that others want them to.
An individual's social wellbeing will be good if they have access to a range of different professionals and services where they meet new people and meet up with their friends and family. They will feel positive and confident about themselves and are therefore more likely to feel confident about trying different services. They will view meeting new people as exciting, enjoyable and an opportunity to learn about others and perhaps develop new relationships.

- **Emotional wellbeing**: an individual's emotional wellbeing may be poor if they have experienced a stressful event in their life, such as being bereaved of a close relative or being diagnosed with a life-threatening condition. They may feel low in themselves and anxious about how they are going to manage. They may therefore find it difficult to act positively when around others, and may be less likely to maintain the relationships they have or build new ones. An individual's emotional wellbeing will be better if they are supported to manage the bereavement they've experienced or the life-threatening condition they've been diagnosed with, by accessing support from professionals such as counsellors and from a support group. They are more likely to feel that they are coping well with events that they have no control over, and will feel more in control of their life. This in turn will mean that they will reflect how they feel when they interact with others, such as their friends or family, and therefore opportunities to develop relationships will increase, because other people are more likely to want to contact them and engage with them.

- **Cultural wellbeing**: an individual's cultural wellbeing might be poor if, for example, they are living in a shared house with people they do not have much in common with and do not share similar beliefs with. The individual will not have a sense of belonging and may feel unsettled and isolated from other people. An individual's cultural wellbeing will be good if they are being supported by professionals who show a genuine interest in who they are, their background, history, beliefs and values and take their unique needs into account. The individual will feel content, proud and secure about who they are, and will be more likely to share their culture with others and in doing so develop different relationships in which they can also learn about others' cultures.

- **Spiritual wellbeing**: an individual's spiritual wellbeing is poor if they do not know who they are or they feel that they no longer have a purpose in life because of, for example, losing capacity or independent skills as a result of an illness. They may find it difficult to engage with others if they doubt their ability to do so and whether others want to engage with them.

An individual's spiritual health will be good if the care and support provided to them reflect their unique strengths and needs and what they want to do, as well as their aspirations for the future. The individual will gain a greater insight into themselves, their strengths and abilities; they are more likely to welcome others getting to know them for who they really are. You could also promote an individual's spiritual health by supporting them to follow spiritual practices such as meditation or prayers, to help them gain a greater insight into their true selves and be able to connect with others around them.

- **Intellectual wellbeing**: an individual's intellectual wellbeing will be poor if, rather than being supported to do things for themselves, they are having things done for them. The individual will become more dependent on others and may feel that they cannot manage on their own. They could lose their sense of hope and achievement, and this will be reflected in what they think about themselves and how they relate to others.

  An individual's intellectual wellbeing will be good if family, friends and professionals providing care and support ensure that they maintain the individual's skills by encouraging them to participate in tasks that they can do, and encouraging them to do as much as possible for themselves when they find it difficult to do so. The individual will view themselves more positively and their behaviours towards others will reflect this, as will their relationships, because these will be highlighting their strengths and abilities rather than focusing on their weaknesses and difficulties.

- **Economic wellbeing**: an individual's economic wellbeing will be poor if, for example, due to their physical health deteriorating they do not have access to sufficient resources to meet their needs and live the life that they want. They may feel fearful about what the future holds and very anxious about how they are going to manage on a day-to-day basis. This stress can impact negatively on them, and they may feel frustrated or even angry; their behaviours towards others may also be full of anger and frustration, making it more difficult for others to want to approach the individual or think about maintaining a relationship with them.

  An individual's economic wellbeing will be good if they have been able to access the resources they require to live a happy and comfortable life, including creative ways for improving their current situation. The individual will have further developed their resilience, which will in turn increase their self-belief and make them more likely to act in ways that will mean that others can engage with them and offer additional support, suggestions and advice.

- **Physical wellbeing**: an individual's physical wellbeing might be poor if, for example, they are in pain on a daily basis as a result of an accident. They are less likely to want to meet or interact with other people because they may feel that they do not want to be a burden to others or appear negative about their life.

  An individual's physical wellbeing will be better if the pain they are experiencing is being carefully managed through the services of a pain management clinic; that includes the provision of physical support (pain medication) as well as emotional support (pain management techniques with a psychologist). The individual may get temporary relief from their pain and develop techniques that can help them manage it better, and they will be more likely to have a positive outlook on their life, their relationships with others and their future.

- **Mental wellbeing:** if an individual's mental wellbeing is poor because they are experiencing a mental illness, they may find it difficult to communicate how they are feeling and be less able to interact with others.

  If an individual's mental wellbeing is better because they are accessing counselling services, then the individual will feel that they have the skills to manage their mental wellbeing. They will gain a greater insight into the impact of their mental wellbeing on their behaviours and relationships, and they will be more likely to engage in positive behaviours that are more conducive to maintaining and developing relationships with others.

The case study below gives you the opportunity to think about how an individual's wellbeing can affect their behaviours and relationships.

Case study

1.7 Wellbeing and its impact

Adele is 71 years of age and lives with her partner at home; Adele has seven grandchildren, a sister and several close friends who live nearby. Adele has pancreatic cancer and has also recently been diagnosed with dementia. Over the last few months, Adele has been feeling sick more often, particularly after eating, and has also been feeling very tired. Adele's partner has been trying to get the local GP to visit Adele at home to see if anything else can be done to make her more comfortable, but this is proving difficult as, due to sickness and leave, there is only one GP working at the local surgery.

At the same time, Adele has been waiting for a referral from her GP to come through so that she can access support from a dementia nurse to help her manage her physical and mental wellbeing better, as she is feeling very low in herself and is fearful of how she is going to manage. Adele's partner has noticed that Adele's family and close friends are visiting less often as her cancer and dementia progress, because they are finding it too upsetting to see her deteriorate and not always recognise who they are, and is worried that they will soon stop visiting.

Discuss:

1. What is affecting Adele's wellbeing?
2. How is Adele's wellbeing affecting her behaviours? Why?
3. How is Adele's wellbeing affecting her relationships? Why?
4. How is Adele's wellbeing affecting Adele's partner? Why?
5. What could be done to improve Adele's wellbeing? What would be the impact of doing so on her behaviours and relationships with her family and friends?

Evidence opportunity

1.7 Wellbeing, behaviours and relationships

Discuss with a colleague or your assessor how an individual's wellbeing may affect their behaviours and relationships with themselves and others. Provide examples of the effects of the individual's wellbeing, as well as how and why they can influence their behaviours and relationships.

6Cs

Care

Supporting an individual's wellbeing is essential for providing high quality care and for ensuring you fully meet an individual's needs, as not doing so could impact negatively not only on them but also on the way they interact with others.

Commitment

You can show your commitment to individuals by supporting them to access a range of services and resources that are available to them. Spending time finding out about the services and resources available and ensuring that they meet individuals' needs will mean that individuals will be more likely to want to use them, which will in turn help to improve their wellbeing.

LO2 Know how to monitor individuals' health

Getting started

Think about the individuals you provide care and support to in the care setting where you work. How do they monitor their own health and wellbeing? Do some of them require support to do so? Have you experienced an individual's physical or mental health deteriorating? What happened?

AC 2.1 Describe ways to engage individuals in monitoring their own health and wellbeing

Engaging individuals in monitoring their own health and wellbeing will involve you supporting and empowering them to make informed decisions to minimise the risk of ill health and ill-being. Below are some of the different ways you can do this; remember every individual is unique and so what suits one individual may not suit another.

Raise individuals' awareness of the importance of their own health and wellbeing by discussing this with them. For example, this could involve having a structured one-to-one discussion with the individual about one or more aspects of their health and wellbeing, such as the benefits of eating a balanced diet with more fruit and vegetables and fewer foods that contain sugar and saturated fats. You could ensure that the basis of your discussion is supported with factual information such as that included in the NHS Eatwell Guide, which states that to have good health and wellbeing people should try to:

- eat at least five portions of a variety of fruit and vegetables every day
- base meals on higher fibre starchy foods such as potatoes, rice, pasta or bread
- include some dairy or dairy alternatives such as soya drinks
- eat beans, pulses, fish, meat, eggs and other protein
- eat small amounts of unsaturated oils and spreads
- drink plenty of fluids (at least 6 to 8 glasses, ideally of water, a day).

Support individuals to access a range of services and resources to monitor their own health and wellbeing. For example, you could support an individual to attend their free NHS Health Check at their local GP surgery by explaining to them what this involves, ensuring that you provide them with all the necessary information so that they can make their own informed decision:

- It will take between 20 and 30 minutes.
- It will be conducted by a nurse, doctor, pharmacist or healthcare assistant.
- You will be asked questions about whether you have any close relatives who have had the illnesses they are checking for.
- You will be asked questions about your lifestyle, including how much you smoke, drink alcohol and do physical activity.
- Your weight and height will be measured to check that you are a healthy weight for your height.
- Your blood pressure will be taken.
- You will have a blood test done either before or after the Health Check.
- You may also have blood taken from your finger during the appointment to check your cholesterol level and in some cases your blood sugar level too.
- You will be given the results during the appointment: you will be given a cardiovascular disease risk score, which describes the likelihood of you getting heart disease or having a stroke within the next ten years, as well as your risk of developing kidney disease and diabetes.
- Depending on your risk score, you will be given advice on how to make lifestyle changes to reduce the risk of developing these illnesses, for example losing weight or stopping smoking. You may be referred as a result to local services to help with these lifestyle changes, such as stop smoking and physical activity services.
- If you are 65 years of age and over, you will be told the signs and symptoms of dementia to look out for.
- Depending on your results, you may be asked to come back for further tests such as to check for diabetes or high blood pressure.
- Your NHS Health Check results will be recorded in your confidential medical records, which can be accessed by your GP and other healthcare professionals who may need to access them. You will also be given access to a copy of your records.

Support individuals to participate in health and wellbeing support or self-help groups. For example, you could encourage an individual who is experiencing mental health issues to monitor and be in control of their own mental health by finding out the mental health support groups that are available in the local area. You could tell the individual about the type of support the groups provide, so that they can make their own informed decision about whether they would like to try to participate in one of these. You could explain to the individual why a mental health support or self-help group may help them:

- to meet up with others who are also living with mental health issues, where you can share openly how you feel, your thoughts and emotions
- to have somewhere safe where others will understand you and not judge you for your mental health issues
- to share ideas for how to manage your mental health better
- to learn new coping skills for how to manage your mental health better.

Provide individuals with information or signpost them to resources in monitoring their health and wellbeing. For example, if an individual in your care setting approaches you to say that they have been diagnosed with Alzheimer's and that they would like to find out more about this condition, you could:

- talk them through the information and/or resources available within your care setting, e.g. there may be staff who have specialist skills in working with individuals with Alzheimer's that they could speak to, or there may be social groups or activities that they could participate in that others with Alzheimer's also attend.
- talk them through the information and/or resources available outside of your care setting. For example, the Alzheimer's Society provides factsheets on a wide range of topics such as key facts and aspects about dementia, emotional and practical guidance, an online community, and other practical dementia support services such as dementia cafes where people can speak to others going through similar experiences. Dementia support workers can help individuals to understand more about their condition, the help and support available to them and how to access it.

Enable individuals to monitor their own health and wellbeing by referring them to another professional or service. For example, if an individual in your care setting tells you that they would like to stop smoking, you could refer them to:

- their GP
- their pharmacist
- their local stop smoking service.

The individual could then access a range of support and resources to give up smoking through, for example, one-to-one sessions with a smoking advisor, group sessions, drop-in sessions, and stop smoking aids such as nicotine replacement patches, gum, tablets, mouth or nasal spray.

You may also find it useful to review your previous learning in AC1.3 of this unit, where you learned about the range of services and resources available to support an individual's wellbeing.

Evidence opportunity

2.1 Engaging individuals to monitor their own health and wellbeing

Develop a case study of an individual who has care and support needs. Write an account that describes the different methods that you could use to engage them in monitoring their own health and wellbeing. What skills do you think you need to do this successfully? Remember to take into account the individual's strengths, abilities, preferences and needs.

AC 2.2 Identify the early indicators of physical health deterioration

AC 2.3 Identify the early indicators of mental health deterioration

Monitoring individuals' health also involves recognising the early indicators of physical health and mental health deterioration, also referred to as 'soft signs' of deterioration; this involves you observing individuals and responding to any changes that you notice. Doing so means that you will be playing an active role in preventing individuals' health and wellbeing worsening, and enabling individuals to access the treatments and support they require in a timely manner. The two diagrams in figure 9.2 include some of the main early indicators of physical and mental health deterioration to look out for; have you come across any others?

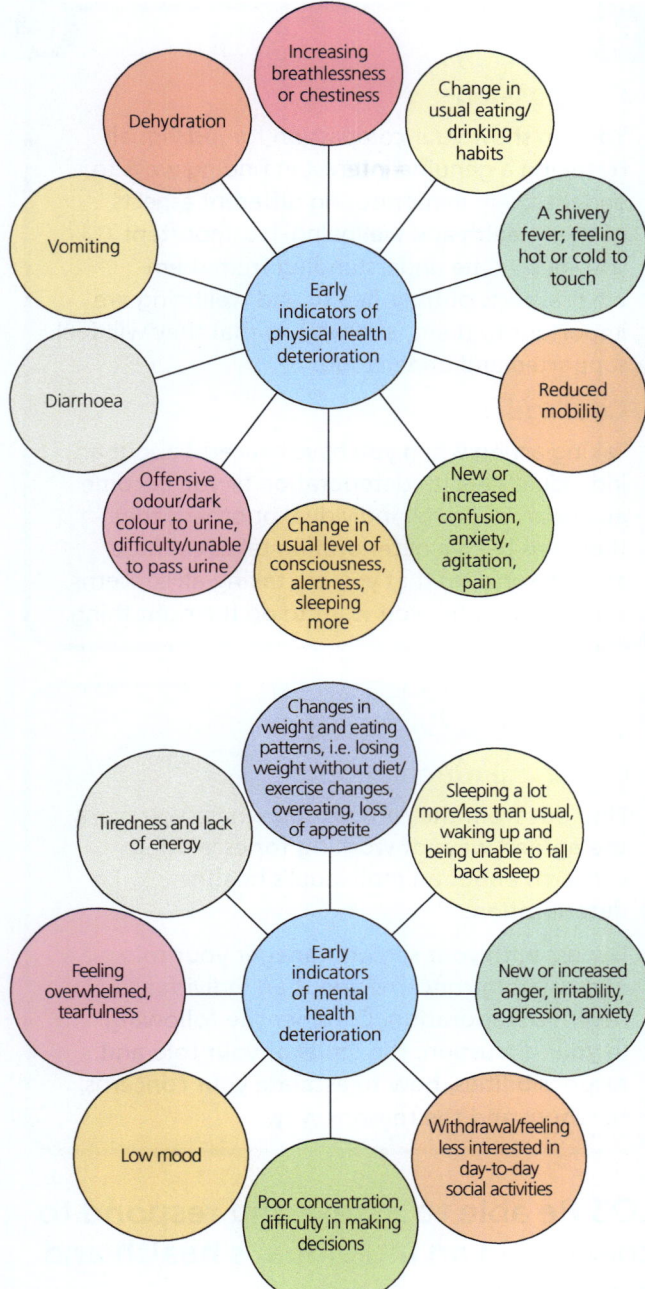

Figure 9.2 Early indicators of physical and mental health deterioration

If you notice one or more of these soft signs of physical or mental health deterioration in an individual, don't ignore your instincts about what you can see and what you know about the individual. Doing nothing is not an option: you must take action and in AC2.4, below, you will learn more about how to respond to health deterioration.

Reflect on it

2.2, 2.3 Soft signs of health deterioration

Reflect on the benefits of knowing the soft signs of physical and mental health deterioration that may occur in individuals that you care for and support.

Evidence opportunity

2.2, 2.3 Soft signs of health deterioration

Discuss with a colleague the main soft signs of physical and mental health deterioration that may occur in individuals.

AC 2.4 Explain how to escalate concerns about an individual's health deterioration, and to whom

As you will have learned in ACs 2.2 and 2.3 of this unit, responding to an individual's physical and/or mental health deterioration is part of your duty of care towards them; it is essential for promoting their rights to access care, support and treatment when they need it to prevent their health from worsening. Below are some tips on what to do if you have concerns about an individual's health deterioration; remember that you must always follow your organisation's policies, procedures and agreed ways of working at all times and act within the limits of your job role and responsibilities.

1 If you have concerns about an individual's health deterioration, **don't ignore this** instinct; **raise the alert** within the care setting/service you work in. It is your duty to promote individuals' rights to good health and wellbeing. Depending on the care setting where you work, you will have to **report your concerns to someone in a more senior position** than you so that the appropriate action can be taken quickly, e.g. this might be to a senior carer/support worker, registered nurse or your manager.
2 **Keep a record of your observations** of the individual, including the changes you have noticed in their health, so that these can be communicated clearly and factually and can be

referred to by other care and health professionals so that they can build a picture of the changes that the individual has experienced. Having this information is particularly useful when the professional involved, such as a hospital doctor, does not know the individual like you do, or when the individual involved cannot speak up for themselves in relation to their health deterioration. You will learn more about recording observations of individuals' health and wellbeing in LO3, ACs 3.4 and 3.5 in this unit.

3 Ensure that, when recording your observations of the individual, you use the appropriate tools as set out in your care setting/service's agreed ways of working, such as **NEWS2** or a NEWS2-based system such as **RESTORE2**, so that you capture all the required detail. You will learn more about what these tools are and how to use them in LO3, AC3.3 in this unit.

4 Ensure that, when reporting your concerns about an individual's health to a healthcare professional such as a nurse, GP or 111, you use the communication tool **SBARD** so that your report, whether it is verbal or in writing, is clear and contains all the necessary information. You will learn more about what this tool is and how to use it in LO3, AC3.3 in this unit.

5 After reporting your concerns, continue to observe the individual to ensure that you are still keeping them safe and comfortable; follow the guidance given to you by the person you escalated your concerns to, e.g. this could be a senior person in the care setting where you work or a healthcare professional outside of your care setting.

Key terms

NEWS2 refers to the second version of the National Early Warning Score tool that was developed by the Royal College of Physicians to identify and respond to clinical deterioration in patients early. It is used across NHS services in England, including in hospitals and ambulances.

RESTORE2 is a physical deterioration and escalation tool for care homes and nursing homes. It is based on early recognition: soft signs, NEWS2 and structured communications (SBARD).

SBARD (Situation, Background, Assessment, Recommendation, Decision) is a communication tool used to escalate concerns about an individual's health deterioration quickly and fully; it can be used for both verbal and written communications.

6Cs

Compassion

You can show your compassion for individuals by taking a genuine interest in finding ways to engage them in monitoring different aspects of their health and wellbeing. It's important you spend time understanding from them what aspects of their health and wellbeing are important to them, and why, so that they will feel supported and understood.

Courage

Taking action when you have concerns about an individual's health deterioration or you become aware, through the individual or others, that there has been a deterioration takes courage and also ensures that you are taking all concerns seriously because you want to do the right thing.

Evidence opportunity

2.4 Escalating concerns

Find out from the care setting where you work the agreed ways of working for escalating concerns about an individual's health deterioration.

Discuss with your senior/manager your role in escalating concerns about an individual's health deterioration. Consider the following in your discussion: the limits of your role and responsibilities, how to escalate your concerns, to whom and the reasons why.

LO3 Be able to assess and respond to changes in an individual's health and wellbeing

Getting started

Think about an occasion in the care setting where you work when you noticed changes in an individual's health and wellbeing. What actions did you take and why? What did you say to the individual and why?

AC 3.1 Engage individuals in understanding their health and wellbeing

Enabling individuals to have a good understanding of their health and wellbeing means that they will gain a greater insight into who they are and will be empowered to use their understanding and knowledge of themselves, and therefore more likely to want to get involved in monitoring their health and wellbeing.

To engage individuals in understanding their health and wellbeing, it is essential that you know the individual and how to engage them. For example, the individual may have a visual impairment and if so, it is important that you know how this affects them and what communication methods they prefer, for example written communications in large print or Braille, or verbal rather than written communications, or a technological aid such as computer software with different coloured screens. Ensure that you know which communication methods the individual prefers and how to use them, so that you can get their attention and engage them; if you're unsure, you can get additional support or advice from someone who knows the individual well, such as another colleague, the individual's family, or their advocate if they have one.

Once you know how to engage the individual, you need to think about how you are going to develop their understanding of their health and wellbeing. To do this, you need to explore with them the knowledge they have: for example, do they understand the importance of health and wellbeing? Do they understand what you mean by health and wellbeing and the different aspects this involves? Do they understand the links between their health and wellbeing and their quality of life? Sometimes, it is easier to initiate the discussion with them by thinking about which aspects of their health and wellbeing they have spoken about or referred to previously; for example, perhaps they have mentioned that they would like to improve their social health by having more opportunities to meet others socially, or that they would like to further explore their spiritual wellbeing or develop their intellectual wellbeing by participating in activities that stimulate their mind. Whichever aspect of their health and wellbeing they decide to explore with you will be a good starting point.

Engaging individuals in understanding their health and wellbeing will require you to demonstrate patience and empathy so that the individual feels that they can be honest with themselves and you about any aspects of their health and wellbeing that they are worried about or having difficulties with; this may be in relation to their mental or cultural wellbeing. The individual can then begin to explore the positive and negative influences on their wellbeing and whether they want to access further support to improve these.

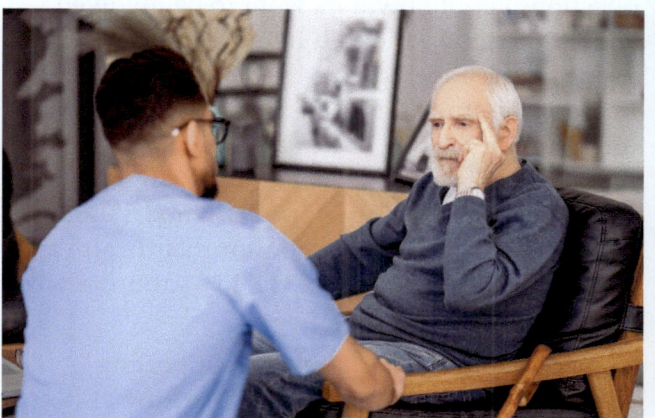

Figure 9.3 What skills do you use when engaging individuals in understanding their health and wellbeing?

AC 3.2 Involve individuals in monitoring their health and wellbeing

To involve individuals in monitoring their health and wellbeing it is essential that you take a step back and do not make any assumptions about how they want to be involved. Instead, ask individuals how they want to be involved; if they're reluctant to at first, then do your best to find out why. Perhaps they do not know how they can be involved, haven't got the confidence to be involved, or are anxious that they might make a mistake or the wrong decision. If so, you will need to explain to the individual why you want them to be involved and how this will benefit them and enable them to make informed decisions and be in control of their health and wellbeing; after all, they are the real experts about their care and support.

The individual may also need reassurance from you that they have the ability to make their own decisions and choices. You could also seek support from the individual's advocate if they have one, or from another person who knows their strengths and abilities.

Involving individuals in monitoring their health and wellbeing will require you to keep an open mind. Every individual is unique and therefore their levels of involvement will also vary, and how you involve one individual will not necessarily be the same for another individual. For example, you might have a discussion with one individual and be able to ask them direct questions about how they want to be involved and let them take the lead in monitoring their health and wellbeing. Another individual might find questioning and discussion difficult, and might prefer for you to explain to them the different ways that they could be involved so that they can choose their preferred method. Another individual may prefer to monitor their health and wellbeing alongside others, i.e. in a group or with another individual.

Knowing the individual you are supporting will make an enormous difference to how successfully you can engage and involve them in understanding and monitoring their health and wellbeing. Remember too that supporting individuals with their health and wellbeing is not something that is done on one occasion or even two, it is something that is continuous and is part of day-to-day life.

6Cs

Competence

Engaging and involving individuals in their health and wellbeing involves having a good knowledge of individuals including their needs, preferences, strengths and abilities as every individual is unique and will require you to support them in different ways.

Reflect on it

3.1, 3.2 My skills

Reflect on the key skills you have that help you to engage and involve individuals in understanding and monitoring their health and wellbeing. Are there any that could be developed further? If so, how are you going to do this?

Evidence opportunity

3.1, 3.2 Engaging and involving individuals with their health and wellbeing

For these ACs, you will be observed. You will need to show your assessor how you engage individuals in understanding their health and wellbeing and involve them in monitoring their health and wellbeing. Think about how you are going to do this. Could your assessor observe you conducting a one-to-one support session with two different individuals, or a group session with several individuals? Remember to demonstrate the skills you have when supporting individuals with different aspects of their health and wellbeing.

AC 3.3 Demonstrate the use of appropriate tools to monitor and report changes in health and wellbeing

As well as using your skills and knowledge of individuals, and those around them who also know them well, to assess and respond to changes in their health and wellbeing, there are a range of tools available that can help with monitoring and reporting changes. The tools available to you will depend on your job role and the agreed ways of working in the care setting/service where you work. Table 9.5 includes some examples of these, and in the activities that follow, you will have an opportunity to consider the tools available to you in the care setting/service where you work.

Table 9.5 Tools to monitor and report changes in health and wellbeing

Examples of tools for monitoring and reporting changes in health and wellbeing	What the tool is and how to use it
Stop and Watch	A tool that can be used by everyone that helps with identifying the warning signs that a person's condition is deteriorating, to prevent the person's conditioning from worsening, becoming fatal or causing disability or organ failure. It consists of 11 prompts to help spot signs of deterioration early. It is designed to support your gut instinct and to help you explain to others what your concerns are. If you identify an important change in an individual (any of the ones below) or someone who knows the individual, such as a family member or visitor, tells you that they've noticed one of these changes, don't ignore it and ensure you report it before you end your shift. **S**eems different to usual: however small the change you notice, think Stop and Watch. **T**alking or communicating less: are they communicating less effectively? This could be a sign that they are becoming confused, depressed or tired. **O**verall needs more help: are they asking for or needing more help to mobilise or with day-to-day activities? This could be a sign of lower energy levels because of an infection or a deterioration in a medical condition. **P**ain new or worsening; participating less in activities: look for non-verbal clues. Are they restless, agitated, not wanting to move? Pain is often a sign that something's wrong. **A**te less: look for a change in eating patterns. Are they eating less or avoiding certain foods? A lack of appetite could be a sign of a medical condition. **N**o bowel movement in 3 days or diarrhoea. This could be a sign of ill health. Monitoring bowels, including the frequency and colour of stools, is important. **D**rank less: it can be difficult to spot if someone is dehydrated. Monitoring their fluid intake and output by using a hydration chart and observing the colour of their urine is important. **W**eight change: are they losing weight without trying to? This could be a sign of ill health. **A**gitated or more nervous than usual: are they more restless, aggressive, tearful or withdrawn? This could be a sign that something is wrong. **T**ired, weak, confused, drowsy: do they appear to have less energy, be weaker, confused? This could be a sign that something is wrong. **C**hange in skin colour or condition: do they have dry skin? This could be a sign of dehydration. Do they have a rash? This could be a sign of an infection. Do they have yellowing of the skin and whites of eyes? This could be a sign of liver failure. **H**elp with walking, transferring or toileting more than usual: do they need more support with their daily living activities such as washing/dressing/toileting and generally getting about? This could be a sign that something is wrong.

Table 9.5 Tools to monitor and report changes in health and wellbeing *continued*

Examples of tools for monitoring and reporting changes in health and wellbeing	What the tool is and how to use it
NEWS2	National Early Warning Score (NEWS2) is a tool developed by the Royal College of Physicians to standardise the assessment and response to acute illness in an individual so that their deterioration is responded to rapidly. NEWS was originally developed in 2012 and updated with the second version in 2017. It has been formally endorsed by NHS England and NHS Improvement as the early warning system for acutely ill patients, including those with sepsis, in hospitals in England. NEWS2 is based on allocating scores to physiological measurements taken routinely when individuals arrive at hospital or are being monitored in hospital. It includes the following six physiological measurements: ● Respiration rate – the number of breaths taken per minute; i.e. in a healthy adult, approximately 12–20 breaths are taken per minute. ● Oxygen saturation – how much oxygen is travelling through the body in the red blood cells; i.e. in a healthy adult the oxygen saturation rate is between 95 and 100%. ● Systolic blood pressure – how much pressure the blood is exerting against the artery walls when the heart beats, recorded as the top number of a blood pressure reading; i.e. in a healthy adult it is 120/70. ● Pulse rate – the number of times the heart beats in one minute. Heart rates vary from person to person and are higher when you exercise and lower when you rest; i.e. a resting heart rate for a healthy adult ranges from 60–100 heart beats per minute. ● Level of consciousness or new confusion – level of consciousness refers to how alert and aware a person is of their surroundings and how they respond to attempts to get their attention. Confusion refers to how disorientated a person is, i.e. that makes it difficult to reason with the person, for the person to provide a medical history, for the person to participate in a medical examination. ● Temperature – body temperature of a healthy adult is usually 37°C. A body temperature of 37.8°C or higher usually means you have a fever and you may feel warm, cold or shivery.
SBARD	A tool for communicating information about an individual accurately. SBARD can be used in a variety of settings, including in care homes and hospitals, and helps to ensure that important information is communicated to others concisely and effectively. Its use is recommended by the World Health Organization and the NHS. SBARD consists of five sections to ensure information is communicated in a standardised way. It can be used when communicating information verbally, in person or over the telephone, as well as in writing via emails and reports. It encourages assertive and focused discussions about the individual: **S**ituation – briefly describe the situation; give a concise overview of what's happened and what your concerns are. Provide details of who you are, i.e. your job role, care setting/service, contact number.

Table 9.5 Tools to monitor and report changes in health and wellbeing *continued*

Examples of tools for monitoring and reporting changes in health and wellbeing	What the tool is and how to use it
	Background – briefly state the individual's relevant history and how you got to this point, i.e. the individual's medical condition, whether they are taking any medication, whether they are receiving treatment or have had any investigations or visits to their GP recently, how their condition has changed. **A**ssessment – summarise the facts only; what do you think is going on with the individual? Describe how you've supported the individual, whether you've given them any medication such as pain relief, whether you know what is wrong with them or not, why you are concerned. **R**ecommendation – what are you asking for? What needs to happen next? For example, asking for the individual to be visited, asking how you can help, e.g. by continuing with your observations of the individual's health and wellbeing, or escalating your concerns to emergency services. **D**ecision – summarise the decision made, what you have agreed, for example who will do what, what actions will be taken, by whom and when. For example, this might be that you will call emergency services if there is no improvement in the individual's condition or there is a continued deterioration.
RESTORE2	A deterioration and escalation tool that was specifically designed for residential care homes, nursing homes and the domiciliary care sector, RESTORE2 can be used to recognise when an individual is deteriorating or is at risk of physical deterioration and to ensure this is communicated effectively to others such as healthcare professionals in hospitals, ambulance staff or the GP. It uses the following techniques that are recognised and used by health and care professionals: ● **Soft signs** – recognises soft signs of deterioration such as increased breathlessness, a rash, changes in skin colour. See ACs 2.2 and 2.3 in this unit for more information. ● **NEWS2** – the National Early Warning Score to standardise the assessment and physical deterioration of an individual, and a communication and escalation pathway to ensure the individual gets the correct help early/promptly. See above for more information. ● **SBARD** – Situation, Background, Assessment, Recommendation, Decision tool to ensure concerns about an individual's health are communicated effectively. See above for more information.
Technological aids	There are many technological aids available to monitor and report changes in individuals' health and wellbeing. Below are some examples of the different types: ● Assistive technology; e.g. drinking cups with sensors that monitor how much an individual has had to drink can help to prevent dehydration; mood tracking software helps with tracking of moods and triggers for ill-being and wellbeing. ● Wearable technologies, e.g. a wearable device for a person with diabetes that takes a glucose reading that is then tracked via an app; a wearable patch that measures a person's pulse, respiratory rate.

Table 9.5 Tools to monitor and report changes in health and wellbeing *continued*

Examples of tools for monitoring and reporting changes in health and wellbeing	What the tool is and how to use it
	• Mobile applications, e.g. mobile apps that monitor a person's condition such as their heart rate and oxygen levels; sleep-tracking apps that monitor your sleep cycles and stages. • Websites; e.g. the NHS website's page 'Live Well' offers information and advice on healthy living, including what a healthy weight is and how to lose weight; the mental health charity Mind's website offers a five-step guide to mental health and wellbeing.
Physiological measurements	Physiological measurements focus on assessing the function of the body's major organ systems and are essential for accessing treatments quickly, thus promoting good health and wellbeing. There are eight areas of physiological measurement: • Audiology, i.e. hearing and balance assessments • Cardiac physiology, i.e. cardiovascular disease interventions • Gastrointestinal physiology, i.e. upper and lower intestine tract assessments • Neurophysiology, i.e. diagnosis of conditions affecting the central and peripheral nervous system • Opthalmic and vision science, i.e. investigations of disorders of vision and diseases of the eye • Respiratory physiology and sleep physiology, i.e. diagnostic tests and services for people who have respiratory diseases and sleep-related breathing difficulties • Urodynamics, i.e. assessments that investigate bladder and urinary tract function • Vascular technology, i.e. investigation and monitoring of diseases of the arteries and veins.

Reflect on it

3.3 Tools at work

Reflect on the different tools that are used in the care setting/service where you work to monitor and report changes in individuals' health and wellbeing. Make a list of the tools you've used, including when you've used them and why.

Evidence opportunity

3.3 Monitoring and reporting changes in health and wellbeing

Your work practices will be observed for this AC.

Discuss with your manager the tools you use in your current job role to monitor and report changes in individuals' health and wellbeing. Make arrangements for your assessor to observe you using these with an individual(s). Ensure that you can show why you use the tools and how you are working within the scope of your job role and in line with your employer's agreed ways of working.

AC 3.4 Demonstrate how to record observations of health and wellbeing

Recording observations of health and wellbeing is not just something that is done daily or weekly; it is a continuous process and essential for ensuring that there is always an up-to-date record of the individual's health and wellbeing in place. This is essential for ensuring that the individual is receiving the care and support they need and also for ensuring that the information gathered can then be communicated clearly and accurately to another healthcare professional who may need it, such as a doctor or mental health nurse.

Observations of health and wellbeing can be recorded in many different ways depending on what information is being recorded and the agreed ways of working in the care setting/service; you must always ensure that you follow the agreed ways of working in the care setting/service where you work for recording observations. For example, in a hospital setting, observations of an individual's respiration rate, pulse rate and temperature may be recorded on a chart. In a care home, observations of an individual's fluid intake and output may be recorded electronically. An individual living at home and accessing domiciliary care may have observations of their mental health and wellbeing documented in their care plan.

It is also important to remember that observation records of health and wellbeing are legal documents that form part of your job role and responsibilities as well as a permanent record of what has happened. Therefore, you must ensure that you complete these records accurately and effectively so that you can demonstrate that you are complying with your duty of care and responsibilities in relation to handling information as well as with legal and organisational requirements that are in place.

> ### Reflect on it
> #### 3.4 Maintaining records
> Reflect on your previous learning in Unit 305, Handling information in adult care settings/services, and discuss with a colleague how to maintain records that are up to date, complete, accurate and legible.

The case study below provides you with an opportunity to consider the different aspects to take into account when recording observations of health and wellbeing.

> ### Case study
> #### 3.3, 3.4 Recording observations of health and wellbeing
>
> Jasmine is a senior carer in a residential care home providing accommodation and personal care support for 18 older adults. Jasmine has supported Cynthia, one of the residents, with her personal care this morning, and she has some concerns about the changes she has noted in Cynthia's mental and physical wellbeing. In line with the home's procedures, Jasmine has completed their SBARD communication tool prior to the nurse visiting the home this morning, so that she can explain her concerns about Cynthia clearly and accurately to the nurse:
>
> **The SBARD Communication Tool for Hyperion Care Home**
>
> My name is Jasmine Knight and I have worked as a senior carer in Hyperion Care Home for 8 years. I am concerned about one of the residents, Cynthia Beech, whose mobility has been deteriorating over the last couple of days and who seems to be sleeping more. Cynthia was admitted to hospital after a fall in her room a month ago and was also treated by her GP about a week ago for a urinary tract infection for which she was prescribed a course of three days of antibiotics.
>
> This morning (25/10/22) I have checked the following for Cynthia:
>
> 1. Temperature – 37.5C
> 2. Blood Pressure and Pulse – 124/80
> 3. Urinary Tract Infection is suspected – No
> 4. Breathing is – 19 breaths per minute
> 5. Any changes in levels of confusion? – A little disorientated when mobilising and seems low in mood, which is unusual.
> 6. Complaints of being in pain? – Yes, a headache.
> 7. Any recent falls? – Yes, on 25/09/22.
> 8. Bowels were last opened on: 25/10/22 – Texture constipated.

9 Sleep pattern is: increased fatigue, sleeping more during the day.
10 Food and fluid intake is: good
11 Oxygen stats are: 96%

Recommendation:
I need a visit from a healthcare professional to provide further advice.

Decision:
After discussion with my manager, it is agreed that the nurse who is attending the Home today on 25/10/22 will visit Cynthia and that we will seek further advice from her before contacting Cynthia's GP.

Date: 25/10/22
Time: 08.05am
Name: Jasmine Knight

Discuss:
1 How Jasmine used the SBARD tool to record her observations of Cynthia. Why was this important?
2 The aspects of Cynthia's health and wellbeing that were recorded and the reasons why.
3 Were Jasmine's observations recorded fully, accurately and clearly? Why?

6Cs

Communication

Responding to changes in individuals' health and wellbeing requires you to be an effective communicator. This means that you must be clear in your communications not only with individuals but also with others you work with to ensure that changes in individuals' health and wellbeing are recorded and reported accurately and in a timely manner. Doing so will mean that you will be able to support individuals and promote their health and wellbeing.

Evidence opportunity

3.4 Recording observations

You will be observed for this AC. You will need to show your assessor how you record observations of health and wellbeing in the care service/setting where you work. You must ensure that the tool you have used to record the observation is appropriate and within the scope of your job role and responsibilities.

You could also include a witness testimony from your manager and the observations of health and wellbeing you recorded as supporting work product evidence of the skills you have in this area.

AC 3.5 Explain when and how to take appropriate action if an observation result is concerning

Knowing how to report and record observations of health and wellbeing is not enough on its own to respond to changes in an individual's health and wellbeing: you will also need to know when and how to take appropriate action if an observation result is concerning. It could be that you've observed the individual, or a colleague tells you about an observation result that is concerning. The actions you take will depend on your role, the agreed ways of working of the care setting/service you work in, as well as the specific change in an individual's wellbeing, i.e. whether it's a medical emergency or whether the individual has a pre-existing condition that affects their mental or physical wellbeing, for example.

If you have any reason to think that an observation result is concerning, then you must trust your gut instinct and you must show courage by always acting on it; doing nothing is not an option. This may involve referring your concerns to a more senior colleague, your manager or even to another organisation such as the NHS or MIND. Where the individual concerned is also the employer, you will need to familiarise yourself with the roles and responsibilities that are set out in your contract of employment as well as the local authority's procedures that are in place for the care setting/service where you work.

Figure 9.7 explains the key actions to take and when they should be taken if an observation result is concerning.

Do not ignore your gut instinct that an observation result is concerning

| Not taking action immediately would mean that the individual's condition may worsen | Doing nothing will mean that you will not be complying with your care setting/service's agreed ways of working |

↓

Ensure the individual's health and wellbeing comes first by reporting your or others' concerns to the named person in the care setting/service where you work

| Reporting your concerns as soon as you notice them will mean that others can take the necessary action. This may also involve the named person speaking to the individual and/or the individual's family | Reporting your concerns to the named person will mean that they can advise you on what action to take next and whether you require further support such as medical assistance from a GP or ambulance |

↓

Keep secure all evidence you have of your or others' concerns. Record the observation results and the concerns as soon as possible and with full details

| Keeping the observation records secure will mean that you will be following your agreed ways of working to ensure all observation results are preserved | Recording observation results promptly will mean you will be more likely to record all necessary information so that it can be acted on and the individual's health and wellbeing can be promoted |

Figure 9.4 Appropriate action to take when an observation result is concerning

Reflect on it

3.5 Dos and Don'ts

Reflect on the Dos and Don'ts when taking appropriate action if an observation result is concerning, including why it is important to take action promptly and how to do so in line with your care setting/service's agreed ways of working.

Evidence opportunity

3.5 Taking appropriate action

Discuss with your supervisor or manager when and how to take appropriate action if an observation result is concerning. Think about the consequences of not doing so for the individual, you, and the care setting/service where you work.

LO4 Be able to promote individuals' health and wellbeing

Getting started

How would you describe yourself? What are your 'positives'? For example, your personality, kind nature or sense of humour? How would others describe you? What do they say are your positives? Do you agree with what others say about you? Why? How can what others say about you impact on how good you feel about yourself? Can you think of an example of when this happened?

As well as what others say about you, what other things affect how you feel about yourself? How can your physical health affect how you feel emotionally? How can your emotional health affect your physical health? For example, if you feel unwell does this make you feel more positive or negative? Why?

AC 4.1 Support individuals in a way that promotes their sense of identity, self-image and self-esteem

For this assessment criterion you will be observed demonstrating how to support an individual in a way that promotes wellbeing.

Supporting individuals' wellbeing is also dependent on ensuring that the environment around them also promotes their wellbeing. This includes the following.

- **Physical environment:** rooms in a care setting, layout in a health service, such as a GP surgery, access to the garden, the individual's personal belongings
- **Social environment:** the atmosphere in a care setting or service, the quality of the working relationships in a service.

Reflect on it

4.1 Physical and social environments

Reflect on the differences there are between the physical and social environment. Reflect on the aspects that are important to you in terms of physical and social environments and the reasons why.

How can you ensure that the physical environment promotes an individual's wellbeing?

- **Furniture and furnishings:** ensuring furniture and furnishings are clean and attractive can make individuals feel good. Ensuring that furniture is maintained and not broken can promote individuals' safety and therefore wellbeing.
- **Personal belongings:** ensuring individuals' personal belongings are placed in their rooms and other areas in a care setting will make individuals feel at home and will help to promote a sense of wellbeing.
- **Temperature:** ensuring rooms and environments are not too hot or too cold; both have the potential to make individuals feel uncomfortable. Checking with individuals if the temperature is about right will make them feel comfortable and promote their wellbeing.

AC 4.2 Demonstrate ways to contribute to an environment that promotes wellbeing

How can you ensure that the social environment promotes an individual's wellbeing?

- **Items and pictures:** ensuring rooms contain items and pictures that are representative of individuals' diverse backgrounds (for example, in relation to their ages, genders and cultures) will ensure that individuals feel a sense of belonging and therefore can promote wellbeing.
- **Management of a care setting or service:** an environment that is managed well and where all staff comply with agreed ways of working will be less likely to place individuals in danger or at risk of harm or abuse and so will promote feelings of security among individuals and in turn a good sense of wellbeing.
- **Atmosphere:** an atmosphere that is welcoming and inviting will promote feelings of wellbeing. A stimulating atmosphere will ensure individuals' needs are met, for example organising the provision for activities or the availability of adult care workers with special areas of expertise. In turn, this will promote a sense of wellbeing as the individuals will feel valued.

Research it

4.2 Adapting physical and social environments

Research how the physical and social environment can be adapted to meet the needs of an individual who has dementia. Discuss your findings with a colleague.

You may, for example, find it useful to refer to the Alzheimer's Society website www.alzheimers.org.uk for information on adapting the environment for people with dementia.

Evidence opportunity

4.2 Ways to contribute to an environment that promotes wellbeing

Identify an individual who has care or support needs, for example this could be an individual with learning or physical difficulties, hearing or sight loss, dementia or a heart condition. Show your assessor how you contribute to an environment that promotes their needs.

Write a case study listing the individual's needs and the different ways that you can contribute to an environment that promotes the individual's wellbeing. Remember that you cannot include personal details about individuals in your portfolio.

AC 4.3 Demonstrate a person-centred approach to working with individuals to improve health and wellbeing

Working in a person-centred way to improve individuals' health and wellbeing is essential for ensuring that the care and support you provide to the individual is appropriate, and for supporting them to be in control of their life and the decisions they make. You will find it useful to review your previous learning in Unit 306, LO3 around working in a person-centred way with individuals.

You can demonstrate a person-centred approach to working with individuals to improve their health and wellbeing by:

- keeping the individual at the heart of everything you do, for example maintaining the individual's health and wellbeing as the focus when working with them by ensuring the support you provide reflects their unique needs and preferences in relation to all aspects of their wellbeing.
- treating individuals kindly and supporting them to be their own person, for example by supporting them to make their own decisions as to what aspects of their health and wellbeing they would like to work on and improve.
- promoting individuals' rights, for example by helping individuals to access the range of resources and services that are available to support their health and wellbeing. You will find it useful to review your previous learning in LO1 of this unit around accessing services and resources available to support wellbeing.
- enabling individuals to make their own choices, for example by providing them with all the necessary information about their health and wellbeing without bias, including the options that are available if they would like to make improvements in any areas.
- showing respect for an individual's privacy, for example by respecting their personal information in relation to their health and wellbeing. This includes information shared verbally in discussions, as well as written information in records. You will find it useful to review your previous learning in LO3 of this unit around recording observations of health and wellbeing.
- enabling individuals to be independent, for example by encouraging them to do as much for themselves as possible and to be in control of their health and wellbeing by supporting them to act on any early indicators of deterioration and involving them in monitoring their own health and wellbeing. You will find it useful to review your previous learning in LO2 of this unit around monitoring individuals' health.
- showing individuals dignity and respect, for example by respecting individuals' views and preferences in relation to their health and wellbeing, such as the aspects that are important to them, those that they want to improve and those that they don't, even when they are different to yours. Valuing individuals' differences and respecting that they are their own experts of their health and wellbeing is a big part of treating individuals with dignity and respect.
- providing care and support that meets individuals' needs, for example by ensuring you involve individuals in understanding their health and wellbeing by communicating with them in ways that they understand, including using their preferred methods of communication and presenting information clearly and in a way that considers their needs. You will find it useful to review your previous learning in LO3 of this unit around engaging individuals in monitoring their health and wellbeing.
- providing care and support to individuals with compassion, for example by showing kindness, consideration, empathy, dignity and respect when working with them to improve different aspects of their health and wellbeing, by listening to their concerns around their health and wellbeing and not dismissing them.
- providing care and support to individuals with courage, for example by working with individuals in a way that is morally acceptable. This could mean not ignoring any observation results that are concerning or standing up for an individual when you have escalated concerns about a deterioration in their health and wellbeing and these have not been acted on.
- effective communication, for example by actively listening to individuals and acting on what they have communicated so that they know that you are promoting their health and wellbeing and that they can trust you with addressing any concerns or with making any improvements that they want to make.
- showing competence when working with individuals, for example, by ensuring you have the necessary knowledge, skills and expertise to support them with their health and wellbeing, including understanding what their needs are and how to meet them.
- working in partnership with individuals, for example by ensuring you work alongside individuals so that they remain at the heart of their care and support and in control of their health and wellbeing.

Reflect on it

4.3 Improving individuals' health and wellbeing

Reflect on the benefits of working in a person-centred way with individuals to improve their health and wellbeing. What impact will this have on the individual and on their health and wellbeing? Why?

Evidence opportunity

4.3 Working in a person-centred way to improve health and wellbeing

You will be observed for this AC. You will need to show your assessor that you use a person-centred approach when working with individuals to improve their health and wellbeing. What methods of working do you think you will need to demonstrate and why? How are you going to show your assessor that you work consistently across different individuals, using a person-centred approach?

You could also collect a witness testimony from your manager or from another senior colleague who has observed your working practices and can provide supporting evidence of the person-centred ways of working you apply to your day-to-day practices.

AC 4.4 Demonstrate approaches to working with others to improve an individual's health and wellbeing

As you will have learned, working with individuals using person-centred ways of working to improve their health and wellbeing is important and can make a positive difference to their lives. Working with others to improve individuals' health and wellbeing, such as with individuals' families, your colleagues and other care and health professionals outside of the care setting or service where you work, is also important and essential for being able to show that you can work as part of a team and in the best interests of the individual. You will find it useful to review your previous learning in LO1 of Unit 300 around the importance of working in partnership with others as well as the skills and approaches used.

You can demonstrate approaches to working with others to improve an individual's health and wellbeing by:

- effective communication, for example by communicating with others clearly and ensuring you clarify information received to avoid any misunderstandings, such as in relation to the advice you received from a dietician after escalating your concerns about an individual's weight loss. You will find it useful to review your previous learning in Unit 304, LO1 and LO3 around using effective communication skills.
- understanding others' roles, for example by finding out about how others will be involved in improving an individual's health and wellbeing, their strengths and limitations and ensuring that you also discuss your role and responsibilities with others so that you can all work together in the best interests of the individual.
- valuing others, for example by treating others respectfully including respecting views and opinions that may be different to yours, being polite and honest in your communications with others, and being open and supportive of others even when something has gone wrong, so that you can show others that you are professional, responsible and trustworthy.
- being supportive, for example by sharing ideas, skills, knowledge and expertise with each other, or by supporting an individual's family member or a colleague of yours who is finding it difficult to discuss the individual's mental wellbeing. Displaying support for others in this way will help with creating strong professional working relationships with others.

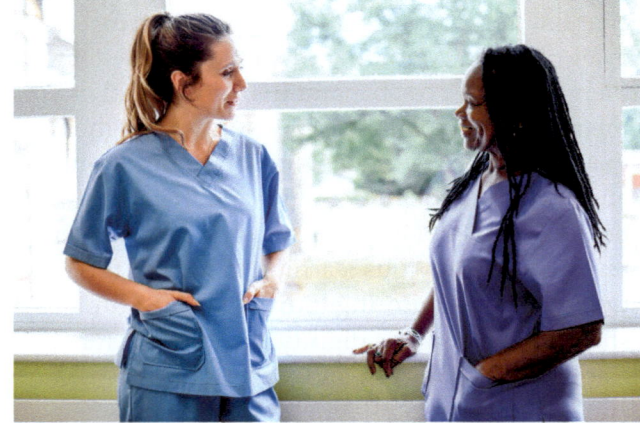

Figure 9.5 How do you work in partnership with others reflectively?

Research it

4.4 Working approaches

Research the different approaches to working with others when improving an individual's health and wellbeing. You could conduct your own research in the care setting/service where you work by discussing this with your colleagues, manager and other care or health professionals who visit and support the individuals you work with, or you could research best practice examples you may have heard about or read about in the media, perhaps an article you've read or a documentary you've watched.

Produce an information hand-out that describes the different working approaches you've found out about and their benefits.

Evidence opportunity

4.4 Working with others

You will be observed for this AC. You will need to show your assessor different approaches you use when working with others to improve an individual's health and wellbeing. When planning for your observation, ensure you show your assessor how you work with a range of others to improve individuals' health and wellbeing. This may include people from within and outside the care setting/service where you work.

You could also collect a witness testimony from your manager or from another senior colleague who has observed your working practices and can provide supporting evidence of the different approaches you use when working with others to improve an individual's health and wellbeing.

Legislation	
Relevant Act	**Key points**
Data Protection Act 2018	Personal information must be recorded, used, stored and shared according to a set of principles or rules to ensure the individuals' rights are protected and the security of their personal information is maintained. This includes when recording observations of their health and wellbeing and reporting any changes that may occur.
The Human Rights Act 1998	Everyone in the UK is entitled to the same rights and freedoms. This includes individuals who have care and support needs. The Act supports the promotion of individuals' rights, including the promotion of their health and wellbeing.
The Mental Capacity Act 2005	This Act supports person-centred working by supporting individuals' rights to make their own decisions in relation to their health and wellbeing, including being provided with the necessary support to do so. It also protects the rights of individuals who lack capacity by providing guidance on who can make decisions about them and how to plan ahead for this in case it arises in the future.
The Care Act 2014	This Act promotes a person-centred approach to care planning. It also defines the concept of wellbeing and outlines how adult care workers can promote individuals' wellbeing. Also see the Government publications: • *Personalised Health and Care 2020*, which sets out how technology and data can be used to improve health and the way health and social care services are delivered. • *The Adult Social Care Outcomes Framework Handbook of Definitions*, which measures how well care and support services achieve the outcomes that are the most important to people.

309 Promoting equality, diversity, inclusion and human rights in adult care settings/services

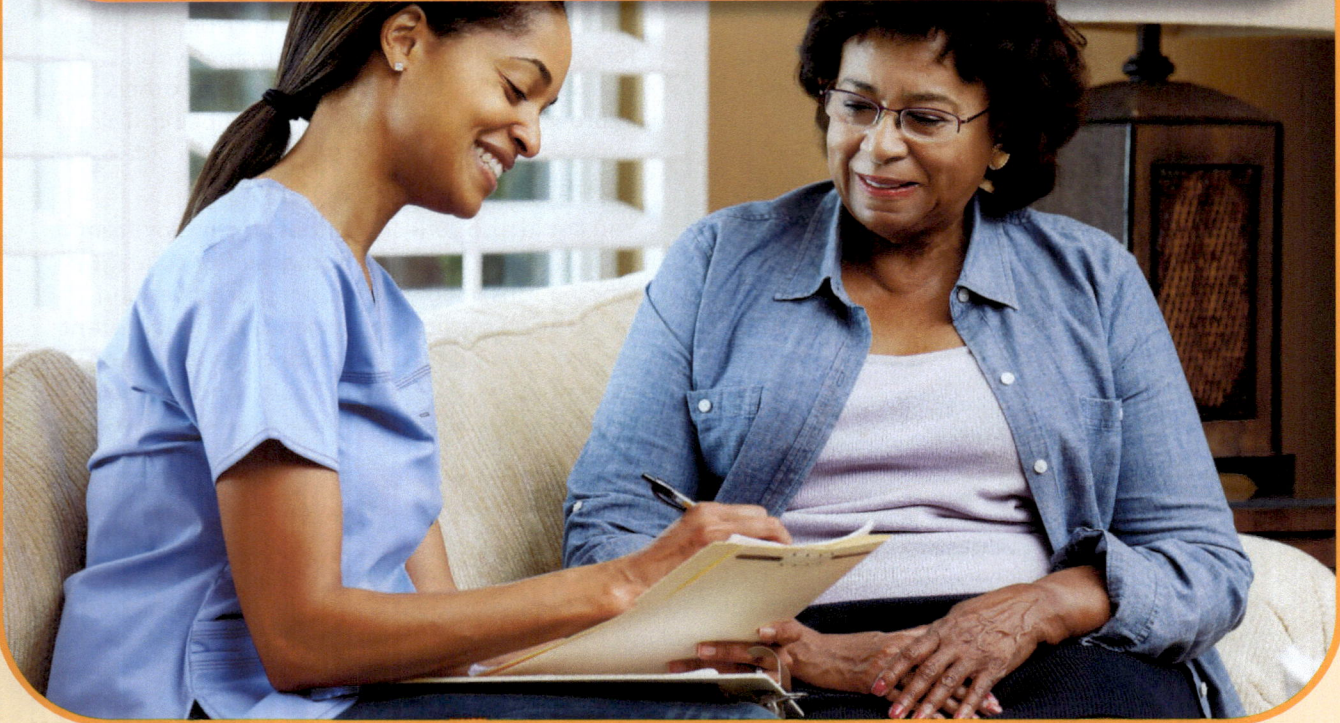

About this unit

Credit value: 2
Guided learning hours: 18

Promoting **equality, diversity, inclusion and human rights** in care settings is essential for delivering safe, good quality care and creating a positive, caring and fair environment. In this unit, you will learn about the meaning and importance of equality, diversity, **inclusion** and human rights, the reasons why these concepts are important to your role as a Lead Adult Care Worker or Lead Personal Assistant, and how they can enable you to reduce the likelihood of **discrimination** occurring.

Being able to practise in an inclusive way involves you complying with relevant legislation, policy and codes of practice, all of which you will find out about in this unit, including how you can apply them as part of your job role and responsibilities. You will be able to practise your skills for showing respect for individuals' beliefs, culture, values and preferences and positively challenging discrimination when it occurs.

Being an effective leader involves modelling inclusive practice and supporting others to promote equality and rights; this unit will provide you with the knowledge to develop these skills as part of your day-to-day working practices and support you to challenge discrimination in ways that promote change.

Learning outcomes

By the end of this unit you will:

LO1: Understand influences on working practices to promote equality, diversity, inclusion and human rights

LO2: Understand the importance of equality, diversity, inclusion and human rights within own work setting/service

LO3: Know how to promote equality, diversity, inclusion and human rights

LO4: Be able to work in an inclusive way

LO1 Understand influences on working practices to promote equality, diversity, inclusion and human rights

AC 1.1 Identify current legislation, codes of practice and policy linked with equality, diversity, inclusion and human rights

AC 1.2 Explain how legislation, policies and codes of practice apply to and influence own work role

It is important that as a Lead Adult Care Worker you know about the main laws, policies and codes of practice so that you can work in an inclusive way and support others to do the same. It is also essential that your knowledge and practices are up-to-date in relation to understanding individuals' and others' rights to equality and diversity and your and others' responsibilities to prevent **discrimination**. UK and international laws relating to equality, diversity and discrimination set out the rights that people have as well as the responsibilities that you and others have to protect and uphold these.

The following laws are the main ones that relate to supporting equality, diversity, inclusion and preventing discrimination (it is important to note, however, that there may be changes to legislation as a result of the United Kingdom leaving the European Union).

Legislation related to equality, diversity, inclusion and human rights and how it applies and influences your role

The Human Rights Act 1998
This establishes the human rights and freedoms that everyone in the UK has. It promotes fairness, dignity and respect and protects these human rights from being infringed. You and others who work in adult health and social care will work in line with this Act which establishes the following rights and freedoms:

- Right to life: you and others will not deprive a person of their life.
- Freedom from torture: you and others will not subject a person to torture or to inhuman or degrading treatment or punishment.
- Freedom from slavery and forced labour: you and others will not hold a person in slavery or servitude or require them to carry out forced or compulsory labour.
- Right to liberty and security: you and others will not deprive a person of their liberty or make the person feel unsafe.
- Right to a fair trial: you and others will uphold a person's right to a fair and public hearing within a reasonable time that will be carried out both independently and impartially.
- Freedom from punishment without law: you and others will support a person's right to not be tried or convicted of a criminal offence under a retrospective law.
- Right to respect for private and family life: you and others will respect a person's privacy, family life, home and correspondence.
- Freedom of thought, conscience and religion: you and others will respect a person's right to have their own thoughts, beliefs and values, be able to practise these and change these.
- Freedom of expression: you and others will respect a person's views and opinions and to have information provided to them in an impartial and unbiased way.
- Freedom of assembly and association: you and others will uphold a person's rights to peaceful assembly and association with others such as a person's right to join a trade union.
- Right to marry: you and others will uphold a person's right to marry and found a family.
- Freedom from discrimination: you and others will uphold a person's rights to not be discriminated against when exercising their rights and freedoms under this Act.
- Right to protection of property: you and others will not deprive a person of their possessions or of their enjoyment of their possessions.
- Right to education: you and others will not deprive a person of accessing education in line with their beliefs.
- Right to free elections: you and others will uphold a person's right to express their opinions freely and take part in elections.

The Data Protection Act 1998
This promotes people's rights to be treated fairly in relation to their information and data. It also safeguards people from having their information and data misused or obtained unlawfully. You and others in adult health and social care will work in line with this Act which establishes the following rights:

- Right to have information and data processed fairly and lawfully: you and others will ensure

that an individual's permission has been sought before information is obtained from them and will only be shared with those who have the right or need to know it such as in emergency situations.
- Right to have information and data only used for the purpose it was intended: you and others will ensure that information gathered is only used for the purpose for which it was intended.
- Right to have only adequate and relevant information and data obtained: you and others will only obtain and use information that is relevant and needed.
- Right to have information and data kept up to date: you and others will ensure the information held about a person is accurate and up to date by verifying this with them.
- Right to have information and data kept only for as long as necessary: you and others will ensure that when information and data is no longer needed it is destroyed in line with your employer's agreed ways of working.
- Right to have information and data used in line with their preferences: you and others will ensure that a person knows what information is being held about them and how it is going to be used and you and others will support their rights to prevent their information being used when they no longer want it to be used.
- Right to have information and data kept secure: you and others will maintain the confidentiality of a person's information and data and ensure that it is kept secure in line with your employer's agreed ways of working.
- Right to not have information and data transferred to other countries: you and others will not transfer a person's information to other countries if a person has not given their permission because other countries may not have in place the required data protection requirements to keep information and data secure.

Data Protection Act 2018

The Data Protection Act 2018 is the UK's implementation of the EU's General Data Protection Regulation (GDPR) 2018. The Data Protection Act 2018 gives individuals greater rights over their personal information, stating the following:

- Organisations will have to demonstrate how they have obtained individuals' consent when handling information.
- Individuals will have the right to give and to withdraw their consent for processing information.
- Individuals' rights and interests must be safeguarded when information is being processed, for example to rectify inaccurate personal data.
- All public authorities must have a named data protection officer who is responsible for ensuring the organisation is complying with the Data Protection Act 2018 and is the main point of contact.

Special Educational Needs and Disability Act 2001

This promotes the rights of people with disabilities to have reasonable adjustments made by schools, colleges, universities, adult education providers, statutory youth services and local education authorities. It sets out the rights that people with disabilities are entitled to:

- Right to equal opportunities: to be offered the same opportunities and choices that people who do not have disabilities are offered.
- Right to support: to be offered support to make choices and participate such as through the provision of a specialist support person for an individual with a learning disability or the provision of teaching and learning materials in alternative formats such as in Braille for individuals who have sight loss.

You should also research the SEND Code of Practice 2014 which details legal requirements that you must follow without exception and statutory guidance that you must follow by law unless there is good reason not to.

The Mental Capacity Act 2005

This protects and promotes the rights of those people who are unable to make their own decisions due to a condition or disability, for example dementia, a learning difficulty or a head injury. It sets out the following rights that you and others who work in adult social care must protect and promote:

- Right to presumption of capacity you and others must not assume that an individual is unable to make their own decision (unless it is proven otherwise) because they have a condition or disability.
- Right to support for decision making: you and others must provide an individual with the support they require to make their own decisions, such as by providing information in a language or format that the individual understands, for example Braille or Makaton.

- **Right to making unwise decisions:** you and others must support an individual's right to make their own decisions that may be different to your own, even if you and others think they are unwise.
- **Right to best interest decisions:** you and others must make decisions on behalf of an individual who lacks capacity that are in their best interests only and be able to evidence why the decisions made are in the individual's best interests.
- **Right to least restrictive decisions:** you and others must ensure the decisions you make on behalf of an individual who lacks capacity are reasonable and the least restrictive option in terms of their rights and freedoms; for example, providing support to an individual who is prone to falling and requests to go a for a walk on their own in the garden is the least restrictive option as opposed to locking the garden door so that the individual cannot access their garden.

Note: Decisions must be made in the best interests of individuals where they lack capacity to make their own decisions about specific actions. Assessments are usually carried out by staff trained as Best Interest assessors.

Best interests are also mentioned in Unit 303 Understanding duty of care. You may find it useful to refer to that unit.

The Equality Act 2010

This protects people's rights to be treated fairly and safeguards people from being discriminated against because of their individual differences. It also promotes equality of opportunity. You and others who work in adult health and social care will work in line with this Act which establishes the following rights:

- **Right not to be discriminated against:** you and others must not discriminate either directly or indirectly against a person because of a protected characteristic; these are: age, disability, gender reassignment, marriage and civil partnership, pregnancy and maternity, race, religion, sex, sexual orientation. This includes the right not to be discriminated against because the person is associated with someone who has a protected characteristic.
- **Right to equal opportunities:** you and others must support a person's right to access goods, services, education, employment, housing and transport without being discriminated against. Pay secrecy clauses in employment are also unlawful.
- **Right to reasonable adjustments:** you and others must support the rights of a person with a disability to have adjustments made by service providers such as installing a ramp so that a person who uses a wheelchair can access the service.
- **Right to breastfeed in public:** you and others must support the rights of a woman to be able to breastfeed in public.
- **Right to take positive action:** you and others must support the rights of a person with a protected characteristic by taking positive action such as by encouraging a person to apply for a job where people with the same protected characteristic are under-represented.

The Care Act 2014

This protects the rights of those people who have care or support needs and their carers when being assessed and when being provided with care and support. It sets out the rights that you and others who work in adult social care must promote:

- **Right to wellbeing:** you and others must support the rights of a person to have their wellbeing promoted when making a decision such as their physical, mental, emotional, social and economic wellbeing.
- **Right to be in control:** you and others must support the rights of a person to be in control of their care or support, for example by involving them in all decisions made and empowering them to lead the decision-making process through for example an independent advocate.
- **Right to being safeguarded from abuse and neglect:** you and others must work together with other professionals and agencies to prevent abuse and neglect and learn from mistakes made.
- **Right to preventative services:** you and others must support the rights of a person to access services that help with reducing or delaying the need for care and support such as counselling and physiotherapy.

> ### Reflect on it
>
> **1.1, 1.2 Are you supporting people's rights?**
>
> Reflect on your and others' responsibilities to ensure that you are supporting people's human rights under relevant equality and diversity legislation. What legal responsibilities do you have? What moral responsibilities do you have? Why?

Local and national policies and how they apply to and influence your work role

Legislation forms the basis of local and national policies that are available in the UK and in the different settings where adult care services are provided. The setting where you work will have in place agreed ways of working for promoting equality and diversity and preventing discrimination in your day-to-day work. For example, there will be policies and procedures in place that relate to equal opportunities, confidentiality, equality and diversity, inclusion, confidentiality and safeguarding. These are essential for preventing discrimination and ensuring everyone is treated fairly and in line with their individual preferences and needs. They also help you and others where you work to carry out your job role and duties to a high standard and in line with best practice, and ensure that you and others are working within the requirements of the laws that are in place.

> **Research it**
>
> **1.1, 1.2 Agreed ways of working**
>
> Research your employer's agreed ways of working for promoting equality, diversity, inclusion and human rights. What do they say about discrimination?
>
> Discuss how you comply with these agreed ways of working in your day-to-day work.

The following are some examples of a range of national policies and initiatives that aim to promote a good understanding of equality, diversity, inclusion and human rights and to prevent discrimination from taking place in the UK.

Innovate UK: diversity and inclusion 2017
This initiative is between Innovate UK and The Prince's Trust and is aimed at engaging and inspiring young innovators from disadvantaged backgrounds to succeed in business. It provides young people from diverse backgrounds with support, advice and resources to succeed and contribute to the UK's business community and economy.

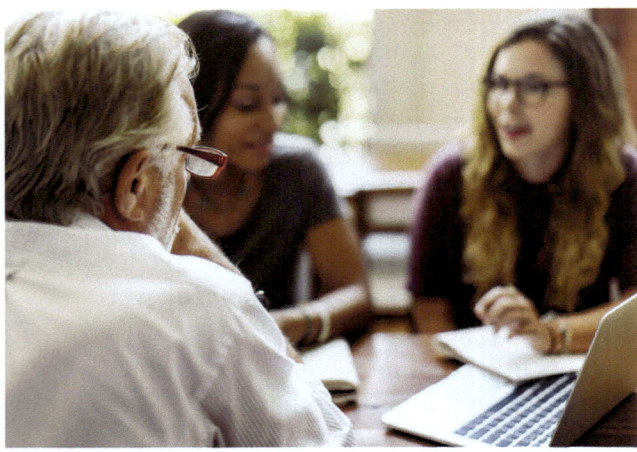

Figure 10.1 How do you and your team comply with equality and diversity legislation?

Disability Confident Employer Initiative 2014
This Department for Work and Pensions government-led initiative is a scheme that is designed to support employers to recruit and retain people with disabilities and encourage all employers to provide opportunities to ensure that people with disabilities and those with long-term health conditions are able to fulfil their potential at work. Its aim is to ensure that workplaces are open, diverse, accessible and inclusive.

The Care Certificate 2014
The Care Certificate is a set of standards that sets out the knowledge, skills and behaviours expected of specific job roles in the health and social care sectors. It is made up of 15 minimum standards. Standard 4 relates specifically to Equality and Diversity and covers understanding the importance of equality and inclusion, working in an inclusive way, as well as accessing information, advice and support about diversity, equality and inclusion. The Care Certificate was developed jointly by Skills for Care, Health Education England and Skills for Health.

Mindful Employer Initiative 2004

This established initiative is UK-wide and run by the Devon Partnership NHS Trust. It includes aspects such as being committed to ensuring that people who have mental health needs are not discriminated against during their recruitment and/or employment. For more information go to www.mindfulemployer.net

In addition, across the UK there are external organisations that are involved in regulating and inspecting health and social care services; one of their roles includes ensuring that these providers are delivering equal, diverse and inclusive services that are free from discrimination. For example, the Care Quality Commission (CQC) is the regulator of health and social care services for England. It registers, licenses, monitors and inspects services to ensure that they meet the standards of care required by law. These standards are known as the fundamental standards and they cover, among others, person-centred care, dignity and respect, safety and safeguarding from abuse.

> **Reflect on it**
>
> **1.1, 1.2 Local policies**
>
> Reflect on a local policy or initiative you have heard about that aims to increase awareness of equality, diversity, inclusion and human rights and prevent discrimination from taking place. Perhaps you heard about this on the radio or on television, or read about it online or in the newspaper. How successful was it? Why? Provide a reflective account.

The Equality and Human Rights Commission (EHRC) is a useful source of information and advice for both individuals and organisations in relation to their rights and responsibilities under equality law; it can also demand that organisations fulfil these. The National Institute for Health and Care Excellence (NICE) provides information, guidance and advice to the NHS and health and social care services on how to continuously improve their delivery.

Codes of practice and how they apply to and influence your work role

Codes of practice are sometimes also called codes of conduct. In this section we are referring to the codes of practice or conduct that provide guidance to help all those who work in health and social care, including those in positions of responsibility such as Lead Adult Care Workers, to comply with best practice and agreed ways of working relating to promoting equality and diversity and reducing and challenging discrimination. By following these codes of practice, you can aim to improve the quality of services being provided and establish the level and quality of care and support that everyone who uses these services can expect to receive.

Some organisations, such as Skills for Health and Skills for Care, have developed specific codes of conduct for their workforce that set out the agreed and expected standards of all those who work in health and social care. Other organisations, such as care providers, usually develop their own codes of conduct that they expect their employees to comply with. Perhaps you could find out if the care setting where you work has one in place and if so, what it says about equality, diversity, inclusion and discrimination. Below are some examples of codes of conduct that are in place for all those who work in adult care settings.

Code of Conduct for Healthcare Support Workers and Adult Social Care Workers in England

This is overseen by Skills for Health and Skills for Care and established the following principles for all those who work in health and adult care settings. It advises that all adult care workers should:

- be accountable for their actions or omissions, for example by ensuring all care or support provided to individuals is documented clearly, fully and accurately
- promote and uphold the privacy, dignity, rights, health and wellbeing of individuals and their carers who use care and support services at all times, for example by ensuring

your day-to-day work practices take into account their individual preferences and needs in relation to, for example, their communication, participation in activities, type of care or support
- work in partnership to ensure the delivery of high quality, safe and compassionate care and support by working together with your colleagues and employer
- communicate openly and effectively to promote individuals' and their carers' health, safety and wellbeing, for example by asking individuals and their carers how they want to be supported rather than make assumptions about what they require or what may meet their needs best
- respect a person's right to confidentiality, for example by supporting them to meet with their visitors in private
- be committed to continuing professional development to improve the quality of care and support provided, for example by attending an equality and diversity training update and supporting others to do the same
- promote equality, diversity and inclusion, for example by following best practice when providing care or support to individuals, supporting care workers to provide care or support to individuals or when monitoring their work practices.

Mental Capacity Code of Practice 2005

This supports the Mental Capacity Act 2005 and its five key principles. The Code of Practice provides guidance on how the five key principles of the Mental Capacity Act 2005 should be applied to those workers (like you) who work with or care for people who can't make decisions for themselves.

> **Evidence opportunity**
>
> **1.1, 1.2 How legislation, policy and codes of practice apply to and influence your role**
>
> Produce a leaflet that explains how you comply with equality, diversity and discrimination legislation, policy and codes of practice in your day-to-day work role. Make sure it explains how legislation, policy and codes of practice relating to equality, diversity and discrimination apply to your work role.

Fundamental standards

The CQC has some fundamental standards which individuals' care must never fall below. The standards state that individuals have the right, for example, to expect person-centred care (care that meets their unique needs and preferences), to be treated with dignity and respect, have their privacy maintained, to be treated equally and have their **social inclusion** promoted so that their independence is promoted.

AC 1.3 Explain how external factors influence own work role in relation to equality, diversity, inclusion and human rights

External factors can also influence working practices to promote equality, diversity, inclusion and human rights. These can range from **social movements**, campaigns, periods in modern history to family, friends, personal experiences, education and the media. The following table provides some examples of how external factors can influence your job role and working practices:

> **Key terms**
>
> **Social inclusion** means providing opportunities for individuals to participate and be involved in their wider communities so that they feel included, have a role and are part of society. This might be through accessing public transport, socialising with friends, accessing a course at a local college or participating in a local cultural event.
>
> **Social movements** refer to a group of people who come together to champion a cause and promote or prevent social, political, economic or cultural change, for example by engaging in demonstrations or picket lines.
>
> **National Dignity Council** is the lead body for the Dignity in Care campaign and supports Dignity Champions. It is made up of different organisations including health and social care organisations.
>
> **European Convention on Human Rights** protects the human rights of people that belong to the Council of Europe; it has 47 members and the UK is one of them.
>
> **European Court of Human Rights** is the Council of Europe's law court and it is based in Strasbourg, France.
>
> **Treaty** refers to a legally binding international agreement.

Table 10.1 Examples of external factors that can influence your work role

Examples of external factors	Examples of how external factors can influence working practices
Social movements	- The UK Women's Suffrage movement – a movement for gender equality that began in the mid-19th century and promoted the rights of women to vote and run for office. This movement has influenced working practices by making gender equality a human right. - The UK LGBTQ + movement – a movement for the rights of lesbian, gay, bisexual, transgender and queer people that raises awareness of the importance of equality and diversity and, for example, led to same-sex marriage being legalised in the UK in 2014. This movement has influenced working practices by raising awareness of issues of historical abuse and the rights of lesbian, gay, bisexual, transgender and queer people. - The Black Lives Matter movement – a movement set up in 2013 for the rights of Black people to live free from racism and violence. This movement has influenced working practices by raising awareness of the racism, discrimination and inequality experienced by Black people.
Campaigns	- The Dignity in Care Campaign – a campaign that was launched in 2006 and led by the **National Dignity Council** that aims to put the values of dignity and respect at the heart of UK care services. This campaign has influenced working practices by promoting the human right of dignity for everyone who accesses care services and improving the quality of care received. - The Disability Confident Campaign – a campaign that launched in 2014 to work with employers to remove barriers to employment for people with disabilities by improving how employers recruit, retain and develop people with disabilities. This campaign has influenced working practices by challenging attitudes towards people with disabilities so that people with disabilities can have the opportunity to access employment opportunities and reach their full potential.
Periods in modern history	- 1940-1950s period – in 1948 the Universal Declaration of Human Rights was established and set out the rights and freedoms that everyone is entitled to. It provided the foundation for the human rights that are protected in the UK today. It formed the basis in 1950 of the **European Convention on Human Rights** that was in turn incorporated in UK law by the Human Rights Act 1998. - 1960s period – in 1966 the UK granted people the right to take their cases of human rights breaches directly to the **European Court of Human Rights** in Strasbourg. In 1998, with the Human Rights Act incorporated into domestic law, people who lived in the UK could take their cases of human rights breaches directly to the British courts instead of to the courts in Strasbourg. It raised awareness of people's human rights. - 21st century period – in 2008 the UN Convention on the Rights of Persons with Disabilities (UNCRPD) was the first human rights **treaty** to be established in the 21st century. It raised awareness of the human rights of people with disabilities to become full and equal citizens.
Family, friends, others	- Family – family can influence your work role and practices in terms of your family background and upbringing with respect to culture, beliefs, values such as respect, trust and inclusion. - Friends – friends can also influence your work role and practices in terms of diverse opinions, views and the development of friendships through mutual trust, respect and inclusion. - Others – others such as your colleagues, peers, managers and professionals from other services can have an impact on your work role and work practices by working with you and demonstrating best practice in relation to how to promote equality, diversity, inclusion and human rights in the work setting.

Table 10.1 Examples of external factors that can influence your work role *continued*

Examples of external factors	Examples of how external factors can influence working practices
Personal experiences	• A positive personal experience – seeing how a family member you've cared for when they were unwell has benefited from your respectful care and support will highlight how important it is to promote human rights in care and the difference it makes. • A negative personal experience – being treated unfairly and discriminated against will influence how you carry out your job role as your experience will give you an insight into the negative effects that not promoting equality and inclusion can have on an individual. • A negative personal experience – being excluded from a service will influence how you carry out your job role, as your experience may make you mistakenly believe that it is not possible to promote inclusion in services for everyone.
Education	• Training – participating in equality and diversity training arranged by your employer in the work setting can influence your job role and work practices by ensuring you understand what is involved in promoting equality, diversity, inclusion and human rights. • Courses, policies and procedures – furthering your knowledge and understanding by undertaking courses and reading your employer's policies and procedures on equality and diversity can improve your knowledge and understanding in this area of up-to-date practices. • Learning from others – others in your work setting such as an experienced colleague or your manager can be sources of good support in relation to responding to any concerns or questions you may have in relation to promoting equality, diversity, inclusion and human rights.
The media	• TV/Radio/Newspapers – these media sources can raise your awareness of the promotion of equality, diversity and inclusion by sharing people's experiences (both negative and positive) as well as organisations leading by example. What you see, hear and read about will influence what you do. • Social media – social media platforms such as Facebook, YouTube and Instagram can highlight the importance of issues in relation to equality, diversity, inclusion and human rights through campaigns and by getting people to chat, engage and share their views, opinions and experiences. The social media you engage in will in turn raise your awareness of current issues that may be impacting on your community and work setting. • Billboards, leaflets, posters – these sources are usually designed and promoted by organisations to draw your attention to important issues in relation to equality and diversity and make you think about how you can help. These may also be displayed in your work setting and can therefore impact on your job role and work practices.

Reflect on it

1.3 External influences on work practices

Reflect on your work practices in relation to promoting equality, diversity, inclusion and human rights. Identify the three external factors that influence your work practices the most. Think about how they influence you. How do they impact on the care and support you provide?

Evidence opportunity

1.3 External factors and your role

Discuss with your manager how external factors influence your work role in relation to equality, diversity, inclusion and human rights.

LO2 Understand the importance of equality, diversity, inclusion and human rights within own work setting/service

> **Getting started**
>
> Write a profile about yourself that explains what makes you unique. Now write a profile for two other people you know well; these could be friends or members of your family. Describe three ways you are all different and three ways you are all similar. For example, you may be from different backgrounds and have different interests or you may be of similar ages and have similar personalities.
>
> Why do you think differences are important? How can differences enhance your relationships with others?

AC 2.1 Define the meaning of: a) diversity, b) equality, c) inclusion, d) discrimination, e) unconscious bias, f) protected characteristics, g) human rights

AC 2.2 Explain the relevance to own practice of: a) diversity, b) equality, c) inclusion, d) discrimination, e) unconscious bias, f) protected characteristics, g) human rights

A) Understanding diversity in adult care settings

People are varied in many different ways, such as in where they live, how they look, how old they are, what interests they have, what their family background is, what experiences they have, what opinions they have, what skills they have, and what beliefs they hold. Adult care settings are part of the UK's diverse society and are therefore also diverse. For example, there are:

- a wide range of different types of adult care settings, such as residential care homes, nursing homes, supported living schemes and individuals' own homes
- different services provided in these, such as healthcare and social care
- different individuals accessing these, such as adults, children, young people and individuals from different backgrounds with different needs, abilities, preferences, cultures, beliefs and values
- different people working in these with different skills, knowledge, levels of expertise, qualifications, job roles, backgrounds and from different cultures.

Your job role will mean that you will need to be able to provide care and support to individuals with different needs and abilities and support others to do the same. In order to do this effectively you will need to recognise that all individuals are unique and have their own specific preferences, cultures, beliefs and values; these will not only differ to those of other individuals but may also be different to your own. This is true whatever your nationality, religion, race, gender or sexuality. You will need to be able to develop the ability to put your own beliefs and values to one side and support others to do the same so that you and others can genuinely promote individuals' right to be different – the basis of all high-quality care and support.

We are living through a pivotal time in history, a social revolution, especially with regards to the rights of lesbian, gay, bisexual, transgender and queer (LGBTQ+) people. This renewed awareness of the importance of diversity and equality has led to same-sex marriage being legalised in the UK in 2014 and the first same-sex marriages taking place in the same year, as well as an increase in the open discussion of women's rights and issues around historical abuse. These discussions are now occupying an important place in the political arena and are crucial to social change.

Your job role will also involve you working alongside people with differing levels of expertise; some of your colleagues will be more experienced than you, others will not and will look to you for guidance and support. You will need to be able to adapt your working practices and approaches so that you can listen and learn from your colleagues but also be able to provide support, guidance and advice when it is needed from you. The colleagues you work with will be from a range of different backgrounds and cultures and may have beliefs and values that are different from your own. Recognising and valuing these differences will mean that you will be able to work effectively together and learn from one another because everyone will feel valued and respected. Not doing so will make working relationships between you and others difficult and will create tension within the team as a whole.

B) Understanding equality

Equality involves valuing people as individuals and treating people fairly. It involves showing your respect for people's individuality and respecting their rights as well as ensuring that they are provided with equal access to life opportunities. Treating people equally does not mean treating everyone the same.

In the UK equality did not always exist until the government brought in laws to prevent people from being treated unequally and therefore unfairly. (This unfair treatment of people is referred to as discrimination. You will learn more about what this involves later on in this section and about the associated legislation in AC 2.1).

Inequalities in the UK still unfortunately form part of our society. For example, only recently did the media report that some women doing the same jobs as men as television presenters were being paid less than their male colleagues. This led to companies investigating the **gender pay gap** in their organisations to look at the difference between the earnings of men and women. Older people also continue to be treated less favourably with, for example, the government making cuts to their care funding. Equality in the UK is essential for everyone to be able to exercise their rights and improve their lives.

> **Key term**
>
> The **gender pay gap** refers to the difference in the hourly earnings between men and women.

> **6Cs**
>
> **Commitment**
>
> You will need to be committed or dedicated to promoting equality, diversity and inclusion in the setting, and working in a person-centred way in order to uphold the individuality and rights of the individuals and others you work with, ensuring that their experiences of care and support and working with you are positive. This is important so that individuals and others feel valued, are able to live according to their preferences and can fulfil their job roles and responsibilities effectively. You can show that you are committed to promoting equality, diversity and inclusion as well as person-centred values, by treating each person with respect and showing a genuine interest in their preferences, experiences, and background.
>
> How do you show that you work positively alongside individuals with care or support needs? How do you show that you work positively alongside other team members? What qualities do you show when working together with your colleagues? How can working with diverse individuals further develop your knowledge and skills?

Equality in adult care settings

Equality underpins all high-quality care and support provided in adult care settings. You can treat individuals fairly and respectfully, for example, by ensuring that you find out about and respect their unique needs and preferences in terms of, how they communicate, the choices they make with respect to their daily living tasks and how they live their lives. You can ensure that individuals have access to the life opportunities available to everyone else by not making assumptions about what they are capable of or not and by focusing on their strengths. Treating individuals in a way that denies their rights to individuality and does not respect their differences will make them feel devalued and isolated and will subject them to unfair and unequal treatment.

Equality must also underpin your current work practices and associated job role responsibilities in order to comply with your employer's agreed ways of working and all relevant legislation. You can treat the people you work with fairly and respectfully by ensuring that the way you communicate and interact with them is polite and takes account of their needs and views, which may be different to your own. For example, you may work with an individual's family who are from a different culture to yours. It is important that you find out from them about their culture and beliefs rather than make assumptions as they may have their own practices and customs that are unique to them. In this way, you can ensure that your behaviour and actions are not offensive or misinterpreted by other people.

Remember that promoting equality and diversity is one of the standards and behaviours expected of you as a Lead Adult Care Worker or Lead Personal Assistant; you will find it useful to review your knowledge about this in Unit 313 Continuous development when working in an adult care worker role, AC 2.1. Maintaining equality in the care setting where you work, in the community where you live and in society in general will mean that you will be contributing to an environment where instability and misunderstandings are avoided and instead positive feelings and relationships are created.

C) Understanding inclusion

Inclusion involves creating an environment where people are, and feel, involved in day-to-day life. This can only happen when people feel their differences are valued, treated fairly and respected and they are supported to take part in aspects of living that they enjoy, are interested in or want to be involved in. Inclusion is not about finding reasons why people are unable to take an active part or why people need to be excluded but rather it is about finding the best ways to provide people with the right type and amount of support that they need to do what they want to do. Being included is something everyone aspires to because it is part of our human nature – most of us do not want to live our lives in isolation but instead enjoy sharing our lives with others such as our families and friends. Being included creates feelings of warmth and gives us a sense of belonging and purpose. Being excluded leads to people being discriminated against and marginalised as well as communities and society being deprived of diverse people, knowledge, skills and experiences. You will learn more about discrimination and its associated effects in LO3.

Inclusion in adult care settings

Your role as a Lead Adult Care Worker or Lead Personal Assistant involves creating a sense of inclusion for all those you work with. In terms of the individuals with care or support needs that you work with it is important that you are committed to providing the support they need to have a sense of purpose or meaning to their lives, and that you are able to support other team members to do the same. For example, when a newly recruited team member confides in you that they are finding it difficult to fit in because everyone else in the setting knows each other, you can act as a good role model by empowering them to play an active part in the team by ensuring they are given opportunities to share their ideas and contributions in discussions and team meetings and are not excluded by others in these. You may also decide that you can actively support them by ensuring that they work alongside the members of the team who will give them the confidence to be themselves and feel they belong.

D) Understanding discrimination

Discrimination is what occurs when equality, diversity and inclusion have not been promoted or successfully implemented. Discrimination involves treating individuals or groups of people unfairly or unequally. It occurs when people:

- **stereotype:** this involves having beliefs about, or making generalisations or assumptions about people that are negative and not based on fact, for example that all young people are lazy, or all older people are frail

- **label:** this involves placing negative labels on people that single them out from others and make them feel unworthy or devalued, for example 'gingers' (based on people's hair colour), or offensive labels based on people's race and ethnicity or gender
- **are prejudiced:** this involves having an untrue, biased, preconceived opinion about people that is not based on facts or reason but is based on people's belonging in a certain group, for example all immigrants are thieves, or all adults with autism cannot communicate
- **are denied their rights:** this involves preventing people from having and exercising the rights they are entitled to, for example privacy, dignity, respect, and to live safely free from harm and abuse
- **are oppressed:** this involves the misuse of power, for example a Lead Adult Care Worker misusing their position of authority to ensure an individual does not refuse their medication, or a Lead Personal Assistant misusing their position of authority to prevent an individual from complaining about their care
- **are disempowered:** this involves the loss of control over one's life, for example not providing individuals with choices, or not taking into account a team member's opinions when agreeing on a new way of working.

It is important that we are aware of our own prejudices because we all have some and they will affect how we think about other people and therefore how we treat them.

> ### Reflect on it
> #### 2.1 Your prejudices
> Reflect on the prejudices you think you may have and where you think they have come from. Why are these negative? What steps can you take to ensure that they do not affect your interactions with others, or impact on your working practices in negative ways?

Types of discrimination
In the UK, it is unlawful to discriminate against a person based on their age, gender, marital/civil partnership status, being pregnant or on maternity leave, their disability, race including colour, nationality, ethnic or national origin, religion, belief or lack of religion/belief or sex and sexual orientation. These characteristics are referred to as the 'protected characteristics'. There is more on this in AC 2.1F.

The following types of discrimination are recognised in the UK and everyone is protected from these by the Equality Act 2010.

- **Direct discrimination:** treating someone with a protected characteristic unfairly and less favourably than others. For example, excluding an individual from a service because of their disability.
- **Indirect discrimination:** putting rules or procedures in place that apply to everyone, but that put someone with a protected characteristic at an unfair disadvantage. For example, offering Christian church servises in a care setting will exclude individuals who follow different religions or no religion.
- **Harassment:** unwanted physical, verbal or non-verbal behaviour linked to a protected characteristic that violates someone's dignity or creates an offensive environment for them. For example, ridiculing a person in front of others because they are changing gender/identifying with a different gender.
- **Victimisation:** treating someone unfairly because they have complained about discrimination or harassment. For example, excluding an individual's family member from a meeting for all individuals' families because they have complained about a team member's negative behaviour towards their relative.

Source: *Discrimination: your rights: How you can be discriminated against – GOV.UK*

Discrimination in adult care settings
Adult care settings are environments where individuals with care and support needs live and people work; everyone in adult care settings has a right to live and work safely and be free from being discriminated against. If you become aware that a person with a protected characteristic in the care setting where you work is being discriminated against then you have a duty of care to support them; this is referred to as taking positive action and is lawful under the Equality Act 2010. Taking positive action involves

employers helping people with a protected characteristic if they:

- are disadvantaged from accessing employment or their active participation is low
- are disadvantaged from accessing training or their active participation is low
- have specific needs that are different to people without their protected characteristic.

Employers can reduce the potential for people with a protected characteristic being discriminated against by, for example, offering them a work placement or providing them with additional support to access and participate in training. As a Lead Adult Care Worker, you will also be expected to follow your employer's agreed ways of working for taking positive action. How effective you are will depend on how committed you are to taking positive action and ensuring that you are able to prevent people from being discriminated against. For example, if an individual with a physical disability told you that they were refused entry to a cinema because the lift was not working, what positive action could you take? Perhaps you could support the individual to write a letter of complaint to the cinema or suggest to the individual that they request a meeting to discuss their experience with the cinema's owners. What would you do and why? How would the actions you take prevent the individual from further discrimination?

You need to be aware of 'institutional racism' that exists in institutions such as care settings and society more generally before you can try to tackle it.

E) Understanding unconscious bias

Unconscious bias involves unfairly showing favouritism or prejudice towards a person or group. It occurs when we make generalisations or assumptions about people that are negative and not based on fact, i.e. stereotypes. You will find it useful to refer back to the earlier section 'Understanding discrimination' that details more about stereotypes, labels and prejudices, including what they are and how they are created.

Although you may think of yourself as a fair person and not prejudiced, unconscious bias can happen to everyone because you may have been exposed to stereotypes. For example, you may have been exposed to what it means in society to have a good education level, i.e. higher education or a degree and these ideas may have also been reinforced by others such as your family, friends and teachers. These ideas can then influence your decisions and make you decide whether a person has a good education level, i.e. anything lower than a degree you may disregard.

Types of unconscious bias

Unconscious bias can take many forms and by improving your awareness of these you'll gain a greater insight into your own personal biases. Some of the common types of unconscious bias are included in the following list:

- **Affinity bias:** being favourable towards a person because they share similarities with you such as in relation to age, personality, skills or background. For example, you spend more time with a colleague during training because they are of a similar background.
- **Attribution bias:** attributing a person's successes to external factors rather than to them which can lead to you not recognising their achievements and instead focusing too much on their faults. For example, you consider a colleague's achievement on a course as luck rather than because they studied and worked hard.
- **Beauty bias:** making assumptions about a person's personality and skills based on their physical appearance. For example, you believe that an individual who looks untidy will be difficult to work with, when the opposite may be true.
- **Conformity bias:** when your decisions are influenced by the views and opinions of others instead of making your own judgements. For example, you agree with your colleagues over how to best support an individual to mobilise when your opinions of how to do so differ.
- **Confirmation bias:** when you make judgements and draw conclusions about another person based on your own personal experience and views rather than looking at the person as a whole and considering the facts. For example, you observe an individual on one occasion being verbally abusive towards a colleague and so you assume that this individual is aggressive; then every time you support this individual you actively look for signs that they may become aggressive through for instance their body language or tone of voice.

- **Contrast effect:** when you form an opinion by comparing two or more similar things rather than considering each one based on their own merits. For example, when involved in recruiting a member of staff you look at the applications of two applicants who have similar levels of experience of working in the health and social care sector and compare their application forms for spelling and grammatical errors rather than consider which applicant is most suitable for the role.
- **Gender bias:** showing your preference for one gender over another. For example, when recruiting participants for a new knitting group you subconsciously think that a woman will be more interested in this activity and so specifically seek out women through your recruitment campaign.
- **Halo effect:** focusing on a single positive aspect of a person and viewing everything about the person as positive without considering other information about them such as negative aspects. For example, seeing a senior colleague as perfect in everything they do may skew your opinion of them and of any bad practices they carry out.
- **Horns effect:** focusing on a single negative aspect of a person and viewing everything about the person as negative without considering other information about them such as positive aspects; the opposite of the halo effect. For example, seeing a senior colleague as incompetent in everything they do may skew your opinion of them and of any good practices they carry out.

Unconscious bias in adult care settings

Unconscious bias is unfair and can lead to making false assumptions about people that can in turn result in negative outcomes for them. Being aware of unconscious bias and how stereotypes, even if we don't believe in them, can subconsciously influence our decisions by being present in the world around us will enable us to be in control of our actions and the decisions we make.

As a Lead Adult Care Worker or Lead Personal Assistant you can overcome unconscious bias and support others to do the same by identifying stereotypes, biases and assumptions when they occur and by putting them to one side when providing care and support to individuals. Instead, you must focus on the individual and get to know and understand the individual; this way of working is referred to as the person-centred approach and you will learn more about this concept in Unit 306 Promoting and implementing person-centred practice. The person-centred approach puts individuals at the very heart of the care and support they receive, helping them to feel in control of their lives and promoting their rights to make their own choices and decisions. In this way, you can ensure that the care and support provided meets individuals' unique needs, views and preferences and leads to positive outcomes for them.

F) Understanding protected characteristics

The Equality Act 2010 safeguards and protects people by making it unlawful to discriminate and treat people unfairly because of their characteristics or aspects of their identity. Under the Equality Act there are nine protected characteristics:

- Age, including any age group
- Disability, including physical or mental impairment
- Gender reassignment, including anyone who is planning to undergo, is undergoing or has undergone the process for reassigning their sex
- Marriage and civil partnership, for example whether or not a person is married or in a civil partnership
- Pregnancy and maternity
- Race, for example ethnic background
- Religion or belief, including any religion, religious or philosophical belief, as well as no religion or belief
- Sex, for example that women should not be treated differently from men
- Sexual orientation, – who someone is attracted to

Source: Gov.uk, Equality Act 2010, Sections 5-12.
www.legislation.gov.uk/ukpga/2010/15/section/5

These nine protected characteristics are important because they mean that discrimination or unfair treatment because of any of these is against the law. However, there are legal exemptions under the Equality Act 2010, for example for occupational requirements for a certain role only to be open to men.

Protected characteristics in adult care settings

As you will have learned, it is unlawful to discriminate against a person on the basis of their protected characteristics and as a Lead Adult Care Worker you have a duty of care to support anyone in the care setting where you work with a protected characteristic from being discriminated against, e.g. an individual, an individual's family, a colleague, a professional from another service and/or visitors.

For more details about how this relates to your own practice you will find it useful to refer back to the section 'Discrimination in adult care settings' as well as your employer's agreed ways of working for supporting people with protected characteristics against discrimination, i.e. referred to as taking positive action.

G) Understanding human rights

The Equality and Human Rights Commission defines human rights as:

- the basic rights and freedoms that belong to everyone from birth until death irrespective of where you are from, what you believe or how you choose to live your life
- the basic rights and freedoms that can never be taken away
- the basic rights and freedoms that are based on values such as dignity, fairness, equality, respect and independence

Source: The Equality and Human Rights Commission, What are human rights?

www.equalityhumanrights.com/en/human-rights/what-are-human-rights

The Human Rights Act 1998 established the human rights and freedoms that everyone in the UK has and protects all of us from having our rights and freedoms abused; if they are, then we have a right to defend our rights in the UK law courts. For more details about the rights and freedoms we have under the Human Rights Act you will find it useful to refer back to AC 1.1, 'The Human Rights Act 1998'.

Human rights in adult care settings

As a Lead, you must ensure that you and others respect everyone's human rights in the care setting where you work; in this way you will be creating a positive and welcoming environment where individuals can live and others can work free from discrimination and abuse. Another important way you can get involved in protecting and actively promoting individuals' human rights where you work is by ensuring that you take their rights into account when making decisions about their day-to-day lives. For example, when providing an individual with support you can act as a positive role model by asking them how they want to be supported. In this way, they are in control of how their needs are met and you can show that you are respecting their views and right to make their own choices. The support you provide to individuals will also be underpinned by a set of values, commonly referred to as person-centred values that will actively promote their human rights. You will learn more about person-centred values and their relevance to your own practice in Unit 306, Promoting and implementing person-centred practice.

> **Evidence opportunity**
>
> **2.1 Equality, diversity, inclusion and human rights**
>
> Discuss with your assessor what is meant by equality, diversity, inclusion and human rights in the care setting where you work. Think about the meaning of diversity from the perspective of:
>
> 1. the individuals you work with
> 2. your colleagues, and
> 3. others who visit the care setting where you work, such as individuals' families and other professionals.
>
> Provide a written account to document your discussion or if you haven't discussed this, then just provide an explanation of what is meant by each one.

AC 2.3 Explain how inclusive practice and cultures promote equality, diversity, inclusion and human rights within own work setting/service

AC 2.4 Explain how the promotion of equality, diversity, inclusion and human rights can lead to improved outcomes for individuals

Inclusive practice and cultures are essential for preventing discrimination from taking place because working in inclusive ways promotes equality and diversity by supporting people's human rights to be treated fairly and have their differences taken into account and valued so that they can be included.

Below are some examples of the different ways that inclusive practice and cultures can promote equality, inclusion and human rights. You will learn more about how you can promote a culture that supports inclusive practices in AC 4.2.

Promoting equality and human rights

Inclusive practice and cultures can promote equality and human rights by:

- **Upholding people's human rights:** for example, to be treated fairly; not to be discriminated against or harmed; to privacy; to dignity.
- **Respecting people:** for example, as citizens living in the UK; as experts in their own care and support; by understanding and valuing their differences.
- **Fostering equal opportunities:** for example, by familiarising yourself with your work setting's equal opportunities or equality policy; by providing information and training for people in a format that they can understand; by adapting working practices when a person's needs change.
- **Not tolerating or engaging in discrimination:** for example, by challenging and reporting discrimination in line with agreed ways of working; by using inclusive working practices. You will learn more about how to challenge discrimination positively in AC 3.3.

> **Reflect on it**
>
> **2.3 Your working practices**
>
> Reflect on your last week at work. How many examples can you think of where your working practices promoted equality in the setting where you work? Were there any occasions where you found this difficult to do? Why? What needs to be put in place to address these areas of inequality?

Promoting diversity and inclusion

Inclusive practice and cultures can promote diversity and inclusion by:

- **Being committed to inclusive practice:** for example, by working in ways that promote equality and diversity; by familiarising yourself with your work setting's diversity policy; by participating in diversity training.
- **Encouraging opportunities for diversity and inclusion:** for example, by actively finding out about people's differences; by encouraging people to talk about their differences and how they can be supported; by involving individuals in planning their care or support.
- **Promoting diversity:** for example, by providing information and training to people in diverse ways such as through the use of diverse images in the setting's marketing information; by taking into account people's differences such as their beliefs, values and preferences.
- **Providing high-quality care or support:** for example, by ensuring all care and support is centred on the individual and fulfils your duty of care.

Improved outcomes for individuals

Promoting equality, diversity, inclusion and human rights can lead to improved outcomes for individuals by:

- **Creating an inclusive environment:** i.e. an environment where everyone feels included, valued, has their differences respected and is able to reach their full potential.
- **Building positive relationships:** i.e. by instilling confidence, trust, mutual respect and by developing effective communication.
- **Developing effective team work:** effective team work means that individuals will be placed at the heart of their care and support, i.e. where everyone feels like they belong, have a purpose, work together and learn from each other.
- **Developing effective working practices:** effective working practices means that individuals will benefit from a range of skills, knowledge and best practices, i.e. where new skills, knowledge and working approaches are shared, discussed and developed and where new ideas are actively encouraged.

Evidence opportunity

2.3, 2.4 Inclusive practice and cultures in your setting

Produce a short presentation that explains how your work setting/service promotes equality, diversity, inclusion and human rights through inclusive practice and cultures and is in line with your employer's agreed ways of working.

Case study

2.1, 2.2, 2.3, 4.1, 4.2 Promoting equality, diversity, inclusion and human rights

Rachel is a Lead Personal Assistant and is responsible for managing the staff work rota. Rachel ensures that she takes into account wherever possible the needs of both staff and individuals when developing the staff rota. In terms of staff needs, Rachel takes into account that Personal Assistant Nina has requested to not work Sunday mornings because she attends church, Personal Assistant Michael has requested time off this month to support his partner, and Lead Personal Assistant Monica has requested to work only mornings so that she can support her sister with the care of their father.

In terms of supporting Josh who has autism with his needs, Rachel ensures she takes into account, when developing the staff rota, Josh's preferences to be supported by Michael when he goes swimming on a Saturday afternoon and to have two personal assistants support him when he visits his family in East London as he finds the train journey very stressful.

Rachel is also responsible as a Lead PA for handling any concerns and complaints that are received about Josh's care and support. Josh has spoken to Rachel in confidence and has informed her that he feels uncomfortable when Nina works on a Sunday afternoon because she talks a lot about going to church on a Sunday and keeps asking him whether he would like her to take him to her church. Josh has asked Rachel to speak to Nina because he does not want to offend her by saying 'no', but also does not want her to keep on talking to him about her church.

Discuss:

1. How is Rachel supporting diversity and inclusion?
2. How is Rachel promoting equality and human rights?
3. How can Rachel address Josh's concerns? How are Nina's actions affecting Josh?
4. What should Rachel say to Josh?
5. What should Rachel say to Nina?

AC 2.5 Describe how own service promotes equality, diversity, inclusion and human rights

Your work setting will have in place agreed ways of working for promoting equality, diversity, inclusion and human rights. For example, there will be policies and procedures in place and codes of practice that relate to treating individuals and others fairly and preventing discrimination. You will find it useful to refer back to LO1, ACs 1.1 and 1.2, that details examples of these. In addition, services can also promote equality, diversity, inclusion and human rights in the following ways:

- Providing information – services can provide individuals and others with training to inform them about the legislation that is in place.
- Raising awareness – services can make individuals and others aware of the policies, procedures and codes of conduct that are in place through for example information updates, discussions in meetings, leaflets and posters.
- Having a responsible person in place – services can have a named person in place who has responsibility for the promotion of equality, diversity, inclusion and human rights in the work setting.
- Monitoring practices – services can monitor people's working practices and also their own in relation to how the service operates when selecting individuals and recruiting team members and others for the setting.
- Consulting with individuals and others – services can actively seek individuals' and others' feedback, ideas and suggestions for improving the promotion of equality, diversity, inclusion and human rights.

> ### Reflect on it
>
> **2.5 Promotion of equality, diversity, inclusion and human rights in your work setting**
>
> What's your work setting doing? Reflect on your service and the different ways it promotes equality, diversity, inclusion and human rights. What does it do well? How does this impact on your job role? How does this impact on individuals and others?

> ### Evidence opportunity
>
> **2.5 How your service promotes equality, diversity, inclusion and human rights**
>
> Produce a short presentation that details the type of service you work in and how it promotes equality, diversity, inclusion and human rights.

AC 2.6 Describe own role in promoting equality, diversity, inclusion and human rights

This AC requires you to show your understanding of how your role promotes equality, diversity, inclusion and human rights. It is important that you know how to do this because as a Lead Adult Care Worker or Lead Personal Assistant you will be expected to be a good role model and demonstrate your knowledge and expertise in promoting equality and rights and supporting others such as team members, colleagues, individuals, their families, carers and advocates to do the same.

Below we discuss some of the things you will need to instil so you can support others to promote equality, diversity, inclusion and human rights.

> ### Reflect on it
>
> **2.6 Discrimination and promoting equality and human rights**
>
> Reflect on how you would feel if you were being discriminated against at work. Why? Now imagine that when you reported your concerns you were not treated seriously and continued to be discriminated against. How do you think you would feel?
>
> Now think about the importance of ensuring that no one at work is discriminated against. How do you promote equality at work? How do you promote human rights at work?

Promoting equality, diversity and inclusion

Be aware of your own prejudices

To be able to promote equality, diversity and inclusion effectively you must be aware of your own prejudices and ensure that these do not affect the ways you work. Openly acknowledging that you have prejudices and that you are aware of your own prejudices can encourage other team members and individuals' families, carers and advocates to do the same. In this way, you and others can work together to find effective ways of not letting your own prejudices affect your practices. For example, you may discuss with individuals' families whether and how they would like to be involved in their relative's care or support rather than make assumptions that may be not true or unfair about which families would like to be involved.

Lead by example
You can support others to promote equality, diversity and inclusion by leading by example. If you treat others fairly by valuing their individuality, then you will earn their respect and trust and you will be more likely to instil in them a desire to do the same. You can show that you value a person's individuality by not making any assumptions about what they like, need or prefer.

Respect differences
You can also provide support to others by showing that you respect their differences. For example, you can show how you take these into account when communicating with individuals by using their preferred means of communication or by ensuring you ask your colleagues how they would like you to take into account any customs or practices they follow as part of their background and culture. Again, individuals will then be more likely to do the same because they will see you doing this in your day-to-day work.

Say when equality, diversity, inclusion and human rights are not being promoted
Supporting others to promote equality, diversity and inclusion also involves having the **courage** to say when this isn't happening. For example, if you observe a carer or family member using discriminatory language towards an individual then you must inform them that this is not acceptable. You may feel awkward in doing so, however, you should not worry about the views of others if you are challenging discrimination. It is essential you take action because if you do not then the carer may continue to practise in this way, unaware that their practices are not promoting equality and the individual may believe that you do not support equality because you haven't said anything or taken any action. You will learn more about how to challenge discrimination in a way that promotes change in AC 3.3.

Promoting human rights, equality, diversity and inclusion

Set a positive example
You can support others to promote human rights by ensuring that you set a positive example in respecting the human rights of individuals and all those you work with at all times. As you will have already learned, this is part of providing person-centred care and support. You may want to refer to Unit 306 Promoting and implementing person-centred practice, where this concept is explored in detail. You can do this in your day-to-day work activities, for example by supporting individuals to do tasks for themselves rather than doing these for them. You should also ensure that achievements are celebrated to further promote the self-esteem and wellbeing of individuals.

Lead by example
You can lead by example by supporting people's human rights not to be discriminated against and to be treated equally, inclusively and as unique individuals. You can do this, for example, by supporting individuals to speak up when they are being discriminated against. This may involve you supporting the individual to write a letter or to arrange a meeting to discuss their concerns. By doing this, you are empowering them to take control and to be confident, which in turn can reduce their vulnerability and the likelihood of discrimination occurring. It also creates a positive working environment where anti-discriminatory practices are supported and encouraged and therefore where discrimination is less likely to occur.

Understand difference
It is important that you understand the factors that make people different and how they may be discriminated against because of these differences. This will involve you making an effort to understand what people's human rights are and what your duties are with respect to promoting

equality, inclusion and diversity in the care setting where you work. This means that you will be able to understand and follow the agreed ways of working that are required for ensuring that discrimination does not occur.

Your manager, supervisor or employer is a good source of advice and support, particularly when you have to report discriminatory practices. They can also help when you want to clarify your understanding of your role and responsibilities in relation to supporting others to promote equality and rights. Keeping your knowledge and skills up to date as a Lead Adult Care Worker or Lead Personal Assistant in relation to promoting equality will ensure that you are able to support others in line with current best practice. For example, you may attend an equality training update in your work setting or read an article about best practice when promoting equality with individuals who have care and support needs. You could then share the knowledge and skills you have developed with others through team meetings, one-to-one and group discussions and by contributing to your employer's training updates and/or agreed ways of working. In this way you can ensure that you and others are working consistently and in line with current best practice. You can make arrangements for training through your manager and during the supervision process as part of the personal development plan (PDP) process. You may want to refer to Unit 313 Continuous development when working in an adult care worker role, where this is discussed in more detail.

Specialist organisations such as the Equality and Human Rights Commission (EHRC) provide useful information, advice and support on promoting diversity, equality and inclusion. They may be able to share with you their ideas and/or case studies that demonstrate best practice. You can seek advice from their specialist advisers and read about best practices in the adult care sector and current legislation. Third sector and voluntary groups such as the Alzheimer's Society, Mind, Age UK and local support groups for individuals with care or support needs can also provide useful information, advice and support for ensuring that you are able to support individuals' rights to diversity, equality and inclusion. Individuals may need support to access information provided in leaflets about their condition, or to attend a support group for people who have the same condition.

6Cs

Courage

Courage refers to ensuring that you positively challenge any discriminatory practices you see and that you know may impact negatively on individuals and others you work with. You can do this by not ignoring them and by ensuring that you report them as soon as they happen. Being courageous in supporting equality and inclusion will mean that you will be contributing to a discrimination-free environment. This is because you will be doing everything you can to challenge it and prevent it from occurring again.

Competence

Competence refers to effectively applying the knowledge and skills you have learned consistently and accurately so that you are able to provide good quality support to others in line with agreed ways of working. It is important that you know what to do if you are unable to promote equality, diversity, inclusion or human rights during your day-to-day working practices and that those you are supporting know that you are doing your best to work in inclusive ways and support their human rights to be included and treated fairly. In this section, you can show that you know the process to follow for accessing information, advice and support from your work setting, and that you can support others to promote equality and rights. You can do this by following the advice that is offered here, as well as discussing this with your manager and colleagues.

> **Research it**
>
> **1.1, 1.2, 2.6 Sources of support**
>
> Being aware of all the different sources of information, advice and support available on diversity, equality, inclusion and human rights is essential for supporting others to do the same. Remember that you can refer to colleagues, the individual or their representative and to your setting's agreed ways of working. You should also ensure you stay up to date with such information, research ways that will enable you to access this information and impart this knowledge to others.
>
> Research the sources of support you have available to you that will enable you to provide support to others in relation to the promotion of equality and rights. Think about the people where you work and other people outside of work who may be able to provide you with support. Draw a spider diagram of the different sources of support that there are available to you both within and outside of your workplace and discuss for each one how they enable you to support others to promote equality and rights.

> **Evidence opportunity**
>
> **2.6 Promoting equality, diversity, inclusion and human rights at work**
>
> Produce a short presentation that describes your role in promoting equality, diversity, inclusion and human rights in line with your employer's agreed ways of working.

Whatever information you access, and direct others to access, make sure it is up to date (out-of-date leaflets may include telephone numbers and email addresses that no longer work), relevant, and that individuals can easily access/read the information. Check that the information is appropriate for the reasons they have requested it and that it is in a format or language they can understand. Ensure that you give the information to them in a timely fashion, that is when they need or request it and are able to make use of it.

LO3 Know how to promote equality, diversity, inclusion and human rights

AC 3.1 Explain the potential effects of discrimination on: a) individuals, b) those who inflict discrimination, c) the wider community and society

Discrimination has many negative effects and can impact on the lives, not only of those individuals being discriminated against but also on their families and friends, those who carry out the discrimination as well as on wider society. The effects of discrimination do not occur in isolation and may last for both the short term and long term irrespective of how often the discrimination has occurred (once or repeatedly) or the type of discrimination (direct, indirect, harassment or victimisation).

A) Effects on individuals

Being discriminated against can affect different aspects of individuals' wellbeing including their physical, emotional and social health. Each of these aspects of individuals' wellbeing are inter-related because, as the example that follows shows, one aspect can impact on another. Physically, an individual may suffer bruises, cuts and burns if physically abused by another person. This may lead to a deterioration in the individual's physical health which may have fatal consequences for some individuals. An individual's emotional wellbeing may also be affected as a result of being subjected to this abuse and discrimination; the individual may experience high levels of anxiety and/or anger as a result of their maltreatment. Their emotional health is bound to negatively affect their physical health because feeling this way could lead to the individual becoming increasingly stressed, which ultimately may lead to physical illness. Emotionally, the individual may also be very vulnerable because they will be left feeling devalued, humiliated, upset and traumatised by the experience. This in turn will affect how they think and view themselves – they may blame themselves for what has happened, which will affect the value they put on themselves (self-esteem) as well as their personal confidence.

This negative experience will also impact drastically on the individual's social health, because with low personal confidence and high levels of anxiety the individual may decide to withdraw from social situations where they meet others for fear of being discriminated against. They may mistrust others and therefore be less likely to make friends and become isolated. Social isolation may lead to high levels of anxiety, causing high blood pressure and poor emotional health including feelings of helplessness and depression. As is demonstrated in this example, the effects and consequences of discrimination are all linked to one another, so it is important that you understand all the effects.

Being discriminated against may also mean that the individual will find it difficult to gain employment as they may not have the confidence to be able to do so. If the individual's physical and emotional health is affected, then these will become additional barriers to the individual finding or maintaining employment and therefore earning an income. In turn this could impact negatively on their health. The effects and consequences are therefore linked to one another, so it is important you understand the various effects and issues here.

Being discriminated against can also have a devastating effect on the families or friends of the individual. Imagine that a family member told you they were being harassed by some of their colleagues at work. How would you feel? You may experience feelings of disgust, anger or anxiety or a mixture of all three. You may also feel guilty or blame yourself that you have been unable to prevent this from happening to them. Knowing that someone you care about is being treated unfairly and in a way that is unacceptable can make you feel disempowered and can cause you to experience high levels of anxiety in case they continue to be hurt. This could have potentially detrimental effects on your physical and emotional health. You may become extremely protective towards your family member, which may lead to your relationship becoming strained and difficult. The effects that discrimination can have on the families or friends of individuals is very much underestimated but as is shown here there can be many, some of which can last a long time and continue to impact on people's lives even after the discrimination has stopped.

B) Effects on those who inflict discrimination

People who inflict discrimination on others do not go unaffected themselves. Some of those who inflict discrimination may have been discriminated against themselves. They may as a result of their own negative experience feel very angry and upset. They may think that putting others through the same negative experience, or showing others the pain and suffering they experienced, will make them feel more powerful. Unfortunately, however, this is rarely the case. Often individuals who inflict discrimination continue to feel angry about their past experiences and the pain and suffering they felt does not go away; in fact, it may worsen and impact on their wellbeing. You should try and understand how those who discriminate feel, and why they discriminate, as well as the feelings of those who are discriminated against in order to be a compassionate and empathetic adult care worker.

C) Effects on the wider community and society

Discrimination can also impact negatively on the wider community and society because it prevents communities and work settings from being effective. For example, discrimination leads to ill-feelings and therefore an unpleasant environment that makes it difficult for people to value each other's differences and respect each other. This in turn will have a negative impact on how people communicate and relate to each other because discrimination can lead to some people being excluded from, for example, community activities. As you have learned, this causes people to be labelled in a negative way, not only resulting in feelings of distrust and creating untrue perceptions but also may lead to those people who are discriminated against withdrawing from their communities and becoming physically and emotionally unwell. They may even begin to believe the label they have been given and therefore become less economically active, which is not beneficial for the community or wider society. This concept is referred to as a 'self-fulfilling prophecy'.

Similarly, where discrimination occurs in work settings this may mean that these settings do not have a diverse workforce with different skills to draw on when recruiting for job roles. This can lead to individuals' needs not being met because the work setting will not have the workforce with the right skills, as people from diverse backgrounds will not be recruited. In addition, employees may not want to work in these settings as they may feel unwelcome or afraid of being excluded or discriminated against if they do. Fostering diversity, equality and inclusion is essential for ensuring that the wider society continues to thrive.

> **Research it**
>
> **3.1 Self-fulfilling prophecy**
>
> Research the meaning of the term 'self-fulfilling prophecy'. You may find the link below useful:
>
> www.psychologytoday.com/blog/psychology-writers/201210/using-self-fulfilling-prophecies-your-advantage
>
> Discuss how self-fulfilling prophecy can impact negatively on individuals who have been discriminated against and on the wider community and society.

> **Reflect on it**
>
> **3.1 Consequences of lack of diversity**
>
> Reflect on the consequences of your work setting not consisting of a diverse team. What impact would this have on the individuals with care or support needs? What impact would this have on individuals' families and friends? What impact would this have on you and your job role? Why?

> **Evidence opportunity**
>
> **3.1 Effects of discrimination**
>
> Identify one type of discrimination that can occur in the setting where you work. Develop a case study to describe the effects on the individual, the family or friends of the individual, the person inflicting the discrimination and on the wider community and society. Remember the rules around confidentiality and protecting the individual's details if you include the case study as part of your portfolio.

AC 3.2 Analyse how unconscious bias may affect own and others' behaviours

As you will have learned, unconscious bias involves being prejudiced towards a person or group and occurs when generalisations or assumptions are made about people that are negative and not based on fact, i.e. stereotypes. Unconscious bias can happen to everyone because you have been exposed to prejudices for example in your childhood, at home, in school, at work and in society as a whole. You will find it useful to refer back to the earlier section 'Understanding unconscious bias' that details the common types that exist and how they may occur in adult care settings.

Unconscious bias affects how we perceive others and this in turn can influence your and others' behaviours and make you and others behave in unfair and negative ways. Below are some examples of how unconscious bias may affect your and others' behaviour:

The stereotypes you and others may have

Unconscious bias involves forming a false opinion of a person based on a general idea of who they are, or who you think they are, because of the groups that they belong to. As a result, you and others may stereotype people because of their gender. When you stereotype someone, you form your opinion of them based on a general idea of who they are, or who you think they are, because of the 'groups' that they belong to. You might stereotype people because of their gender, sexuality, race or religion.

People usually stereotype when they do not understand people that may be different to them. People who stereotype do so because they have not interacted with people from these other groups. Their views (both negative and positive) may be shaped by a very limited interaction they may have had, or by the ways in which certain groups are depicted on television, in films and on the news. Stereotypes can be both positive and negative. You might expect a person to be nice and friendly because they come from a certain country, but then be suspicious of someone and have a negative opinion of them because of their background and the way they look.

It is very easy to stereotype, to see a group of people in simple terms as 'all the same'. However, you should avoid this. Viewing people in these ways can lead to positive behaviour towards some people and discrimination against others, whether you do this knowingly or unknowingly. To stop this from happening, as a Lead Adult Care Worker you will need to make an effort to understand people on an individual basis, and know that while people may belong to different groups, people are not all the same. They have differing needs and preferences.

Labelling others

Stereotypes can lead one set of people to label another group of people. These labels are usually negative and are placed on people to devalue them. For example, young people may be called 'lazy', migrants may be called 'thugs', travellers 'thieves', older people 'useless'. These labels are untrue and negative and have the potential to cause even more harm if the person that has the label placed on them starts behaving like the label. For example, a young person may not see the point of applying for jobs if they believe that others view them as lazy and therefore incapable of finding a job. A traveller who is labelled a thief may decide to commit theft and live up to their reputation if they think that others view them like this anyway.

Reasons why unconscious bias can affect own and others' behaviours

Unconscious bias can affect behaviours in work settings for many reasons; understanding and respect for differences can overcome most of these.

Not getting to know the person

Not spending time getting to know individuals you and others provide care or support to means that you and others will be unaware of their unique likes, dislikes and preferences. This could lead to discrimination, both deliberate or unintentional. This could also happen if as the Lead you have not asked a new team member how you can help them become part of the team. The new team member may not feel comfortable because their colleagues have a lot more experience than they do.

Not respecting one another's differences

In adult care settings, individuals and others may be from a diverse range of backgrounds and not respecting these differences may lead to some individuals being stereotyped (as discussed earlier). One example may be thinking that all those who are Muslim will want to pray at the same times every day and participate in fasting, rather than checking first with each person as to their preferences for praying and fasting. Another example might be that all young people are only interested in going out with their friends to socialise and are lazy when they have to study or work.

Insufficient knowledge

It is possible that both individuals and others may never have worked or lived as part of a group in a care setting where they would have gained experience of other individuals and adult care workers from different cultures and backgrounds with different beliefs and values to their own. As a result, you and the individuals you work with may not be aware of your own prejudices. For a (Lead) Adult Care Worker, it is important that you learn about different practices and take some time out to reflect on your own prejudices and seek feedback from others – such as your manager at work or your partner at home – who know you well and may be able to provide you with further information about your own prejudices. Just working with different individuals (and others) will help to build your knowledge of different people. You should also encourage positive interaction between individuals which will help to break down any negative assumptions, and create understanding between individuals (and others) from different backgrounds. As a (Lead) Adult Care Worker, you must also continue to update your knowledge about anti-discrimination practices throughout your career.

Dos and don'ts for anti-discrimination practices	
Do	See people as individuals with different needs and preferences
Do	Respect people's individuality
Do	Treat people as individuals and understand that just because people belong to a particular group this does not mean they are all the same
Do	Value people's differences
Don't	Treat all people the same. Think about how you would feel if people focused on a certain characteristic about you, for example your race or your religion
Don't	Make assumptions about people
Don't	Stereotype people
Don't	Label people

> **Reflect on it**
>
> **3.2 Preventing negative, discriminatory behaviours in the work setting**
>
> Think about what your opinions of certain groups of people are. You may think about gender, races and religions.
>
> - What positive opinions do you have of these groups?
> - What negative opinions do you have of these groups?
> - Why do you think of these people in these ways?
> - What can you do to make sure you do not have any 'stereotypical' views?
>
> Then reflect on your responsibilities as a (Lead) Adult Care Worker for ensuring that discrimination does not occur in your work setting.
>
> Perhaps you could reflect on what you can do to fulfil your duty to provide good-quality care to individuals and support to others that is free from discrimination and how you are keeping your knowledge and practices up to date.

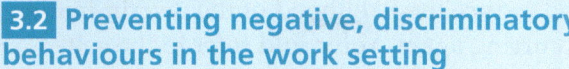

> **Evidence opportunity**
>
> **3.2 Unconscious bias**
>
> Think about how unconscious bias can influence you and others' behaviours in work settings. For three types of unconscious bias that you have learned about, produce an information handout that details how and why they can occur in the work setting. Remember to include different examples of the ways they can occur as well as the reasons why and how they can be overcome.

AC 3.3 Describe how to respond to and challenge discrimination in a way that promotes positive change

As you will have learned, being able to promote diversity, equality and inclusion in your work setting is an important part of your role as a Lead Adult Care Worker or Lead Personal Assistant. It is also important for you to lead by example by working in inclusive ways and knowing how to challenge those not doing so constructively and positively.

Working in an inclusive way involves being able to:

- **recognise practices that are discriminatory:** these may be deliberate or unintentional and can occur for different reasons, such as a lack of clear understanding or knowledge about equality, diversity and/or inclusion; a lack of awareness of own and others' behaviours at work and towards individuals; or fear or a lack of confidence over how to respond to an individual's needs, for example when they display behaviour that challenges or have a condition such as dementia
- **know what to do if you become aware of or see discrimination taking place:** this may occur either in or outside of the care setting where you work
- **challenge discrimination positively:** this involves making others aware of their behaviours that are discriminatory and ensuring that they are provided with the support and information they require to address these and prevent them from happening again.

It is very important that your practices promote diversity, equality and inclusion because as a Lead Adult Care Worker or Lead Personal Assistant you are accountable for your actions. If you do discriminate either deliberately or unintentionally you can be disciplined for this by your employer and you could be dismissed from your job. In addition, your employer could be held responsible for your actions.

When challenging discrimination, it is important that you do this in a way that promotes change. Not doing so may:

- **lead to the discrimination becoming worse and occurring more regularly:** if you do not make others aware that their behaviours are discriminatory then they may continue practising in this way, thinking that they are working in line with best practice
- **inadvertently reinforce these negative unwanted behaviours:** individuals may think that you are encouraging the discrimination to continue and may therefore feel that you too are being discriminatory – this will impact negatively on your relationship with the individual
- **mean that you will be failing in your duty of care towards the individuals you provide care or support to:** you may wish to refer to Unit 303 Understanding duty of care for more information on this topic.

Research it

3.3 Agreed ways of working for responding to and challenging discrimination

Research your employer's agreed ways of working for responding to and challenging discrimination where you work. What does it say about your role and responsibilities? What actions are you required to take in the event of discrimination occurring? How do these actions compare with those in the dos and don'ts table? Discuss your findings with your manager or employer.

Responding to and challenging discrimination in a way that promotes positive change involves being positive, supportive and constructive, leading by example and modelling inclusive practice. You can do this by:

- having a discussion with the person responsible so that they understand why their practices are discriminatory; this involves answering any questions they may have and providing reassurance that they will be supported with addressing these behaviours so they do not occur again
- suggesting self-reflection to increase their awareness of and insight into their behaviour, and reduce the likelihood of the discrimination occurring again. You could refer to the self-reflection process in Unit 313 Continuous development when working in an adult care worker role, LO3
- suggesting further training so that they can update their knowledge about inclusive and anti-discriminatory practices
- suggesting shadowing more experienced colleagues so that they can observe and learn about good ways of working when supporting individuals in inclusive ways
- accessing an advocate and others who do not work in the setting to ensure individuals are supported to challenge discrimination when it arises
- ensuring that you voice your suggestions and discuss them with your manager or employer so that these become part of the setting's agreed ways of working for everyone to follow
- empowering individuals and encouraging the active participation of individuals so that they can themselves challenge discrimination and any barriers they may come across.

	Dos and don'ts for responding to and challenging discrimination and promoting change
Do	Act straightaway to make it clear that it will not be tolerated.
Do	Support others to act straightaway to make it clear that it is unacceptable.
Do	Report all incidents so that the necessary actions can be taken.
Do	Record all incidents to ensure the details of the incident are documented. This includes who was affected and what actions were taken. This document can be referred to at a later stage if necessary.
Do	Keep up to date with good practices so that you can constructively challenge discrimination in a way that promotes change.
Do	Ensure you know your work setting's agreed ways of working for constructively challenging discrimination.
Don't	Accept it.
Don't	Ignore it.

Case study

3.3 Skills for responding to and challenging discrimination

Challenging discrimination in a way that promotes positive change is not easy and requires you to be consistent as well as constructive and supportive. Read through Case study 3.3 and think about the skills that you will require to be able to respond to and challenge discrimination in a way that promotes positive change.

Ken works as a Lead Support Worker and this morning witnessed Scott, an older man with care and support needs tell Malachi, an older woman with mental health needs, that she could not sit at the same table at breakfast time because she could not speak English fluently. Upon witnessing this Ken immediately approached Scott in a calm manner and assertively explained to him that what he had said to Malachi was not fair, was discriminatory and would not be tolerated because it is every individual's right to choose where they want to sit at breakfast time, irrespective of their differences.

Scott immediately apologised to Ken for his behaviour. Ken explained that Scott needs to also apologise to Malachi. After Scott had done so, Ken asked Malachi how Scott's behaviour had affected her. Malachi explained that she was very hurt by his comments and felt unwanted. Scott again apologised to Malachi and invited her to sit with him at the table to have breakfast and offered to fetch her a cup of tea. Malachi accepted Scott's apology and cup of tea.

Ken informed his manager and the rest of the team at the next staff meeting about what had happened between Scott and Malachi and how he had addressed it immediately, showing **care** and **compassion**. Ken added that he also reviewed the tenants' handbook with Scott to ensure that he fully understood that discrimination would not be tolerated as part of his tenancy and that any repeat incidents may result in him losing his tenancy. Ken suggested that Scott attend a tenant information day about equality, diversity and inclusion so that he could raise his awareness of what discrimination is and why it must be avoided, including how to promote equality and rights, and Scott agreed to attend.

Discuss:
1. Which skills do you think Ken has?
2. Why are these useful for responding to and challenging discrimination?
3. How did Ken support Scott to develop his skills for responding to and challenging discrimination?
4. Are there any other skills you think Scott needs to further develop? Why?

6Cs

Compassion

Compassion involves you showing concern for the wellbeing of individuals if they are being discriminated against and caring enough to challenge it. This will not only show that you are taking a stand against discrimination in the setting and saying that it will not be tolerated, but also shows your regard and respect for the rights of the individuals for whom you provide care. You can show compassion by supporting individuals who have been discriminated against and recognising the impact this has had on them personally. Allowing yourself to empathise with the individual will help you understand how they are feeling, find a solution that will bring about long-term change and make a positive difference.

Care

Care, in this section, involves doing what you can to ensure that if an individual is discriminated against, then you are able to do what you can to improve the situation and have their wellbeing as the focus. It is about showing that you can make a positive difference to an individual's life through your role. Again, you can show this by:

- positively challenging all discrimination you may come across
- showing that you care through your communication
- making sure that individuals know that you have their best interests at heart.

This is important for ensuring that individuals trust you to support them and promote their rights to live in a way that is free from discrimination.

Evidence opportunity

3.3 How to challenge discrimination in a way that promotes positive change

Develop a verbal presentation to describe to some of your colleagues how to challenge discrimination in a way that promotes change. Or you could provide a written description.

AC 3.4 Explain how to report and record any discriminatory or excluding behaviour within own work setting/service

Sometimes discrimination at work cannot be prevented and you may find that you are discriminated against or that you witness discrimination taking place in your work setting.

Doing nothing is not an option. It is important that you act straightaway by reporting and recording any discriminatory or excluding behaviour to prevent it from continuing and/or worsening and to make it clear that it will not be tolerated. Your work setting or service will have in place agreed ways of working for how to report and record any discriminatory or excluding behaviour and it is important that you follow these.

The following list contains some additional information about the process to follow in work settings for reporting and recording discriminatory or excluding behaviour:

1 By making an informal complaint:
   - Talk to your employer about what has happened or write to them explaining what has happened. By making an informal complaint first you are giving your employer an opportunity to listen to your complaint and resolve it.
   - Your work setting's agreed ways of working will detail who to make your informal complaint to, i.e. your manager or someone else if your complaint is about your manager.
   - Your work setting's agreed ways of working will also detail how to record your complaint, i.e. by completing an informal complaint record, by recording full details such as what happened, date, time, why you think it's discrimination, any evidence you have and how you would like the issue resolved.
   - If you want to speak to someone about any discriminatory or excluding behaviour a meeting can be set up so that you can discuss your complaint in private and without any interruptions.
   - You could also ask your employer if you can bring someone with you to the meeting for support such as a colleague or a union representative; your employer doesn't have to agree to this as this is an informal complaint. Ensure the meeting is recorded; you or your employer can do this. If your employer does this ensure that you have a record of what has been said and agreed. If your employer does not provide you with a record write to them with your record and ask them to agree to this. This is important because you will need this record if you take the matter further, i.e. by making a formal complaint.

2 By making a formal complaint:
   - If you do not hear back from your employer or your employer does not do what they agreed to in the meeting, or you are not satisfied with your employer's response to your informal complaint, you can make a formal complaint called a grievance, which is a complaint in writing to your employer. Making a formal complaint is important so that the discrimination does not continue.
   - You must follow your employer's agreed ways of working for making the formal complaint, which will detail how you must do this.
   - The written grievance is the start of a formal complaints procedure where your employer will invite you to a grievance meeting to discuss your complaint. Your employer will then investigate your complaint and provide you with a written decision of the outcome of their investigation. If you do not agree with your employer's decision you can appeal and your employer will set out in their written response to you how this can be done, i.e. in writing, within agreed timescales.

3 By going to a tribunal:
   - If your employer is not able to resolve the issue then you can take legal action by taking your complaint to an employment tribunal.
   - If you decide that you want to take your complaint to an employment tribunal then you must do this within three months of when the discrimination occurred; this is what the law says.
   - You will need to make available all evidence you have of the discrimination, including any notes of meetings or records of correspondence with your employer, so that your case an be heard.

Research it

3.4 Agreed ways of working - discrimination

Research your work setting's agreed ways of working for reporting and recording discrimination. What does it say about the process that you must follow?

> **Evidence opportunity**
>
> **3.4** Reporting and recording discrimination in your work setting
>
> Consider how you would report and record discriminatory or excluding behaviour you witnessed in your work setting. Produce a flow diagram to explain the key actions to take and the reasons why they must be taken.

LO4 Be able to work in an inclusive way

> **Getting started**
>
> Think about an occasion when you or someone you know observed a person being treated unfairly. How did this make you and the person feel? What actions were taken? Why? What would have been the consequences of taking no action?

AC 4.1 Demonstrate interaction with individuals and others in a way that respects their lifestyle, beliefs, culture, values and preferences

This AC requires you to demonstrate or show that you work with individuals in a way that respects their beliefs, cultures, values and preferences. It is important that you know how to do this because as a Lead Adult Care Worker or Lead Personal Assistant you may have to support others who you work with to do the same and it is important therefore that you are a good role model for them and show them ways that promote equality and respect diversity and inclusion.

What are your lifestyle, beliefs, culture, values and preferences?

Having your own lifestyle, beliefs, culture, values and preferences is part of who you are; they are what make you unique. Being aware of what your own lifestyle, beliefs, culture, values and preferences are is the first essential step for respecting those of the individuals you care for and support. This is because everyone is different and so being able to accept individuals' differences can only happen if you ensure that you do not let your own lifestyle, beliefs, culture, values and preferences **prejudice** the ways you work.

For example, you may hold a strong belief that people should lead by example and that they should treat others how they want to be treated themselves. As a Lead Adult Care Worker or Lead Personal Assistant this may involve being kind and considerate when working with individuals, being empathetic and compassionate and above all else being open and transparent when you or others make mistakes and their care and support goes wrong. You can review your knowledge of your duty of care and candour when working in adult care in Unit 303 Understanding duty of care.

Your preferences will be determined by your lifestyle, beliefs and values and they may be in relation to how you like to spend your time when not at work, what you like to eat, what music you like to listen to, where you prefer to live and what job role you prefer.

Your culture refers to the traditions or customs of the country you originate from; these will not be the same for everyone and will vary in how they are applied by different people and families. For example, depending on the country you originate from and what traditions and customs you and your family follow, you may have specific preferences about what foods you eat and don't eat, what you wear, and what religion and associated rituals you follow.

How can you interact with individuals and others in ways that respect their lifestyle, beliefs, culture, values and preferences?

Once you are aware of your own lifestyle, beliefs, culture, values and preferences you can then begin to understand how important it is that you work in ways that are respectful of the different individuals you work with.

You can interact in ways that show respect for individuals' and others' lifestyles and beliefs by:

- **showing a genuine interest:** this involves spending time with individuals and others, getting to know them and finding out from them about their lifestyles and beliefs by asking them what these are rather than making any assumptions about what these may be so that they feel valued. For example, perhaps they follow some religious practices that affect how they dress, how they want to be cared for, who they want to be cared for by and/or what they eat. Working in these ways will mean the individual will feel valued.
- **not making assumptions:** this involves not making assumptions about individuals' and others' lifestyles and beliefs even when they are from a similar background or culture. Everyone is different and therefore how you take into account their lifestyles and beliefs must also be different and suited to them to gain their trust.
- **planning and preparing yourself:** this involves taking the time to understand what individuals' and others' lifestyles and beliefs are, and checking with them that you have understood how they, the individual, want you to take these preferences into account before you do your day-to-day work.
- **being tolerant:** this involves accepting that individuals' and others' lifestyles and beliefs may be different to your own and reflecting on the prejudices you may have.

Reflect on it

4.1 Your beliefs and values

Reflect on your beliefs and values. What are they? How do they affect your life? How do they affect your work? Now reflect on your culture, lifestyle and preferences. How do they impact on your day-to-day life? How do they impact on your day-to-day work life? What can you do to ensure they do not prejudice the ways in which you work with individuals?

Alternatively, you could think about the different cultures represented by individuals and colleagues in your setting. Do you know what the associated customs and beliefs with each of these are?

6Cs

Communication

Good communication involves building good working relationships with individuals that instil mutual trust and respect. This is because communicating well can make individuals feel that they are being listened to and that their thoughts and opinions are valued. Good communication makes individuals feel respected and involved. You can ensure that you communicate well by showing that you are aware of individuals' and others' lifestyles and beliefs and can show respect for these during all your communications. You may also like to refer to Unit 304 Effective communication in adult care settings/services.

You can interact in ways that show respect for individuals' and others' culture by:

- **getting to know the person:** this involves finding out about their background and culture. There are different ways you can do this, for example by talking to the person about their culture or by finding out about their culture from those who know the person well such as their family, friends or advocate. You may also decide to carry out your own research about the person's culture. If you do this, remember not to make assumptions about the person's culture and associated practices. Interacting in these ways will mean that you will be able to show your understanding of how diverse every person is and your commitment to respecting their differences.
- **enabling the person to take the lead:** this involves providing opportunities for the person to show you how they would like you to respect their culture. It is important that you listen attentively and if there is something you are unsure about or do not understand that you ask them about this. Interacting in these ways will mean that you will be able to respect every person's culture.

You can interact in ways that show respect for individuals' and others' values by:

- **asking the person about their values:** this involves finding out from them what they hold as important to them. Interacting in these ways will mean that you will be respecting the person and empowering them.

- **not making judgements:** this involves not making judgements about the person's values, particularly if they are different to yours or you do not agree with them. It is important that you always ensure that the person's values are at the centre of all your interactions with them. You may find it useful to refer to Unit 306 Promoting and implementing person-centred practice.
- **not influencing the person's values:** this involves ensuring that your values do not influence them. It is important that you remain fair and **objective** at all times so that you can show your respect for the person's values, so that they feel empowered to make their own decisions and choices and have their self-esteem raised.

You can interact in ways that show respect for individuals' and others' preferences by:

- **empowering the person:** this involves not only finding out about the person's preferences but also enabling them to share their preferences with you. To be able to do this the person needs to feel able to approach you and talk to you. It is important that you create an environment where the person feels relaxed and where you can spend time with each other without any interruptions or distractions. You may find it useful to revisit Unit 304 Effective communication in adult care settings/services.

> **Key term**
>
> To be **objective** is to be fair, and not influenced by your own feelings or beliefs.

- **taking into account the person's preferences:** you will need to do this at all times. To do this effectively you must ensure that you have agreed on ways to do so with the person. Do not assume that the person's preferences will remain the same – they may change on a daily basis, or from time to time, depending on the person. It is good practice therefore to always check with the person how to take their preferences into account before doing so and after doing so to clarify with them whether how you have taken their preferences into account has been effective. You may find it useful to refer to Unit 313 Continuous development when working in an adult care worker role.

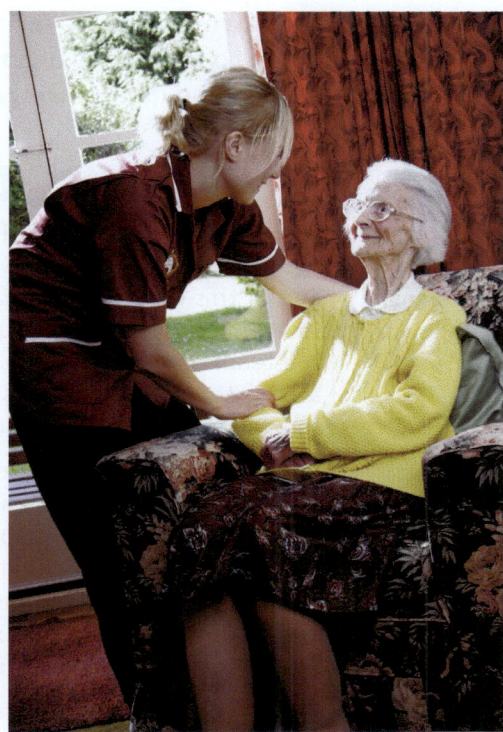

Figure 10.2 How do you ensure you respect an individual's values?

- **not imposing your preferences on the person:** this involves supporting and enabling the person to speak up about who they are, what their preferences are and how they want you to support them to ensure their preferences are upheld. You can show respect for the person's preferences by ensuring you do not let your own preferences influence theirs; this involves you being aware of what your own preferences are. It is important that you enable the person to take the lead by ensuring that they communicate their preferences to you and that you listen to what they are saying.
- **being aware of how you interact with the person:** this involves observing the person through your interaction to check how they are receiving your interaction, for example by what they say, what they don't say and their body language. This involves being aware of how you interact with them, for example whether you are using non-discriminatory language and what your body language is showing to them. For example, is it showing that you are genuinely interested? Is it showing that you are listening attentively? You will find it useful to refer to Unit 304 Effective communication in adult care settings/services, in relation to verbal and non-verbal communication.

The reflective exemplar provides you with an opportunity to explore the consequences of not interacting with individuals and others in a way that respects their lifestyles, beliefs, culture, values and preferences.

Reflective exemplar	
Introduction	I work as a Lead Adult Support Worker providing support to adults with mental health needs. I lead a team of five support workers.
What happened	Earlier this week, two individuals with mental health needs, Jane and Jules, were referred to the team for support. Both Jane and Jules have chronic depression. I gave the team an overview of both Jane and Jules, including how their chronic depression affects them and the types of support they will require. I also informed the team that Jane lives with her husband and that Jules shares a flat with a friend.
	I received a call from Monica, one of the support workers who visited Jane, who explained that she was unable to support Jane with her personal hygiene this morning because Jane was not happy that Monica had refused to allow Jane's husband to assist her with her personal hygiene. Monica explained to me that she thought it was inappropriate for Jane's husband to help with the morning routine because he was male. Monica went on to explain that, as a result, Jane became very agitated with her and told her to leave. Monica added that she respected Jane's wishes to leave.
	I explained to Monica that she must always ensure that she respects the individual's values and preferences. It is Jane's right to have her husband assist her with her personal hygiene routine if this is what is important to her and what she prefers. I explained to Monica that she must take into account the individual's lifestyle, values and preferences at all times.
	At this week's team meeting the support workers who visited Jules indicated that they were unsure about how best to support Jules with his nutrition because of his Jewish culture and beliefs, as he does not like the pre-prepared kosher meals. Because of this, the support workers explained that they did not order any meals for him and had agreed instead with Jules that he would go food shopping with his friend who he shares the flat with.
	Later in the week, I received a telephone call from Jules who explained that he was not happy because he was not being supported by the support workers with his culture and beliefs in relation to food shopping and cooking as agreed and how instead he had been told to go shopping with his friend. Jules added that his friend is not happy to do this because he feels it should be done by his support workers. I reassured Jules that I and the team of support workers would be respecting his culture and beliefs when providing him with support and I agreed to visit him so that he could complete a food shop and cook an evening meal.
What worked well	I think that I informed the team about how chronic depression personally affects Jane and Jules as individuals. I was assertive when I received the phone call from Monica and made it clear that she must take into account individuals' lifestyles, values and preferences at all times and not let hers influence theirs.
	I thought I was proactive in handling the conflict that had arisen with Jules and managed to prevent the situation from worsening. Jules appreciated me visiting him the same day that he phoned the office. I used the opportunity to ask Jules all about his Jewish culture and beliefs and built up a very good picture about how he would like the team and me to support him in relation to his dietary requirements and needs.

→

	Reflective exemplar
What did not go as well	When I gave the team the information about Jane and Jules, I should have also provided them with information about how Jane's and Jules' needs may also be affected by the people they live with, particularly in relation to how they are both supported. Doing this would have ensured that the team of support workers could have shown their respect for both individuals' lifestyles, beliefs, culture, values and preferences at their first support visits.
	In relation to what I said to Monica, I should also have explained the consequences of not respecting individuals' lifestyles, values and preferences as well as the potential impact these may have on the individual and on the development of a good working relationship with the individual.
	In relation to Jules, I haven't yet fed back to the team about my visit to Jules and the information I found out. I need to document this and ensure this is available to the whole team.
What I could do to improve	I think I need to hold another team meeting as a matter of urgency in relation to ensuring the whole team understand how best to support Jane and Jules.
	The information I collate about individuals' beliefs, cultures, values and preferences needs to be done in a lot more detail and I need to review how I document this and communicate this to the team. Perhaps I can speak to my manager about further support and training in this area.
	I think the team and I would benefit from some more training in relation to how to ensure we are working in an inclusive way. After this training we could then, as a whole team, undertake a review of the individuals we currently support to determine how effective we are in respecting their unique lifestyles, beliefs, cultures, values and preferences.
Links to unit's assessment criteria	ACs: 2.3, 4.1

Key terms

Kosher refers to foods that are permitted to be eaten under Jewish dietary laws and that can be used as ingredients in the production of additional food items.

Evidence opportunity

4.1 Interacting with individuals and others in ways that respect them

Your practices will be observed for AC 4.1. Make arrangements to be observed for interactions with two different individuals and others that you work with. (Ensure you plan this with your assessor in advance.)

For example, you may arrange to be observed meeting with an individual to review an aspect of their care or support or to discuss an issue with a colleague that is important to them or worrying them. For each person, ensure you show how you respect their unique lifestyle, beliefs, culture, values and preferences.

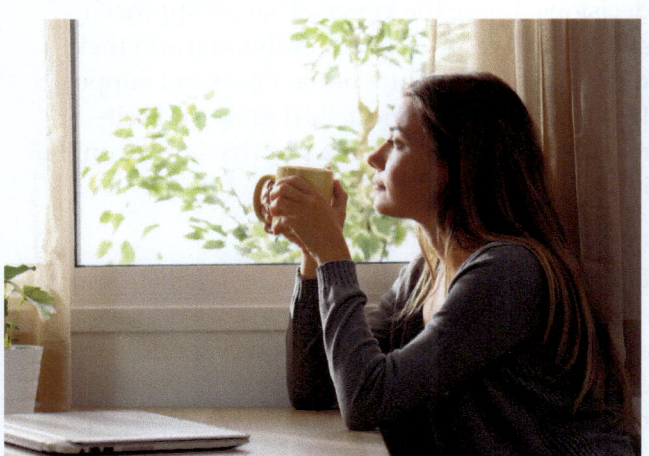

Figure 10.3 Are you an effective reflector?

AC 4.2 Model inclusive practice

This AC requires you to demonstrate that you are able through your job role to promote a culture that supports inclusive practices. It is important that you know how to do this because, as you will have learned in AC 2.4, inclusive practice has many benefits for individuals and can lead to improved outcomes for them as it prevents them from being excluded and isolated. Inclusive practice also enables individuals to feel valued and promotes a sense of belonging because it recognises that every individual has a right to make their own choices and be an active participant in day-to-day life, both in their community and in wider society.

Inclusive practice in adult care

Inclusive practice provides individuals with the opportunity to lead their life as they wish and to access the care and support they require to do so. The implementation of the Care Act 2014 made it a requirement (there was only guidance in place previously) for local authorities to offer personalised care and support planning. Best practice in health and social care involves working in ways that are inclusive and there are many examples in the adult care sector of approaches and strategies that model inclusive practices; below are some examples.

Personalisation

Personalisation is an approach that involves recognising that every individual has abilities, strengths and preferences and has the right to be in control of their care and support, including how it is delivered and which services they would like to use. This is also referred to as 'self-directed support'. It involves the provision of person-centred care that involves recognising individuals as leaders of their own care and support and supporting individuals to make their own choices and decisions in everyday activities. It involves providing and designing care and support around the unique needs and preferences of individuals rather than developing care and support and/or services that individuals are required to fit into.

You can model the personalisation approach by ensuring that individuals are the focus when providing care or support. This means treating individuals with respect and believing that they are able, with the correct type of support, to make their own choices and decisions. For example, you can ask the individual about their strengths and abilities; do not assume you know what these are. Finding out directly from the individual and/or their representative what these are will mean that you are enabling the individual to share with you what they can do for themselves and what they would like to continue to do for themselves.

Similarly, you can model the personalisation approach when developing and providing the care or support the individual needs. For example, you can establish with the individual what aspects of their everyday life, including future goals, they require support with; who they would like to provide this support and the reasons why; what type of support they require and why; and when and how long they require support for. In this way you can ensure that the individual's choices and preferences inform the development and provision of their care and support and that the care and support provided not only meets their needs but also enables them to maintain as much control as possible over their everyday activities.

There are numerous benefits for using this approach. For example, not only does it mean that you and your colleagues can work in ways that reflect best practice but also that you and your colleagues are playing an important role in empowering individuals to reach their full potential by making their own choices and decisions. Using the personalisation approach shows your respect for the individual and their right to be at the centre of their care and support. It promotes the individual's dignity and self-respect which in turn has a positive impact on the individual's wellbeing.

Direct payments

Direct payments are provided by local authorities and enable individuals who have been assessed as requiring assistance from social services to arrange and buy the care services they require themselves. Direct payments can be used to pay for employing a personal assistant or a carer as well as for other services they may need, such as support with preparing meals, going shopping or maintaining personal hygiene. Direct payments are means tested and therefore it depends on the individual's financial situation whether they have to pay towards the cost of their care and support. If the individual uses direct payments for employing carers themselves there is support available to help the individual do this safely and fairly. This means that the individual can employ carers who they want, feel that they can trust and are comfortable with. If the individual lacks capacity and cannot make their own decisions, then someone who knows them well such as their carer or a family member can apply for direct payments and manage the direct payments on the individual's behalf, if the local authority is satisfied that this person will act in the individual's best interests.

Personal budgets

Personal budgets are an agreed amount of money offered by the local authority following an assessment of people's care and support needs to ensure individuals' and their carers' needs are met. Personal budgets enable individuals and their carers to have full control over how their needs are met but unlike direct payments do not require the person to become an employer; they can, however, also be received in the form of a direct payment.

Personal budgets enable people to have full control over how the money allocated to them is spent in relation to their care and support. They empower individuals to understand how their care and support needs can be met and how much money they have to spend towards these. Your role may involve supporting the individual to choose the care and support or the services that are best for them and that meet their needs. You can model inclusive practice by ensuring that you continue to provide individuals with the support they need to be in control of their lives. This may include empowering them to make their own daily choices, as well as encouraging them to having a positive view of themselves so that they feel interested in leading their own care and support.

> **Evidence opportunity**
>
> **4.2 Inclusive practice**
>
> Show your assessor or manager how you promote a culture that supports inclusive practice with two different individuals who have care and support needs. For example, you could choose a specific aspect of their life or the care and support that you provide.
>
> Ensure your assessor or manager is able to witness you working in this way and ask them for feedback afterwards. How effective were you in supporting inclusive practice? Were there any aspects of your practice that you could have improved on?

AC 4.3 Reflect on own practice in promoting equality, diversity, inclusion and human rights

AC 4.4 Make recommendations for developing own practice in promoting equality, diversity, inclusion and human rights

You can reflect on your working practices for promoting equality, diversity, inclusion and human rights by raising your awareness of your own beliefs, culture, values and preferences by reflecting on what these are. You need to be very honest to be able to establish how these affect you, not only personally but also professionally in your day-to-day work. It may be a good idea to obtain feedback from those who know you well so that you can find out whether your preferences are affecting your work; this may be a colleague who knows you well or your manager. If you work on your own, this may be the individual with care and support needs or someone who knows the individual well, such as a member of their family or their advocate. It is also important to be aware that these preferences may change over time, so reflecting on these should not be done on just one occasion but throughout your career.

Other ways to raise your awareness may include attending training updates as these will further develop your knowledge and increase your awareness of what best practice consists of.

Discussions with others at work may also be a good way to gain a greater insight not only into yourself but also into how you come across to others. In this way you can ensure that you promote equality, diversity and inclusion and remain respectful (towards the human rights of individuals and others in your work setting).

Once you've had time to reflect on the feedback you've received from others and the insights you've gained, you need to act on your reflections so that you can continue to develop your practice in promoting equality, diversity, inclusion and human rights. For example, you may find out that you have made assumptions about a team member's beliefs because they are from the same culture as you. You may in this instance make a conscious effort to speak to this team member and actively find out about their beliefs and how they want you to take them into account in day-to-day working activities. This will develop your practice in this area because you will be actively putting your assumptions to one side so that you can be open to this team member and treat them fairly and in line with their unique preferences. Similarly, you may find out in a training update that you attend that you had forgotten about the broad range of human rights individuals and others have or you may come across a topic you are unfamiliar with or know little about. You may therefore decide to take on further research or reading in this area so that you can further develop your knowledge in these areas and ensure it is up to date.

Reflect on it

4.3, 4.4 Your practice and how to develop it

Reflect on your working practices in relation to promoting equality, diversity, inclusion and human rights. Which of these reflect best practice? Why? Are there any of your practices that you'd like to further improve? Why? How could you develop your working practices further? How will developing your working practices impact on you, individuals and others? Why is this important?

Evidence opportunity

4.3, 4.4 Reflecting on and improving your practice

Write a reflective account on how you promote equality, diversity, inclusion and human rights in the care setting you work in. What areas of your practice could be further improved and developed? Make recommendations for how you plan to continue to develop your practice.

Legislation and Codes of Practice	
Act/Code of Practice	**Key points**
The Human Rights Act 1998	Everyone in the UK is entitled to the same basic human rights and freedoms. This includes individuals who have care and support needs. It promotes fairness, dignity and respect and protects these human rights from being infringed.
The Data Protection Act 2018	People have rights to be treated fairly in relation to their information and data. It also safeguards people from having their information and data misused or obtained unlawfully.
Special Educational Needs and Disability Act 2001 Children and Families Act 2014 and the Special Educational Needs and Disabilities (SEND) Code of Practice 2014	People with disabilities have rights to have reasonable adjustments made by schools, colleges, universities, adult education providers, statutory youth services and local education authorities. The Children and Families Act 2014 introduced a range of new legislation regarding adoption and family justice. Part 3 includes a new Special Educational Needs and Disabilities (SEND) Code of Practice. This supersedes the Code of Practice from 2001 (but does not replace the Special Educational Needs and Disability Act 2001). You can find more information here: www.gov.uk/government/publications/send-code-of-practice-0-to-25

Legislation and Codes of Practice	
Act/Code of Practice	**Key points**
The Mental Capacity Act 2005	Individuals have the right to make their own decisions for as long as they are able and to be supported to make arrangements for a time in the future when they may lack the capacity to make their own decisions due to a condition or disability such as dementia, or a learning difficulty; for example, in relation to their care and support.
The Equality Act 2010	It is unlawful to discriminate against individuals in respect of the nine protected characteristics, i.e. age, disability, gender reassignment, marriage and civil partnership, pregnancy and maternity, race, religion or belief, sex, sexual orientation. It also protects people's rights to be treated fairly and safeguards people from being discriminated against because of their individual differences.
The Care Act 2014	People who have care or support needs and their carers have rights when being assessed and when being provided with care and support. It also introduced the wellbeing concept as the basis of all person-centred care that all individuals and carers are entitled to when being provided with care and support.
Code of Conduct for Healthcare Support Workers and Adult Social Care Workers in England	Outlines a number of principles that must be followed by those who work in health and adult care settings. For example, promoting and upholding the privacy, dignity, rights, health and wellbeing of individuals, promoting equality, diversity and inclusion.
Mental Capacity Code of Practice 2005	The five key principles of the Mental Capacity Act 2005 should be applied by those who work with people who can't make decisions for themselves and those who care for people who can't make decisions for themselves. It provides guidance on what certain people must do and think about when they act or make decisions on behalf of people who can't act or make those decisions for themselves.

See AC 2.1 for more information on legislation and codes of practice.

310 Promoting health and safety in adult care settings/services

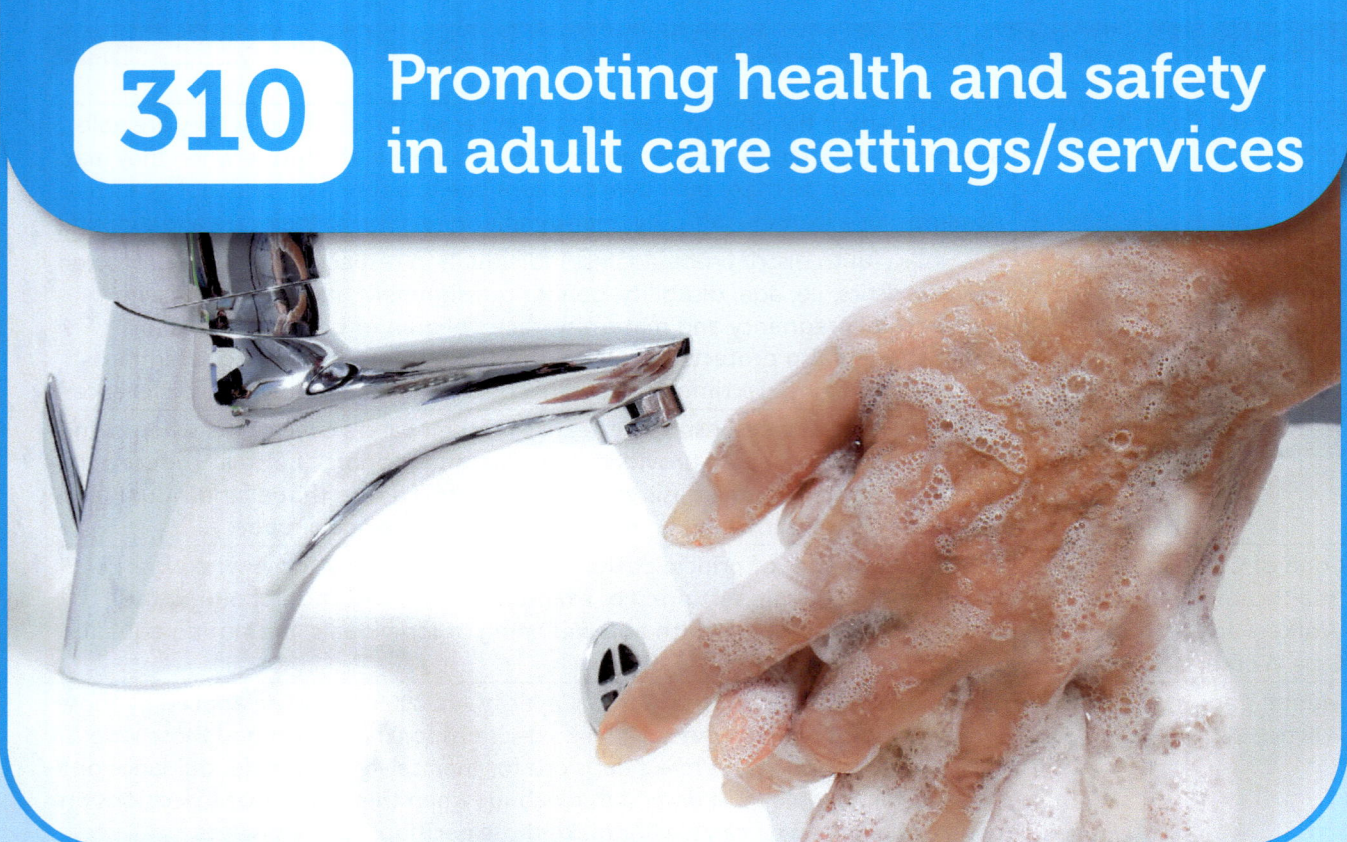

About this unit

Credit value: 3
Guided learning hours: 20

Health, safety and wellbeing in care settings is everyone's responsibility and promoting it on a day-to-day basis is both interesting and challenging. Health and safety is more than just accident prevention and assessing risks; it involves ensuring care settings are safe environments where individuals feel at home and workers enjoy coming to work.

In this unit you will learn about the various aspects that are involved in making sure the environment you work in is a safe one. You will also find out about the various aspects that are involved in making sure that you keep yourself, the individuals you work with and others safe.

Learning outcomes

By the end of this unit, you will:

LO1: Understand own responsibilities, and the responsibilities of others, relating to health and safety in the work setting/service

LO2: Understand procedures for responding to accidents and sudden illness

LO3: Be able to carry out own responsibilities for health and safety

LO1 Understand own responsibilities, and the responsibilities of others, relating to health and safety in the work setting/service

> **Getting started**
>
> Think about the importance of being healthy and staying safe. How do you maintain your health and minimise falling ill? How do you keep safe and free from danger? Why is this important? Discuss with a colleague in a similar lead role to you how you both promote people's health and wellbeing where you work. Then think about people's safety where you work – how do you both promote their safety? How does your employer promote you and your colleagues' health and safety?

AC 1.1 Outline current legislation relating to health and safety that applies in own care work setting

Care settings are environments where accidents, injuries and illnesses can occur and so knowing about and practising general health and safety at work is important for protecting all those who live in, work in and visit these from danger as the statistics below show:

- 1.3 million workers were suffering from a work-related illness (new or longstanding) in 2015/16
- 0.5 million workers were suffering from work-related **musculoskeletal disorders** (new or longstanding) in 2015/16
- 0.5 million workers were suffering from work-related stress, depression or anxiety (new or longstanding) in 2015/16.
Source: *Health and Safety Executive (2016) 'Health and safety at work: Summary statistics for Great Britain 2016'*

With many more individuals living in their own homes, you may be providing care to individuals on your own so it is very important that you are aware of how to maintain your own health and safety as well as that of individuals and others who may visit their home while you are there.

As a lone worker, unlike residential-based workers who always work alongside team members, you will for the most part be visiting individuals' homes on your own and will therefore have to know how to manage and respond to different types of situations, such as finding that an individual's hoist or security alarm isn't working or dealing with a family member who does not agree with the care you are providing. As a lone worker it is your responsibility to ensure you deal with all situations effectively; taking no action is not an option. If you were a lone worker, how would you deal with each of the situations mentioned above?

For example, if you are a lone worker and you find an individual's hoist or security alarm isn't working, it would be your responsibility to contact the manufacturer and explain this; whereas, if you work in a residential setting you would report this to the **health and safety officer** or to your manager, whose responsibility it would be to contact the manufacturer. If you come across a family member who does not agree with the care you are providing, as a lone worker you would have to discuss their concerns directly with them, whereas in a residential setting you would report this to a more senior colleague or to your manager, who would discuss this with the family member.

You would need to report these and record the actions you've taken.

In care settings, individuals may be more likely to have accidents, sustain injuries and develop illnesses because they may, for example, have:

- difficulties when walking or moving that may result in them slipping and tripping
- vision loss that may result in them having falls
- weak **immune systems** due to health conditions that may result in them becoming ill.

Adult care workers and others who visit individuals, such as their families and friends, may also be more likely to fall ill and have accidents because:

- they are working closely with individuals who may be unwell
- they are carrying out tasks that involve being in contact with individuals' **body fluids**
- they are carrying out tasks that may be complex, for example using a hoist to move individuals from one position to another
- the environment may generally pose risks and hazards to everyone if it is not maintained.

> **Key terms**
>
> **Musculoskeletal disorders** refers to injuries, damage or disorders of the joints or other tissues in the upper and lower limbs or the back.
>
> **Immune system** is the body's natural defences that work together to fight disease and infections.
>
> **Health and safety officer** refers a named person in an organisation who is responsible for overseeing all health and safety matters, for example reviewing health and safety procedures and investigating accidents at work.
>
> **Body fluids** refers to any fluid that circulates around the body or is expelled from the body, such as blood, urine, sputum and vomit.

Did you know that the Health and Safety Executive (HSE) is the **regulator** for workers in England, Scotland and Wales and also for individuals in Scotland and Wales and that, in England, from April 2015 the Care Quality Commission (CQC) took over the responsibility for individuals' health and safety for health and social care providers that are registered with them?

Legislation is also in place to ensure that everyone's general health and safety is safeguarded. This includes safeguarding all those who live in, work in and visit care settings.

Legislation

As a Lead Adult Care Worker or a Lead Personal Assistant you will be expected to play your part in ensuring that your work practices and those of others you work with are safe and that you promote health and safety at all times where you work. There are specific pieces of legislation in place that set out what is required in terms of health and safety and that underpin your employer's agreed ways of working:

Health and Safety at Work Act (HASAWA) 1974

The main piece of legislation that is relevant to care settings is the Health and Safety at Work Act (HASAWA) 1974. This Act forms the basis of all other current health and safety regulations and guidelines in work settings. The main purpose of health and safety regulations is to amend or supersede current laws.

- It is the basis of all current health and safety legislation and is known as the 'enabling' Act because it enables other health and safety regulations to be made.
- It established the Health and Safety Executive (HSE) as the regulator for the health, safety and welfare of people in work settings in the UK. You need to know about the HSE because it is a useful source of information and guidance about your specific responsibilities and those of others you work with such as your employer and your colleagues; you will learn more about health and safety responsibilities in AC 1.3.
- It aims to protect the health and safety of everyone in a work setting, i.e. in the setting where you work; this includes individuals, your colleagues and other team members as well as visitors such as individuals' families, their carers, advocates, and other professionals such as GPs, social workers, chiropodists and contractors.
- It established the key duties and responsibilities of all employers and employees in work settings.
- It requires both employers and employees to work together in promoting a safe work environment and reinforces that health and safety is everyone's responsibility.

Management of Health and Safety at Work Regulations (MHSWR) 1999

- It requires employers and managers to assess and manage risks by carrying out risk assessments such as in relation to a work practice or activity. You will learn more about how to manage risks safely where you work in LO3.
- It requires work settings to have arrangements in place including appointing competent people to manage general health and safety; for example, this may be the manager in a care setting or you. All people appointed will have received the necessary training to be able to carry out their role effectively.
- It requires work settings to have procedures in place for emergency situations, for example in relation to fire safety or in the event of an accident occurring. You will have an opportunity to explore your own work setting's policies and procedures in more detail in AC 1.2.
- It requires employers to provide information, training and supervision so that work activities can be carried out safely, for example a training day on health and safety at work. This means you

and other employees are required to undertake training when asked by your employer so that you can ensure that your and others' work practices are safe and reflect current work practice.

Workplace, (Health, Safety and Welfare) Regulations 1992

- This regulation requires workplaces to be environments where risks to general health and safety are minimised. You will learn more about how this can be done in the setting where you work in LO3.
- It is concerned with the safety of the working environment. This relates not only to making sure that there are no hazards present that may pose a danger to you and others, but also to ensuring that the environment is one in which it is safe and comfortable to work, for example in relation to temperature (not too hot or too cold), lighting (avoiding poorly lit areas) and ventilation (avoiding poorly ventilated areas such as kitchens and bathrooms) and making sure that floors are safe to walk on and not slippery.
- It requires the safety of the actual building where you work, both inside and outside. This will include ensuring windows and doors can be closed securely, ensuring that areas such as bathrooms have non-slippery floors and that carpets are not worn.
- It requires the availability of welfare facilities for all employees. This will include ensuring that there is access to separate areas for employees to eat and drink, as well as clean and well-lit toilets supplied with hot and cold water, soap, washbasins and hand drying facilities.
- It requires the maintenance of a healthy and safe work environment such as by making sure all areas are cleaned regularly, ensuring that all spillages are cleaned and removed immediately and that all types of waste are disposed of safely. You will learn more about safe waste disposal practices in Unit 312 Implementing health and safety in adult care settings/services.

Manual Handling Operations Regulations 1992 (as amended 2002)

- It requires risks associated with moving and handling activities to be eliminated or minimised by employers, for example avoiding hazardous activities such as lifting heavy equipment and using risk assessment for managing moving and handling tasks safely.

It is important that you are aware of the legal responsibilities your employer has so that you can ensure that you are only following safe agreed ways of working and do not undertake any moving and handling tasks that you are not trained or competent to do. You will learn more about the legal and organisational requirements for moving and handling equipment and other objects safely in Unit 312 Implementing health and safety in adult care settings/services.
- It requires employers to provide information, training and supervision about safe moving and handling, for example instructions on how to use a ceiling hoist safely or guidelines on how to move an individual from one position to another.

Provision and Use of Work Equipment Regulations (PUWER) 1998

- It is concerned with the safety of work equipment used in work settings. This can include any type of equipment that you and/or others may use such as cleaning equipment or kitchen appliances that require employees to operate and use equipment safely.
- It requires employees to receive training before using work equipment, i.e. training in its use and the safety precautions to take. Undertaking this training forms part of your responsibilities as an employee and shows compliance with your employer's agreed ways of working for promoting health and safety.
- It requires work equipment to have visible warning signs and for employees who use work equipment to understand what these mean. This will form part of the training you receive. It is important that you ask if you are unsure about what any signs mean; you can also check the equipment manufacturers' instructions. You will learn more about moving and handling equipment in Unit 312 Implementing health and safety in adult care settings/services.

> ### Reflect on it
> #### 1.1 Work equipment safety
> Think about the different work equipment you and others operate as part of your day-to-day responsibilities. What are the consequences of not complying with legal requirements in terms of the safety of yourself and others?

Lifting Operations and Lifting Equipment Regulations (LOLER) 1998

- It is concerned with the safety of lifting equipment used in work settings; in care settings this may include hoists and other mobility aids.
- It requires lifting equipment to be maintained and used solely for the purpose it was intended for, in order to ensure it is used safely and to avoid injuries or accidents. This requires you to be vigilant that others are using equipment safely and also requires you to follow your employer's agreed ways of working for use of lifting equipment.
- It requires that all lifting operations must be planned, supervised and carried out in a safe manner by people who are competent, i.e. the employer must ensure that employees are trained and competent when using lifting equipment such as hoists. It is important than you are aware of both your rights and responsibilities so that you can ensure that you're complying with relevant legislation.

Personal Protective Equipment at Work Regulations (PPE) 1992

- It is concerned with the provision of **personal protective equipment (PPE)** such as aprons and gloves to provide protection against infections when changing an individual's dressing, assisting an individual with their personal hygiene or when handling food. You will find out about how to safely use different types of PPE in Unit 311 Supporting infection control and prevention and control in adult care settings/services, LO2.
- It requires employers to provide PPE free of charge. Did you know that it is a legal requirement for your employer to do so?
- It requires PPE to be maintained in good condition so that it is effective, otherwise it will not provide protection as intended from infections being transferred from one person to another. Being able to reduce the spread of infection is a topic you will explore in Unit 311 Supporting infection control and prevention and control in adult care settings/services.
- It requires training to be provided in the use of PPE, i.e. when, why and how to put it on and dispose of it.

> **Key terms**
>
> **Personal protective equipment (PPE)** is worn by care workers to prevent infections from spreading. PPE includes disposable gloves and plastic aprons. You will be expected to know the different types of PPE and their correct and appropriate uses in your work environment. Appropriate use may, in some cases, mean that after consideration PPE is not required.
>
> **Dangerous occurrences** are incidents that do not cause injury but have the potential to do so.
>
> **Hazardous substances** are substances that have the potential to cause harm and illness to others, for example cleaning detergents, medication, acids and bodily fluids such as blood and urine.
>
> **Hazardous materials** are materials that have the potential to cause harm and illness to others, for example used dressings or PPE that has come into contact with body fluids.

Reporting of Injuries, Diseases and Dangerous Occurrences Regulations (RIDDOR) 2013

- It requires employers to report and keep records for three years of work-related accidents that cause death and serious injuries (referred to as reportable injuries), diseases and **dangerous occurrences** (incidents with the potential to cause harm). Do you know the reporting and recording requirements of the setting where you work in relation to RIDDOR?
- It requires work settings to have procedures in place for reporting injuries, diseases and incidents. Are you complying with your employer's agreed ways of working?
- It requires employers to provide information and training on reporting injuries, diseases and incidents. Do you understand your employer's responsibilities?

Control of Substances Hazardous to Health (COSHH) 2002

- It requires employers to carry out a risk assessment to prevent or control exposure to **hazardous substances**, or **materials**; in care settings this includes cleaning materials. This is to ensure that you and others are working in safe environments and undertaking tasks safely.
- It classifies hazardous substances under the following types: very toxic, toxic, harmful,

corrosive and irritant. You will explore these types in more detail in Unit 312 Implementing health and safety in adult care settings/services, LO2.
- It requires employers to have procedures in place for safe working with hazardous substances, for example wearing PPE and carrying out a risk assessment.
- It requires employers to provide information, training and supervision so that work activities can be carried out safely, for example by monitoring workers' practices to ensure they are safe.

Electricity at Work Regulations 1989
- It is concerned with ensuring that the electricity and electrical appliances that are used in work settings are safe by ensuring they are maintained. What checks are carried out in your setting to ensure that electrical appliances such as kettles, toasters, heaters and televisions are safe to use?
- It requires that all electrical equipment installed is made safe by being tested both on and after installation, and by being clearly marked that it has been tested. How do you know if electrical equipment has been tested in the setting where you work?
- It requires employers to provide training to employees in carrying out safety checks on electrical equipment, including how to report faulty equipment and how to carry out tests on electrical equipment. What safety checks do you (or others where you work) carry out? What do they involve?

Regulatory Reform Order (Fire Safety) 2005
- It requires fire risk assessments to be completed by the person responsible for the premises; in care settings this could be the manager or employer. This should have been explained to you as part of your induction in the setting where you work.
- It requires fire equipment to be provided and maintained, for example fire extinguishers and fire blankets.
- It requires fire escape routes and exits to be provided. How do you and others ensure these are kept clear at all times? Why is this important?
- It requires employers to provide training to employees in relation to fire safety, for example what actions to take if there is a fire. As part of this process it is also important to familiarise yourself with the layout of the building where you work. Are you confident that you know where the fire escape routes are?

Health and Safety (First Aid) Regulations 1981
- It requires the provision of first aid to be made available to employees.
- It requires employers to have an appointed person in the work setting who is responsible when an emergency arises. Are you a qualified first aider? If not, who is a qualified first aider where you work?
- It requires the provision of first aid facilities, for example a first aid box and trained first aiders. Do you know what should be in the first aid box where you work?

Food Safety Act 1990
- It requires that good personal hygiene is maintained when working with food so that it is safe to eat.
- It requires that records are kept of where food is from so that it can be traced if necessary.
- It requires that any unsafe food is removed and an incident report completed. Do you know what information is required from you to complete the incident report?

Food Hygiene (England) Regulations 2006
- It requires that food safety hazards are identified. Have you been trained to do so?
- It requires that food safety controls are in place, maintained and reviewed. Do you know what these are? Do you feel confident to show others what these are?
- It requires that environments where food is prepared or cooked are kept clean and in good condition.

Civil Contingencies Act 2004
- It requires that organisations work together to plan and respond to local and national emergencies.
- It establishes how organisations such as emergency services, local authorities and health bodies can work together and share information.
- It requires that risk assessments are undertaken and emergency plans are put in place. Are you aware of whether there are arrangements in place for emergency planning in the setting where you work?

Health and Social Care (Safety and Quality) Act 2015
- It requires that adult social care providers share information about a person's care with other health and care professionals so that

safe and effective care can be provided. This promotes individuals' wellbeing and safety.
- It reduces the risk of harm and abuse by making provision for removing people convicted of certain offences from the registers kept by the regulatory bodies for health and social care professions. You can learn more about safeguarding individuals in Unit 301.
- Adult social care organisations should use a consistent **identifier** (for example the NHS Number) when sharing information about a person's care.

Research it

1.1 Health and Safety Executive (HSE)

Research some key facts and statistics specifically related to accidents, injuries and illnesses that occur in care settings. The health and social care services page on the Health and Safety Executive's website is a useful source of information:

www.hse.gov.uk/healthservices/index.htm

Provide a written account of your findings.

Key terms

An **identifier** is a tool (for example an NHS Number) used to match people to their health records.

Evidence opportunity

1.1 Health and safety legislation

With your assessor, discuss how six pieces of health and safety legislation are relevant to where you work. You could also provide a written account identifying current legislation relating to health and safety in your care setting.

AC 1.2 Explain the main points of the health and safety policies and procedures agreed with the employer as applied in own work role

Every adult care setting is required to have in place policies and procedures that set out how to put into practice safe working practices in ways

Research it

1.2 Policies and procedures

Research what the Health and Safety at Work Act 1974 says about health and safety policies. You will find the link below to the Health and Safety Executive's website a useful source of information:

www.hse.gov.uk/legislation/hswa.htm

Explain in your own words the key points that a health and safety policy and procedure must include and the reasons why. You may find it useful to refer to your own work setting's health and safety policy and procedures.

that comply with the health and safety legislation and regulations that you learned about in AC 1.1. Health and safety policies and procedures therefore set out how people's health, safety and wellbeing will be safeguarded. This may be in relation to how to keep your workplace safe, how to maintain your own safety as well as that of individuals and others you work with, or knowing what to do in an emergency, such as a fire, at work.

An employer with five or more employees is required to have a health and safety policy in writing that includes:

- a statement that indicates the policy's purpose, i.e. to provide a safe workplace
- who is responsible for the policy and for health and safety activities, i.e. the employer's, employees' and others' responsibilities
- the arrangements in place to achieve the policy's purpose, i.e. the health and safety procedures to follow.

The policy may also include procedures for identifying and reporting health and safety hazards, how to record and report accidents and incidents, and the evacuation procedures to follow.

Health and safety policies and procedures are important because they:

- reinforce the importance of health and safety to everyone
- increase everyone's understanding of safe working practices
- reduce the occurrence of injuries, accidents and illnesses.

> **Reflect on it**
>
> **1.2 Your setting's policies and procedures**
>
> Reflect on the consequences of not understanding the health and safety policies and procedures that are in place in the adult care setting where you work.
>
> How could this affect your working practices? What impact could it also have on your colleagues? The individuals you provide care or support to? Those who visit the care setting?

> **Evidence opportunity**
>
> **1.2 H&S policies and procedures agreed with the employer**
>
> Read a copy of the health and safety policy that is in place in the care setting where you work. Discuss with your manager or assessor how three main points that it explains are important in relation to health and safety. Make sure you also discuss procedures. (If you discuss this with your manager, you will need a witness testimony or voice recording to be used as evidence.) You could also provide a written account explaining the main points of health and safety policies and procedures agreed with your employer.

AC 1.3 Explain the main health and safety responsibilities of: a) self, b) the employer or manager, c) others in the work setting

The health and safety policy and procedures in the care setting where you work are essential for ensuring that it is a safe place for you, your colleagues, the individuals you provide care or support to, their families, carers, advocates and any other visitors and contractors. Maintaining health and safety is therefore everyone's responsibility.

Your responsibilities

Under the Health and Safety at Work Act (HASAWA) 1974 you are responsible for the following:

- Taking reasonable care of your own and others' health and safety, for example by reporting any hazards that you see such as a wet floor that may lead to someone slipping over. This might also mean ensuring that your clothing and dress does not pose a danger: jewellery can pose hygiene concerns, for example.
By not reporting the hazards you see your actions may place others in danger; this will mean that you will not be fulfilling your responsibilities as a Lead Adult Care Worker or Lead Personal Assistant. It is important that you report hazards as soon as you identify them and that you are able to alert others to the dangers they pose so that they do not cause any harm to others.

- Taking reasonable care to not put yourself and others at risk, for example by not coming into work when you have the flu, as this may lead to you spreading your illness to others. The individuals you provide care or support to may be frail and so this may lead to their conditions worsening. By not being responsible and taking care of your own health you may inadvertently affect the health of others by spreading illness to colleagues or team members. Your actions have serious consequences because it may mean that they have to take time off work. This in turn means that there will more pressure on the staff remaining in your work setting as they will have to cover for colleagues who are unwell; this may lead to them feeling stressed which can then impact on the quality of the service they provide to individuals they care for.

- Co-operating with your employer on all health and safety information, training and procedures to follow, for example by attending health and safety training and by wearing, using and disposing of protective clothing in line with your employer's agreed ways of working. By not doing so you will not be fulfilling your duty of care to maintain your own health and safety as well as that of others. You will also not be complying with your employer's agreed ways of working which will mean that not only will you not be setting a good example to others in your team but you may also be in breach of your contract of employment, which may ultimately lead to your dismissal.

- Understanding the meaning of safety signs and following these, for example if a contractor is carrying out some work in an area of the care setting and there is a 'do not enter' sign then you must respect this as not doing so may put you and others in danger.

Carrying out your responsibilities in this way is essential if you want to be a good role model for others in your team – if they see you complying with safety signs then it is likely they will do the same. Not doing so will mean that you and others will not be fulfilling your duty of care.

- Not misusing first aid facilities, for example not accessing these without authorisation or using the contents of the first aid box for other work activities, such as for crafts.

  It is very important that you don't misuse first aid equipment because this may mean that in the event of a health emergency they will not be available to those who really need them. This could lead to a person's pain or distress being prolonged or, worse, having fatal consequences. For example, not having quick access to a dressing when someone is bleeding may mean that you cannot apply as much pressure to the area as you would like because you may have to use your hand instead.

- Using the welfare facilities provided, for example using the hand-washing and drying facilities.

  These facilities are made available so that you and others are able to maintain good personal hygiene routines, thus minimising the spread of infection, and follow good practice when carrying out your duties and responsibilities. In Unit 311 you will have an opportunity to learn more about the recommended method for hand washing.

- Using equipment provided in accordance with instructions and training, for example ensuring the hoist is clean and in working order before using it and ensuring it is returned to its storage area after use.

  In this way you will be able to set a good example to others in ensuring that you do not spread infection between yourself and others. You will learn more about effective ways of working to reduce the spread of infection in Unit 311.

- Taking reasonable care that you follow safe working practices, for example by complying with all risk assessments in place, following your employer's agreed ways of working and not carrying out a task that you have not been trained to do.

  Complying with all risk assessments in place will mean that you will not be placing any individuals or colleagues at risk by, for example, working in a way that is unsafe. Following your employer's agreed ways of working for health and safety will mean that you will be working in ways that are in line with your employment contract and organisation's requirements. By only carrying out tasks that you have been trained to do you will ensure that you are not placing yourself and others at risk of being harmed or injured.

- Reporting all accidents, injuries and diseases to your employer, for example by completing the accident book and/or incident form.

  Not following reporting requirements will mean that your employer will not be aware of what has happened and therefore will be unable to put in place the necessary safeguards to prevent these accidents, injuries or diseases from occurring again. It is also a legal requirement for employers to keep a record of accidents, injuries and diseases that have occurred; not doing so may mean that you have acted unlawfully. This may put not only your job but also your career at risk.

- Informing your employer if your ability to work is affected. For example, you may be unwell and therefore unable to assist an individual to move, or you may be taking medication, meaning that you will not be able to operate moving and handling equipment such as a hoist.

  Not communicating with your employer when you are unwell may mean that you may have an accident at work, for example while operating equipment such as a hoist. If you feel unwell while carrying out a moving and handling activity you could injure yourself or the individual, or a colleague if they are assisting you with the move.

You should remember that in addition to your responsibilities, you have employee rights. These include the right to receive health and safety equipment such as PPE to carry out your role, the right to work in a safe environment, and the right to report any concerns you may have. These are examples; you can find out more information about your rights from organisations such as the HSE and from your contract of employment, as well as directly from your employer or manager.

> **Reflect on it**
>
> **1.3 Your responsibilities**
>
> Reflect on your health and safety responsibilities in the care setting where you work. Think about an occasion when you took care of your own and others' health and safety. What happened? What actions did you take? Why?
>
> What might the consequences have been had you not taken those actions: for you, for others and for the setting where you work?

Your manager's or employer's responsibilities

Under the Health and Safety at Work Act (HASAWA) 1974 your manager or employer is responsible for the following:

- Providing a workplace that is safe for everyone, for example by ensuring that any hazards, such as a damaged wheelchair or a frayed carpet, are removed and replaced.
  Not doing so may lead to others inadvertently using the wheelchair, this may then lead to the individual or your colleague being harmed. Similarly, not replacing the frayed carpet may lead to you or others tripping over it and being harmed.
- Ensuring the workplace is free from risks, for example by carrying out risk assessments to identify any risks and taking the necessary actions to reduce them, such as providing adequate lighting.
  In this way there will be no areas that are poorly lit so the risk of individuals falling over or slipping is minimised, for example.
- Providing information, training and supervision around health and safety, for example by making health and safety policies and procedures and training available to employees.
  In this way you and others will have received the necessary information and guidance about how to work in safe ways and follow good practice when carrying out work tasks, as well as how to support others to do the same.
- Providing safety signs, for example to alert employees that the floor may be slippery as it is being cleaned.
  This type of equipment makes the work environment a safe place to work in. Your employer must provide you with training and guidance on the meaning of safety signs and why they are used.
- Providing adequate first aid facilities, for example a first aid box and a room for first aid. First aid facilities are a legal requirement and a good way of ensuring that appropriate first aid treatment can be provided quickly in the event of an accident.
- Providing adequate welfare facilities, for example access to clean hand-washing facilities and a separate area where food and drinks can be prepared.
  This ensures that you and others you work with can maintain good personal hygiene routines, thus minimising the spread of infection.
- Providing PPE free of charge, for example aprons and gloves.
  In this way, you and others will be able to use PPE as and when you need to, for example when assisting individuals with their personal hygiene routine, handling used laundry or preparing food.
- Providing equipment free of charge, for example a hoist or a bed lift.
  Along with the provision of equipment your employer will also provide you with training and guidance on how to operate each piece of equipment. You must only use equipment and show others how to use it if you have been trained in doing so yourself and are competent to do so.
- Assessing risks and taking precautions against risks of injury, for example assessing the risks of moving an individual from one position to another and taking the necessary precautions, such as using lifting equipment.
  This will also form part of the risk assessment process that in your role as Lead Adult Care Worker or Lead Personal Assistant you will have an opportunity to contribute to. Remember that the Health and Safety Executive is the regulator whose aim is to prevent workplace injuries, deaths and illness by helping work settings to manage and control risks that arise.
- Reporting accidents, injuries, diseases and dangerous occurrences to the appropriate authority, for example the reporting of falls, fractures, **hepatitis C** and the failure of equipment while being used, such as a hoist.
  In this way the occurrence of accidents, injuries and diseases can be monitored, and measures can be put in place to prevent them or stop them from recurring.

Employers have a responsibility to ensure all of the above. In addition, they should ensure that they report any accidents and incidents to the Health and Safety Executive (HSE). They must ensure that machinery and equipment are safe to use and that there are emergency procedures in place, for example evacuation procedures to follow in the event of a fire. They must also ensure that you do not come across anything that is detrimental to your health including substances or equipment that may pose dangers (electrical equipment for example), and that the environment that you work in is a safe one. These are just a few examples; your manager/employer will be able to provide a more comprehensive list.

Others' responsibilities

Under the Health and Safety at Work Act (HASAWA) 1974, others in the work setting are responsible for:

> **Research it**
>
> **1.3 Training**
>
> Research the health and safety training that your employer has planned for you and the team, including the reasons why it is necessary. How and why will it be different from/similar to last year's training? Your manager will be a useful source of information.
>
> What would be the consequences of not attending, or not complying with the training? If there are any aspects of the training you do not understand, what should you do?

> **Key terms**
>
> **Hepatitis C** is a term used to describe inflammation of the liver caused by the hepatitis C virus. This is usually spread through blood-to-blood contact with an infected person.

- Following safe health and safety practices; for example visitors may be required to wash their hands when entering the care setting as part of its infection control procedures, sign a register upon entering and leaving the building and comply with fire emergency procedures.
  This may mean that if you see an individual's family member or a professional not washing their hands upon entering or not signing the register when entering or leaving, you must ask them politely to do so. Explaining the reasons why you are asking them will not only enable them to understand why you are asking this of them, but will also show them that you are a competent professional who understands the importance of health and safety at work.
- Complying with health and safety procedures, for example not smoking on the care setting's premises and reporting any visible hazards that may pose a danger, such as a frayed carpet or a door that will not close.
  For example, if you see an individual or a carer or advocate smoking then you must ask them not to do so, and explain your reasons why. You must also report this to your manager or employer so that this can be recorded and the situation monitored closely so that it does not happen again.
- Not misusing anything that is provided in relation to health and safety, for example the first aid box and the fire extinguishers.
  If you do see a team member misuse fire or first aid equipment you must report this as soon as possible to your manager or employer so that they can speak to the team member about their actions and replace the item if necessary.
- Maintaining a safe environment, for example not entering a care setting if you are unwell and not behaving in an aggressive way towards the workers in the care setting.
  Keeping the environment safe for you and everyone must be one of your main priorities and helping others to do the same will not only assist you in fulfilling your duties but will also mean that you will be leading by example in relation to practising in safe and non-aggressive ways.

> **Research it**
>
> **1.3 Responsibilities**
>
> You will find it helpful to refer to the Health and Safety Executive's (HSE) website:
>
> www.hse.gov.uk/workers
>
> This includes links to information on:
>
> - workers' rights and responsibilities
> - employer's responsibilities.
>
> Explore the differences between your employer's responsibilities and your own. What are the main differences and similarities? Why? Discuss with your manager or employer.

What if you don't have policies and procedures in place?

If you work with an individual who uses direct payments and there are no formal policies and procedures in place then it is important to find out from your employer and/or their representative what is in place to ensure that your work environment is safe and how to ensure that you carry out your role safely.

> **Evidence opportunity**
>
> **1.3 Health and safety responsibilities**
>
> Compare and contrast your responsibilities with those of your employer/manager and two others, and provide a written account.
>
> For your analysis, consider the similarities and differences that exist between your responsibilities and those of others, including the reasons why and the consequences of not following these.
>
> If you are a lone worker, how would you and your employer share responsibility for health and safety? You might need to agree how to deal with different health and safety emergencies that may arise.

> **6Cs**
>
> **Competence**
>
> You should feel able and confident to carry out health and safety tasks, such as moving and handling. You can only do so competently if you have received the necessary training, have understood how to carry out the task and are able to do so safely. You can only show others how to carry out health and safety tasks safely if you are practising safely yourself. How safe a practitioner are you?

AC 1.4 Describe specific tasks in the work setting that should not be carried out without special training

As part of your health and safety responsibilities there are some work tasks that require special training and must not be carried out until your employer has trained you to do so. It is the responsibility of your employer to provide you with the training for these tasks and it is your responsibility to attend this training and only agree to carry out the tasks if you feel **competent** to do so.

As procedures change and evolve, you must ensure that you receive up-to-date training. You cannot simply trust the training you previously received to still be relevant. Instead, your employer should arrange for training to be in line with new procedures, legislation and regulations. Think about the requirements that were introduced in health and social care settings because of Covid-19, such as wearing face coverings and social distancing to keep individuals and staff safe. These changes required employers to provide training and information.

Only carrying out health and safety tasks that you are competent in and have been trained to carry out is essential for:

- providing high-quality care or support; i.e. attending training means that you have kept your knowledge and practices up to date and based them on current health and safety legislation and your employer's agreed ways of working
- avoiding putting yourself and others at risk; for example ensuring that you only carry out moving and handling when you have been trained to do so will mean that you will use safe practices when moving an individual from one position to another thus reducing the risks to you (such as a back injury) and to the individual (such as a fall). Remember that this can be dangerous, so if there are any new procedures you have not received training in you must receive training in these, whether it involves equipment you have used before or not. See the legislation relating to the Manual Handling Operations Regulations 1992, Lifting Operations and Lifting Equipment Regulations (LOLER) 1998 and Provision and Use of Work Equipment Regulations (PUWER) 1998 on pages 387–388.
- carrying out your health and safety responsibilities competently – complying with the health and safety policy and procedures available in the care setting where you work means that you will be carrying out your job role and responsibilities to the best of your ability.

Reflect on it

1.4 Training

Reflect on a task that you were required to carry out in the care setting where you work that required special training. What was it? Why did it require special training? Did you feel competent to carry it out? Why?

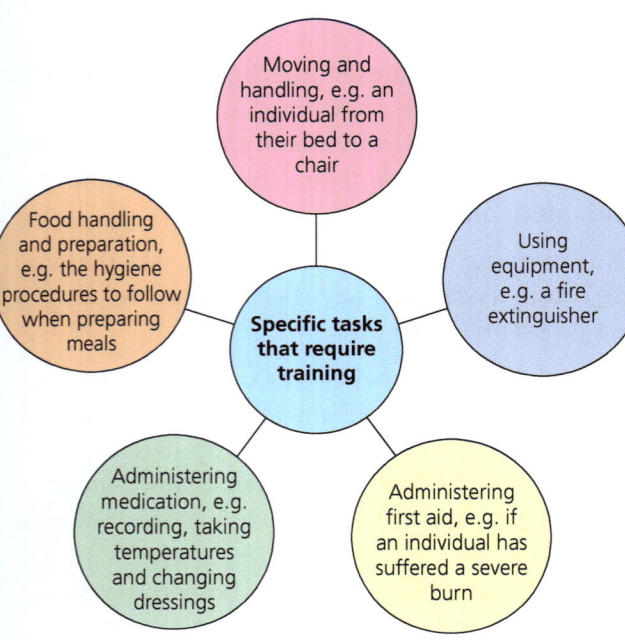

Figure 11.1 Health and safety tasks that should not be carried out without training

Tasks that you should not carry out without special training

Tasks that you should not carry out without special training may include those relating to:

Use of equipment

Using equipment such as moving and handling equipment requires special training. You must make sure that you receive training because not doing so may mean that you use the wrong type of equipment for an individual who wants to be hoisted from their bed to a chair. For example, using the wrong size sling may result in you injuring the individual or yourself.

First aid

You must never carry out first aid without having received training first because doing so may mean that you cause the individual unnecessary pain or harm. For example, if an individual has a broken limb it is important that you ensure they do not move the limb. If you are not aware of this you may not only cause the individual pain but could cause additional injuries.

Medication

You have a duty of care towards the individuals you provide care and support for. Administering medication is a highly skilled task because you need to know, for example, how it is administered correctly, including any special precautions to take and any observations you may need to carry out. Administering medication without any special training may result in you administering medication to an individual ineffectively; this may have fatal consequences for the individual.

Health care procedures

Health care procedures such as changing used dressings or taking individuals' temperatures and blood pressure requires special training. You must not carry out health care procedures without training because doing so may result in an individual's blood pressure not being obtained or recorded correctly, for example. This may mean that an individual's condition deteriorates without you and/or others noticing.

Food handling and preparation

Handling and preparing food is a skilled task and must not be undertaken without special training as doing so may result in you causing individuals to fall ill. For example, providing individuals with food that has not been cooked to the right temperature could result in them being poisoned with harmful bacteria; this may lead to individuals becoming ill and may even lead to fatalities.

Evidence opportunity

1.4 Tasks that require special training

Discuss with a senior colleague or your assessor the range of health and safety tasks that you both carry out in the care setting where you work and that require special training. What differences are there between your health and safety responsibilities and those of your senior colleague? Write a self-reflective account of your findings.

LO2 Understand procedures for responding to accidents and sudden illness

> **Getting started**
>
> Think about an occasion when you or someone you know became unwell or had an accident. Discuss what happened. Why do you think the illness/accident happened? Could anything have been done to prevent it from happening? What treatment was provided? Who provided it? When? Why?

AC 2.1 Identify different types of accidents and sudden illnesses that may occur in own work setting / service

Accidents and sudden illnesses may occur when hazards and risks have or have not been identified or minimised through the risk assessment process.

In work settings, accidents and sudden illnesses can happen and can range from being relatively minor to very serious. In adult care settings, there are some types of accidents and sudden illnesses that occur more frequently than in other work settings because of the work activities that adult care workers carry out on a day-to-day basis. These include supporting individuals with care tasks including eating, drinking, personal care and moving and positioning individuals, as well as supporting individuals who may have conditions that affect their physical and mental health. The statistics below from the Health and Safety Executive (HSE) illustrate the more common types of accidents and illnesses relating to care workers in adult care settings.

The HSE reports that each year for the health and social care sector:

- 5 per cent of workers suffer from an illness they believe to be work-related – of the illnesses reported, 44 per cent are stress, depression or anxiety, 37 per cent are musculoskeletal disorders and 19 per cent are other illnesses
- 2 per cent of workers sustain a work-related injury – of the non-fatal accidents reported by employers in 2015/16, 27 per cent are slips, trips and falls, 25 per cent are lifting and handling and 21 per cent are physical assault.

Source: *Health and Safety Executive (2016) 'Statistics for the Health and Social Care sector'*

> **Reflect on it**
>
> **2.1 HSE statistics**
>
> Reflect on the statistics reported by the HSE above. Did any surprise you? Why? Were there any that you were expecting to see? Why? How did your current knowledge compare to this?

Common types of accidents in adult care settings

- **Slips, trips and falls:** slips, trips and falls may be caused by hazards in the work setting that have not been identified or assessed correctly, or because individuals with care or support needs are more susceptible to having accidents if, for example, they have sight loss or difficulties with their mobility. These types of accidents may lead to fractures, back injuries, cuts, bruises and bleeding.
- **Lifting and handling:** lifting and handling in adult care settings may involve both supporting individuals with moving and positioning as well as moving items or equipment such as hoists, beds, wheelchairs and furniture, for example when cleaning. If you do not follow your agreed ways of working you may injure your back or cause an individual to fall. You will learn more about safe practices for moving and handling items and equipment in Unit 312, LO1. Lifting and handling equipment may also cause injuries, for example electric shocks may occur if equipment is faulty and choking may result if equipment such as hoists and slings are not used correctly.
- **Physical assault:** physical assault is more commonly experienced by workers in the health and social care sector than by workers in other sectors and can be the cause of stress as well as physical injuries. Physical assault may result because of the needs of an individual whose behaviour challenges, medical conditions or frustration with not having their care or support needs met.

Common types of illnesses in adult care settings

- **Stress, depression and anxiety:** working long shifts, providing support to meet the needs of an individual whose behaviour challenges, such as an individual with mental health needs or dementia on a day-to-day basis, can lead to adult care workers being placed under additional stress. If this is left untreated then it can lead to individuals feeling low in themselves and even to the development of depression and anxiety. See Unit 314 Understanding personal wellbeing, LO4 for more information on stress.
- **Musculoskeletal disorders:** poor working practices when supporting individuals to move from one position to another, such as over-stretching and lifting, can lead to repetitive strain being placed on the back, arms and legs, which can result in disorders that cause pain and restrict the body's movements.
- **Other illnesses:** medical conditions, such as type 2 diabetes, asthma or heart disease can be the cause of sudden illnesses. For example, diabetes can lead to a diabetic coma where the individual loses consciousness, asthma can lead to severe breathing difficulties and heart disease to a heart attack or cardiac arrest. Epilepsy can lead to seizures. A stroke may occur when a blood clot obstructs the flow of blood and oxygen to the brain (ischaemic stroke) or when there is bleeding in or around the brain (haemorrhagic stroke). This may result in the person's face drooping on one side, not being able to lift and keep both their arms up, their speech being slurred or having difficulties understanding what you're saying to them. Poor working practices, such as lack of good hygiene, may lead to the spread of infections and illnesses such as food poisoning. You will learn more about how to reduce the spread of infections in Unit 311.

Research it

2.1 Diabetes

Research the 'BIG 3 signs of diabetes'. Write down your findings.

You will find it useful to visit the Diabetes.co.uk website for more information on the big three signs of diabetes.

Would you know what to do if an individual with diabetes became unwell? Does your employer have a policy in place for dealing with medical emergencies? If so, what is it?

Evidence opportunity

2.1 Accidents and sudden illnesses

How many different types of accidents and sudden illnesses do you know about that have occurred where you work, or may occur? Produce a written account describing these. What do you think were the causes? Discuss them with your assessor or manager and record the conversation (if you can) or obtain a witness testimony from them.

Now reflect on the illnesses that you know have been experienced by the individuals and staff in your work setting. How many different types were there? Do you know their causes? Discuss them with your assessor or manager, as above.

If you are a lone worker, how would you keep a record of the different types of accidents and illnesses that have occurred and why? You might need to record these in an individual's care plan and in a separate section, whereas in a residential setting you may have to record accidents and illnesses that have occurred in an accident book, for example, or using specific documents.

AC 2.2 Describe procedures to be followed if an accident or sudden illness should occur

When an accident or sudden illness occurs in a work setting everyone has a role to play and that includes you! Providing first aid, as you have learned, is a task that cannot be carried out without special training. Therefore, it is important if you have not been trained in first aid that you do not provide first aid treatment to a person who has had an accident or sudden illness in your work setting. Doing so may have serious consequences because you may cause the person further pain or discomfort and may make the situation worse. You will also not be complying with your own work setting's agreed ways of working and so you may be disciplined by your employer.

If you work in a residential care home, then it is unlikely you will have to take the lead in a health emergency as you will be working as part of a team; instead you may need to seek assistance from a more senior colleague who is a trained first aider. If, however, you are working on your own as a personal assistant with an individual who lives in their own home then it is likely that as well as seeking help from emergency services you will need to take action yourself. However, you will need to ensure that you have received the relevant training.

Just because you are not a trained first aider does not mean that you cannot play an important role in providing assistance when an accident or sudden illness has occurred by following your work setting's procedures.

Provide assistance and reassurance

You can provide the casualty with support; kind words and reassurance are in high demand when you are in pain. Remember what you have learned about person-centred care and ensure that you listen to the individual and do what you can to respect their privacy. It may be that they do not want others to see them in this way, and so you could find a way to ensure that others do not come near the scene. Of course, dealing with the situation first is key.

Working in this way will ensure that you are fulfilling your duty of care and respecting individuals' rights. Being considerate towards individuals and others will help to calm the situation down and will mean that you will be able to act professionally and competently.

Call for help

Do this as quickly as you can because not doing so may mean that the person's condition worsens because they have not had access to medical help. This may mean calling 999 for an ambulance or paramedic, or locating a qualified person in your setting. This will depend on where you work. If the incident is in someone's home you will need to call 999 first; if in a care setting, again the emergency services will be the best point of contact. However, you may also need to alert another staff member who is more qualified to deal with the situation, depending on what the situation is; there may even be a medical professional available. If you are working in a hospital there will be medical professionals around you that you can seek for immediate help. The key thing is to get help immediately.

Provide first aid

The section below covers this, but the important thing to remember is that you should only provide first aid if you have received the proper training and feel confident in carrying this out.

If you have not received the correct training and you carry out first aid, you may cause the person more pain and distress and your actions may inadvertently lead to the person developing more serious injuries. For example, if you move an individual who has fallen downstairs and landed on their back, rather than ensure that you make them comfortable and that they do not move, you may cause further damage to their back. This may even lead to irreversible damage, and them being never able to walk again.

Make the area safe

Make sure the area around the individual is safe, and that there is nothing that has the potential to cause further harm either to the individual or to those who may also be in the area. At the same time, do not attempt to remove anything that may cause further harm until the emergency services arrive. Make sure that others do not come near the scene if this will cause harm. You may even need to put a sign up if there is one available. This will also ensure that you are doing your utmost to protect the individual's privacy.

Assist others

You can provide assistance to the qualified first aider. Make sure you do as the qualified first aider instructs. They will tell you what they need and what to do, and you should do as they say. Not doing so may mean that your actions may be negligent. You may, for example, need to call for help or an ambulance, or find a blanket to keep the casualty warm. You may need to ensure the area is kept safe as mentioned above, for example by asking other individuals not to approach the casualty so as to protect the casualty's privacy and dignity. Remember that when you are telling others about the situation, whether it is someone on the scene or the emergency/ambulance services, speak clearly, remain calm and answer all the questions they ask you. In this way they will be able to take the correct actions quickly and provide the casualty with the help they need.

Also provide reassurance to others who may be concerned or distressed about what has happened, especially if the incident has been an upsetting one. Inform them of the facts, at the same time as reassuring them. You should also seek support if you have also found the situation distressing. This will need to be done after the incident, but it is important to remember to do this so that you can share your feelings, feel supported and are therefore in a position to support others. Not doing so may mean that you will find it difficult to support others because you will be feeling too upset and/or stressed.

Reflect

Make sure you take the time to reflect on what has taken place. Could this incident have been prevented? How? How did you deal with the situation? What did you do well? What could you have improved? How would you support others to deal with a similar situation?

Ensure your training and knowledge is up to date

You can keep your knowledge and skills up to date by attending training and reading through your work setting's procedures for what to do in the event of an accident or sudden illness. Keeping yourself up to date is very important because by doing so you can ensure that the methods you are using reflect current good practice and ensure that you are complying with your manager or employer's agreed ways of working.

Suggest changes and improvements

In light of the accident, illness and procedures followed, is there anything that could be improved to better the procedures, or make the environment safer to prevent further accidents in the setting, home or community? Make sure that you discuss this with your manager, or the individual that you care for if you are working in their home. This will lead to improved care and support and a safer environment.

First aid procedures

Although you may not be a qualified first aider it is still useful to have some knowledge of basic first aid when attending an accident or sudden illness. These are stressful situations that you may come across in your work setting and so having an understanding of what to do can help you feel more able to handle them. It will also enable you to be an effective role model for others to whom you may need to provide support and/or additional information.

You can use **DR's ABC** as a good way of helping you to remember what to do when you come across an accident or sudden illness.

- **D** (Danger): Look around you and check for any risks or signs of danger. Never put yourself in any danger.
- **R** (Response assessment): Assess all casualties. Check whether they are conscious by calling their name, tapping them on their shoulders, observing whether they are breathing normally.
- **S** (Shout for help): Call an ambulance or get someone else to do this for you. Ask them to come back and tell you that they have done this.
- **A** (Airway): Check that the casualty's airway is open and not blocked. Check that help is on its way.
- **B** (Breathing): Check whether the casualty is breathing normally. If the casualty is breathing normally place the casualty in the recovery position. If the casualty is not breathing, start CPR only if you have been trained to do so. Check that help is on its way.
- **C** (Circulation): Once you've established the casualty is breathing check for any signs of severe bleeding. If the casualty is bleeding apply direct pressure to the wound. If the casualty is not bleeding and unresponsive keep them in the recovery position until help arrives. Continue to monitor the casualty and check that help is on its way.

Reflect on it

2.2 How you can help

Reflect on an occasion when you witnessed an accident or someone becoming suddenly unwell.

How did you feel? What did you do? Why?

Now think about the other ways of helping that you learned about by following your work setting's procedures. Is there any other action you could have taken? Why?

Research it

2.1, 2.2 First aid

Research the basic first aid treatment for two accidents and two sudden illnesses. Write down your findings.

You will find a current first aid book a useful source of information. There should be one available in your work setting – ask your manager if you can reference it. Your work setting's first aid procedures will also be useful.

Research it

2.2 First aid

Research how to treat three conditions that individuals may have with first aid and discuss your findings with a colleague. The St John's Ambulance information page 'First Aid Tips, Information and Advice' is a useful source of information:

www.sja.org.uk/get-advice/first-aid-advice/?parentId=12265&categoryId=12349

It is important that you have an understanding of the different first aid procedures and that you receive training for these before you perform them.

Tables 11.1 and 11.2 outline some useful sources (mainly St John's Ambulance and the NHS) that will explain some of the first aid procedures you will need to know. They are helpful sources of knowledge and information, although they will not replace training.

Of course you are not expected to know all of the medical procedures. However, it is useful to be trained in first aid so that you are equipped with the knowledge and skills that you may need until the medical services are at the scene.

You will also find it useful to research and learn more about the first aid procedures for the following:

- **Anaphylaxis (or anaphylactic shock):** www.nhs.uk/conditions/anaphylaxis and www.nhs.uk/conditions/anaphylaxis/treatment are useful sources of information.
- **Drowning:** www.sja.org.uk/get-advice/first-aid-advice/breathing-difficulties/drowning/ is a useful source of information.
- **Difficulty breathing:** www.nhs.uk/conditions/shortness-of-breath may be a useful source of information.
- **Hot and cold conditions:** www.sja.org.uk/get-advice/first-aid-advice/effects-of-heat-and-cold/ is a useful source of information.
- **Loss of consciousness:** www.nhs.uk/conditions/first-aid/ may be a useful source of information.

The NHS web page, www.nhs.uk/conditions/first-aid/, is a good source of information for the different types of accidents and illnesses discussed above (you may need to scroll down to see each type).

You will also need to know how to place a casualty in the recovery position, as you will need to do this when dealing with various emergencies. Go to www.sja.org.uk/get-advice/first-aid-advice/unresponsive-casualty/how-to-do-the-recovery-position/ to understand the procedure.

The information on these websites will not replace training. You must ensure that you attend all first aid training courses that you are advised to attend. You and your employer are responsible for ensuring you receive the training and guidance that you need.

Table 11.1 Accidents, signs and symptoms and useful sources of information

Type of accident	Signs and symptoms	Useful source of information
Fracture	• Swelling • Oddly positioned limbs • Pain around the fractured area	www.sja.org.uk/get-advice/first-aid-advice/bones-and-muscle-injuries/broken-bones-and-fractures/
Cut	Large or small amounts of blood	Cuts and grazes: www.sja.org.uk/get-advice/first-aid-advice/minor-illnesses-and-injuries/cuts-and-grazes/
Bleeding	Large or small amounts of blood	Severe bleeding: www.sja.org.uk/get-advice/first-aid-advice/bleeding/severe-bleeding/ Nose bleeds: www.sja.org.uk/get-advice/first-aid-advice/bleeding/nosebleeds/
Burn/scalds caused by heat/flames/hot liquids/chemicals/electrical currents	• Swollen or blistered skin • The person may be in severe pain or shock	www.sja.org.uk/get-advice/first-aid-advice/burns-and-scalds/
Poisoning caused by chemicals, plants or substances like drugs and alcohol	• The person may be unconscious • The person may be in severe pain • Swollen or blistered skin around the mouth and lips	www.sja.org.uk/get-advice/first-aid-advice/poisoning/
Electrical injuries caused by low voltages (e.g. electrical appliances such as a kettle or heater)	• The person may have burns • The person may have had a cardiac arrest	www.sja.org.uk/get-advice/first-aid-advice/minor-illnesses-and-injuries/low-voltage-electrocution/

Table 11.2 Sudden illnesses, signs and symptoms and useful sources of information

Type of sudden illness	Signs and symptoms	Useful source of information
Cardiac arrest is caused by a heart attack, shock or electric shock	• The person has no pulse • The person is not breathing	Cardiac arrest: www.sja.org.uk/get-advice/first-aid-advice/heart-conditions/cardiac-arrest/ Heart attack: www.sja.org.uk/get-advice/first-aid-advice/heart-conditions/heart-attack/
Stroke is caused by blood clots that block the flow of blood to the brain	• The person may have an uneven face • The person may not be able to raise and hold both arms • The person's speech may be confused	www.sja.org.uk/get-advice/first-aid-advice/stroke/
Epileptic seizure is caused by changes in the brain's activity	Involuntary contraction of muscles. This is also referred to as a convulsion or a fit	www.sja.org.uk/get-advice/first-aid-advice/seizures/seizures-in-adults/

Table 11.2 Sudden illnesses, signs and symptoms and useful sources of information *continued*

Type of sudden illness	Signs and symptoms	Useful source of information
Choking and difficulty with breathing usually caused by food becoming stuck in the throat	• Coughing, gasping • Difficulty breathing (gasping) • Difficulty speaking	www.sja.org.uk/get-advice/first-aid-advice/choking/adult-choking/
Shock is caused when blood is not flowing round the body effectively	• Cold, clammy and/or pale skin • Fast pulse • Fast breathing • May feel sick	www.sja.org.uk/get-advice/first-aid-advice/bleeding/shock/
Loss of consciousness is caused by a faint or a serious illness	Not being responsive, either partial or total unresponsiveness	www.sja.org.uk/get-advice/first-aid-advice/unresponsive-casualty/how-to-do-cpr-on-an-adult/ This website has information on what to do when dealing with an unresponsive breathing adult. There is also information on 'responsive adult' on this website; the NHS website may also be useful.

Some important points to remember:

- Make sure you receive training in first aid and remember its importance.
- Only carry out the actions that you have been trained in and are able to do safely without causing the individual harm.
- Do not attempt to treat an individual if you do not have the right training or take any actions that you do not have understanding of, as this could harm the individual.
- Make sure you get help as fast as you can and support the individual as best you can.
- Make sure the area around the individual is safe and free of any dangerous objects.
- Support the person who is dealing with the situation, for example a medical professional.
- Seek the advice of a medical professional first if possible.
- Remember the Data Protection Act 2018 when you record the incident and when you record details about the individual.
- The actions you take will vary depending on your setting. For example, in a care setting you will be able to seek the advice of colleagues, although they may not be doctors or medical professionals. If you are working in someone's home it may be that you will need to seek help from medical professionals or emergency services in situations where you do not have the expertise and have not received training.

Evidence opportunity

2.2 Procedures to follow if an accident or sudden illness should occur

Identify one accident and one sudden illness that may occur in the care setting where you work. Explain to your assessor the procedures that must be followed when responding to these. Provide a written account to document your discussion.

AC 2.3 Outline the records that must be maintained relating to accidents, incidents and sudden illness

You must report and record accidents and sudden illnesses. You should ensure that you report them immediately to your manager, a senior member of staff or a first aider.

After an accident, incident or sudden illness, you must ensure that all the information is recorded even if it was minor. This is a legal requirement as set out by RIDDOR. Make sure that you record what happened by completing the accident book or incident form. Record details of:

- the individual
- date
- time
- place of the accident/sudden illness

- their injury/illness
- what you witnessed
- any information you received
- your actions taken in response and the actions taken by others (when you sought help, what time help arrived on the scene, whether you needed any equipment or medication to deal with the situation)
- the outcome of the incident
- your name and signature.

This covers the main points you will be expected to record but this might vary depending on your setting.

It is important that this is all recorded so that the information can be shared with your manager, if you work in a setting, or an inspector. It may even be needed by medical or legal professionals, so it is important that you record as much detail as possible.

> **Evidence opportunity**
>
> **2.3 Records**
>
> Discuss with a colleague the records that must be maintained in your work setting for accidents, incidents and sudden illness.

LO3 Be able to carry out own responsibilities for health and safety

> **Getting started**
>
> Think about an occasion when you identified a hazard in the care setting where you work. This may have been in relation to unsafe practices or a high-risk activity. How did your employer manage this risk? What was your role? Did you access any additional support? If so, from whom, where and why? Why was it important that your employer's health and safety agreed ways of working were followed?
>
> Reflect on the situation you described above. Looking back, would you do anything different next time?

AC 3.1 Demonstrate the use of policies and procedures or other agreed ways of working that relate to health and safety in care settings/services

Employers' health and safety policies and procedures and agreed ways of working will vary across different adult care settings but they will all contain the same main points that detail what the policy is about and its purpose as well as the procedures to follow in practice. Below are some examples of some of the main points included in an adult care setting's policies and procedures; you will need to follow these when you use them as you will be observed doing so for this AC.

Moving and handling

Moving and handling policy: The purpose of this policy is to promote safe ways of moving and handling at work so that the risk of injury is reduced and to ensure that all employees follow agreed ways of working in line with legal requirements.

The work setting must be committed to ensuring that all moving and handling activities are carried out safely and that all employees receive training, instruction, support and guidance to be able to carry out all moving and handling activities competently.

This policy applies to all employees and sets out areas of responsibility for everyone including care workers, Lead Adult Care Workers, the manager and the chief executive. For example, care workers must attend moving and handling training, Lead Adult Care Workers must monitor work practices of care workers to ensure their safety and report any concerns to the manager, the manager must ensure risk assessments are carried out for all moving and handling tasks and the chief executive must ensure that all the moving and handling equipment that is required is bought for the setting.

> **Reflect on it**
>
> **3.1 Agreed ways of working for moving and handling**
>
> Reflect on your employer's agreed ways of working for moving and handling. What procedures do you use in your work setting? How do these compare to the ones above? Why? Are there any individuals who have moving and handling guidelines specific to their needs? Why are these necessary?

Moving and handling procedures: These procedures are for all employees and must only be used after a risk assessment has been completed with the individual and you have referenced the individual's moving and handling guidelines and plan of care.

For example, to assist an individual to stand up from sitting in a chair, you will need to refer to the individual's risk assessment to find out if the individual requires assistance to stand or can do so independently. If you want to enable the individual to safely stand independently, then ask the individual to move forward to the edge of the chair, place their feet apart, one foot in front of the other and their hands on the arms of the chair. Ask the individual to look ahead and to lean forwards and ask them to stand up on the command 'stand' (e.g. 'ready, steady, stand.'). If the individual requires assistance then you must position yourself on one side of the individual, facing towards their side. Then bend your knees and place your feet apart, adopting a wide base, with one foot level with the individual's feet. Place one hand on the small of the individual's back and the other hand on the individual's shoulder. Follow the process for assisting an individual who is independent and then on the word 'stand', transfer your weight from one leg to the other in the direction of the individual standing through your forearm so that you can assist the individual to stand safely.

Fire policy

Fire policy: The purpose of this policy is to prevent fires from happening and in the event that a fire does occur, to ensure that all employees know what to do and how to respond quickly and safely.

The organisation/setting where you work must be committed to ensuring that the risks of fires occurring are minimised and that all staff receive regular training in what to do in the event of a fire.

The named fire officer, which may or may not be you, will be responsible for calling the fire brigade and liaising with them upon their arrival to ensure everyone can be accounted for. If you identify that someone is not accounted for then let the fire officer know.

Fire procedures: These procedures are for all employees. In the event of a fire or the fire alarm going off, or being triggered, staff must go to the nearest fire assembly point. Remain calm. When asked to evacuate, if possible assist others such as individuals, visitors, other staff. Do not re-enter the building once evacuated until you've been told it's safe to do so and do not stop to collect valuables and personal possessions.

> **Research it**
>
> **3.1 Fire safety procedures**
>
> Read through the fire safety procedures that you use in your work setting. If you work with individuals in their own homes, then compare these to a fire procedure used in a residential setting or vice versa. How do these compare and contrast? Why?

First aid

First aid policy: The purpose of the policy is to be able to provide first aid support to a person who has been injured or become unwell.

The setting where you work must be committed to ensuring that qualified first aiders are able to attend all incidents quickly, provide support and take necessary actions.

First aid procedures: These procedures are for all employees, individuals and visitors. In the event of a minor injury, report it to a named first aider. Follow the first aider's advice. Record the minor injury in the accident book as soon as possible. The first aider will also report the accident to their manager or employer so that a risk assessment can be completed to find out why the accident occurred and how it can be prevented from happening again.

> **Evidence opportunity**
>
> **3.1 Using policies and procedures that relate to health and safety**
>
> Think about an occasion when you had to refer to your employer's health and safety procedures or agreed ways of working. Why did you refer to these?
>
> If you work in a setting, find a colleague who is working at the same level as you and ask them to observe you carrying out a task using your setting's agreed ways of working/procedures in relation to health and safety. Ask your colleague whether they thought you practised in line with this. If not, ask them why. What improvements do you need to make to your practices? Do you think you're able to show others how to use policies and procedures and agreed ways of working in relation to health and safety? Arrange for your assessor to observe you or obtain a witness testimony from your manager or employer if you are a Lead Personal Assistant.

AC 3.2 Demonstrate how to support others to understand and follow safe practices

As a lead, your role will involve providing support to others and ensuring they follow safe working practices too; after all there is no point in you working safely and others not doing so. You will be observed supporting others to work in ways that are safe.

> **Reflect on it**
>
> **3.2 Why accidents and illnesses occur**
>
> Reflect on the reason why accidents and illnesses may occur in your work setting. For example, it may be that the individuals you support have mobility difficulties and are prone to tripping and slipping; perhaps they have dementia and are therefore not aware of dangers in the environment; or they have behaviours that challenge that can result in them injuring themselves and/or others.

You can support others by:

- **Empowering others:** providing others with information that they can understand in relation to health and safety so that they can take responsibility for their own health and safety. For example, an individual with a learning disability may require information to be produced using words and photographs; a team member may require you to explain aspects that they don't understand and how it will affect their practice; an individual's family member may have questions about how they can contribute to health and safety. Useful sources of information include the Health and Safety Executive (HSE), your employer, the named person responsible for health and safety in the setting where you work, and training courses. It is important that you empower individuals by talking to them about health and safety, complete risk assessments for them and ensure that they understand how they can take responsibility for their own health and safety.

- **Recognising and taking action over unsafe practices:** supporting others in relation to health and safety will involve making them aware when they have not practised in a safe way so that they understand what they must do to take care of their own and others' health and safety. For example, you may see a colleague not following an individual's guidelines when assisting them to use a hoist or a mobility aid – you must not ignore this. You must ask the colleague to stop and explain to them constructively why their practices are unsafe; you can do this by sitting down with them away from the individual and speaking to them about their actions and ways to improve how they practice. If you do this constructively, your colleague will listen to you and be committed to improving the way they work. They may also request that you supervise them so they can ensure they have understood how to practise safely.

- **Being a positive role model:** following safe health and safety practices yourself will encourage others to follow your lead. You can, if you are working alongside others, explain to them what practices you are following and expecting them to follow and the reasons why. This will help them to understand why they must work in safe ways and the consequences of not doing so.

> **Research it**
>
> **3.2 Skills for supporting others**
>
> Research the skills that are required by lead practitioners such as yourself to support others to understand health and safety and follow agreed safe practices. You may find your manager or employer a useful source of information.
>
> Assess the skills that you already have to support others and discuss your assessment with your manager or employer. Did they agree? Do you need to take any further action? Why?

> **Evidence opportunity**
>
> **3.2 Supporting others to understand health and safety**
>
> Identify a team member or colleague who requires your support with following agreed safe practices. Ask your assessor to observe you providing this support.
>
> You could also accompany the observation with a written account explaining how you support others' understanding of health and safety and follow agreed safe practices.
>
> If you are a lone worker how would you explain health and safety to a family member visiting an individual? You might need to have a discussion with them or explain some current best practices such as in relation to hand washing and infection control, whereas in a residential setting you would not have to do this directly, you would report it to a more senior colleague or to your manager.

AC 3.3 Demonstrate how to minimise and manage potential risks and hazards

Identifying health and safety hazards and associated risks on their own is not sufficient for protecting the safety of everyone in your work setting. All identified health and safety risks must also be reported so that they can be eliminated or minimised and not continue to pose a danger to those who may be affected by them. It is one of your responsibilities as a care worker to report any unsafe situation or anything that poses a risk.

Once the risks have been assessed, your setting/employer will need to make sure that they put measures in place to control and reduce these risks. If it is established that the hazard cannot be eliminated then it will be considered how the level of risk can be reduced to minimise the likelihood of harm occurring. For example, this may include wearing PPE when handling soiled laundry to minimise the risk of infection to you and others or ensuring two carers support an individual to mobilise to minimise the risk of the individual falling and/or the carers injuring their backs.

The health and safety policy in the care setting where you work will include information and guidance about how and when to report potential health and safety risks that you have identified or that others, such as individuals or visitors, have reported to you.

You must report potential health and safety risks as soon as you have identified them or others have told you about them. Not doing so may result in others being put in further danger or harmed. In the first instance you should report these to your manager. Your manager will then guide you to ensure that the risk poses no further danger or harm and show you how to record the risks you have identified.

The Management of Health and Safety at Work Regulations (MHSWR) 1999 mean that employers and managers are legally required to assess and manage risks by carrying out risk assessments. Figure 11.3 shows an example of how to report in writing the health and safety risks you have identified. What documents do you use in your work setting?

> **Reflect on it**
>
> **3.3 Reporting risks**
>
> Research the procedures that you are expected to follow for reporting health and safety risks that have been identified in the care setting where you work. Confirm your understanding of these with your manager. Write a short reflective account.

Minimising and managing potential risks and hazards

Being able to minimise and manage potential risks and hazards means that, as a Lead Adult Care Worker or Lead Personal Assistant, not only will you need to be aware of your own practices but also those of others and the work environment that you and others work in. It is important that you are able to do this because you will be observed minimising potential health and safety risks so that you and others can take the necessary actions to prevent them from becoming a danger. You can minimise and manage potential risks and hazards by:

- **ensuring a safe environment:** as part of your work role you may need to complete regular health and safety checks. For example, you may be required to walk around the premises and do visual checks of every area. For example, in the bathroom – are there any slippery floors? In the kitchen – are there any electrical appliances that have not been checked for safety? In the hallway – are there any loose rugs? On the stairs – is there any loose carpet? Corridors – are there any items blocking the walk-through areas? In this way you will be showing your vigilance and ensuring that all areas are kept safe for you and everyone else who uses them.
- **following safe practices:** as part of your work role you must also know what to do when you have identified any potential risks so that you can prevent them posing any dangers to others. As well as recording them and reporting them to your manager and employer there are other specific actions you can take. For example, if you see a slippery floor in the bathroom ensure you wipe it dry and consider whether a different type of floor covering may be more appropriate, such as one that is non-slippery and designed especially for bathrooms, or perhaps a non-slippery bath mat is needed. If there is an electrical appliance in the kitchen that hasn't been safety tested, find out why, report it immediately and remove it from the area so it cannot be used by others who may end up being injured. You will also need to place the appliance in a safe storage area and put a label on it to warn others of the danger and to ensure it is not used.

> **Evidence opportunity**
>
> **3.3 Minimise and manage potential risks and hazards**
>
> You will be observed minimising and managing potential risks and hazards.
>
> Discuss with your assessor how you minimise and manage potential health and safety risks in your work setting. Obtain feedback from your manager about the skills and knowledge you demonstrated in relation to how you minimise and manage potential risks and hazards. What areas did you do well in? Why? What areas do you need to further improve on? Why?

AC 3.4 Use risk assessment in relation to health and safety

Taking risks is not easy but this should not prevent you from doing what you want to do. Taking risks is part of everyday life and when risks are taken in a positive manner they can bring about many benefits. An essential part of the health and safety responsibilities you and all those in the care setting where you work have involves being aware of how hazards and risks can occur.

Hazards

Hazards are dangers that have the potential to cause harm; i.e. they can be items in the work setting or situations or particular activities that may be the cause of accidents, injuries, ill health, deaths or damage.

Work setting

Hazards in the work setting can include the following:

- Wheelchairs, if not stored away securely when not in use, can be trip hazards.
- Walking aids, if not checked to be safe to use, can lead to individuals falling over.
- Broken furniture, if not replaced or fixed, can lead to individuals injuring themselves.

Situations

Situations in the work setting that pose dangers include the following:

- An individual becomes distressed and throws a chair at a window that results in it being broken.
- An adult care worker forgets to wipe a spillage clean on the floor resulting in their colleague slipping over and hurting their back.
- A visitor leaves their bag in the middle of the hallway resulting in an individual tripping over and fracturing their leg.

> **Research it**
>
> **3.4 Common hazards**
>
> Research the common hazards that are posed by adult care settings. You can base your research on the care setting where you work. You may also find the HSE's information page, 'Sensible risk assessment in care settings' a useful source of information:
>
> www.hse.gov.uk/healthservices/sensible-risk-assessment-care-settings.htm
>
> Also research some of the regulations that require risks to be assessed. These include the Noise at Work Regulations 1989 and Control of Asbestos at Work Regulations 2002. Some are also mentioned in AC 1.1 (Personal Protective Equipment at Work Regulations 1992 and Control of Substances Hazardous to Health Regulations 2002). What other regulations can you find out about that require risk assessments to be carried out? How do these relate to you? Write notes on what you find.

Particular activities

Activities can also pose dangers. These can include the following:

- An adult care worker cleans the floor and then forgets to lock the detergent away securely after use. This could lead to it being swallowed accidentally by a child visiting an individual at home.
- Supporting an individual with their personal hygiene requires the effective wearing, use and disposal of PPE such as an apron and gloves; not doing so can lead to contact with body fluids that can spread illness and result in ill health.
- An adult care worker who does not follow an individual's moving and handling guidelines could cause an injury to themselves and the individual they are supporting.

Risks

Risks are the likelihood of harm occurring as a result of a hazard. The risks may be high, medium or low in terms of their likelihood of occurring and their impact on you, the individuals and others you work with. For example:

- There may a high risk of a broken chair in the lounge causing an injury to anyone who sits on it if it is not removed immediately.
- There may be a medium risk when moving an individual from their bed to their chair with one adult care worker supporting as the individual is a little unsteady on their feet; two adult care workers may be required to avoid any accidents from happening.
- There may be a low risk of an individual who prepares their own meal in the evening forgetting to turn off the oven after they have used it.

The risk assessment process

Risk assessment processes involve the five key steps listed below.

1. Identify the hazards of an area (such as a kitchen) or a work task (such as assisting an individual to move from one position to another).
2. Identify those who may be harmed by the hazards (individuals, you or your colleagues or visitors).
3. Evaluate the risk by deciding whether it is a high, medium or low risk. Then evaluate how the risks can be controlled or reduced.
4. Record the risk assessment to ensure there is a written record of the risks identified and the methods that have been agreed to control or reduce them, so that this can be referenced by all those involved.
5. Review and update the risk assessment to ensure any changes to the level of risk or hazards identified in an area, or work task, are recorded and updated. This means that the risk assessment is an accurate record that can be referenced and used by all those involved.

Assessing health and safety risks

Assessing health and safety risks forms part of the responsibilities that you and your employer have in the care setting where you work. This process is commonly referred to as risk assessment. Risk assessment is a requirement of the Management of Health and Safety at Work Regulations 1999. The risk assessment process involves five steps, as shown in Figure 11.2.

In addition to the points mentioned in Figure 11.2, when carrying out a risk assessment, remember to question what the purpose of the risk assessment is, who will undertake it, who is at risk, what it is that you should be assessing and when this should be done. You should also consider what the potential benefits of taking the risk are. These are all important considerations to take into account.

Assessing health and safety risks (such as those you learned about that are posed by your work setting, situations or particular activities), is very important because it is part of the provision of good care. It shows that you want to make a positive difference to individuals' lives by ensuring their safety at all times. Assessing health and safety risks is also important because it:

- **protects the safety of everyone,** i.e. to prevent you, your colleagues, the individuals you provide care or support to and others who visit, from being placed in danger, harmed or becoming unwell
- **enables potential and actual dangers to be identified as well as their associated risks.** This enables you to decide on the measures that are needed to either eliminate or reduce risks that could be dangerous, harmful or cause illness

- **enables your employer, and you and your colleagues as employees, to comply with the health and safety legislation that is in place,** for example the Health and Safety at Work Act (HASAWA) 1974 and the Management of Health and Safety at Work Regulations (MHSWR) 1999.

Once the risks have been assessed, your setting/employer will need to make sure that they put measures in place to control and reduce these risks. This may include making sure that there are policies in place if a spillage has occurred, or training is given to employees. If you are working in someone's home, then it may be that you can merely advise them about hazards and risks rather than actually make changes to their home.

How risk assessment can help address dilemmas between rights and health and safety

Risk assessment is, as you know, essential for protecting everyone's safety. However, in adult care settings it can also be a useful process for helping to ensure that individuals' rights to be in control of their lives are supported alongside your and your employer's responsibilities to ensure their safety. Supporting an individual's rights against health and safety risks is a dilemma all too often faced by adult care workers because good care and support involves supporting individuals to make their own decisions, including taking risks, but it also involves protecting individuals' safety.

Ultimately, measures to protect people's safety may affect or change the way that they live. For example, an elderly person with mobility issues may not want to have a stair lift installed in their home because of the way it will affect the layout of their home, and they have a right over how their home should look. However, this poses a safety issue as climbing and coming down stairs may be dangerous for them. Another example may be if an individual has been abusive to their family and poses a threat to their safety. In all cases, a risk assessment will be carried out and measures put in place to manage those risks.

Risk assessment can help address dilemmas between individuals' rights and health and safety risks. You can do this by:

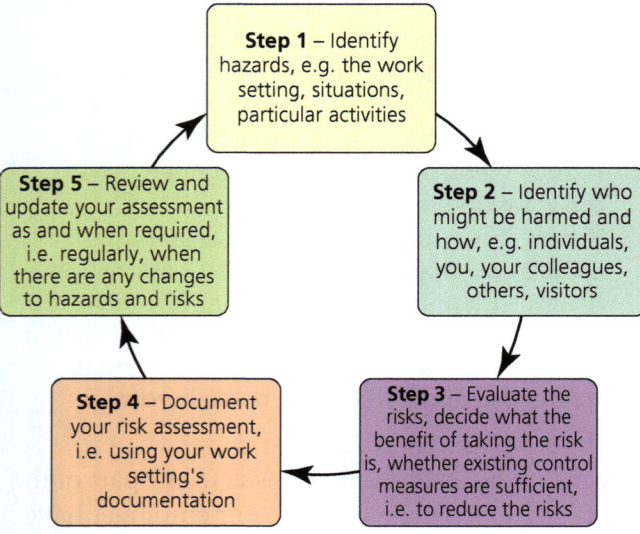

Figure 11.2 Assessing health and safety risks

6Cs

Care

Care, in this section, refers to showing that in your day-to-day responsibilities you are maintaining your responsibility to protect individuals from any dangers or harmful situations that may arise. (The risk assessment process is part of this.) You can show you are doing this by co-operating with your employer when the risk assessment process is being carried out.

- encouraging individuals and adult care workers to talk about the dilemmas and what can be done to address them
- supporting individuals to understand what dangers there are and how these can be balanced against their preferences. Sometimes all you may be able to do is advise them on the best course of action
- making positive decisions with individuals about taking risks.

A risk assessment could be used to address the following examples of dilemmas that may arise in an adult care setting.

- Two people with learning disabilities wish to have a romantic relationship. You could have a discussion with each individual about their wishes, including what type of relationship they would like to have and their understanding of what this may involve. For example, you could discuss the benefits as well as the risks of relationships with others. You could explore the rights of both individuals with each of them; both individuals, for example, have a right to have a relationship and to also refuse to be in a relationship. You could all make a decision that balances the safety and rights of both individuals.
- An individual who is experiencing difficulties with their mobility due to gaining weight wishes to have two desserts rather than one every lunch time. You could explore the impact this will have on the individual's weight and mobility and on the additional support needed from staff. This will need to be discussed in a compassionate way as it is a sensitive issue. You could also discuss the individual's wishes to lose weight and to be more mobile. You could also discuss how this makes them feel. You can then support the individual to make their own decision after balancing the risks to their health and wellbeing against their preferences.
- An individual who has recently moved into a care home wishes to bring with them three large items of furniture and have these placed in their room. The care home manager is concerned that doing so will mean there will be very little space for the individual and staff to move around in her room which in turn may lead to injuries or falls. You could discuss the dangers of doing so with the individual and also discuss the staff's wishes to ensure the safety of everyone. A decision could be made that balances the safety

and rights of both, such as agreeing with the individual for one item of furniture to be placed in her room and for the other two items to be placed in a communal area in the home.

A positive risk assessment process, if done well, can be a very effective way of addressing the dilemmas that may arise between people's rights and their ability to live safely.

> **Reflect on it**
>
> **3.4 Concerns**
>
> Reflect on how you would feel if someone had concerns over your safety in relation to you carrying out an activity that you wanted to do. Would you see this as a positive or negative? Why?

The benefits of positive risk taking for those not in residential care

Positive risk taking also benefits individuals who live in their own homes and who access community-based services because it means that these individuals will feel more confident in themselves in terms of their abilities and potential. This in turn will mean that these individuals will develop their resilience and become more independent in their thinking when making decisions about their own lives.

Risk assessments in reablement practice

Reablement is an approach that is different to the provision of traditional care at home because it enables individuals to do things for themselves by supporting them to regain their independence. It is an approach that not only identifies the individual's strengths and areas for development but also finds out from the individual what their hopes are. It is an approach that provides holistic support to individuals so that they can re-learn how to do things for themselves; the process takes place with the individual. For example, an individual may have stopped making their own hot drinks because the last time they did they had a fall. Now they fear that they will have another fall, so they have been relying on family members to make drinks since their fall. A reablement risk assessment will identify with the individual the benefits of them making their own hot drinks. For example, they can make them as often as they want, it gives them a reason to move around and therefore maintain their mobility, and they could make drinks for their visitors.

> **6Cs**
>
> **Compassion**
>
> Compassionately discussing a sensitive issue with an individual involves showing that you care about them and how they are feeling. You can show this by being aware of your body language: are you, for example, leaning towards them when speaking to them? The tone of your voice: is it gentle and polite? What you say: are you using kind and thoughtful words?

The risk assessment will also consider the individual's overall wellbeing. For example, an individual's mental and emotional health may be improved by referring them to their GP for counselling; this may be to help them manage their fear of falling again. Other practical ways of managing the risk of falling can also be discussed with the individual, such as using a kettle tipper to avoid the individual losing their balance when pouring hot water from the kettle, and placing their drink on a walker tray for safety. The individual will be provided with support to use these aids and both you and they will monitor what worked and what didn't. The situation can be assessed again until the individual has reached their goal to make their own drink.

Using health and safety risk assessments

There is no point in having a risk assessment in place if you do not use it and for this AC you will be observed using a risk assessment. In order to use a risk assessment effectively you must be able to find it, understand the information it includes and know how to put it into practice. For example, this may be in relation to a specific individual you work with or a work task you carry out. For example:

- **An individual:** An individual with mental health needs who lives on their own and does not have capacity wishes to smoke in bed before going to sleep. A risk assessment is in place because the individual also takes sleeping tablets before going to bed and there is a risk that the individual may fall asleep while smoking in bed, which may lead to a fire and have fatal consequences. The risk of this occurring has been assessed as high. The risk has been explained to the individual but at times the individual's desire to smoke overrides their concern for their safety. In order to reduce the risk, it has been agreed with the individual that no cigarettes will be left in the house with the individual on their own – as the carer buys the cigarettes with the individual's shopping, the individual will only smoke in the presence of the carer in the evening before they complete their visit. It has been agreed with the individual that this will be monitored closely and reviewed every two weeks to ensure that the individual is still happy with these arrangements.

- **A specific work task:** The main front door of a residential care setting has a password code that is used by staff to open it. One of the residents found out the password by observing staff and visitors entering and leaving the building. The individual has dementia and used the password to let themselves out of the building, and a member of staff found the individual walking along the main road. A risk assessment was developed because of the risk this poses not only to this individual but also to others in relation to them leaving the building without being supported by staff. As there is a busy main road nearby this may result in an individual being injured as they may be unaware of the dangers of fast moving traffic. There is a risk of them becoming disorientated and getting lost; another risk could be from the general public who may identify the individual as vulnerable and exploit them or take advantage of them. The risk assessment means that a new password code is being used and all staff have been made aware not to show it to others and to be vigilant when using it to ensure no one else can see it. For additional security the password will be changed every week. In relation to the individual who wanted to go out, their advocate and family members were informed of the incident and together they have agreed to take it in turns to assist the individual to go out so that their need to socialise with others, go shopping and go out for walks can be fulfilled in a manner that is safe and does not put the individual in any danger. It has been agreed that these actions will be monitored and the outcomes reviewed within two weeks to ensure their effectiveness.

Reflect on it

3.4 Consequences of not assessing risks

Reflect on the consequences if risks in your work setting were not being assessed. How could this impact on your work activities? On the wellbeing of the individuals you provide care or support to? On working as a team?

Evidence opportunity

3.4 Risk assessment in relation to health and safety

You will be observed using risk assessment in relation to health and safety.

Before you do so, find a risk assessment that is in place for an individual you work with or for an activity you complete. Where did you find it? Why is it important that you make reference to it? Before using it, discuss it with your colleague and ensure you explain the following: its purpose, what the risk is, who has assessed the risk, what actions have been agreed and why, and how effective it is. Now use the risk assessment in relation to a health and safety task; ask the person observing you to provide you with feedback afterwards.

AC 3.5 Monitor potential health and safety risks

Monitoring risks

Monitoring risks is important because risks arise on a continuous basis and can change from hour to hour, day to day. You will be observed for this AC monitoring potential health and safety risks. Monitoring risks involves:

- **keeping a close check on the environment**, the work activities you and others carry out, the equipment you and others use and the individuals you work with. For example, you may notice that a spillage of a hot drink has occurred in the corridor, the brakes on an individual's wheelchair are not working, an individual's family member becomes unwell or a contractor has a fall. Make sure that you are aware of the different hazards where you work. This will include environmental hazards such as a torn carpet; hazards posed by those you work with, such as individuals who may display behaviours that challenge or those visiting the setting; or hazards posed by the equipment you use being faulty or damaged.
- **taking action so that any risks identified can be dealt with quickly.** You will learn more about reporting the risks you've identified on the following pages. Doing nothing is not an option.
- **reviewing actions agreed so that you and others can ensure that the methods you have agreed on are working effectively.** Risk assessments must be reviewed to ensure that they are working. If they are not, then you can always change them, but you can only do this if you know they are not working! You should also review risk assessments if they are no longer effective, or there have been any accidents or near misses or there have been changes that could lead to new risks arising such as a new staff member or equipment used. For example, you may have agreed with your employer that when an individual you work with displays behaviours that challenge others, you will assist the individual to their room where they can calm down. However, when reviewing their risk assessment, if you find that the individual is taking longer and longer to calm down when going to their room or is attempting to self-harm, then you and your employer will have to find other ways of managing this situation. For example, perhaps one of you can sit with the individual until they calm down or perhaps they may benefit from going for a walk. It is also important to remember to update your risk assessment record with these changes, so that it is up to date and can be used by everyone in the team to provide consistent support to the individual.

Reflect on it

3.5 How you monitor risks at work

Reflect on how you monitor risks at work. Think about a situation that changed and that required you and others to change your ways of working. How effective was your monitoring of this situation? Are there any improvements that could be made should this situation arise again?

The Reporting of Injuries, Diseases and Dangerous Occurrences Regulations (RIDDOR) 1995 (amended 2008) means that you are legally required to report such concerns. You can report any health and safety concerns you have directly to the Health and Safety Executive (HSE). Your manager will need to report these, as well as deaths, to the HSE, your local authority's environmental health department for food hygiene concerns, the Care Quality Commission for failures in individuals' care. These will be recorded and tracked so that if there are regular occurrences of such incidents, they can be acted upon. If it is found that these are occurring on a large scale across the country, it can become an issue for government to deal with.

Research it

1.1, 3.5 RIDDOR

Research what the Reporting of Injuries, Diseases and Dangerous Occurrences Regulations (RIDDOR) 2013 says about the reporting and recording of work-related accidents that cause death and serious injuries (referred to as reportable injuries), diseases and dangerous occurrences (i.e. incidents with the potential to cause harm).

You will find the link below to the HSE's information page on their website, RIDDOR – Reporting of Injuries, Diseases and Dangerous Occurrences Regulations 2013, a useful source of information:

www.hse.gov.uk/riddor

Discuss your findings with a colleague. Explain to your assessor some examples of how you have minimised potential health and safety risks.

Reporting risks

Sometimes you may not be able to effectively deal with a risk you have identified. This may be because you have never dealt with the type of risk before and therefore do not feel competent to do so, it may be because the actions you have agreed with your manager or employer have not been effective or it may be because the situation has changed. In these situations, it is always best to report this immediately to your manager or employer who will be able to take the necessary action. For example, you may have identified that the garden is very uneven and likely to cause individuals to trip or that an individual's mobility aid is no longer working.

Reporting risks involves:

- **reporting them immediately to your manager or employer.** You will need to explain what the risk is and the danger(s) it poses. It is also a good idea to discuss the actions you have taken already and whether they were effective or not; this includes whether you have made the area safe in the meantime. For example, in the event of the garden being uneven, you could lock the doors that lead out to the garden and put a notice on them to explain why they are locked. In the case of the individual's faulty mobility aid, you could place it in a safe storage area with a label on explaining why it is not to be used; you should also explain the situation to the individual and to others in the team who may want to use it.

- **recording the risk fully.** Your work setting will have specific ways of recording risks – there may be a specific form to use or a Word file to access and complete. Whatever method you use to record the risks you have identified you must record them clearly, identifying what they are, the date and time you noticed them on, the potential dangers they may cause and the actions you took when you identified the risks as being a danger. It is important to record all these details fully because this will be a permanent record that may be reviewed at a later date and referred to for information, for example by the HSE, if your employer is required to report it to them. You will learn more about recording fully and accurately and reporting in Unit 305 Handling information in adult care settings/services. Remember to consider confidentiality when recording details. Your setting will have policies and procedures for recording and reporting (e.g. whether this is in a risk assessment book) that you will need to know.

Research it

3.5 Reportable injuries and diseases

Although we are discussing risks here, remember that the reporting of accidents, injuries, diseases and dangerous occurrences is a legal requirement.

Find out which injuries, diseases and dangerous occurrences are reportable. You may find it useful to look at the Health and Safety (HSE) website and the section on RIDDOR:

www.hse.gov.uk/riddor

Do you know how to record and report these? For example, do you know where the accident report book is kept and what you will need to record? Do you know who to go to when reporting these?

Risk assessment record Date of risk assessment: 27/01/23					
What is the hazard?	Who might be harmed and how?	What is being done to control this risk?	Who needs to take these actions?	When do these actions need to be taken?	Have these actions been completed?
The front door of the care home does not lock securely consistently.	J has dementia and may leave the care home with no one noticing. Staff and individuals could be harmed if an intruder gains access to the home. Individuals' and staff's possessions may be stolen and/or damaged if an intruder gains access to the home.	The contractor has been contacted and will be arriving to repair the door within the next three hours. In the meantime, members of staff are taking it in turns to keep the front door secure by remaining in the hallway at all times.	The manager has phoned the contractor the care home uses. All staff members are to monitor the security of the care home.	Immediately and until the contractor has repaired the front door.	Yes: Signed (manager): Date: No: Are any further actions needed? If so, by whom? If so, when?

Figure 11.3 Recording the health and safety risks that have been identified

> ### Evidence opportunity
>
> **3.5 Monitor potential health and safety risks**
>
> With your manager, employer or assessor, complete a walk around of an area where you work and where you have identified potential health and safety risks. Review the risks you identified (you will need your previous recordings of these to help you). Discuss: has anything changed? If so, what? Does this alter the risks originally identified?

AC 3.6 Access support or information relating to health and safety

There may be occasions when you are carrying out your health and safety responsibilities and you are unsure about whether you are carrying out a task correctly or have understood the health and safety procedures relating to the task. This might be something as simple as knowing the technique to use when washing and drying your hands or how to dispose of your apron and gloves safely after use. In these situations it is important that you are able to access further support and information so that you can continue to carry out your health and safety responsibilities effectively.

For this AC you will be observed in your work practices doing this. You have already learned about some useful sources of information, such as health and safety legislation and the policies and procedures of the care setting where you work. There are many more sources of support and information available to you both within and outside the care setting where you work.

Sources of support and information

- Your manager can be a valuable source of support and information in terms of providing you with guidance and information to ensure you understand how to comply with the work setting's agreed ways of working. For example, this could be in relation to knowing what to do in the event of a fire in the work setting.
- Your colleagues can also provide you with support, particularly in relation to supporting you to follow best practice when carrying out health and safety tasks. They may also provide you with information and show you how to use safe techniques. For example, this could be in relation to carrying out health and safety checks such as checking that windows are secure and smoke alarms are in working order.

- Your **trade union representative** will be able to provide you with support and information if you have any health and safety concerns, for example in relation to observing unsafe practices in your work setting or not feeling competent to carry out a work task that you have been trained to carry out.
- Your health and safety officer in the care setting where you work (this may be your manager or another senior member of staff) can provide you with useful and relevant information and training. For example, this could be in relation to changes to health and safety legislation and their impact on your working practices.
- The Health and Safety Executive (HSE) provides useful publications about maintaining health and safety in health and social care settings.
- The Care Quality Commission (CQC) provides useful information about the health and safety standards that are expected in adult care settings.
- **Sector Skills Councils**, such as Skills for Care and Skills for Health, provide useful information about maintaining good quality, safe working practices and also the standards that are expected from the adult care sector's workforce, i.e. the Care Certificate.
- Additional information sources can include books and journals.

Accessing support and information

When you access support and information relating to health and safety you need to think about the following:

- What do my work setting's procedures say about accessing support and information in relation to health and safety?
- Which sources are available to me in my work setting? What process must I follow and why? In what situations can I access these?
- Which sources are available to me outside of my work setting? What process must I follow and why? In what situations can I access these?

In most care settings, you would approach your manager or health and safety officer in the first instance. You can do this formally during supervision with your manager or informally, through discussion for example. This could be a good opportunity to refer to Unit 313 and read about sources of support that are available for personal development where you work.

Reflect on it

3.6 Support and information

Reflect on an occasion when you or one of your colleagues accessed support or information in relation to health and safety. Why was this necessary? What was the outcome?

Key terms

Trade union representative refers to a member of an organised group of workers who speaks up for the rights and interests of the employees of an organisation, for example in relation to safe working conditions.

Sector Skills Councils are organisations led by and for specific employment sectors, for example Skills for Care for the adult social care workforce and Skills for Health for the healthcare workforce.

Research it

3.6 Support and information

Research the roles of two organisations that you can access for support and information about health and safety. Write down your findings.

Evidence opportunity

3.6, 1.4 Accessing support and information

Select a task that you must not carry out in your work setting without special training. Think about an aspect of this work task where you will need to access additional support or information. Follow the procedure in your work setting and do so. Did you ask your employer or your manager? Why? Ask your manager/employer for their feedback on the process you followed for seeking their support or information from them. Did you follow your employer's agreed ways of working? Are there any areas for improvement?

Legislation	
Act/Regulation	**Key points**
Data Protection Act 1998	The right to privacy in relation to personal information must be upheld. Personal information about the individuals and others you may come across, such as individuals' families and your colleagues, must be kept confidential.
Data Protection Act 2018	Also see Unit 304 for more information on the Data Protection Act 2018.
Health and Safety at Work Act (HASAWA) 1974	The health and safety of everyone in a work setting must be protected – in a care setting this includes individuals, adult care workers and those who visit. It also established the key duties and responsibilities of all employers and employees in work settings.
Management of Health and Safety at Work Regulations (MHSWR) 1999	Employers and managers must assess and manage risks by carrying out risk assessments. It requires employers to provide information, training and supervision so that work activities can be carried out safely.
Workplace (Health, Safety and Welfare) Regulations 1992	The working environment must be safe in relation to the building, its facilities and housekeeping and it must be healthy in relation to temperature, lighting and ventilation.
Manual Handling Operations Regulations 1992 (as amended 2002)	Risks associated with moving and handling activities must be eliminated or minimised by employers. It also requires employers to provide information, training and supervision about safe moving and handling.
Provision and Use of Work Equipment Regulations (PUWER) 1998	Work equipment used in work settings must be safe. It requires employees to receive training before using work equipment and requires work equipment to have visible warning signs.
Lifting Operations and Lifting Equipment Regulations (LOLER) 1998	Lifting equipment used in work settings must be safe. It requires lifting equipment to be maintained and used solely for the purpose it was intended for. It also requires that all lifting operations are planned, supervised and carried out in a safe manner.
Personal Protective Equipment at Work Regulations 1992	Personal protective equipment (PPE) to provide protection against infections must be provided free of charge by employers. It requires PPE to be maintained in good condition and requires training to be provided in the use of PPE.
Reporting of Injuries, Diseases and Dangerous Occurrences Regulations (RIDDOR) 2013	Employers must report and keep records for three years of work-related accidents that cause death and serious injuries (referred to as reportable injuries), diseases and dangerous occurrences (i.e. incidents with the potential to cause harm). It requires work settings to have procedures in place and to provide information and training on reporting injuries, diseases and incidents.
Control of Substances Hazardous to Health (COSHH) 2002	Employers must have procedures in place for safe working with hazardous substances and provide information, training and supervision so that work activities can be carried out safely.
Electricity at Work Regulations 1989	Electricity and the electrical appliances that are used in work settings must be safe. It requires employers to provide training to employees in relation to carrying out safety checks on electrical equipment.
Regulatory Reform Order (Fire Safety) 2005	Fire risk assessments must be completed by the person responsible for the premises and requires the provision of fire equipment, fire escape routes and exits, as well as fire safety training.
The Health and Safety (First Aid) Regulations 1981	First aid and first aid facilities, including trained first aiders, must be provided.

Legislation	
Act/Regulation	**Key points**
Food Safety Act 1990	Good personal hygiene must be maintained when working with food so that it is safe to eat. It requires that records are kept of where food is from so that it can be traced if needed.
Food Hygiene (England) Regulations 2006	Food safety hazards must be identified and food safety controls put in place, maintained and reviewed so that environments where food is prepared or cooked are safe.
Civil Contingencies Act 2004	Organisations such as emergency services, local authorities and health bodies must work together to plan and respond to local and national emergencies. It requires that risk assessments are undertaken and emergency plans are put in place.

311 Supporting infection prevention and control in adult care settings/services

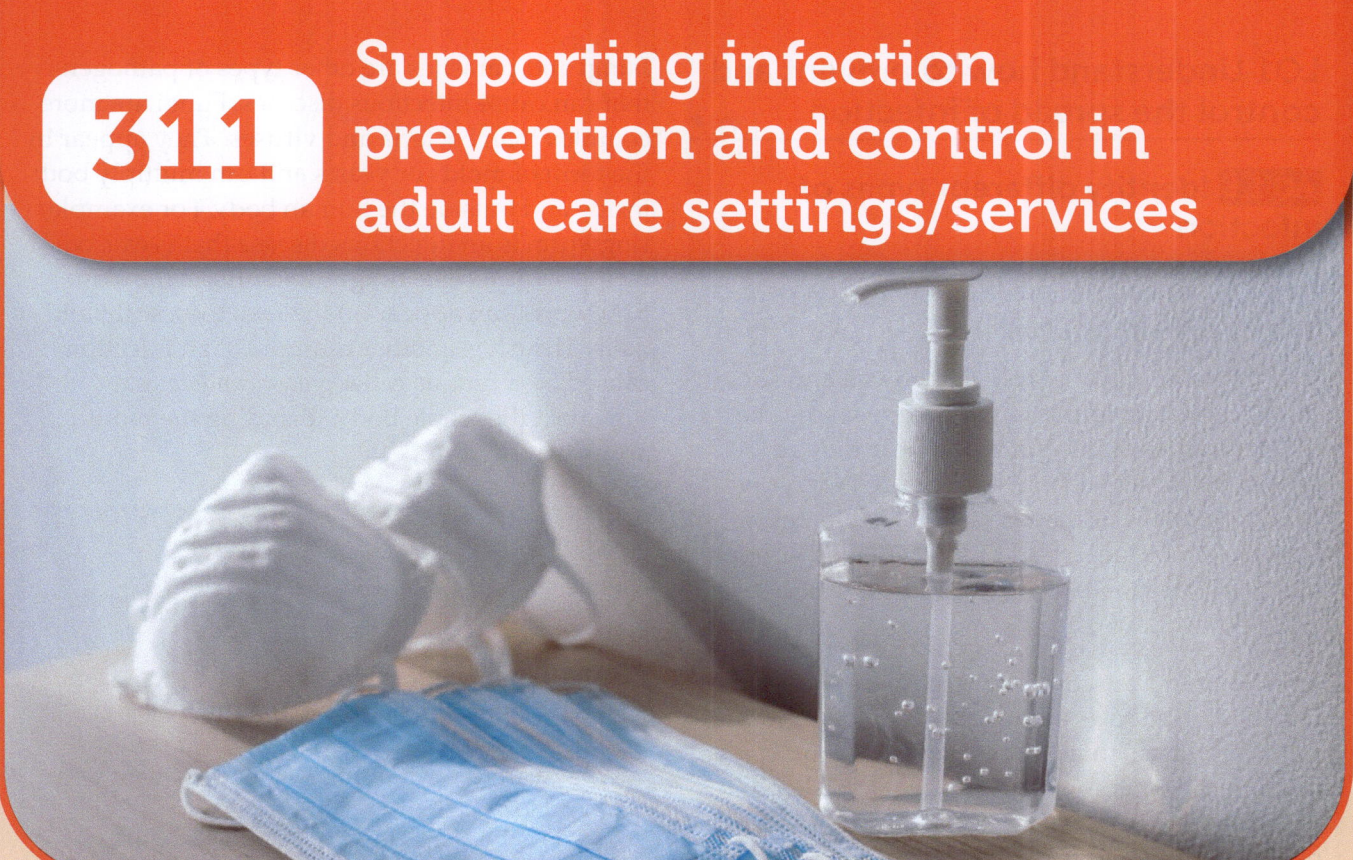

About this unit

Credit value: 2
Guided learning hours: 15

Infections can occur anywhere and can affect everyone in care settings/services. In this unit you will learn about how to prevent and control the spread of infection by developing your knowledge and understanding of the different types of infections that exist, who is at risk and how they can spread. You will also explore your responsibilities for the cleaning of environments and equipment as well as the measures you can use for preventing and controlling infections including the use of risk assessment, personal protective equipment and recommended techniques and products for hand hygiene.

Learning outcomes

By the end of this unit, you will:

LO1: Understand how to prevent and control the spread of infection

LO2: Be able to contribute to the prevention and control of the spread of infection

LO1 Understand how to prevent and control the spread of infection

AC 1.1 Identify different types of infection

AC 1.2 Describe how different types of infection are spread

Infections can make people feel unwell and some can be fatal. It is important you know about the different types of infections and how they're caused because as a Lead Adult Care Worker or Lead Personal Assistant you will need to know how to reduce the spread of infection and support others in infection prevention and control.

What are the causes of infection?

Infections are caused by harmful disease-causing germs referred to as pathogens. Pathogens are microorganisms that can cause disease, and can be found everywhere, such as inside our bodies and in the air, and they can be spread from person to person. Microorganisms can also cause secondary infections in other parts of the body.

There are many different types of pathogens, but the two main types are bacteria and viruses. Bacteria release toxins into our bodies and viruses can damage our bodies' cells which can lead to serious infections. Table 12.1 provides you with some information about each type including the differences between the two.

Table 12.1 The differences between bacteria and viruses

Bacteria	Viruses
Bacteria reproduce in large numbers to cause infections.	Viruses are smaller than bacteria in size and can reproduce in small numbers to cause infections.
Bacteria can multiply outside of the human body.	Viruses can only multiply within the human body.
Bacteria can be treated with antibiotics.	Viruses cannot be treated with antibiotics.
Examples of infections caused by bacteria include: gastroenteritis, tuberculosis, cholera.	Examples of infections caused by viruses include: flu, measles, chicken pox.

Fungi and parasites are other types of pathogens that can cause infectious diseases. Fungi are more complex than bacteria and viruses. They appear in the form of molds or yeasts and can multiply both inside and outside the human body. For example, ringworm is an infectious disease that is caused by the *dermatophyte* fungus and affects the skin. Ringworm can appear on the feet, toes, scalp and nails. Thrush is another example of an infection caused by a fungus called yeast *candida* that can affect the whole body, including the mouth, armpits and groin.

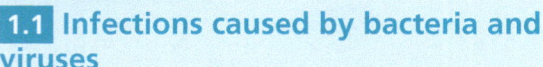

Reflect on it

1.1 Infections caused by bacteria and viruses

Reflect on the infections caused by bacteria, viruses, fungi and parasites. Have you or someone you know experienced any of these? What were the symptoms? What treatment was provided?

Key terms

MRSA stands for methicillin-resistant *Staphylococcus aureus* and is often referred to as a 'superbug' because it is difficult to treat. It is a bacterium that can cause serious infections.

Norovirus is an infection of the stomach that causes diarrhoea and vomiting.

Cross infection is the spread of infection from person to person, from contaminated objects, through air, food, animals and insects.

How can infection spread in care settings?

Care settings are environments where infections can spread easily because:

- **they are places where there are large numbers of people**, some of whom may be unwell and therefore carrying an infection, for example an individual who has **MRSA**, an adult care worker who has gastroenteritis or a visitor with the **norovirus**. Infections may therefore spread from one person to another in a process called 'cross infection'.
- **the work activities that take place are at high risk of carrying infections**; for example, supporting individuals with care needs

involves being in contact with their body fluids. Activities such as assisting individuals with eating, drinking and personal care, handling food, disposing of waste and cleaning areas and equipment can pose high risks of infection. Infections can also be caused by food that is consumed. Food can become contaminated and infected by bacteria such as *E. coli* and *Salmonella*. This may be due to use of equipment that has not been cleaned properly or bacteria on hands. It may also occur when food is not heated, cooked or cooled properly.

- **individuals may be more vulnerable to infections**; for example, older individuals and individuals who are unwell cannot fight off infections as easily as someone who is healthy because their bodies' ability to fight off infections has been weakened due to their age or damaged through other illness.

> ### Research it
>
> **1.2 Spread of infection**
>
> Research examples of two care settings where the spread of infection was not prevented. Write down what happened and how it affected all those involved in the care setting.
>
> You will find the internet and local newspapers useful sources of information.

Infections can spread in care settings in different ways, such as when you have physical contact with a person who has an infection (e.g. MRSA) or through food that has become contaminated with pathogens (e.g. *Salmonella*), from pathogens present in the air you breathe (e.g. chicken pox) as well as through contaminated objects such as bed linen and work surfaces.

Infections spread in care settings through six key stages. These stages are often referred to as the 'chain of infection' and they are identified in Figure 12.1.

The chain of infection shows that infections can quickly spread from person to person if the conditions are right. For example, the perfect environment for bacteria to grow is one where food and moisture is available. This could be leftover food as well as body fluids such as urine and faeces. It could be where the temperature is warm and the environment is constant giving the bacteria time to multiply, for example a waste bin that has not been emptied for two days.

Similarly, infections can only spread from person to person if they have transport and a route through which to enter and exit our bodies, for example an uncleaned toilet seat or hands that have not been washed (indirect contact) or through coming into contact with an individual's body fluids from coughing or from minor cuts (direct contact).

> ### Evidence opportunity
>
> **1.1, 1.2 Causes and spread of infection**
>
> Using the chain of infection that you have learned about, develop a written account that describes the main causes of infection, the different types and how they can spread in the care setting where you work.

1. Pathogen causes infection
2. Environment allows pathogen to multiply
3. Transport allows the pathogen to move
4. Route into the body allows the pathogen to enter
5. Route out of the body allows the pathogen to exit
6. The pathogen then enters the body of another person

Figure 12.1 The chain of infection

> **Research it**
>
> **1.2 The cause and spread of infection**
>
> Research how infection enters the body. Find out about 'endogenous', 'exogenous' and environmental pathogens.
>
> For example, how can pathogens in the body spread to other organs, from one person to another (through sneezing, for example) and from the environment (such as bacteria on equipment)?
>
> Find out about how infections can be passed on through direct and indirect contact. For example, they may be passed on via direct contact such as from one person to another, or indirect contact through used disposable gloves, for example, or airborne such as through sneezing and coughing, or via arthropods such as flies and mosquitos. Infections can enter the body in different ways including natural openings such as the mouth and ears and other openings such as a cut in the skin or a surgical wound.

AC 1.3 Describe how to minimise the spread of infection in care settings/services

AC 1.4 Explain how to identify individuals who have or are at risk of infection

AC 1.5 Describe actions to take to minimise the risks of infection to individuals and others

Who is more likely to get an infection? Who is a more 'susceptible' host?

Some groups of people are more susceptible to infections than others – they may be more 'susceptible hosts'. For example, babies and children have immature immune systems which means they have less protection against infection. Older people's immune systems become less effective with age and therefore their bodies are more susceptible to infections and less effective when fighting these. People who are ill may have had their immune systems damaged by illness and therefore their immune systems do not work as effectively.

Preventing the spread of infections and taking action to minimise the risks of infection

In AC 2.2 you will learn about one of the key ways to prevent the spread of infection. However, there are a number of other measures you can take to break the chain of infection. Some of these will be covered in ACs 2.4 and 2.5 but a few things to remember are:

- **Wear protective clothing:** see AC 2.2 for information on personal protective equipment (PPE).
- **Wear gloves:** you will need to ensure you wear gloves when you come into contact with bodily fluids, when you are dealing with broken skin or rashes for example. You will also need to wear them when disposing of waste including soiled bedding or dressings. You will learn more about how to put gloves on in AC 2.2. Where there are serious illnesses or infections like MRSA you will need to follow your setting's policies and procedures, so it is important that you know what these are.
- **Carefully dispose of waste so that you or others do not come into contact with any germs or harmful substances:** you may need to wear gloves and aprons when disposing of waste and make sure you follow your setting's procedures for doing so. Remember that standard precautions such as effective hand washing and wearing aprons and gloves create a protective barrier to help prevent the spread of infection; it is important that you and others are aware of their importance in reducing the spread of infections. Often there are procedures for disposing of waste in different bags based on whether they are used for waste that is clinical, soiled or recyclable.
- **Make sure a healthy environment is maintained and equipment is cleaned:** different individuals and staff may come into contact with equipment (for example, hoists or chairs). Make sure that the setting is working to ensure that equipment is cleaned correctly and that you are doing your utmost to do so. Of course, you are not always responsible for the cleaning of equipment, but you should consider this in your practice and look for it in others'. There will be measures in place in your setting to make sure you and others maintain cleanliness, for example anti-bacterial gel dispensers placed around the setting so that there are opportunities to clean your hands.
- **Make sure that your health and hygiene does not lead to spread of infection:** see AC 2.5 for more information.

Promoting health and safety in an individual's home

For domiciliary care workers, promoting health and safety in an individual's home is important but there may be other considerations to take into account. For example, in an individual's home you may not have separate waste bins for disposing of household waste (such as paper) and clinical waste (such as used dressings). Effective precautions can still be taken to prevent the spread of infection, for example by ensuring that all waste is placed into a bag and then sealed rather than left open in a black bin bag. There may not be a separate utility area in an individual's home for washing soiled linen; precautions can be taken by ensuring soiled linen is washed separately in the washing machine and on a high setting to destroy any bacteria.

6Cs

Compassion

You can show your compassion by being empathetic towards individuals who have or are at risk of infections. You can do this by ensuring that you identify which individuals may be more susceptible to infections and the reasons why. You can also show your compassion by respecting individuals' concerns about the spread of infections and showing your understanding of how they may feel.

Courage

Showing courage means taking action to minimise the risks of infection to individuals and others, and involves ensuring that individuals' rights to live safely and free from harm are respected. You can show your courage by following best practice at all times in your day-to-day working activities such as by wearing PPE, using safe disposal methods for waste and maintaining a clean and healthy environment.

Evidence opportunity

1.3, 1.4, 1.5 Minimising infection

For the care setting where you work write an account that:

- details three ways in which you minimise the spread of infection
- includes examples of two individuals who are at risk of infections and the reasons why
- describes three ways in which you minimise the risks of infection to individuals and others.

AC 1.6 Outline own role and responsibilities in identifying, or acting upon the identification, of an outbreak or spread of infection

Your role and responsibilities when there's an outbreak or spread of infection

As you will have learned, preventing the spread of infections is an integral part of your job role; but what would you do if there was an outbreak or spread of infection in your work setting?

An outbreak of infection in your work setting refers to when two or more people have the same infection or similar symptoms around the same time or within days of each other. Although the signs and symptoms of infections vary there are some general signs and symptoms that may indicate that a person is suffering with an infection including:

- Feeling feverish
- A raised body temperature (i.e. above 37°C)
- Swelling of an area
- Redness of an area
- Discharge of pus
- Enlarged glands, i.e. in the neck, armpits or groin
- Pain
- Lack of appetite
- Vomiting
- Diarrhoea
- Changes in behaviour such as feeling confused, agitated, restless.

Reflect on it

1.6 Signs and symptoms of infection

Think about an occasion when you or someone you know had an infection. What signs and symptoms did you/they have? How did it affect you/them? How long did it take to recover?

If you notice any of these signs and symptoms in yourself or others you must report them as soon as possible to prevent the infection spreading even further. The manager of the care setting where you work will be responsible for managing the outbreak and so it is important that you report a suspected outbreak to the manager or authorised person so that they can telephone the **UK Health Security Agency (UKHSA)** to discuss the outbreak and agree on the actions required.

The UKHSA will ask the manager or authorised person for details of the outbreak including the total numbers of people affected, the symptoms people have experienced and when their symptoms started. The UKHSA will then undertake a risk assessment of the outbreak based on the information provided and the type of infection identified and provide advice to the care setting on the actions to take. It is your responsibility to ensure that you follow the actions identified by the UKHSA, which may for example include reinforcing infection prevention and control measures that are already in place in the care setting and supporting others to do the same, or temporarily reducing mixing with those identified as experiencing symptoms. For example, a staff member could be asked to remain at home and not return to work until feeling well again.

6Cs

Competence

You can demonstrate your competence by having the knowledge and understanding of what to do if there is an outbreak of infection in your work setting. Acting promptly and fulfilling your role to the best of your ability will mean that you will not only safeguard individuals from the prevention of infection but also yourself and others in your work setting.

Evidence opportunity

1.6 Infection outbreaks

Find out about the infection prevention and control measures that are in place in the care setting where you work. What do they say about your role and responsibilities when there's an outbreak or spread of infection?

Produce an information leaflet that sets out the actions you must take when there is an outbreak or spread of infection in the care setting where you work. Explain why it is important that you take these actions.

Key terms

UK Health Security Agency (UKHSA) is a UK government-led organisation that replaced Public Health England in 2021 and is responsible for public health including protecting the public from infections and disease.

Clinical waste bins are bins where waste that is contaminated with body fluids (for example used dressings, bandages and disposable gloves) is disposed of as it poses a risk of infection. These are usually located in bathrooms and laundry areas.

AC 1.7 Outline own role in supporting others to follow practices that reduce the spread of infection

In your work setting both you and your employer have a vital role to play in ensuring that **infections** are prevented because they can affect everyone. When infections do occur because an individual is unwell, for example, you and your employer are responsible for ensuring that your actions prevent the spread of these infections to other individuals, your colleagues and others who visit the care setting where you work.

To be able to support others effectively to follow practices that reduce the spread of infection you must be aware of your own responsibilities and those of your employer.

Your responsibilities as an employee in infection prevention and control

As an employee, you are responsible for ensuring your work practices are safe and that they protect you, your colleagues and others from infections. As an employee, you have a responsibility to:

- **follow your work setting's agreed ways of working:** for example, by ensuring you read and understand your work setting's infection prevention and control procedures, such as those in relation to food handling and the use and disposal of aprons and gloves. You will also need to read information updates provided to you by your employer, such as in relation to changes in relevant legislation.

- **attend training:** you must ensure that you learn from the training and information provided by your employer about infection prevention and control. You must ensure that you apply what you have learned from the training you have attended in your day-to-day working practices.
- **record and report:** you must record all infection hazards and risks immediately, such as an overflowing **clinical waste bin** that contains used dressings, or the non-availability of gloves; you must report if you become unwell with an illness such as gastroenteritis.

> **Reflect on it**
>
> **1.7 Information available in your setting**
>
> Reflect on the infection control posters and information that are available in your work setting. Write down all the ones you know about. Discuss this with your manager. Did you find out about any more?

Your employer's responsibilities in infection prevention and control

Your employer is required by law to prevent and control infections in the work setting; most of these legal requirements come under the Health and Safety at Work Act (1974) that you learned about in Unit 310.

Your employer is responsible for ensuring that you and all employees are safe at work and therefore aware of infection prevention and control. They should be aware of the reasons why this is important and relevant to day-to-day work tasks.

Your employer has a responsibility to:

- **provide information:** for example, by displaying information posters such as handwashing posters above sinks; by providing information leaflets for employees and others who visit; and by keeping relevant records, such as accident and incident records and infection outbreak records.
- **provide education:** for example, by developing infection prevention and control policies and procedures and ensuring these are followed. Your employer needs to ensure that you, as care workers, are aware of what to do if you are informed that an individual in the care setting has the **norovirus**. They need to provide training on infection prevention and control, provide updates to changes in procedures and legislation and monitor work practices to ensure agreed ways of working are being complied with.
- **provide equipment:** for example, by making available free of charge aprons and gloves for protection against infections (you will learn more about different types of PPE in AC 2.2). Your employer will need to provide cleaning equipment, such as mops and cleaning agents; provide facilities for the safe disposal of waste, such as used dressings and gloves; and provide welfare facilities, such as separate areas for eating and hand washing. If you are working in an individual's home and the individual you are providing care for is also your employer, then the individual will be responsible for providing you with all the necessary equipment you need to carry out your job safely.

Supporting others

Being an effective role model to others means that you will be demonstrating the current best practices to follow for reducing the spread of infection. For example, by washing your hands using the recommended technique before and after you undertake work activities (you will learn about this technique in AC 2.4), it will be more likely that others will do the same. If you do not do this, others may not see the importance or relevance of having to do so themselves.

You can also support others by answering their questions about infections and infection control. For example, they may be unsure about their role in reducing the spread of infections or perhaps they need your assistance in using a piece of protective equipment effectively.

Supporting others may also involve putting them forward for training so that they can update their knowledge about infection control or suggesting that they shadow you working so that you can model effective practices to follow, such as how to dispose of PPE safely or how to clean a piece of equipment such as a mobility aid and why this helps prevent infections from spreading.

6Cs

Communication

Supporting others to follow best practices for reducing the spread of infection will require you to be an effective communicator because not only may you have to demonstrate best practice but you may also have to explain the importance of the practices you're following to others, including answering any questions they may have. Communicating effectively with others will mean that they will be more likely to look up to you as an effective role model and follow in your footsteps.

Commitment

Supporting others also involves you demonstrating your commitment to preventing and controlling the spread of infection in your work setting. You can do this effectively by role modelling best practice to others and supporting others with any questions or further training needs they may have. Listening to others and showing your genuine support towards them will reflect your determination to make your work setting a safe and clean working environment.

Evidence opportunity

1.7 Roles and responsibilities

Produce an information guide or PowerPoint presentation about your role and responsibilities in the prevention of the spread of infections and supporting others. You could also include the skills, knowledge and qualities you have to carry out your role effectively.

AC 1.8 Describe own responsibilities for ensuring the appropriate cleaning and decontamination of environments and equipment

Your responsibilities for cleaning and decontamination

Maintaining clean environments and equipment reduces the spread of infection because harmful pathogens that cause infections thrive in environments that are dirty. Maintaining a clean environment in the care setting where you work includes not only cleaning the building but also the furniture and fixtures within it. Maintaining clean work equipment that you and others may use is also essential for reducing the spread of infection and includes cleaning equipment such as mops, vacuums and cloths as well as other equipment that may be used with individuals such as hoists and commodes.

You can maintain a clean environment by:

- **carrying out regular maintenance** – maintain and keep clean the building's doors, windows, lights, chairs, tables, wall shelves and cupboards.
- **having in place cleaning schedules** – prevent a build-up of dust and dirt by following weekly and monthly cleaning schedules for cleaning rooms, toilets, bathrooms, kitchens, dining areas, as well as vacuuming carpets and mopping floors.
- **increasing cleaning when needed** – when there is a spillage on the floor, or after an individual has used the shower, toilet or hoist.
- **maintaining cleaning equipment** – prevent the spread of infection from one area to another by regularly changing cloths, washing and changing mop heads, cleaning vacuum brushes and changing their filters, and colour-coding equipment according to the area it has been used in, such as kitchen, bathroom, bedroom, laundry area.
- **following manufacturers' instructions** – promote the safe and effective use of cleaning detergents by following the instructions such as to mix it with warm or hot water, or to rinse it off after it is used.
- **using decontamination techniques** – reduce or remove the spread of infection by using the following three **decontamination** techniques: **cleaning, disinfection** and **sterilisation**. Work equipment and areas must always be clean first before you can disinfect and/or sterilise them because cleaning removes dirt and prevents cross contamination from one surface to another. For example, you can clean a kitchen floor by sweeping it first to remove any surface dust or debris and then by using a mop with hot water and detergent and then rinsing the detergent off afterwards and leaving the floor to air dry naturally. Disinfection must only take place after the area/equipment has been cleaned and is free from dirt; common examples of disinfectants used are **anti-bacterials** and **antiseptics**. For example, you can disinfect a commode by cleaning it first using detergent and warm water and then by using a disinfectant such as Milton to disinfect it and then drying it using paper towels.

Sterilisation must also only take place after the area/equipment has been cleaned and is free from dirt. Sterilisation involves using heat or chemicals and prevents the spread of infection by destroying any harmful pathogens that may lead to disease. For example, items such as syringes or medical instruments that are used for surgery and come into contact with body tissues or fluids are sterilised, by using heat in the form of steam.

The care setting where you work will have a policy in place that sets out the standard expected for the appropriate cleaning and decontamination of the work setting and equipment used within it. It is important that you familiarise yourself with your work policy including the aspects of cleaning and decontamination that apply to your job role.

Key terms

Decontamination means cleaning to a high standard, to remove or reduce harmful pathogens that cause infections.

Cleaning is the decontamination used for low infection risk items such as floors and furniture.

Disinfection is the decontamination technique used for medium infection risk items such as bedpans and bottles.

Sterilisation is the decontamination technique used for high infection risk items, such as medical instruments used for surgery.

Anti-bacterials are agents that destroy and prevent the growth and spread of bacteria.

Antiseptics are agents that prevent the growth of harmful pathogens that can cause infections.

6Cs

Care

Maintaining a work environment that is clean is essential for reducing the spread of infection in your work setting. Carrying out your responsibilities for cleaning and decontamination to the best of your ability and ensuring you follow your work setting's agreed ways of working will ensure that you are doing your bit to maintain an environment that is clean and less likely to contain harmful pathogens or encourage the spread of infection.

Evidence opportunity

1.8 Cleaning and decontamination in the workplace

Find and read through your workplace's policy for cleanliness and decontamination. What are the expected standards for cleanliness where you work? Why is this important?

Make a list of your responsibilities regarding cleanliness and decontamination in the workplace and describe what these are in the form of a written account.

LO2 Be able to contribute to the prevention and control of the spread of infection

AC 2.1 Risk assess infection control measures in a range of situations

In care settings, personal protective equipment (PPE) refers to the equipment that is worn by adult care workers to protect against the spread of infections. PPE can prevent and control the spread of infections because:

- it protects individuals from infections you may be carrying
- it protects you from infections individuals may be carrying
- it creates a barrier between the infection and you which means that the infection is unable to spread from you to others or vice versa, or from a surface or piece of equipment to you and others by, as you have learned, a process known as cross infection.

Sometimes, it may be decided, because you are supporting one individual in their own home and there is no risk of the spread of infection, that PPE is not used. This may, for example, be when you are supporting an individual to get dressed or when supporting an individual living in their own home to prepare a meal.

If this is the case, then it must be recorded that you have agreed this with the individual and the reasons why. It is important to monitor this closely in the event of there being any changes to the individual's condition, or in the event of you or others becoming unwell as this may affect you and the individual's decision to use PPE, so that you do not spread infection to them.

It is important therefore that you risk assess infection control measures in a range of situations because it is part of the provision of good and safe care; you will find it useful to review your previous learning about risk assessment in Unit 310. Risk assessing infection control measures will:

- minimise the risk of you or others becoming unwell
- enable you to decide on the infection control measures that are needed to eliminate or reduce risks that could cause illness
- ensure you are complying with legislative and organisational requirements.

Reflect on it

2.1 The key steps of the risk assessment process

Review your previous learning of the risk assessment process that involves five key steps. What are the key steps involved when you risk assess? What do these mean and why are these important?

Evidence opportunity

2.1 Risk assessments of infection control measures

You will be observed for this assessment criterion. In your care setting, risk assess infection control measures for three of the following situations: personal care, assisting individuals with continence, preparing food and drink, performing clinical skills, providing pressure area care, responding to illness or accidents or any other appropriate work task within a care work setting.

Remember to report and record fully any risks identified in line with your care setting's policies and procedures.

AC 2.2 Use appropriate Personal Protective Equipment (PPE) correctly in a range of situations

To ensure that you are using PPE appropriately and that it is effective in preventing the spread of infections it is important to:

- read what your work setting's PPE policy states about the different types of PPE you will be using as part of your day-to-day work tasks
- always follow the manufacturer's instructions when using PPE
- always wash your hands before using PPE
- always wash your hands after disposing of PPE.

Table 12.2 describes some examples of PPE used in care settings, including the reasons why they are used and examples of when they can be used.

PPE is only an effective tool if you know when to use it and if you know how to put it on and take it off correctly. Table 12.3 provides some guidance on this.

Ensure PPE is effective

Disposable gloves and aprons must be changed every time there is contact with a different individual or when there is a change in task, for example supporting the individual with washing and then with eating and drinking. It is also important to check that all PPE is clean and has no tears before wearing it as this may be an opening for a harmful pathogen to enter and cause infection. If you do find a problem, do not use the PPE and report it immediately to your manager who will be able to provide you with advice and guidance.

Remember that some individuals may find PPE too clinical, not like how it feels or think that it stigmatises them as being dirty so it is important you reassure individuals and explain to them why it needs to be worn.

Table 12.2 Why and when to use PPE

Type of PPE	Why use it	When to use it
Disposable gloves	To provide a barrier for the infections that can be spread through your hands.	For example, when supporting individuals with personal care or with their continence as you may come into contact with an individual's body fluids, such as vomit, urine and faeces. You should wear gloves when dealing with an accident where you may come into contact with an open wound or an individual's body fluids, such as blood and vomit as well as when providing pressure area care and performing other clinical skills. You should also use them when you come into contact with broken skin, rashes or burns for example. When disposing of used or soiled linen or waste, it is also a good idea to wear gloves.
Plastic aprons	To provide a barrier for the infections that can be spread through your clothing.	For example, when handling food as you may come into contact with both cooked and raw foods. You should also wear an apron when carrying out a cleaning task as you may come into contact with a harmful substance. You will also need this when coming into contact with bodily fluids such as when assisting individuals with their continence and when responding to accidents.
Surgical face masks	To provide a barrier for the infections that can be spread through breath from your nose and mouth.	For example, when supporting individuals with personal care, because you will come into close contact with them. You might also wear a surgical face mask if an individual is unwell or recovering from an operation to protect them from the risk of infection from you to them.

Table 12.3 How to use PPE

Type of PPE	Putting it on (donning)	Taking it off (doffing) and disposal
Disposable gloves	Choose the correct size gloves. If they are too big they may slip off and if they are too small they may tear and let harmful pathogens spread. Wash your hands before putting gloves on so you do not spread harmful pathogens into your gloves.	Remove one glove at a time. Hold the outside of the glove with your opposite gloved hand and peel it off so it turns inside out. Place it, balled, in your still gloved hand. Then, taking care not to touch the outside of the glove, place your finger tip inside the other glove and peel this one off so the first glove ends up inside it. Place them in the clinical waste bin. Wash and dry your hands to avoid cross infection.
Plastic aprons	Place the apron over your head and then tie it round your waist to give you maximum protection over any harmful pathogens that may be transported to and from your clothing. Wash your hands before putting plastic aprons on so you do not spread harmful pathogens into your gloves.	Unfasten or break the ties round the waist and then remove the apron by pulling it away from your neck and only touching the inside of the apron while doing so. Roll up the apron and place it in the clinical waste bin. Wash and dry your hands to avoid cross infection from the outside of your apron to your hands and to the environment.

Table 12.3 How to use PPE *continued*

Type of PPE	Putting it on (donning)	Taking it off (doffing) and disposal
Surgical face masks	Choose the correct size face mask. If it is too big, it may slip off: if it is too small and does not fit comfortably over your nose and mouth it may let harmful pathogens spread. Wash your hands before putting it on to prevent harmful pathogens getting onto the mask. Place the mask over your nose and mouth and minimise any gaps between the mask and your face. Avoid touching the front of the mask so you do not spread harmful pathogens onto your mask. Use the ear loops to put it on.	Remove the mask by using one ear loop at the time and moving the mask away from your face. Avoid touching the mask so you do not spread harmful pathogens onto your hands or face. Place and dispose of the mask in the clinical waste bin. Wash and dry your hands to avoid cross infection from the outside of your mask to your hands and to the environment.

Reflect on it

2.2 Consequences of not using PPE correctly

Reflect on the consequences of not changing your disposable gloves and apron when you have finished supporting an individual to have a shower.

What are the consequences for the individual? For you? For others in the care setting where you work?

What actions could you take to minimise these risks to the individual and others in your care setting?

Write a short reflective account detailing your thoughts.

Evidence opportunity

2.2 Using personal protective equipment (PPE)

You will be observed for AC 2.2. Practise donning, doffing and disposing of two different types of PPE that you use in your work setting. Ask your assessor for feedback. How did you do? Are there any areas for improvement?

The reflective exemplar provides you with an opportunity to explore in more detail how adult care workers in care settings can seek further support and advice when they are having difficulties complying with their work setting's PPE policy.

Research it

2.2 Your setting's PPE policy

Research what the PPE policy in your work setting says about the different types of PPE you must use as part of your day-to-day work tasks, how to use them, and when and how to report any difficulties you may identify. Discuss with your manager why and when they are used. Write down details of your discussion.

If you work with an individual and PPE is not required, explain why.

	Reflective exemplar
Introduction	I work as a personal assistant to Joan who requires support with showering, dressing and preparing breakfast. Joan has cerebral palsy and finds it difficult to mobilise.
What happened?	This morning I visited Joan as usual and she told me that she wanted to speak with me. I sat down next to her as she explained that she no longer thinks there is any need for me to wear disposable gloves and an apron while I provide care and support to her in the mornings, given that I have been her personal assistant for over a year now and have got to know her very well. Joan added that she would feel a lot more relaxed if I didn't wear these in her home. I informed Joan that I was required to follow my work setting's PPE policy and would therefore always have to wear them when providing her with care and support. Joan frowned and explained that she didn't feel like getting up this morning and would prefer it if I came back tomorrow. I agreed to come back tomorrow.
What worked well?	The fact that I informed Joan that I have to comply with my work setting's PPE policy.
What did not go as well?	Joan's reaction to the information I gave her, i.e. she does not usually frown.
What could I do to improve?	Perhaps I should have explained the reasons why I must wear PPE to Joan. Perhaps I should have referred Joan's request to my manager. The use of PPE could then have been risk assessed with Joan and the work setting to address how to balance her rights with concerns for health and safety. I think I need to discuss this situation with my manager and refer back to my work setting's PPE policy in relation to what it says about wearing PPE when an individual asks for it not to be used.
Links to unit assessment criteria	ACs 2.1, 2.2, 2.5

AC 2.3 Identify when it is necessary to perform hand hygiene

AC 2.4 Perform hand hygiene using recommended techniques and appropriate products

Hand hygiene – why and when?

Preventing the spread of infection can only be done if one or more of the links in the chain of infection you learned about in AC 1.2 are broken; if the chain of infection isn't broken then infections will continue to spread. One of the most effective ways of preventing the spread of infection in care settings is through hand hygiene, which refers to both hand-washing techniques and the use of appropriate sanitiser.

You must always carry out effective hand hygiene in care settings during your day-to-day work activities because pathogens are likely to be present in the tasks you carry out and can therefore be the cause of infections that can spread.

For example, you must always wash your hands to protect yourself, the individuals and others you work with, as well as the environment, from the spread of germs. You must wash your hands:

- before and after you start work
- before and after contact with individuals who you provide care or support to, i.e. support with eating, drinking, washing
- before putting on and after disposing of gloves
- before preparing and handling food
- before and after eating
- after contact with your own or others' body fluids, or any procedure that means you may come into contact with body fluids
- after going to the toilet
- after coughing or sneezing, or blowing your nose
- after disposing of waste or handling used or soiled linen
- after coming into contact with clinical waste.

The method for hand washing in care settings

The Care Quality Commission (CQC) recommends that workers in care settings use liquid soap and warm water for washing their hands and that they carry out the following hand-washing techniques for approximately 30 seconds, outlined on the NHS's 'Hand hygiene technique for staff' poster (this can be accessed from: www.infectionpreventioncontrol.co.uk/resources/hand-hygiene-technique-for-staff-poster).

> **Research it**
>
> **2.3, 2.4 NHS guidance**
>
> You will also find it useful to refer to the NHS website for up-to-date guidance on hand hygiene: www.nhs.uk/Livewell/homehygiene/Pages/how-to-wash-your-hands-properly.aspx

To summarise:

1&2 Wash your hands under warm running water and apply liquid soap to cover all the hand surfaces.
3. Rub your hands, palm to palm using a circular action.
4. Rub the back of each hand with the palm of the other hand, with fingers interlaced.
5. Rub palm to palm with fingers interlaced.
6. Rub backs of fingers to opposing palms with fingers interlocked.
7. Rub each thumb clasped in opposite hand using a rotational action.
8. Rub tips of fingers in the opposite palm in a circular action.
9. Rub each wrist with the opposite hand.
10. Rinse your hands under warm running water.
11. Use your elbow or a paper towel to turn off the tap.
12. Dry your hands thoroughly with paper towels.
13. Remember that hand washing should take 15-30 seconds.

In addition, it is recommended that staff in care settings also comply with the following hand hygiene practices that are important in the prevention of infections:

- When you provide care to individuals you must roll your sleeves up to the elbows – this is referred to as Bare Below the Elbows (BBE).
- Jewellery must not be worn, for example rings and bracelets.
- Finger nails must be kept clean and short.
- Nail extensions, acrylic nails and nail varnish must not be worn.
- Any cuts or abrasions must be covered with a waterproof dressing.

Hand-washing technique with soap and water

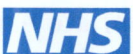

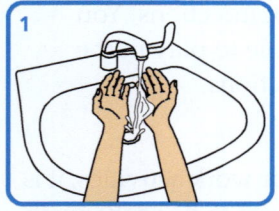
1. Wet hands with water

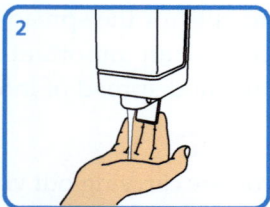
2. Apply enough soap to cover all hand surfaces

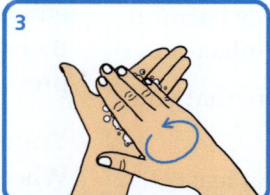
3. Rub hands palm to palm

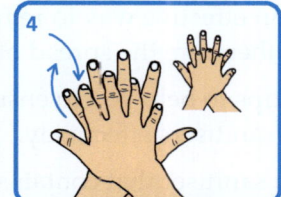
4. Rub back of each hand with palm of other hand with fingers interlaced

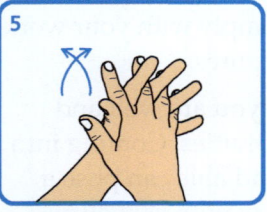
5. Rub palm to palm with fingers interlaced

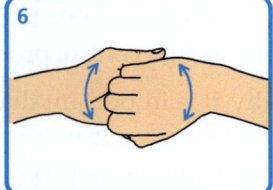
6. Rub with back of fingers to opposing palms with fingers interlocked

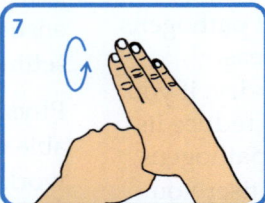
7. Rub each thumb clasped in opposite hand using a rotational movement

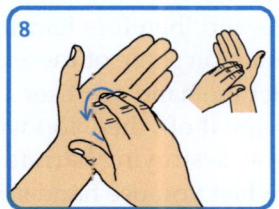
8. Rub tips of fingers in opposite palm in a circular motion

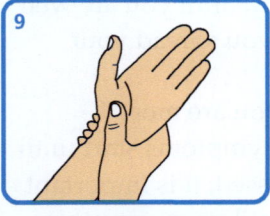
9. Rub each wrist with opposite hand

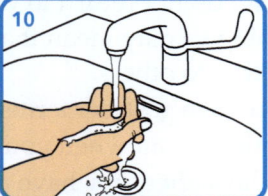
10. Rinse hands with water

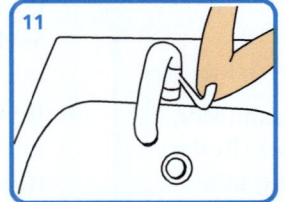
11. Use elbow to turn off tap

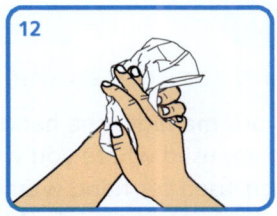
12. Dry thoroughly with a single-use towel

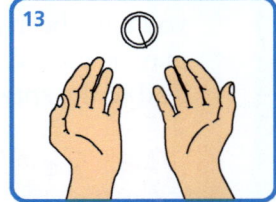
13. Hand washing should take 15–30 seconds

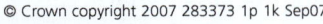

© Crown copyright 2007 283373 1p 1k Sep07

Adapted from World Health Organization *Guidelines on Hand Hygiene in Health Care*

Figure 12.2 Hand hygiene technique for staff

Use of appropriate hand sanitiser

As you know, washing your hands with soap and water whenever possible is the most effective way of reducing and removing harmful pathogens from your hands. If you do not have access to soap and water then hand sanitisers that contain at least 60% alcohol can be an effective way to reduce harmful pathogens and therefore the spread of infections.

Here are some tips to help you to ensure that you are using hand sanitisers effectively:

1. Select a hand sanitiser that contains at least 60% alcohol; if you do not, it may not be as effective at destroying harmful pathogens.
2. Ensure you follow the manufacturer's instructions and use sufficient sanitiser on your hands; if you do not, it may not cover all areas of your hands and therefore harmful pathogens may still remain on some of these areas.
3. Ensure you let the hand sanitiser air dry; if you do not and wipe it off, then you will reduce its effectiveness at destroying harmful pathogens.
4. Ensure that when you use hand sanitiser you apply it to the palm of one hand and then rub it all over the surfaces of both hands until your hands have completely dried.

> **Reflect on it**
>
> **2.3, 2.4 Hand sanitiser in the workplace**
>
> Discuss with your manager the hand sanitising products that are used where you work. Reflect on the products used for hand washing and hand sanitising where you work. Who uses these products? Why?

> **Evidence opportunity**
>
> **2.3, 2.4 Hand hygiene in care settings**
>
> You will be observed for this AC. Practise washing your hands and using appropriate hand sanitiser following the recommended methods and using appropriate products. Ask a colleague or your assessor to observe you while you do this and make a note of any improvements you could make to your practice. Reflect on their feedback and practise washing your hands again. Remember, effective hand washing takes approximately 30 seconds – how long did you take? How many of the 13 steps did you use? Did you use the hand sanitiser effectively?

AC 2.5 Demonstrate ways of working to ensure own health and hygiene does not pose a risk to individuals and others at work

Care settings, as you have learned, are perfect environments for the spread of infections. You therefore have an important role to play in the prevention and spread of infections.

Your health

When you are carrying out your work activities, it is crucial that you are in good health to do so. Being in good health means having both physical and mental wellbeing; you will learn more about how to manage your mental wellbeing in Unit 314 Understanding personal wellbeing. Mental wellbeing is crucial for ensuring that you are able to comply with your work setting's infection control procedures.

Physically, it is important that you are well and able to carry out your work activities. Coming into work when you are not well and able can pose a risk to the individuals you work with as well as to your colleagues and other visitors to the care setting. For example:

- If you have the flu it is important you visit your GP and do not return to work until you are well as doing so may mean that you spread your infection to others.
- If you have gastroenteritis you are most infectious from when your symptoms start until two days after they have passed; it is important therefore to stay off work until your symptoms have stopped for two days.
- If you have a skin rash it is important that you visit your GP and do not return to work until you have been given permission to do so, as this may be passed on to others and therefore can lead to the spread of infections.

> **Research it**
>
> **2.5 Sickness policy**
>
> Research the sickness policy in the setting where you work. Discuss with your manager what types of infections you must report, the reasons why and the procedures for doing so.

Your personal hygiene

Maintaining your personal hygiene to a good standard is not only more pleasant for everyone you come into contact with, but it is also an essential part of the control of infection. As you have learned, hand washing and wearing PPE are integral to ensuring that you prevent the spread of infection and are two key aspects involved in maintaining good standards of personal hygiene. Other important aspects of your personal hygiene for controlling the spread of infections include the following:

- **Hair care:** your hair must be regularly washed, brushed and kept clean to prevent infections such as head lice. If you have long hair it should be tied back to prevent any unwanted hairs from falling into, for example, food that you are preparing. Your hair may also come into contact with individuals which could lead to the spread of infection. It could also be a hazard as it may become caught in equipment or machinery. Likewise, if you wear a head scarf, or head covering, ensure that it is safely tied in place.
- **Hand and nail care:** your nails must be kept clean and short. Nail varnish and nail extensions must not be worn as these may flake and/or fall off while carrying out your work activities and therefore have the potential to spread any harmful pathogens that they contain. Similarly, jewellery such as rings and bracelets can also be potential risks of infection as harmful pathogens may become trapped in these. Good hand hygiene, as you have learned, is essential in your role, particularly when preparing food. Remember that food can be a source of infection if hygiene procedures are not followed.
- **Oral care:** you must brush your teeth regularly to avoid infections or halitosis (bad breath). This can be unpleasant for the individuals and others you work with as you may be in close proximity to them.
- **Body care:** you must wash, bathe or shower every day, wear clean clothes and use deodorant to ensure that you prevent body odour and the risk of infections to others. This can be unpleasant and unhygienic for all those who enter the work environment including visitors to the setting where you work.
- **Skin care:** your skin must be kept moisturised because with frequent hand washing it is likely to become dry and could therefore flake off during work activities and spread infections. If you have open wounds you must keep them covered, and skin rashes must be treated to avoid the risk of cross infection as you may spread infection not only to individuals but to your colleagues that you work with.
- **Clothing/uniform:** you must wash the clothes you wear at work and/or uniform regularly so it is kept clean and pathogen-free. Wearing an apron will protect the front/outside of your clothes from harmful pathogens. Remember, if you wear your uniform outside of the work setting you may be at risk of cross infection, for example if visiting the supermarket during your lunch break or travelling home from work on the bus. In these situations, it may be better to change into and out of your uniform at work. In this way you will ensure that your clothing and uniform do not spread infections from person to person and place to place.

> ### Reflect on it
>
>
> #### 2.5 'Transports' for infection
>
> Reflect on your previous learning in this unit and write a short reflective account about how clothes, jewellery, nails and open wounds can be the 'transport' for infections.

Research it

2.5 The importance of food hygiene

Food can be a source of infection if it is not cooked properly or if you do not follow good hygiene practice. You should remember the things that you have learned in this LO and the rest of this unit when preparing food. Hand hygiene is key. For example, you should remember that if you have a cut, then you should cover this with a bright plaster that can be easily spotted if it comes off while you are preparing food and can be disposed of. It is important that you are aware of how to avoid infection and cross-contamination, how to cook food properly to avoid this from happening, how to ensure that bacteria from food is killed, and the health and safety rules to follow when preparing food.

You will also need to be aware of best before dates, allergies and special dietary requirements and the rules to follow when preparing food to cater for different requirements.

Below are some useful sources of information that you should read with regard to food safety:

www.gov.uk/food-safety-your-responsibilities/food-hygiene
www.food.gov.uk/business-guidance/hygiene-requirements-for-your-business (also available as a PDF)
www.food.gov.uk
www.foodsafety.gov

Evidence opportunity

2.5 Your health and hygiene

Write an account to describe two or three different ways of ensuring that your health and hygiene do not pose a risk to an individual, colleagues, visitors in the care setting where you work. Follow up your written account with a professional discussion with your assessor.

Legislation	
Relevant Act	**Key points**
Health and Safety at Work Act (HASAWA) 1974	The health and safety of everyone in a work setting must be protected – in a care setting this includes individuals, adult care workers and those who visit. It also established the key duties and responsibilities of all employers and employees in work settings.
Management of Health and Safety at Work Regulations (MHSWR) 1999	Employers and managers must assess and manage risks by carrying out risk assessments. It requires employers to provide information, training and supervision so that work activities can be carried out safely.
Personal Protective Equipment at Work Regulations 1992	Personal protective equipment (PPE) to provide protection against infections must be provided free of charge by employers. It requires PPE to be maintained in good condition and requires training to be provided in the use of PPE.
Reporting of Injuries, Diseases and Dangerous Occurrences Regulations (RIDDOR) 2013	Employers must report and keep records for three years of work-related accidents that cause death and serious injuries (referred to as reportable injuries), diseases and dangerous occurrences (i.e. incidents with the potential to cause harm). It requires work settings to have procedures in place and to provide information and training on reporting injuries, diseases and incidents.

312 Implementing health and safety in adult care settings/services

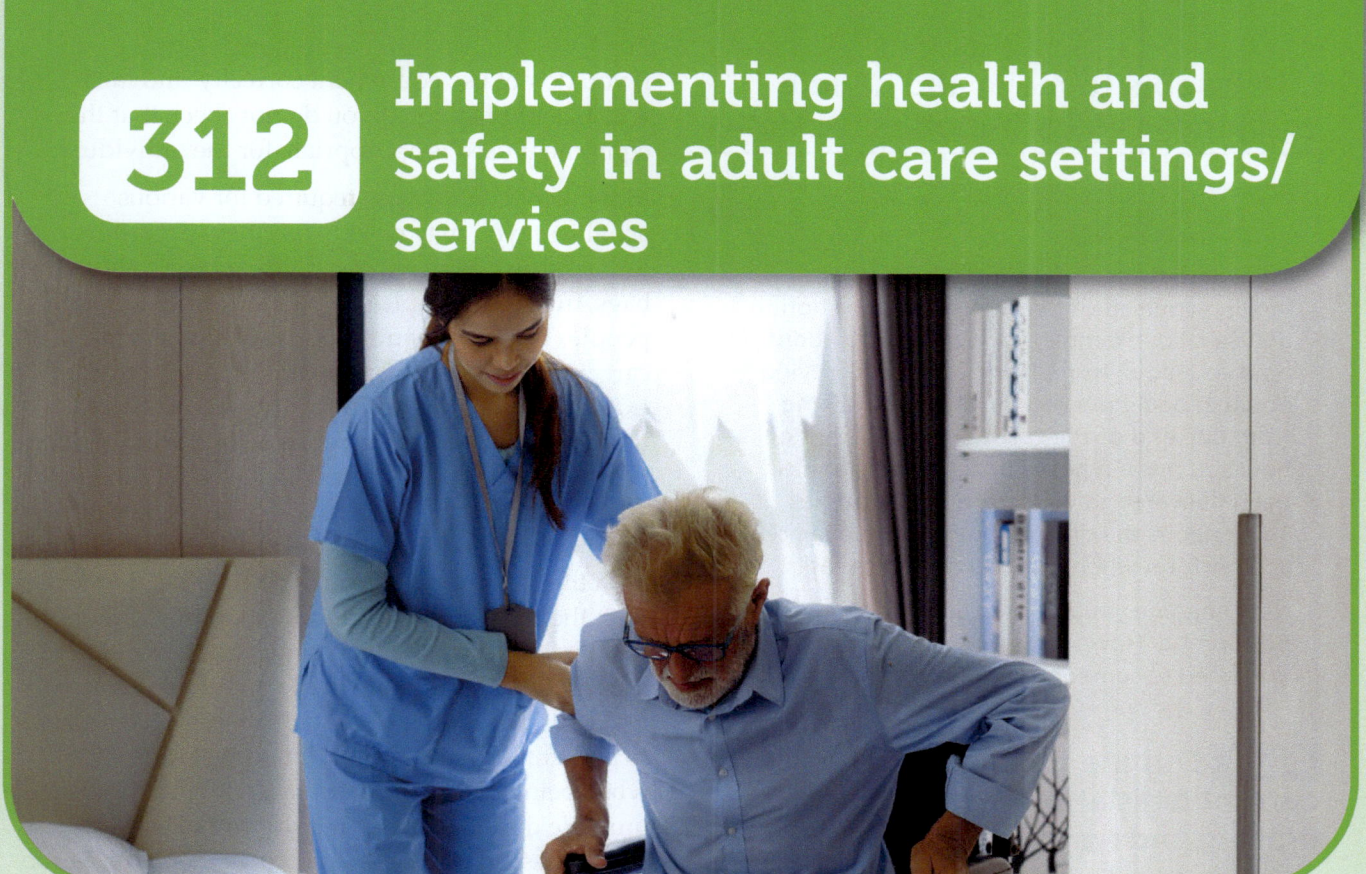

About this unit

Credit value: 3
Guided learning hours: 20

Promoting and implementing health and safety when supporting individuals applies to every task you carry out in the care setting where you work. In this unit you will learn about how to carry out the safe moving and handling of equipment and other objects as well as how to store, use and dispose of hazardous substances and materials safely. This unit will also equip you with the knowledge and skills you need to promote fire safety and implement security measures at work.

Learning outcomes

By the end of this unit, you will:

LO1: Be able to move and handle equipment and other objects safely

LO2: Be able to handle hazardous substances and materials

LO3: Be able to promote fire safety in the work setting

LO4: Be able to implement security measures in work settings

LO1 Be able to move and handle equipment and other objects safely

> **Getting started**
>
> Think about the different steps involved in moving yourself or items from one position to another. For example, you could think about how you move from sitting in a chair to lying down in bed, how you move when walking from one end of the corridor to the other or how you move a heavy boxed item that has been delivered to your front door upstairs. Think about the different range of movements you perform when carrying out these tasks.
>
> Now imagine you need support with moving or positioning. How would you explain the support you need to someone who didn't know you?

AC 1.1 Outline the main points of current legislation that relate to moving and handling

Moving and handling in care settings involves providing support to individuals to be able to move from one position to another as well as being able to handle lifting, moving and positioning equipment, such as hoists, slings, bath lifts, standing transfer aids, and other objects, such as wheelchairs and boxes, safely.

Moving and positioning individuals safely is required for ensuring that:

- individuals are being supported to move and position in line with their plan of care and their specific needs
- individuals do not experience pain or distress
- individuals' independence and dignity are promoted
- the agreed ways of working, policies and procedures that are in place in care settings are being complied with.

Policies and procedures

Agreed ways of working for moving and positioning individuals safely are underpinned by specific legislation that relates to moving and handling so that it is carried out safely and accidents can be avoided. Complying with legal requirements will ensure that you protect yourself, individuals and others from injuries and/or accidents. This will help prevent back injuries, which can occur if you do not use equipment correctly, and falls which could happen if you do not check that the equipment used is appropriate for the individual.

Moving and handling is required for various activities – you may need to use these procedures for tasks such as moving and lifting boxes, shopping bags, furniture, supplies or you may need to move people. You may require special equipment to carry out the moving and handling procedure, for example, a sling. In this case, you should check that the sling used is appropriate for the individual being hoisted. You will need to check the sling is appropriate for the weight, height and shape of the individual, whether the individual requires support with their whole body including their head or just with the trunk and whether their condition causes them pain. Remember that slings come in different shapes and sizes and are made out of different materials depending on what the individual requires to be comfortable and to maintain their dignity when being hoisted. Individuals with profound and multiple disabilities may require you to use adapted techniques such as signs (to involve them during the whole process), adapted equipment and slings.

The following are examples of specific pieces of legislation that relate to moving and handling activities and come under the Health and Safety at Work Act (HASAWA) 1974.

Manual Handling Operations Regulations 1992 (as amended 2002)

These regulations are relevant to moving and handling activities and include lifting, lowering, pushing, pulling and carrying. They require that employers must:

- avoid, as far as is reasonably practicable, any manual handling activity that is hazardous and likely to involve a risk of injury
- carry out a risk assessment of all manual handling activities that cannot be avoided and put control measures in place to reduce the risk of injury*
- provide any equipment necessary for supporting health and safety.

*A manual handling assessment involves five key aspects which can be easily remembered using the TILE (O) acronym:

- **T** – Task (what am I lifting and where am I moving the load to?)
- **I** – Individual (am I capable of lifting the load safely on my own?)

- **L** – Load (how heavy is the load? What shape and size is the load?)
- **E** – Environment (is the load in a small space? Will it be difficult to lift?)
- **O** – Other aspects (do I need to wear PPE?).

As an employee you also have moving and handling responsibilities including:

- maintaining your own safety and those of individuals and others who you work with
- attending moving and handling training provided by your employer
- only carrying out moving and handling activities that you have been trained in
- complying with your work setting's moving and handling procedures and agreed ways of working at all times
- reporting and recording all hazardous moving and handling activities.

Provision and Use of Work Equipment Regulations (PUWER) 1998

These regulations require that all work equipment including moving and handling equipment is used safely. They require that employers must provide moving and handling equipment that is:

- suitable for the intended use
- maintained in a safe condition
- monitored to ensure it is in good working order*
- used only by people who have been trained in its use
- accompanied by suitable health and safety measures, such as emergency stop controls and clearly visible markings
- used in line with the manufacturer's instructions.

*If a risk assessment shows that those handling the equipment are at risk, then employers must make sure that this is checked. Advice can also be sought from the health and safety officer and the manufacturers of the equipment.

Lifting Operations and Lifting Equipment Regulations (LOLER) 1998

These regulations require employers to ensure that lifting equipment used in work settings is safe by requiring that:

- all lifting equipment is used solely for the purpose it was intended for and must be installed correctly to reduce any risks
- all lifting equipment is marked with warning and safety signs to show safe working loads
- all lifting equipment is maintained and monitored for safety and records kept (all equipment used must be safe. It must be monitored and examined regularly, not just when defects are reported, to ensure its safety is maintained)
- all lifting equipment that is unsafe is reported and removed from use until it is repaired or replaced and safe to use again
- all lifting activities are planned, supervised and carried out in a safe manner (that is, only by people who have been trained and are able).

Although it is not mentioned as part of LOLER, you should remember that, as an employee, you are responsible for complying with all information, instruction and training you have received from your employer in relation to moving and handling, and to use all equipment you have been trained in safely and in line with the manufacturer's instructions. If you identify that a piece of equipment is faulty then you must report this immediately to your employer and not use it.

> **Research it**
>
> **1.1 Assisting individuals**
>
> Individuals in care settings may require support with moving and positioning because they may have specific conditions that affect how their bodies move and that can make movements difficult and/or painful. This information is used to risk assess and put into place moving and positioning practices that meet individuals' specific needs and that are safe to use.
>
> Research how the following two conditions may affect individuals' movements and then produce an information handout with your findings.
>
> 1. Brittle bone disease
> 2. Stroke.
>
> You may find the following link on brittle bone disease useful:
> www.brittlebone.org
>
> You may find the following link about an individual who has had a stroke useful:
> www.stroke.org.uk/what-is-stroke/types-of-stroke
>
> You can also find out more about LOLER at:
> www.hse.gov.uk/work-equipment-machinery/loler.htm

> **Reflect on it**
>
> **1.1 Duty of care**
>
> Reflect on your duty of care in relation to safe moving and handling in the care setting where you work. Why is this important? What are the consequences of not fulfilling your duty of care?

> **Evidence opportunity**
>
> **1.1 Moving and handling legislation**
>
> With a colleague, discuss and then write down three moving and handling tasks that are carried out in your work setting. For each task identify the specific legislation that is in place.

AC 1.2 Outline the principles for safe moving and handling

In care settings, a wide range of moving and handling equipment is used to meet the diverse needs of the individuals who require support with moving and positioning. This includes:

- **lifting equipment**, such as mobile hoists that lift and lower individuals from, for example, their bed to an armchair, and bath hoists that lift and lower individuals into and out of the bath
- **moving and handling equipment**, such as slide sheets that move individuals without lifting them up and down the bed and transfer boards that enable individuals to slide from their wheelchair into an armchair
- **moving and handling aids**, such as hand rails that provide support to individuals going up steps or walking frames that support individuals' weight while walking.

You can use moving and handling equipment safely and move other objects safely by following these good practice rules or principles:

- Follow your work setting's agreed ways of working for moving and handling, for example by only carrying out moving and handling activities that you have been trained for. Not doing so may result in you or others being injured.
- Ensure you have read the moving and handling guidelines that are in place for individuals. For example, read through individuals' moving and handling risk assessments before carrying out moving and handling activities or using any moving and handling equipment to ensure the safety and wellbeing of individuals.
- Complete safety checks before using moving and handling equipment. For example, is it clean? Is it working? Have you noticed any faults? Not doing so may result in a serious failure in the equipment as you are using it which may cause unnecessary distress or injury to an individual.
- Prepare to move an object safely by completing safety checks, for example is there enough space in the environment to carry out the move? Is the load too heavy for one person? Not doing so may mean that you will be putting yourself, the individuals and others at risk of being harmed or injured.
- Report any concerns you have when carrying out health and safety checks. For example, you should report if a piece of equipment is not working, or if you witness a colleague using unsafe practices when moving an individual using lifting equipment. Not doing so may mean that unsafe equipment and practices continue in the work setting. Think about stories you may have read or heard about where individuals have been left in their beds, unable to move because no assistance has been provided. There have been bans in some organisations on lifting. If you see such practice, it is important to discuss or report this to your manager.
- Always communicate clearly with those involved in moving and handling activities. For example, explain to the individual how you are going to support them with the move, check that they are not in any pain and that their dignity is not undermined in any way, encourage them to actively participate in the move and check with your colleagues which of you is going to take the lead when carrying out the move. Not communicating with the individual will be disrespectful towards individuals' rights to be actively involved in all care and support activities. Poor **communication** between you and colleagues may result in moves becoming unsafe.

- Use a safe posture when moving objects. For example, keep your legs and feet slightly apart, your knees slightly bent, do not stoop or twist, keep the load as close to your body as possible. Not doing so could result in you injuring your back. At worse you may cause your body irreversible damage and result in you experiencing distress.
- Be honest with yourself. For example, if you are unsure about how to follow any of the above principles, seek advice from your manager. Not doing so could result in you not complying with best practice and therefore not promoting your health, safety and wellbeing as well as that of the individuals and colleagues you work alongside.

Research it

1.2 Moving and handling equipment

Research the different types of moving and handling equipment, lifting equipment and moving and handling aids that are used with the individuals in the care setting where you work. Produce a one-page information handout with your findings.

Reflect on it

1.2 Health and safety checks

Reflect on the importance of carrying out health and safety checks before using moving and handling equipment and moving objects in care settings. How can doing so prevent accidents from occurring?

Evidence opportunity

1.2 Principles for moving and handling

For each of the principles you learned about in relation to moving and handling equipment, discuss with your assessor their importance for health and safety. Remember to consider how the principles can keep you, individuals and others safe.

6Cs

Communication

Good communication when moving and handling is essential for reassuring individuals during moves and for ensuring that you have their permission to carry out the move. Remember the principles of person-centred care that you have learned about. Remember that this is a joint procedure. Good communication enables you to ensure individuals' understanding of how the move will be carried out. It also encourages their active participation, and means that you have considered their rights. Good communication with your colleagues is also essential for ensuring that you work together to enable all moves are carried out smoothly.

AC 1.3 Move and handle equipment and other objects safely

In care settings, moving and handling activities are part of adult care workers' day-to-day work activities. The techniques used involve the use of moving and handling equipment to safely transfer individuals with care or support needs from one position to another, as well as following the general principles you learned about in AC 1.2 for moving objects such as shopping bags, furniture, boxes and supplies safely.

Expressing the total number of musculoskeletal disorder cases in the Health and Social Care sector as a rate, the HSE statistics show that:

'Annually around 1.7% (per 100,000 workers) of workers in the sector were suffering from a musculoskeletal disorder they believed was work-related.

This rate is statistically significantly higher than the rate across all industries (1.3%)'

Health and Safety Executive (2015) 'Health and Safety in the Health and Social Care sector in Great Britain 2014/15' (Source: Labour Force Survey)

> **Research it**
>
> **1.3 Your setting's guidelines**
>
> Research your work setting's moving and handling procedures and discuss with your manager what these say about the equipment and objects you may be expected to move and handle as part of your work activities. Find out if your work setting has any guidelines in place for safe practices when moving and handling individuals. Write down notes to document your findings.

> **Reflect on it**
>
> **1.3 Safety checks**
>
> Reflect on the safety and maintenance checks that are carried out on the moving and handling equipment used in your work setting. How often are these carried out? Why?

Using moving and handling equipment safely

Using moving and handling equipment is a skill and to avoid accidents and injuries to yourself, individuals and your colleagues, you must:

- **be trained in its safe use:** your employer is required to provide you with the training to do so.
- **follow your work setting's moving and handling procedures:** you are required to comply with the safe processes your employer has developed for all moving and handling activities that you carry out. For example, this may involve using the type of equipment appropriate for an individual in line with their height, weight and condition. You may need to use a piece of equipment to move an individual with two staff instead of one.
- **check that the equipment is safe to use:** you are required to do this every time you use a piece of moving and handling equipment. For example, you will need to check the battery is fully charged (not doing so may result in it stopping from working during a move), that there are no visible signs of wear and tear and that it has been tested as per legal requirements.
- **check that the equipment is clean:** you are required to do this every time you use a piece of moving and handling equipment. Not only will this reduce the risk of cross infection but it is also showing your respect and consideration for the individuals you are assisting with moving.

Moving objects safely

From time to time, adult care workers may need to move objects in care settings from one position to another. For example, boxes of PPE are delivered to the front door that need to be moved into the first aid room or a delivery of groceries is made that needs to be moved into the kitchen. Moving objects safely is a skill and using the techniques below will help you with this.

- **Plan how you are going to carry out the move:** for example, consider whether you will need assistance, where you need to move the object to and ensure you have prepared the route you plan to use.
- **Ensure you are in a stable position before carrying out the move:** for example, your feet should be apart to maintain your balance and you should avoid wearing footwear with no support or tight clothing that may make it difficult to move safely.
- **Ensure you are in a safe position when handling the object:** for example, keep and hold the object close to your body, do not stoop when lifting the object, keep your knees, hips and back slightly bent, keep your shoulders facing in the same direction as the hips, keep your head up and look ahead. Put the object down in a smooth movement by keeping hold of it until it reaches the surface you want it on and then slide the object into its desired position.

Moving and handling legislation does not indicate a safe maximum weight limit that can be lifted by a person. Instead, as you have learned in AC 1.1, it places legal duties on employers to risk assess all manual handling activities and situations including the person who will be carrying out the move, such as their physical strength and whether they have any health condition that may affect their ability to lift objects. In other words, it is always better to be safe than sorry when moving and handling! If in doubt, ask your manager to ensure your practice remains safe.

> **Case study**
>
> **1.2, 1.3 Using moving and handling equipment**
>
> Jan, a care worker in a residential care home, is assisting May who is 84 years old with having a bath this morning. As it has been a very busy morning, Jan is running a little late and May is not happy that she will be having her bath a little later than she usually does.
>
> Once Jan agrees with May to assist her to have a bath, Jan carefully reads through May's care plan and moving and handling guidelines. This is to ensure that there have not been any changes to May's care needs and to the moving and handling equipment used to assist her with moving in and out of the bath.
>
> Once Jan has prepared the bathroom and assisted May to prepare herself, Jan supports May to sit in the bath lift. As Jan begins to operate the bath lift so that May can get in the bath, the lift stops working.
>
> *Discuss*
> 1. How could this situation have been prevented?
> 2. What equipment checks could have been done?
> 3. What impact did this situation have on May?
> 4. What support can you provide to Jan?

Moving and handling in an individual's home

Equipment such as hoists may be difficult to operate in an individual's home where the space is confined; for example there may be a small bathroom where it is difficult to manoeuvre. Where possible, risk assessments must take into account the size of equipment and the room available – for instance, two people may be more appropriate to support an individual to mobilise than a large piece of equipment. In all cases you must not put yourself, the individual, or your colleagues at risk. If you have any concerns, do not carry out any actions that you deem to be unsafe.

> **Evidence opportunity**
>
> **1.3 Move and handle equipment and objects safely**
>
> You will be observed in the workplace for AC 1.3 on how to do the following.
>
> In pairs, show how to:
>
> 1. safely use a piece of moving and handling equipment safely, for example a hoist or bath lift
> 2. safely move an object, for example a box of first aid supplies or stationery.

LO2 Be able to handle hazardous substances and materials

> **Getting started**
>
> Look around your home and see how many substances and materials you can find that may cause you to become unwell if you come into contact with them. Why are they potentially dangerous? What impact could they have on your health? Why? You could also discuss your findings with a colleague and see if there are any others that you might not have thought about.

AC 2.1 Identify types of hazardous substances that may be found in the work setting

Care settings are the types of environments where hazardous substances and hazardous materials can be found and therefore it is very important that you know what these are so that you can carry out your duty to promote your own, individuals' and others' safety in the care setting where you work.

Hazardous substances and materials can come in different forms such as liquids, sprays and powder. In a care setting, care workers are likely to encounter these in everyday products such as cleaning detergents, medication and bodily fluids.

> **Key term**
>
> **Nanotechnology** is technology that deals with the understanding and manipulation of atoms and molecules.

There are different types of hazardous substances that you may come across in your work setting and these include for example:

- chemicals such as disinfection chemicals used in a community centre.
- products containing chemicals such as kitchen cleaner if you work in an individual's own home.
- fumes such as carbon monoxide that may be emitted by gas appliances in a nursing home.
- dusts such as from dirt accumulated on surfaces in clinics/surgeries.
- vapours such as flammable vapours that may be emitted by a gas boiler in the kitchen of a residential care home.
- mists such as water mists emitted from a burst hot water pipe in a supported housing's central heating system.
- **nanotechnology** such as that which enables specific tumour sites in the treatment of skin cancer to be targeted in a hospital.
- gases and asphyxiating gases and biological agents such as oxygen (gas), carbon monoxide (asphyxiating gas), and bacteria (biological agent) that can be found in a range of care settings/services.

The Control of Substances Hazardous to Health Regulations 2002 (COSHH) classify hazardous substances into different types depending on the dangers they pose, i.e. toxic, very toxic, corrosive, harmful or irritant.

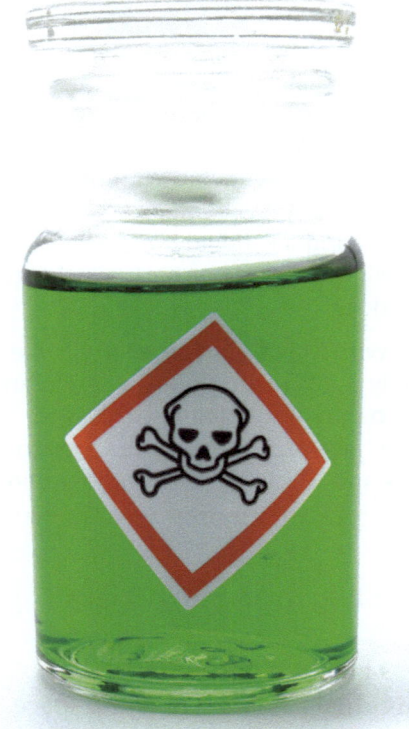

Figure 13.1 Example of a warning label

> **Research it**
>
> **2.1 COSHH Regulations 2002 and labels**
>
> Research the COSHH Regulations 2002 and find out the meanings of the classifications of different types of hazardous substances. Produce a poster with your findings.
>
> Then carry out further research into the different symbols, and find out why they are hazardous. You should also find out what the abbreviations for these are. There is more information in AC 2.2.

> **Reflect on it**
>
> **2.1 Protecting individuals**
>
> Reflect on the different ways you could protect individuals in your care setting from the dangers of the hazardous substances you identified as being present in the care setting where you work.

> **Evidence opportunity**
>
> **2.1 Hazardous substances**
>
> Find examples of hazardous substances present in your work setting. For each one, write down what type they are and the potential dangers they pose.

AC 2.2 Demonstrate safe practices for a) storing, b) using hazardous substances and c) disposing of hazardous substances and materials

For this AC you will be observed using safe practices when storing and using hazardous substances and when disposing of hazardous substances and materials.

Hazardous substances and materials, such as cleaning fluids, medication, bodily fluids and used dressings, have the potential to cause harm and illness to others when stored, used or disposed of incorrectly. This is why the COSHH Regulations 2002 require your employer to have in place procedures for safely storing, using and disposing of hazardous materials and substances.

Below are some examples of the safe practices to follow.

When storing hazardous substances (such as cleaning fluids and medication) check:

- **where they are being stored:** the temperature and ventilation of the area need to be checked by you and your employer. Some cleaning substances can be highly flammable and therefore must be kept in an area that is cool and well ventilated.
- **how they are being stored:** you need to check whether they are being stored in line with the manufacturer's instructions. Hazardous substances need to be stored in their original containers as supplied by the manufacturer, labelled correctly and with their safety lids on and closed. This is so that individuals in care settings do not accidentally mistake them for a drink and swallow them. The COSHH file in your setting will tell you about how to store these substances
- **the precautions to take:** you will need to check whether the necessary storage precautions have been taken to ensure cleaning substances and medication have been stored in secure and appropriate areas. This is to avoid any outbreaks of fires or illnesses, for example. Make sure that you do not change the labels, and that you do not use the same container for storing another hazardous substance.

> **Research it**
>
> **2.2 Safe practices**
>
> Go to www.hse.gov.uk/coshh/basics.htm for more information on COSHH. This requires that all employers control hazardous substances.
>
> You should also go to www.healthyworkinglives.scot/workplace-guidance/safety/hazardous-substances/Pages/common-hazards.aspx to find out more information on safe handling, use and storage of hazardous substances in the workplace.
>
> Make notes detailing what you learned.
>
> What safe practices do you follow in your work setting for storing hazardous substances?

When using hazardous substances (such as cleaning fluids and medication) check:

- **the label:** always remember that before using a hazardous substance you should check the label for the hazard symbol. You will then need to check the COSHH file to find out about what precautions you need to take and follow the procedures that have been laid down by your setting.
- **how to use them:** you need to check whether PPE must be worn. For some hazardous substances, disposable gloves may need to be worn because if they come into contact with your skin they may cause a skin rash or, worse still, burns.
- **the techniques to use:** you need to make sure the techniques you use are safe. Some cleaning substances must be diluted before they are used, others must not. Medication should not be left unattended as doing so may mean that individuals swallow it or even pass it on to others; this in turn may result in illnesses and even fatalities.
- **the precautions to take:** using warning signs to alert others of the dangers when preparing to use a hazardous substance is important so that you are not interrupted while doing so or distracted from the task. In other words, you should alert others beforehand and also alert them just before you are preparing to use the hazardous substance. Remember to report any incorrect labels, containers and lids to your manager, and do the same if you see anyone else using these substances incorrectly or in a dangerous way.

When disposing of hazardous substances and materials (such as cleaning fluids, medication, used dressings and PPE with body fluids) check:

- **where to dispose of them:** the location will vary depending on what the waste is. For example, clinical waste that contains body fluids must be disposed of separately to general waste, otherwise you risk cross infection – the bags must be labelled and the labels must say what they contain. Sharps must be disposed of separately in a sharps box where they cannot cause an accidental injury; they must be sealed and, like the clinical waste, will be incinerated. Leftover cleaning fluids must be disposed of in a separate utility area where they cannot cause any harm. You will need to make sure that you know all the different types of waste and how to dispose of each safely, including how to label them, especially because you will not be the last person to handle these – someone else will then have to handle the bags and containers, so it is important for their safety that you follow the correct procedures.
- **the techniques to use:** you must know how to dispose of hazardous substances and materials safely, for example by wearing gloves and aprons to prevent pathogens from transferring from hazardous waste, wearing a face mask when coming into contact with body fluids or hazardous substances, and by washing your hands after disposing of waste products. These techniques will help prevent cross infection, for example, by preventing pathogens present in body fluids from entering the body through the eyes or mouth.
- **the precautions to take:** you should check whether all necessary precautions for the disposal of hazardous waste have been taken so as to avoid accidents, injuries and cross infection.

Your setting should have a COSHH file that should include clear information on hazardous substances. This will include where they are kept, how they are labelled, the effects they have, the maximum exposure you can have to them while staying safe, and what to do if there is an emergency involving any one of them.

Safe practice when working in an individual's home

In an individual's home, cleaning materials may be in a downstairs or kitchen cupboard instead of being locked away. Always return any cleaning materials you use to their appropriate location. If you feel these may pose a risk to either the individual or someone else who visits their home such as a child, then share your concerns with the individual so the appropriate action can be taken.

> **Research it**
>
> **2.2 COSHH file**
>
> Find out from your manager or employer where the COSHH file is kept in your work setting and the information it contains in relation to storing, using and disposing of hazardous substances and materials. Discuss the key points with your manager.
>
> Does it mention how to store these substances? Does it explain when and in what situations you may need to handle these substances? Does it state the length of time that people should be exposed to these substances? How about the PPE you must wear when handling these substances?
>
> **Good practice when dealing with hazardous substances**
>
> The Health and Safety Executive's website includes a list of points to follow for good practice in the control of substances hazardous to health. They have been included here but you should go to their website to research these further:
>
> www.hse.gov.uk/coshh/detail/goodpractice.htm
>
> 1. Design and operate processes and activities to minimise emission, release and spread of substances hazardous to health.
> 2. Take into account all relevant routes of exposure – inhalation, skin and ingestion – when developing control measures.
> 3. Control exposure by measures that are proportionate to the health risk.
> 4. Choose the most effective and reliable control options that minimise the escape and spread of substances hazardous to health.
> 5. Where adequate control of exposure cannot be achieved by other means, provide, in combination with other control measures, suitable personal protective equipment.

6. Check and review regularly all elements of control measures for their continuing effectiveness.
7. Inform and train all employees on the hazards and risks from substances with which they work, and the use of control measures developed to minimise the risks.
8. Ensure that the introduction of measures to control exposure does not increase the overall risk to health and safety.

Disposal of waste

Research the following waste products and find out how each of these needs to be disposed of. This is important because not disposing of them correctly can lead to illness and infections:

- clinical waste such as dressings
- soiled bedding
- soiled clothing
- recyclable equipment and other instruments
- bodily fluids
- syringes, needles, sharps.

You could go to the following web page to find out more about these: www.hse.gov.uk/healthservices/healthcare-waste.htm

Reflect on it

2.2 Consequences

Reflect on the consequences of not following safe practices for storing, using and disposing of hazardous substances and materials. What impact would this have on you? On your work colleagues, team members, individuals and others? On the organisation or employer you work for?

Evidence opportunity

2.2 Safe practices

Identify two different types of hazardous substances that are present in your work setting and demonstrate how you use safe practice for storing and using hazardous substances, and for disposing of hazardous substances and materials. Ask your assessor or manager to observe you doing so.

LO3 Be able to promote fire safety in the work setting

Getting started

Read the article about the Cheshunt care home fire that left two people dead and 33 people in need of rescue:

www.bbc.co.uk/news/uk-england-39540401

What were your immediate reactions and why?

AC 3.1 Describe practices that prevent fires from starting and spreading

Practices that prevent fires from starting

As a care worker, it is important that you know how to prevent fires from starting as well as the correct actions to take to prevent fires from spreading and causing even more danger and harm.

A fire can only start if it has all three of the following: oxygen (present in the air and can be given off by some chemicals), fuel (any item that can burn, i.e. a solid, liquid or gas) and heat (the cause of the fire such as an unattended cigarette, equipment that has overheated or a trailing electrical wire).

A fire will not start if precautions are taken and safe working practices are followed. These include:

- ensuring that all hazardous materials that may be flammable are stored securely, for example in a locked fireproof cupboard
- ensuring that all hazardous materials that are flammable are kept to a minimum, for example by using non-flammable hazardous materials instead
- ensuring that items that may cause fires are removed and controlled, for example by assessing the risks of individuals smoking and putting in control measures, reporting immediately all defects with electrical equipment
- ensuring that safe working practices are used, and there is regular testing of fire safety equipment such as smoke detectors that can alert you to any fires that may be starting. You will also need to assess any hazards and risks that activities such as cooking may pose.

Remember that it is good practice to remain vigilant. Be aware of electrical equipment that may cause a fire hazard, and ensure that people do not smoke inside the building or in an unsafe area. This will vary if you work in the individual's home, but it is good practice to ensure that you are aware of fire hazards.

The GOV.UK website (www.gov.uk) offers some guidance on fire safety in the workplace. They suggest a five step fire risk assessment:

1. Identify the fire hazards
2. Identify people at risk
3. Evaluate, remove or reduce the risks
4. Record your findings, prepare an emergency plan and provide training
5. Review and update the fire risk assessment regularly.

You can find out more about these at: www.gov.uk/workplace-fire-safety-your-responsibilities/fire-risk-assessments

Practices that prevent fires from spreading

If a fire does start in your work setting it is very important that you follow your work setting's procedures so that you do not put yourself, individuals or others in danger. You will also have received training from your employer in fire safety and have practised what to do in the event of a fire.

There are a number of practices that you can follow to prevent a fire from spreading and therefore minimise the danger, harm and damage that it can cause. For example, ensure that:

- all fitted smoke detectors, fire alarms, sprinklers and fire extinguishers are maintained and in good working order so that they will work quickly and effectively in the event of a fire starting. You can do this by testing them. You should report any defects you or others notice.
- smoke detectors and sprinklers are not obstructed with items that are piled up underneath them so that they work effectively in the event of a fire. You can do this by completing health and safety checks on a regular basis.
- windows and doors are kept closed to keep the fire contained.
- you know what to do when a fire starts and are able to keep the fire contained until help arrives, for example by using a fire extinguisher, but only if you have been trained to do so.

You can find out more information about these practices in your work setting's fire safety procedures.

> **Reflect on it**
>
> **3.1 Your role and responsibilities**
>
> Reflect on your role and responsibilities for preventing fires from starting and spreading. If you are unsure about any fire safety aspects, reflect on who and where you can go to for information and guidance.

> **Evidence opportunity**
>
> **3.1 Practices that prevent fires from starting and spreading**
>
> Discuss with your assessor the practices that you use in the care setting where you work that prevent fires from starting and spreading. Do you feel confident in following these practices? If not, what do you need to do? Perhaps you may need further fire safety training or to read through your work setting's fire safety procedures. Write an account to evidence your discussion. You may wish to do some further research before your discussion.

Your employer's responsibilities

Your employer has responsibilities with regards to fire safety. These include:

- appropriate fire safety guidance and training, which you must attend. You must also ensure you keep your knowledge about fire safety practices up to date
- fire safety procedures clearly displayed, and accessible for all those in the setting
- clear fire exit signs, and fire doors
- fire safety equipment, such as correct fire extinguishers, in the setting
- following legislation and regulation with regards to fire safety, including having a fire drill and confirming the actions to take in the event of a fire.

You should know not only what your personal responsibilities in an emergency are but also who else is responsible and what they are responsible for.

> **Research it**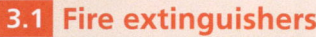
>
> **3.1 Fire extinguishers**
>
> It is important that you know that there are different types of fire extinguishers. These are labelled with instructions and will clearly say whether they contain water, foam or powder, for example, and they will also include instructions on how to use them. While you do not need to know everything about each type of fire extinguisher, it is important to know which ones are in your setting, understand how to use them and receive training in this.
>
> Go to the following website to read about some of the different types of extinguishers, what they are used for, the dangers around using them, how to use them and how they work:
>
> www.fireservice.co.uk/safety/fire-extinguishers
>
> This is not a substitute for training, but it will help you gain an understanding of the different fire extinguishers.

AC 3.2 Explain emergency procedures to be followed in the event of a fire in work settings

Your work setting's fire safety procedures will detail the emergency procedures you must follow in the event of a fire in the work setting. It is important that you read through and understand what these are so that you do not place yourself or anyone else in danger, as these will vary depending on the care setting where you work and your job role.

Most fire safety procedures will include the following points:

1. Raise the fire alarm. Do this as soon as possible. Delaying may allow the fire to spread which could result in fatalities.
2. Call the emergency services on 999 or tell someone else to do this immediately.
3. Make sure you ensure the safety of others and that they are moved away from any danger.

Your setting will have procedures in place dealing with different people, for example how to safely move people who are not mobile. This might include the use of wheelchairs, and how to move bed-bound individuals. Make sure you know about the evacuation procedures.

4. If you have received training, you can use the correct fire extinguisher to put out the fire. You must know where fire safety equipment is kept, to ensure that you can locate it quickly if you need to use it.
5. Go to the designated assembly point. Workplaces have fire drills to ensure that you know where this is and so you understand the procedure of what to do in the event of an actual fire. This is so that you can leave the building quickly in the event of a fire and support others to do the same.
6. Do not return to the building. You will be told when it is safe to do so. Returning to the building may place you in danger and you may not be able to get back out. Someone else would then have to risk their life to try and find you and bring you to a place of safety.
7. Reflect on your practice. You will need to consider what worked well, what didn't and why, and what you can do to improve. This is so that in the event of a fire occurring again you can ensure that you are practising to the best of your ability.

The 'dos and don'ts' table includes some of the key actions to take that apply to all care settings in the event of a fire.

> **Reflect on it**
>
> **3.2 Fire emergency procedures**
>
> Reflect on the importance of being familiar with the fire emergency procedures in place in the care setting where you work. How can this help you in promoting fire safety in the event of a fire? How can this reassure the individuals you provide care or support to?

	Dos and don'ts when there is a fire emergency
Do	Immediately alert others that there is a fire (check what to do in your work setting; it may vary from sounding the alarm to alerting a senior member of staff).
Do	Control and contain the fire (only if you have been trained and it is safe to do so).
Do	Contact the fire brigade (check what to do in your work setting. Some fire alarm systems automatically dial the fire brigade; sometimes only allocated members of staff can contact the fire brigade as they have been trained to do so). The fire brigade will require information from the contact person, such as their name, address and details about the fire, for example where it is, how far it has spread, the type of care setting it is and whether anyone is in danger.
Do	Assist with ensuring everyone is in a place of safety either inside or outside of the building. For example, visitors could be supported to leave the building by the nearest fire escape route, individuals who are unable to mobilise can remain in their rooms providing their doors and windows are closed until the fire brigade arrives.
Do	Try to remain calm and wait until the fire brigade informs you that it is safe to re-enter the building.
Do	Walk calmly when exiting. Assemble outside the building in line with your work setting's agreed ways of working.
Don't	Run, as this may cause others to panic and may lead to slips and falls.
Don't	Stop or re-enter the building for any personal items as this could place you in danger. Others may not know that you have returned and may therefore be unaware that you are in the building. You must assemble outside the building in line with your work setting's agreed ways of working.
Don't	Panic – remember if you stay calm this will be reassuring for others.

Research it

3.2 Your work setting's fire emergency procedures

Research your work setting's fire emergency procedures. Discuss with your manager the steps you are required to take in the event of a fire in the care setting where you work and the reasons why you should take these steps.

Evidence opportunity

3.2 Emergency procedures

Produce a poster explaining the emergency procedures you must follow and actions you must take and not take in the event of a fire in the work setting. Use diagrams and relevant images in your poster.

AC 3.3 Demonstrate measures that prevent fires from starting

Fire safety involves taking preventative action so that fires do not start. As well as the practices described in AC 3.1 that you can follow there are also other practical measures that prevent fires from starting.

It is important that you are aware of these because you will need to demonstrate for this AC that you can put these measures into practice. Some examples of these include:

- **smoke free areas:** restrictions on smoking may vary across different work settings but ensuring that, for example, smoking is only done off the premises, in a designated area, not at night or not in individuals' rooms can reduce the risk of a fire being caused.
- **waste collection:** the accumulation of waste such as paper and dust over time can lead to the build-up of flammable material that may ignite should a fire start. By keeping all areas clean and free from waste, the risk of a fire starting can be minimised.
- **maintenance of electrical appliances:** ensuring all electrical appliances are tested for their safety before they are used. In this way, they will be less likely to cause a fire.
- **sources of heat:** ensuring that portable heaters or electrical fires are not used where possible and that if they are used they are not placed next to, for example, clothes or paper that may ignite and lead to a fire starting.
- **supervision of work activities:** ensuring cleaning and maintenance of all areas are completed regularly and in line with the employer's agreed

ways of working. Ensuring high risk activities such as cooking, for example, are completed safely and are supervised when required so that they do not lead to any fires occurring.

Reflect on it

3.3 Your role in preventing fires

Think about the precautions you take as a lead adult care worker and support others to take to prevent fires from starting. How effective are your practices and those of others? What could you or others do to improve these?

6Cs

Care

You can show that care is at the very heart of what you do by ensuring that you take responsibility for ensuring fire evacuation routes are clear as part of your fire safety checks. Doing so will ensure the environment is kept as safe as possible not only for individuals but also for others who may need to evacuate the building in the event of a fire.

Evidence opportunity

3.3 Demonstrating measures that prevent fires from starting

Identify two team members who would benefit from additional guidance and information about fire safety. Demonstrate to them the measures that prevent fires from starting; give explanations while you demonstrate these measures. At the end of your demonstration ask both team members what their understanding is of the measures they can take to prevent fires from starting.

Make sure you ask your assessor or manager to observe you.

AC 3.4 Ensure evacuation routes are clear

In order to be able to safely exit a building where there is a fire, it is very important that your work setting's fire escape routes are kept clear at all times. If they are not kept clear, this may prevent you and others from evacuating the building, which places you and others in danger and/or may result in slips, trips and falls.

You will be observed for this AC ensuring that you keep evacuation routes clear at all times. This is not just something you demonstrate you can do as a one-off, but will form part of your fire safety checks.

Research it

3.4 Fire escape routes in your setting

Research where the fire escape routes are in the care setting where you work. How many fire escape routes are there? Why? You will find your manager a useful source of information.

You may work in a variety of different work settings, including individuals' homes and residential care homes and so it is very important that you are aware of the escape routes for each setting that you work in because they are the means for ensuring your safety and that of others.

Fire evacuation routes must be:

- clearly signposted, i.e. they must indicate where the fire escape route and exit is
- well lit so that they can be easily located at night or if there is smoke. Well-lit routes can also help individuals with vision loss to locate these
- fitted with fire safety equipment; for example there must be fireproof doors and fire extinguishers
- suitable as an escape route; for example they must not be too narrow and they should be fitted with handrails
- safe to use with no obstructions, such as boxes or mobility appliances, that can make it difficult to escape in an emergency. They must have floor coverings that are not worn or damaged. Wear and tear in floor coverings can cause trips and falls.

Reflect on it

3.4 How can you ensure fire escape routes are safe?

Reflect on how you and others can ensure that fire escape routes are safe to use. You could think about the checks that are carried out.

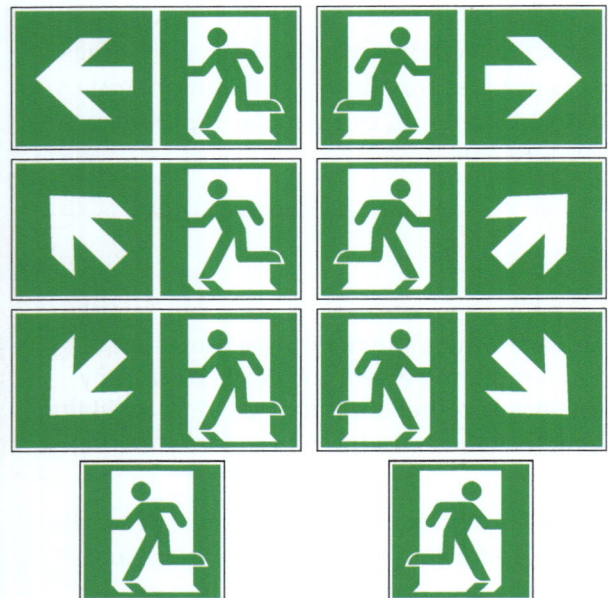

Figure 13.2 Do you know what these fire escape signs mean?

> ### Evidence opportunity
>
> **3.4 Importance of maintaining clear evacuation routes**
>
> Show your assessor or manager how you ensure the evacuation routes of where you work are kept clear.
>
> Produce a one-page information handout about the importance of maintaining clear fire evacuation routes at all times as well as the consequences of not doing so.

LO4 Be able to implement security measures in work settings

> ### Getting started
>
> Think about an occasion when you were visiting a building or premises and you were asked to confirm who you were. What were you asked about yourself?
>
> Think about an occasion when you requested information over the telephone in relation to yourself. For example, this may be in relation to blood test results or a doctor's appointment. How did the person on the other end of the telephone check that you were who you said you were? How did this make you feel?

AC 4.1 Explain the importance of ensuring that others are aware of own whereabouts

The importance of others being aware of your whereabouts

Ensuring that others are aware of your whereabouts is very important when working in care settings in the event of an emergency, such as a fire. Recap your previous learning around the emergency procedures to be followed in the event of a fire, including the reasons why it is important that the fire brigade is aware of everyone's whereabouts.

Ensuring others are aware of your whereabouts is also important in the event of your colleagues requiring your immediate assistance, for example in the case of an individual having a fall or becoming unwell.

It is also important that others are aware of your whereabouts so that they know you are safe. You may be working with individuals who have a history of violence or you may work with individuals in their homes, so there are risks that you may face.

How to make others aware

You can make others aware of your whereabouts by:

- signing in and out every time you enter and leave the premises
- letting your colleagues know if you are working after office hours
- informing a named person of your whereabouts if you are not working on the premises. You may need to inform your colleagues that you will be visiting an individual in their home or meeting with a professional in their office, for example. Make sure they know details of where you will be and what time you will return.

Accessing immediate help can only be done if others are aware of your whereabouts. Ensuring you comply with your work setting's lone working, staff welfare and health and safety policies and procedures is central to maintaining your own security and that of others.

Precautions to take when outside the setting

You will need to make sure that you have some training in how to protect yourself both in the setting and when working alone. This might include self-defence training in the event of a violent situation. The trainers or your manager will be able to support you with advice and ways to address situations where you feel threatened. You will also need to be aware of other precautions that you can take such as carrying a panic button or personal alarm so that you are able to call for help. There may also be a policy where lone workers are required to call or ring in, and there may even be trackers on mobile phones.

> **Research it**
>
> **4.1 Lone working**
>
> Research your work setting's procedures for lone working and personal safety while at work. Produce an information leaflet with your findings.

> **Reflect on it**
>
> **4.1 Consequences**
>
> Reflect on the consequences for you and others if you do not follow your work setting's procedures for maintaining your personal safety while carrying out your day-to-day work activities.

> **Evidence opportunity**
>
> **4.1 Informing others of your whereabouts**
>
> Make a list of the people you inform of your whereabouts during your day-to-day work activities. This could include people from your work setting as well as others you know outside your setting. Write an account of why you should make these people aware of your whereabouts. If you work in an individual's home, who do you inform of your whereabouts?
>
> What agreed ways of working underpin your practices? Where can you find these? Who could you go to if you require additional information about these?

AC 4.2 Use agreed procedures for checking the identity of anyone requesting access to premises and information

Promoting health and safety at work involves putting into practice **security measures**, such as checking the **identity** of all visitors. This is because care settings are environments where individuals who have care or support needs live. Due to their conditions or disabilities, they may be more susceptible to not realising the dangers of bogus visitors claiming to be, for example, contractors or adult care workers. Implementing security measures in care settings, therefore, is everyone's responsibility so we can ensure that all settings are kept safe for you, the individuals you support and others who you work with.

You will be observed for this AC following your setting's procedures or your employer's agreed ways of working for checking the identity of those who want access to the premises and to information.

Requesting access to premises

The agreed ways of working or the procedures to be followed for checking the identity of anyone requesting access to the premises where you work will vary depending on your work setting and job role. For example, you may be required to refer anyone requesting access to the premises to a senior member of staff or you may be required to check the person's identity yourself. Your work setting's procedures will provide you with guidance on what to do. Whatever the procedures, it is important that you safeguard individuals against unwanted visitors and intruders, and protect individuals' private property and information.

> **Key terms**
>
> **Identity** in the context of handling information means confirmation of who a person is, for example their name, who they work for and who they are visiting.

The following are some examples of good practice security measures that you can follow.

Before allowing a visitor access to the premises

- **Stop and think:** before you let the visitor enter into the premises, stop and think. Consider whether the visitor is known to you or anyone else, whether the visitor has got an agreed appointment with anyone, whether you can check this information with anyone, such as with your manager or the person they have an appointment with; if you do check this information with someone else, remember not to let the person enter the premises until you have done so, i.e. politely ask them to wait outside. It is good practice to be vigilant and question anyone that you do not recognise. For example, if you see someone in the setting that you have not seen before, go over to them and ask them if you can help them. If they say they are visiting someone, you could ask them who and why and escort them to where they need to go. Make sure that you stay with them. This is also covered in the section below. You may also need to check the individual's file to see if there are any reasons you cannot allow visitors. This might be for medical reasons, for example, or to safeguard the individual but you will need to be aware of the reasons.

- **Use security measures fitted to the premises:** these can include a spy hole, a door chain, or the intercom system; you could even look through the window to check the identity of the visitor. Your setting may have electronic entrance systems where identity passes are required for access, or a code is required to enter. You may need to use a key safe to enter into an individual's home. These measures are to help to ensure intruders do not enter the premises.

- **Check the person's proof of identity:** if the visitor gives you an identity card, check that the person looks like the person in the photo and their name matches who they say they are; you could even ring the organisation who they say they are from to further confirm their identity.

If you are unsure about the person's identity do not allow them to enter the premises until you have sought advice from your manager explaining what your concerns are. It may be necessary to call the police.

If the individual you support says they do not wish to receive the visitor, then you must deny the visitor access in an assertive but polite tone. Remember the principles of person-centred care that you have learned about. If the person is a family member and still requests access, you must remember that the individual you care for is your priority and you must respect their wishes. You could apologise and explain that if the individual changes their mind, you will give them a call.

After allowing a visitor access to the premises

Once you have confirmed a visitor's identity you can allow them to enter the premises. The following 'dos and dont's' table outlines important points to remember when dealing with visitors.

> **Research it**
>
> **4.2 Unwanted visitors**
>
> Research an occasion reported in the media where an individual with care or support needs was targeted by bogus callers. Share the news story with a colleague and discuss what happened and the impact it had. An example of such a news story is available below:
>
> www.bbc.co.uk/news/uk-scotland-south-scotland-34346274

Requesting access to information

The agreed ways of working or the procedures to be followed for checking the identity of anyone requesting access to information where you work will also vary depending on your work setting and job role. For example, you may be required to pass a request for information from an individual's relative on to the manager or you may respond to an email that has been sent by an individual's advocate in relation to their daily activities.

Under the Data Protection Act 2018 you have a responsibility to ensure that you keep safe and secure all personal information you come across about individuals. This may be in relation to their health, care needs or preferences. You will also need to obtain the individual's permission to do so; unless of course it is an emergency or the information is needed to provide care or support to an individual. Doing so will not only ensure that you respect individuals' rights to privacy but will also mean that individuals will learn that they can trust you and feel able to confide in you. You will find it useful to review your learning of the requirements of the Data Protection Act 2018 in Unit 305 Handling information in adult care settings/services.

Dos and don'ts for dealing with visitors	
Do	Ask them to sign in as a visitor with their full name, the company they are from, the date and purpose of their visit.
Do	Ask them to wear a visitor's badge so that others are aware of who they are.
Do	Explain to them that you have let the person they have come to visit know that they have arrived and that they are expecting them.
Don't	Allow the visitor access to the premises if they have not signed in.
Don't	Allow the visitor access to the premises if they are not wearing their visitor's badge. In some settings, name badges may not be a requirement as this may unsettle individuals but your workplace will have procedures in place with regards to name badges for security purposes. You should check what the policy and procedures are.
Don't	Allow the visitor to walk through the premises unescorted by you.

Research it

4.2 Data Protection Act 2018

Go to the following website: https://www.gov.uk/data-protection

Conduct some research into the Data Protection Act 2018. How does this affect your role when ensuring you uphold security measures and deal with information in ways that protect confidentiality?

6Cs

Commitment

This involves being dedicated to good practice and doing your very best to place the individual's needs first, ensuring that the way you work has their best interests at heart. This is important for the provision of person-centred care and for establishing good working relationships with individuals. You can show your commitment to following good practice by ensuring individuals understand why information is disclosed to others and what efforts you and others have made to keep it private and secure.

The following are some examples of good practice security measures that you can follow.

- **Check that the person requesting the information has a right to know it:** you will need to check with your manager whether you are able to disclose the information requested. If not, you will need to find out the reasons why so that these can be explained to the person requesting access.
- **Check that you have the individual's consent to provide information:** if you do have the individual's consent to provide information then you must always check the identity of the person and the purpose of their request. You may have to do this in person, over the telephone or in an email depending on the nature of the enquiry.

If you have to provide information to others without informing the individual, for example when a health emergency occurs, it is good practice to inform the individual afterwards that you did so and the reasons why. In this way you can show your commitment to upholding the individual's rights.

Reflect on it

4.2 Personal information

Reflect on how you would feel if you told a friend something personal about yourself in confidence and then found out that they had shared this personal information without your consent with the rest of their friends.

Evidence opportunity

4.2 Agreed ways of working for checking identity

You will be observed for AC 4.2. Demonstrate to your assessor how you check:

1. the identity of a contractor requesting access to the premises
2. the identity of a social worker requesting access to an individual's support plan.

This should be in line with your current job role and the agreed procedures to follow in the care setting where you work. Follow up your demonstration with a professional discussion with your assessor.

AC 4.3 Use measures to protect own security and the security of others in work settings

There are a number of measures to protect the security of care workers and others in the care setting. This can include identity checks that you learned about in AC 4.2, such as security passes for access to the setting, a policy of distributing visitor badges, and password and firewall systems to protect digital personal data. Here we discuss some of the measures you can put into place to protect your own security and the security of others in the work setting.

It is important that you know how to put these into practice to protect your own security and the security of others. You will be observed doing so for this AC.

- **Maintain everyday security of the premises:** this can include completing daily health and safety checks, such as checking rooms and communal areas, checking the doors close securely and that windows are not left open at night, checking visitor badges and ensuring that any security codes for entry to the premises or different rooms are changed regularly to keep them safe.
- **Reflect on your day-to-day practices and those of others:** this can include discussing with your colleagues what security checks have been carried out and reflecting on the security checks that require improvement and the benefits of doing so.
- **Follow your agreed ways of working for lone working:** this includes ensuring others know your whereabouts at all times and signing in and out of the premises.
- **Follow your agreed ways of working for security:** this includes ensuring visitors sign both when they arrive and leave the premises and keeping any passwords that you may have, such as on key pads on doors, confidential to protect the security of both the premises and all those on the premises.
- **Follow your agreed ways of working for ensuring the security of individuals' personal property and valuables:** this includes recording what items and valuables individuals have with them in the setting, and knowing what to do when things go missing in the setting.
- **Follow your agreed ways of working for security emergencies:** this includes immediately reporting all security emergencies that may arise, such as lost keys for a filing cabinet that contains individuals' personal records, or a broken window or faulty door latch.
- **Attend training:** this includes accessing training and information provided by your work setting about how to protect your security and the security of others at all times.

Research it

4.3 Daily checks

Research the daily health and safety checks that must be carried out with respect to security in your work setting. Your manager and your work setting's procedures are good sources of information.

Reflect on it

4.3 Lack of security

Reflect on an occasion you or someone you know experienced a lack of security. You can reflect on the impact this had, the reasons why it happened, whether it was addressed and, if so, how.

Lone working

There are procedures in place for all lone workers to ensure their safety is maintained at all times. Working safely as a lone worker involves always ensuring others know your whereabouts so that they can call for help on your behalf if they become aware that you may be in danger. For example, if you are supporting an individual to go out one evening, ensure you check the individual's risk assessment for anything you need to be aware of. For example, the individual's mental health may have deteriorated and you may need to check if it is still appropriate to support this individual to go out with you on your own. If you do go out with the individual, ensure others know what time you are going out, where you are going and how long you are likely to be. You will need to ensure that others can contact you and that you can contact others so you may need to take a mobile phone with you.

Evidence opportunity

4.3 Implementing security measures

You will be observed for AC 4.2. Demonstrate to your assessor how you used two security measures in your work setting to protect your own security and the security of others. Follow up your demonstration with a professional discussion with your assessor.

> **Case study**
>
> **4.2, 4.3 Implementing security measures at work**
>
> Enzo is a care worker in a nursing home for older adults who have a range of different conditions. During the very busy morning shift Enzo hears the front door bell ring. As it is usually the senior care workers' responsibility to answer the front door, he ignores it. Approximately five minutes later the person is still ringing the doorbell. Enzo goes to look for one of the senior care workers on duty; one is on her break and the other is in the middle of the medication round and cannot be disturbed.
>
> Enzo walks past the front door and the person standing on the doorstep looks a little familiar and waves excitedly at Enzo to let her in.
>
> **Discuss**
>
> 1 Do you think Enzo should let the person in? Why?
> 2 What would you expect Enzo to do in this situation if it occurred in your work setting? Ensure your response is in line with your work setting's agreed ways of working.
> 3 What would you say to Enzo? Why?

Legislation	
Relevant Act	**Key points**
Health and Safety at Work Act (HASAWA) 1974	The health and safety of everyone in a work setting must be protected – in a care setting this includes individuals, adult care workers and those who visit. It also established the key duties and responsibilities of all employers and employees in work settings.
Workplace (Health, Safety and Welfare) Regulations 1992	The working environment must be safe in relation to the building, its facilities and housekeeping and it must be healthy in relation to temperature, lighting and ventilation.
Manual Handling Operations Regulations 1992 (as amended 2002)	Risks associated with moving and handling activities must be eliminated or minimised by employers. It also requires employers to provide information, training and supervision about safe moving and handling.
Provision and Use of Work Equipment Regulations (PUWER) 1998	Work equipment used in work settings must be safe. It requires employees to receive training before using work equipment and requires work equipment to have visible warning signs.
Lifting Operations and Lifting Equipment Regulations (LOLER) 1998	Lifting equipment used in work settings must be safe. It requires lifting equipment to be maintained and used solely for the purpose it was intended for. It also requires that all lifting operations are planned, supervised and carried out in a safe manner.
Personal Protective Equipment at Work Regulations 1992	Personal protective equipment (PPE) to provide protection against infections must be provided free of charge by employers. It requires PPE to be maintained in good condition and requires training to be provided in the use of PPE.
Control of Substances Hazardous to Health (COSHH) 2002	Employers must have procedures in place for safe working with hazardous substances and provide information, training and supervision so that work activities can be carried out safely.
Electricity at Work Regulations 1989	Electricity and the electrical appliances that are used in work settings must be safe. It requires employers to provide training to employees in relation to carrying out safety checks on electrical equipment.
Regulatory Reform Order (Fire Safety) 2005	Fire risk assessments must be completed by the person responsible for the premises. It also requires the provision of fire equipment, fire escape routes and exits, as well as fire safety training.
Civil Contingencies Act 2004	Organisations such as emergency services, local authorities and health bodies must work together to plan and respond to local and national emergencies. It requires that risk assessments are undertaken and emergency plans are put in place.

313 Continuous development when working in an adult care worker role

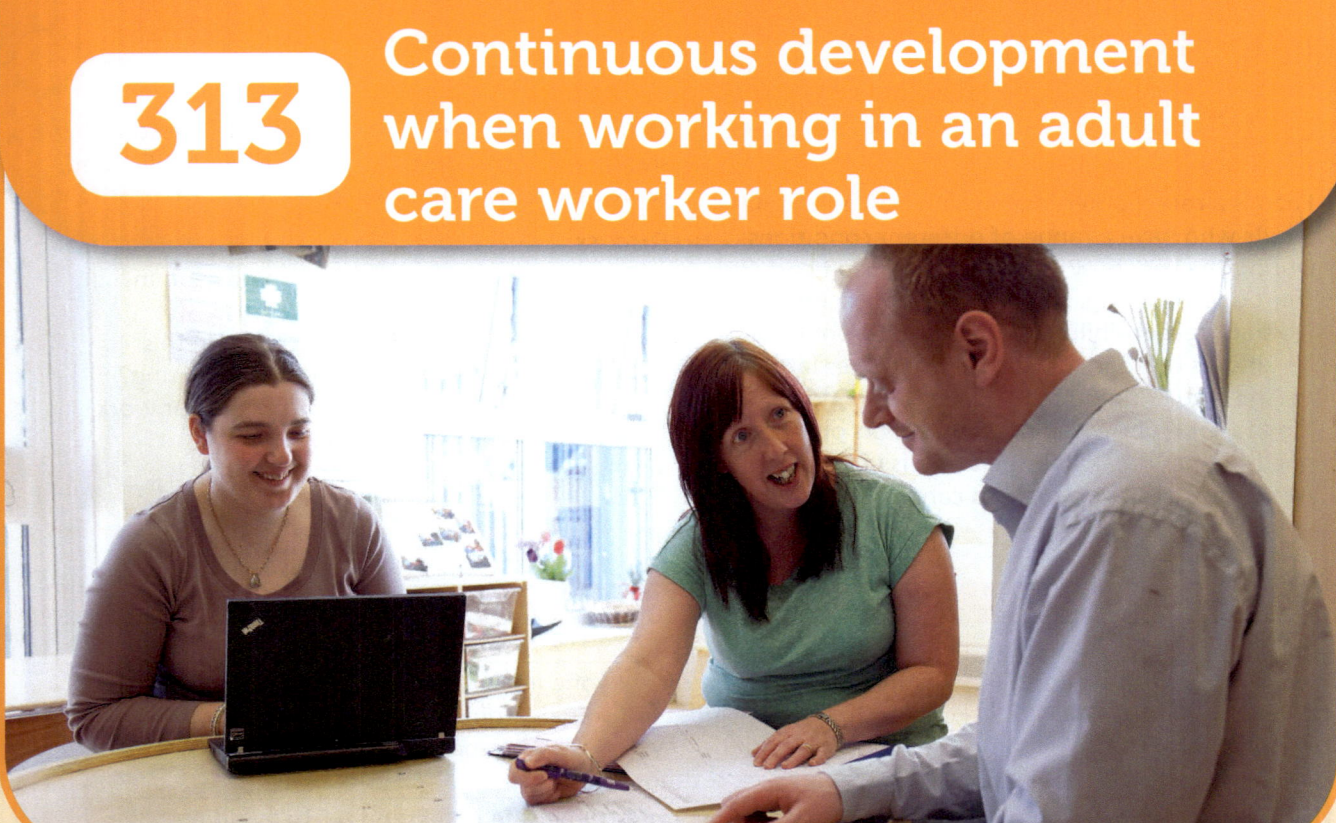

About this unit

Credit value: 3
Guided learning hours: 20

Promoting personal development is not just about developing your own knowledge, skills and practice at work; it involves being a role model for others and showing them why it is important and how it can lead to improved ways of working.

In this unit, you will have an opportunity to explore the duties and responsibilities of your role, the standards that form the basis of your work role and how as a Lead Adult Care Worker or Lead Personal Assistant you can work effectively with others. Being able to reflect on your practice is an essential part of your role and in this unit you will be able to find out how being an effective reflector can improve the quality of the service you and others provide, and ensure that your values, beliefs and experiences do not impact on your work negatively.

Of course, you are not expected to evaluate your work performance on your own so you will learn more about how to use feedback from others, as well as relevant standards to inform the effectiveness of your work practices. Recording your personal development is important and this unit will explore the sources of support available to you, how to work with others to review and prioritise your learning and development and how to agree a personal development plan (PDP) including evaluating learning activities, exploring how reflective practice has led to improved ways of working, understanding why continuing professional development (CPD) is important, and recording the progress you're making.

Learning outcomes

By the end of this unit you will:

LO1: Know what is required to be competent in own role

LO2: Be able to demonstrate commitment to own continuous development

LO3: Understand the value of reflective practice

LO4: Be able to use reflective practice to improve ways of working

LO5: Be able to develop leadership behaviours

LO1 Know what is required to be competent in own role

AC 1.1 Describe the duties and responsibilities of own work role

> **Getting started**
>
> All work roles in health and social care have specific duties and responsibilities. If you read through your job description or profile you will see that it describes the specific tasks (i.e. your work duties) that you are required to complete as part of your job role as well as how you must carry these tasks out (i.e. your work responsibilities). What are the main duties and responsibilities outlined here?

As you enter the adult care profession (or a new role within it) you will be informed of the duties and responsibilities that you will be required to do in your role. All roles in a care setting, including the one you are in, will have a set of knowledge, skills and behaviours that are required and expected from workers. These are essential for:

- ensuring that high quality care and support is provided to individuals by encouraging all Lead Adult Care Workers and Lead Personal Assistants to work in consistent ways
- making clear what is expected from Lead Adult Care Workers and Lead Personal Assistants by ensuring they understand what their day-to-day work tasks involve
- ensuring that all Lead Adult Care Workers and Lead Personal Assistants show the correct attitudes, values and behaviours (such as dignity and respect) towards the individuals they care for.

Table 14.1 provides you with some additional information about the range of duties and responsibilities that are expected of different lead adult care work roles in the health and social care sector.

> **Reflect on it**
>
> **1.1 Your setting's values**
>
> Reflect on your work role and how it fits into the values of the profession more generally. How do the duties and responsibilities of your role relate to those that are expected in the profession more widely?

Table 14.1 Examples of duties and responsibilities in adult care roles

Lead work role	Examples of duties and responsibilities
Lead Personal Assistant (e.g. working with an individual with a sensory impairment living at home)	• Lead the day-to-day work of a small team of Personal Assistants • Provide support and training to the team when required • Support the individual to take part in activities of their choice • Promote the individual's personal choices and rights • Communicate effectively with the individual and their advocate over their care and support needs • Administer medication to the individual safely • Communicate effectively with the individual, their family and friends • Maintain the health, safety and wellbeing of the individual and others at all times • Maintain all information and recording systems relating to the work role • Take responsibility for your own continuous professional development.
Senior Support Worker (e.g. working with adults with mental health needs)	• Co-ordinate and support the day-to-day running of the service by assisting the Service Manager • Supervise and manage the team of support workers • Be a role model to new and less experienced support workers • Provide training to the team of support workers • Support staff by being their first point of contact for information and advice • Safeguard individuals and promote their health and wellbeing • Support individuals to manage all aspects of their daily lives

Table 14.1 Examples of duties and responsibilities in adult care roles *continued*

Lead work role	Examples of duties and responsibilities
	• Promote individuals' rights to live independently • Communicate effectively, verbally and in writing with individuals, their families, and others involved in their lives • Provide a safe and supportive environment for individuals and staff to work together.

6Cs

Competence

Applying the knowledge and skills you have gained in your role is central to providing high quality care and support. As mentioned above, you can show that you are competent in your role by effectively carrying out the duties and responsibilities that you are assigned. This includes being aware of and complying with the policies and procedures in your setting and ensuring you follow best practice to provide the best support you can for individuals and be an effective leader and role model to other members of staff in your team.

Constantly thinking how competent you are in your role and thinking of ways to improve it will also enable you to become a better Lead Adult Care Worker or Lead Personal Assistant as you will be continually trying to progress and achieve high standards of practice and care for individuals.

There are also other legal requirements that inform your duties and responsibilities, and these are explored in AC 1.3.

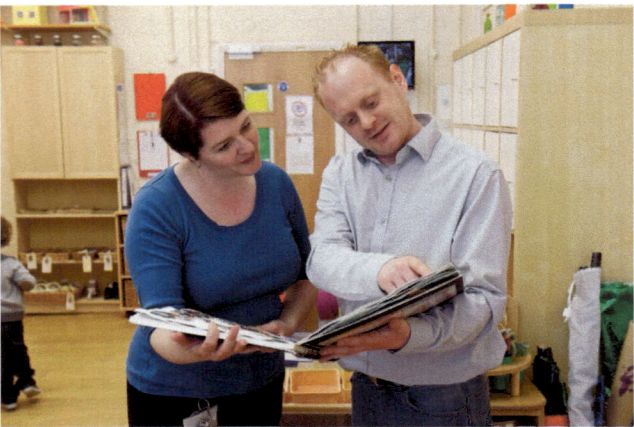

Figure 14.1 How do you support colleagues in your role? What leadership qualities do you have?

Evidence opportunity

1.1 Your duties and responsibilities

Discuss with two colleagues, one new and one experienced, the duties and responsibilities that you are expected to follow in your work role. Describe what these include and how they are different to those of your colleagues. You could also discuss with them what specific skills and knowledge you think are necessary to carry out your duties and responsibilities effectively. Provide a written account detailing your description and discussion.

How you carry out your responsibilities will depend largely on you, your personality, your approach to your work and your passion and interest in carrying out your job to the best of your ability. Your ability to carry out your role well is referred to as competence. If you are competent then you show that you have the correct and expected knowledge, skills, attitudes, values and behaviours and can apply these when you are carrying out your job. If you are not competent then you will not be able to carry out your job role well or effectively and you will not therefore be able to provide high quality care and support. Also remember that there will be other care roles, such as Senior Care Workers, Outreach Development Workers, Care Supervisors, and Supervising Care Workers, and it would be useful for you to find out about the duties and responsibilities of all of these.

AC 1.2 State skills and behaviours required to carry out own work role

As you will have learned in AC 1.1, you will be expected to have a set of skills and behaviours to be able to carry out your role competently and provide quality care. This means that when you carry out your work role you will be able to show that you have the correct set of skills and behaviours and can apply these through your work practices. If you do not have the required skills and behaviours then you will not be able to provide quality care because you will not be able to carry out your work role effectively.

Skills

Skills refer to the expertise you have learned to be able to carry out the tasks required of you in your job role competently. Below are some examples of the skills required of all those working in an adult care worker role when providing person-centred care and support:

1 Good communication skills – this involves being able to communicate clearly with individuals who have different needs, i.e. due to a disability or a condition such as dementia, and others such as individuals' families, colleagues and professionals from other services. You will find it useful to refer to Unit 304 Effective communication in adult care settings/services for additional information about good communication skills.

2 Good observational skills – this involves being willing to take the time to observe individuals and respond to what you are seeing or what they are telling you so that you can recognise early if there are any changes in an individual's physical or mental health or wellbeing, i.e. indicators of being harmed, illness.

3 Good compassion skills – this involves being patient, respectful, supportive, understanding, empathetic and sensitive when providing person-centred care and support to individuals, i.e. when supporting individuals to manage continence, pain or difficult situations such as bereavement.

4 Good organisational skills – this involves having the ability to plan and organise a range of different tasks so that you can ensure that the day-to-day tasks involved in providing person-centred care and support to individuals are achieved, i.e. shopping, completing household tasks, attending appointments.

5 Good flexibility skills – this involves being willing to think on your feet and change any planned activities when unexpected or difficult situations happen, i.e. medical emergencies, an individual becoming distressed.

6 Good continuous development skills – this involves being willing and committed to continuously improve and update knowledge and skills gained to be able to provide quality care.

> **Research it**
>
> **1.2 Your skills**
>
> Research the skills expected for your job role. You will find it useful to refer to your job description and employer's agreed ways of working.
>
> Produce a poster of the key skills expected. Reflect on how they compare to the skills above.

Behaviours

Behaviours refer to the ways in which you act, including towards others such as individuals and their families, colleagues and professionals from other services.

These are the 6 behaviours, also referred to as the 6 C's, that are expected of all those working in an adult care worker role:

1 Care – this means caring consistently and enough about individuals to make a positive difference to their lives.
2 Compassion – this means delivering care and support with kindness, consideration, dignity, empathy and respect.
3 Courage – this means doing the right thing for people and speaking up if the individual you support is at risk.
4 Communication – this means using good communication which is central to successful caring relationships and effective team working.
5 Competence – this means applying knowledge and skills to provide high quality care and support.
6 Commitment – this means improving the experience of people who need care and support to ensure it is person-centred.

You will learn more about how the 6 Cs can be applied in your work role throughout each of the units in this book.

> **Reflect on it**
>
> **1.2 Your behaviours**
>
> Reflect on the behaviours expected from you in your job role. Why are these important?

> **Evidence opportunity**
>
> **1.2 Skills and behaviours at work**
>
> Discuss with your manager the skills and behaviours that you require in your job role when providing person-centred care and support.

> **Key term**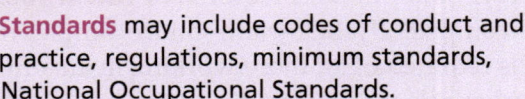
>
> **Standards** may include codes of conduct and practice, regulations, minimum standards, National Occupational Standards.

AC 1.3 Describe expectations of own work role as expressed in relevant standards

What standards are in place for Lead Adult Care Workers and Lead Personal Assistants?

The way you carry out your duties and responsibilities in the care setting where you work is guided by a set of **standards** that establish the knowledge, skills and values that will help you carry out your duties and responsibilities to a high standard. Below are some examples of the different sets of standards that are in place for those who work in the health and social care sector. It is important to get to know these so that you understand the types of things that you need to do in order to follow best practice and provide high quality care, as well as support others to do the same.

Codes of practice

- Codes of practice are agreed ways of working for professions such as Lead Adult Care Workers and Lead Personal Assistants and other organisations that provide services such as care and support. Codes of practice reflect best practice and although they are not a legal requirement, it is recommended that they are followed.
- They are not meant to replace an organisation's or employer's policies and procedures but rather to be used alongside them, such as those in relation to data protection, safeguarding, health and safety.
- Codes of practice set out the care standards expected of Lead Adult Care Workers and Lead Personal Assistants as well as the standards that should be maintained to deliver high quality care and support. Figure 14.2 is an example of a Code of Practice for a Lead Personal Assistant.

Code of Practice – Lead Personal Assistant

Protect the rights and promote the interests of individuals and their carers
- Treat each person as an individual
- Treat each person fairly
- Respect the rights of the individual, for example to dignity, privacy, choice
- Promote the views, wishes and preferences of the individual

Establish and maintain the trust and confidence of individuals and their carers
- Be open, honest and fair
- Be trustworthy
- Be reliable and honour work commitments agreed to
- Communicate in a clear and open way

Promote the independence of individuals while protecting them as far as possible from danger or harm
- Promote the independence of individuals and support them to understand their rights
- Report all abusive and discriminatory behaviour as well as unsafe practices
- Follow safe working practices and support others to do the same
- Support individuals with positive risk taking
- Do not place at risk the health, safety and wellbeing of yourself, individuals, their carers and others

Working practices and accountability for the quality of work
- Ensure that you only carry out tasks that you are competent to do and can carry out safely
- Treat individuals, their carers and others you support and work alongside with respect
- Respect the individual's home and possessions
- Do not smoke when in the individual's home
- Do not harm, abuse, neglect or exploit individuals, their carers or others you work with
- Maintain and respect the privacy and confidentiality of the individual and their carers at all times

Figure 14.2 Example of a Code of Practice

> **Reflect on it**
>
> **1.3 Standards expected of you**
>
> Reflect on the standards expected from Lead Personal Assistants as set out in the Code of Practice in Figure 14.2. How do these compare to the standards expected from you as a Lead Adult Care Worker? What underlying values and principles are being promoted? Why are these important?

In 2013, Skills for Care and Skills for Health developed a Code of Conduct for Healthcare Support Workers and Adult Social Care Workers in England. It established the standards of conduct, behaviours and attitudes that can be expected from all care workers and support workers, including lead practitioners. For example, it states that healthcare support workers and adult social care workers must:

- be accountable by making sure they can answer for their actions or omissions (oversights), for example by being honest about when things have not gone well, and mistakes have been made
- promote and uphold the privacy, dignity, rights, health and wellbeing of the individuals who use health and care services and their carers at all times, for example by supporting individuals' and carers' rights when meeting with them
- work together with their colleagues to ensure the provision and delivery of high quality, safe and compassionate healthcare, care and support, for example by showing your kindness and respect when supporting individuals' preferences
- communicate in an open and effective way to promote the health, safety and wellbeing of the individuals who use health and care services and their carers, for example by involving individuals and their carers when planning their care and support.

Source: *Skills for Care and Skills for Health (2013) 'Code of Conduct for Healthcare Support Workers and Adult Social Care Workers in England'*

Regulations

Rules and regulations that are set in law influence the way that Lead Adult Care Workers and Lead Personal Assistants can carry out different tasks in the care setting where they work. The Care Quality Commission (CQC) is the independent regulator of health and adult social care provision in England.

The CQC checks that the care and support services provided are safe, effective, caring, responsive to people's needs and well led, and documents its findings in a report that is made available for the public to see and read. The CQC was established under the Health and Social Care Act 2008 (Regulated Activities) Regulations 2014 and includes a set of regulations that influence the day-to-day practice of all care workers including Lead Adult Care Workers and Lead Personal Assistants.

Table 14.2 provides additional information about a couple of relevant regulations that influence the expectations of adult care work roles. You will learn more about these regulations and how they influence the work practices of Lead Adult Care Workers and Lead Personal Assistants in Unit 310 Promoting health and safety in adult care settings/services

Table 14.2 Regulations and how they influence expectations about adult care work roles

Regulation	How it influences expectations about adult care work roles
The Control of Substances Hazardous to Health Regulations 2002	Lead workers must ensure the safety of their own and others' work practices in relation to handling substances such as cleaning substances that may be dangerous to their health. For example, they require Lead Adult Care Workers to monitor that others wear protective equipment such as aprons and gloves when using cleaning substances, and lead by example by ensuring cleaning substances are locked away securely after use to prevent them being used by individuals who may not understand how to use them safely.
The Management of Health and Safety at Work Regulations 1999	Lead Workers must lead by example and ensure, for example, that they take reasonable care of their own health and safety and that of others such as individuals and visitors and report any health and safety concerns they have.

The Health and Social Care Act 2008 (Regulated Activities) Regulations 2014 is also a very important piece of legislation to keep in mind and you should look into the various regulations for this. For example, Regulation 9: Person-centred care says that providers of care must work with the individual and support them to understand and make informed choices and decisions about their care and support. Providers must also ensure that they take into account the individual's capacity and ability to consent.

Minimum standards

The minimum standards refer to the knowledge and skills that are required by all those who work in the health and social care sector. As regulator for the sector, the CQC sets the minimum standards that all those who access adult care services can expect and below which the the level of care provided must never fall.

Note that not all services are regulated by the CQC, for instance friends of the individual's family or one of their neighbours might provide informal care to an individual. However, the CQC

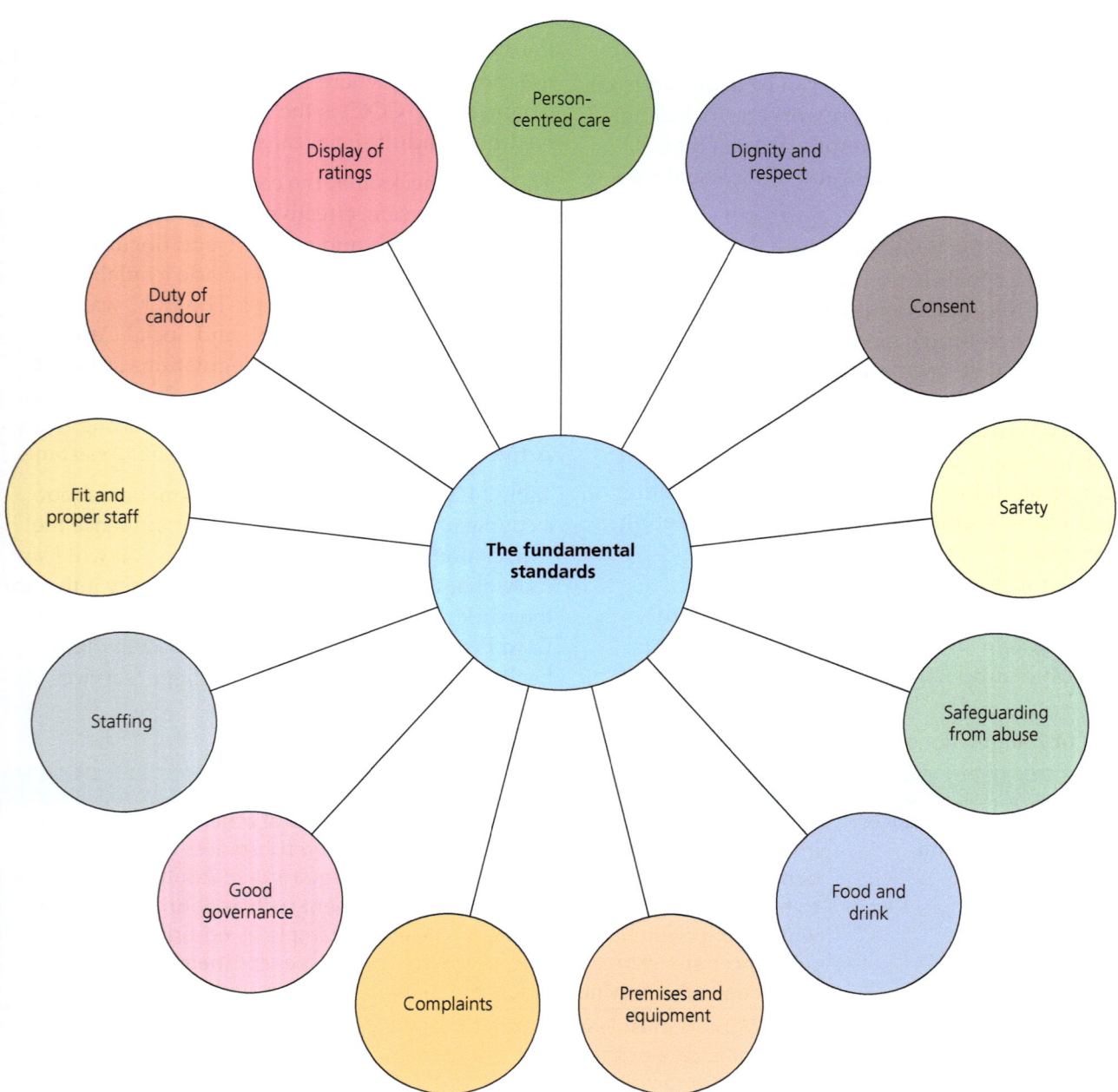

Figure 14.3 CQC's fundamental standards

> **Research it**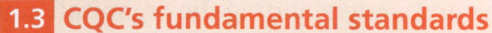
>
> **1.3 CQC's fundamental standards**
>
> Research three of the CQC's fundamental standards; you will find the information contained within the regulation table (Table 14.2) useful as well as the CQC's website that contains more information about the fundamental standards.
>
> For each standard consider the following:
>
> - How do you meet the standard in your day-to-day work activities?
> - Why is this standard relevant to your job role?
> - How do you support others to meet the standard in their day-to-day work activities?
> - Why is this important?
>
> Discuss your findings with your employer.

requirements are still good practice in such cases and should be followed.

All adult social care workers and healthcare support workers in England are also expected to meet the standards set out in the Code of Conduct, published by Skills for Care and Skills for Health. The Code of Conduct outlines the behaviours and attitudes that people who access care and support should expect and how workers should behave in their work roles. They cover the following areas:

1. Being accountable for your own actions
2. Promoting and upholding the rights and wellbeing of individuals and their carers
3. Working together with your colleagues
4. Communicating effectively
5. Respecting individuals' rights to confidentiality
6. Being committed to continuous professional development
7. Promoting and upholding equality, diversity and inclusion

More information on the Code of Conduct is available from here:

www.skillsforcare.org.uk/resources/documents/Developing-your-workforce/Care-topics/Core-Skills/What-are-core-skills-in-social-care.pdf

It is important that you are aware of these minimum standards because in your job role as a Lead you may be supporting and monitoring the practices of adult care workers. For example, you may be supporting adult care workers with their personal development by helping them to identify their learning needs and development areas, or to work in ways that have been agreed by your employer and that reflect current and best practice, such as when providing support to an individual with an activity or communicating with an individual's family member in relation to an individual's care.

Knowing the minimum standards is also important because adult care workers may be reporting to you and seeking information and advice from you on a variety of different aspects of care in relation to their job roles, for example how to adapt the communication methods they use with an individual to ensure that they meet the individual's needs, or what to do if they suspect an individual is being harmed or abused. You may then decide that you need to continue to monitor the adult care worker's practice or recommend that they attend further training to ensure that they meet the minimum standards while carrying out their day-to-day work activities.

It will also be important to know about these minimum standards if, as part of your job role, you also carry out **formal supervision** with adult care workers or complete their induction programmes with them so that you can accurately assess their knowledge and competence in relation to these standards.

> **Key terms**
>
> **Formal supervision** means having regular meetings with your manager, senior or employer to discuss any issues relevant to your job role and receive feedback on what has been going well and what improvements you need to make.

National Occupational Standards

The Health and Social Care National Occupational Standards (NOS) are jointly owned by Skills for Care and Development and Skills for Health. They ensure that all those who work in the adult care sector provide safe, effective and high-quality care and support and that best practice is followed at all times.

The Health and Social Care National Occupational Standards describe:

- the required knowledge, skills and values for health and social care workers in the UK and best practice in different areas of work
- the basis of training and qualifications. For example, the Level 3 Diploma in Adult Care which you are studying is a qualification that is based on the National Occupational Standards and describes the knowledge and skills required of Lead Adult Care Workers and Lead Personal Assistants.
- the standards that every worker in every role in the health and adult social care sector must meet.

For example, the role of a Senior Care Assistant may include developing and reviewing care plans with individuals, leading and supporting other care assistants to comply with the organisation's policies and procedures as well as preventing unsafe practices in the setting, promoting fire safety and supporting others to do the same.

In your role as a Lead you may also be expected to manage your own professional development as well as contribute to the professional development of others. There is a NOS titled 'Manage and develop yourself and your workforce within care services' that sets out the knowledge requirements and competence expected in relation to professional development. This includes:

- reflecting on your work practices and seeking feedback from others such as the individuals you work with and your colleagues, so that you can identify your strengths and areas for development
- keeping your knowledge and skills up to date, for example by reading, undertaking research, participating in training and supervision so that you can practise safely and effectively
- reviewing the work performance of those you supervise to ensure their compliance with relevant standards and codes of practice
- maintaining confidentiality when reviewing the work performance of others to ensure a positive and supportive work and learning environment
- knowing and understanding the legal and organisational requirements in relation to managing and developing yourself and others, such as those on equality, diversity, discrimination, safeguarding, rights, confidentiality and sharing of information
- knowing and understanding the organisational requirements for recording and reporting in relation to your own and others' development, for example by following the security requirements in place for accessing and storing paper-based and electronic records and reports, ensuring that records and reports are written using non-discriminatory language.

Source: *SCDLMCSA1 Manage and develop yourself and your workforce within care services, National Occupational Standards, Skills for Care and Development and Skills for Health*

Research it

1.3 Care Certificate

This is a set of 15 standards commonly used alongside the Code of Conduct for Healthcare Support Workers and Adult Social Care Workers.

It established the standards that health and social care workers are expected to follow in their day-to-day work to be able to provide high-quality care and support.

Workers are introduced to these standards as soon as they begin work as part of the introduction to their role and the care setting where they work. It would be useful for you to research the Care Certificate's 15 standards.

Evidence opportunity

1.3 Expectations about your role as expressed in standards

Discuss with your assessor the standards that are relevant to your job role. For each one explain how it relates to what is expected of you in your current job role by your employer, your colleagues and yourself. Include in your discussion why these expectations about your job role are important and how they impact on the quality of the care and support you provide and the views of others in relation to how you carry out your work role. Provide a written account.

AC 1.4 Explain how continuing professional development supports the provision of quality care

Continuing professional development (CPD) means looking at the skills and what you are learning in your role, making sure that you are keeping a record of what training and learning you have undertaken, for example by keeping records of any certificates you have received for courses you have undertaken, and putting together a CPD folder that includes these. You can also include other evidence such as reflections and witness statements from those who have observed your practices.

CPD also involves continually looking at opportunities and ways to further your development by outlining any new training that you need or other ways to develop, through mentoring sessions for example. As a result, you will have a clear idea of how you are progressing, your goals and where you are headed long-term in terms of your career. If you do not do this, then you may not realise that you are using work practices that are out of date, your skills and knowledge will not develop further as a result and you will not be able to provide individuals with up-to-date, good quality care.

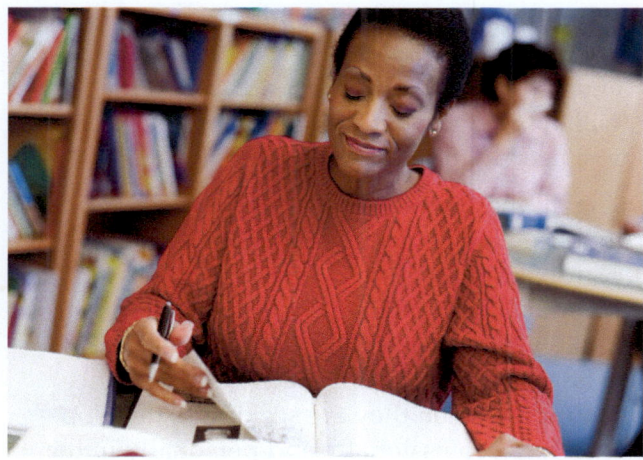

Figure 14.4 Is your CPD up-to-date?

Research it

1.4 Benefits of CPD

Research the benefits of CPD in the adult care sector. You could use your work setting, and organisations such as Skills for Care and CQC as sources of information. Discuss your findings with a colleague.

Maintaining, reviewing and updating your professional development throughout your career is important because doing so will support the provision of quality care by:

- **improving your knowledge and understanding:** your knowledge of specific areas of work will increase because you will have clearly outlined the areas you want to increase your knowledge and understanding in.
- **improving your skills:** your skills will develop because you will have clearly outlined these and identified ways to improve and gain new skills, for example through training. This is not just professional skills and qualities such as being an effective communicator but also personal qualities of **compassion** and empathy that are also required in your role.
- **improving your work practice:** constantly thinking about your practice, how you are progressing and ways to improve will mean your practice is more likely to meet the required standards such as those that we discussed in AC 1.3.
- **helping you apply new working approaches:** as you think about your practice, you may identify new ways of working; you will gain an understanding of new and effective working approaches and how to ensure that these will also impact on individuals in a positive way.
- **helping you adapt your practice:** as you develop you will learn about best practice and how to apply it, including using different skills to change the way you practise to ensure it remains up to date.
- **helping you develop in your job role:** you will increase in confidence when applying the knowledge and skills you have learned; this may lead you to explore different job roles and positions, for example the role of a supervisor.

- **providing you with an opportunity to reflect:** your self-awareness of your knowledge, skills, and behaviours will increase, meaning that you will know what you are doing well and what you need to improve to develop further.

Doing all the above will mean that you will be a good role model for members in your team. If your team see you striving to improve your work practices and being committed to doing so, it is likely that they will do the same. They will also be more likely to approach you for advice and support when they are seeking to develop themselves professionally and personally in the roles that they have been employed to carry out. So, your CPD has an impact on others' CPD – your development will help others to develop and support the provision of quality care.

6Cs

Compassion

Being able to deliver support to individuals and team members with compassion involves doing so with kindness, consideration, dignity and respect. However, it is important not to just be compassionate when working with individuals, but to be compassionate in your relationships with families and your colleagues, even as you offer advice or point out a weakness. For example, you could mention to a colleague that they carried out a task well but also made a mistake and make suggestions on how to improve it, including CPD opportunities they could access and the reasons why. This means that you are thinking about how they may receive the feedback and offer positive as well as negative feedback. Of course, you may not always be able to offer positive feedback, but it is important to be clear about your reasons so that they understand why they are being criticised. This is also showing compassion in your interactions while highlighting the importance of CPD.

Reflect on it

1.4 Your professional development

Reflect on your effectiveness at maintaining and updating your professional development. Are you a good role model? How could you improve?

Evidence opportunity

1.4 Why CPD is important

Read through Case study 1.4 and answer the questions that follow. Use the Case study as the basis for exploring the importance of continuing professional development for supporting the provision of quality care. Explain why continuing professional development is important. What are the consequences of not maintaining your CPD? Provide a written account.

Case study

1.4 The importance of CPD

Miriam is an experienced Lead Personal Assistant and has been asked by her employer to think about how she can further develop her skills in her job role as the last time she attended a training activity was about three months ago.

Miriam is not very happy about this as she feels that her employer is questioning her skills and knowledge believes that she does CPD activities all the time, a mixture of formal and informal ones, and therefore does not need to evidence these or reflect on these anymore.

Discuss:
1. Do you agree with Miriam? Why?
2. What should Miriam do? Why?
3. What can Miriam's employer do to support Miriam?

AC 1.5 Identify sources of support when planning own continuous development needs

There are many sources of support that you can access both within and outside of the setting where you work. It is important that you know about these, their purpose and how to access them as they will be essential for helping you to plan and review your own development. Table 14.3 discusses the main sources of support within the organisation.

Table 14.3 Formal and informal sources of support within the organisation

Formal and informal sources of support within the organisation	Importance for planning and reviewing your development
Supervision and appraisals	• Your manager or employer will meet with you to assess your performance at work. This process is referred to as formal supervision and is there to support you with planning and monitoring your personal development. For example, in the care setting where you work you may have regular performance reviews where you discuss and evaluate your performance at work with your manager; sometimes these may take the form of a meeting instead (for example, if you are a Lead Personal Assistant). • Supervision means you have regular meetings with your manager or employer. This is important for planning and reviewing your development because you will have an opportunity to discuss any issues and receive feedback on what has been going well, and what improvements you need to make. Because they may happen only every few weeks it is a good idea that you prepare before these meetings by, for example, reflecting on and writing down the things that you want to discuss beforehand. This is a good opportunity to discuss specific situations that have happened, staff and individuals you are working with. You can also use these opportunities to demonstrate how well you are doing by noting down all the ways in which you have shown good practice and reflected on your work. You can also discuss career progression and whether you have identified any sources of support and training courses you would like to undertake to inform your development. • Your manager may also arrange some regular formal support meetings for you and your colleagues to discuss any issues you are experiencing in your professional environment such as in relation to new ways of working, individuals' conditions or changes to the service. They may even organise **mentoring** sessions where you will be able to speak with more experienced colleagues and get advice on the issues you are facing at work as well as on career development. • Appraisals are another source of formal support and involve your employer (not necessarily your manager) assessing your performance in your job role with you over a much longer period, for example one year. This provides you with a good overview of your performance as a whole as well as the opportunity to discuss and reflect on your work performance by identifying your strengths; areas for development; what improvements you need to make and how you can progress in your role with training and development opportunities.
Colleagues	• Your colleagues can be the source of both formal and informal support. They can share best practice with you and provide you with their honest views about your strengths and work practices which can be very useful for informing your development. They can also be the people you turn to when you need advice or guidance about your day-to-day work activities. This might be through the formal meetings discussed above, a more informal catch-up at lunch or coffee break, or even some advice or words of encouragement when you are doing your job.
Individuals	• Individuals can be a useful source of support as they will very often show you how your work practices have impacted on them. They can also provide you with their views about the care and support they have received. Individuals are very useful in terms of your development because they can provide you with insight and increase your self-awareness about the impact your practice is having.

Table 14.3 Formal and informal sources of support within the organisation *continued*

Formal and informal sources of support within the organisation	Importance for planning and reviewing your development
Training	• Training (both formal and informal) is an important way to build new skills, understanding and improve your current practice. • You may receive training from your manager in, for example, how to complete supervisions with staff or this may come from colleagues. • It may be that your manager has organised some formal training inside the care setting, where a professional trainer visits you in the setting in relation to changes to health and safety practices at work, for example. • Training can be 'on-the-job' where you learn new skills as an ongoing process as you do your job, for example how to handle medications safely, although you may have training days dedicated to this. • There may be online courses that you can do, for example a course on promoting equality and diversity at work. Although these may be more theoretical, they can still give you an idea of how to apply that theory to your work practices. • To get the most out of training, ensure that you understand what skills you will learn and ask your manager or employer any questions you may have before you attend. It is also worth making notes during the training and keeping any material that you are given for future reference. Telling colleagues about the training once you have completed it can help reinforce what you have learned. For example, the trainer may ask you to complete an activity beforehand and ask for feedback. It is important that you complete all the activities set, ask questions and take part in the presentations or extra activities the trainer provides. This will ensure that you get the most out of the course and you can apply any feedback offered during your training to your work practices. Also ensure that you give the trainer honest feedback on the course, so that they can improve the experience for those who receive the training next.
Assessor	• Your assessor can support you with further development and verification of your knowledge, skills and behaviours in your current job role. They can provide you with access to useful information about best practice and work closely with you so that you are able to provide evidence of your competence at work. This will involve observing your work practices and speaking to others such as your manager, employer and/or colleagues who you work with.
Standards	• The standards in the care setting where you work can be useful sources of information about the level and quality of work practice you will need to provide as evidence in order to be considered as a competent Lead Adult Care Worker or Lead Personal Assistant. As you have read, these can also be used as the basis for when you are reflecting on your work activities. See AC 3.1 for more information.
Agreed ways of working	• The agreed ways of working in the care setting where you work can be a useful source of information and guidance for ensuring that you carry out your duties and responsibilities in accordance with your job description, legislation and the standards that the care setting where you work expects from you.

Table 14.3 Formal and informal sources of support outside the organisation

Formal and informal sources of support outside the organisation	Importance for planning and reviewing your development
Trainers	As discussed, training plays a key role in planning and reviewing your development. Training can be both in the setting and outside the setting. It may mean that you go to a training provider outside of the setting. They can share their knowledge and skills in specific areas of work such as dementia care, planning activities or completing health and safety risk assessments.
Your family and friends	You must not forget the support you receive from your family and friends, for example, financial support when you are studying or help with other personal responsibilities when working long shifts. However, you must not discuss work related issues with your family and friends, especially issues that are confidential to those you work with and support.
Online forums	These provide support and suggestions for how to overcome difficulties you may be experiencing. They are also places where people can share best practice and useful resources such as books and websites they have come across to help further develop their work practices (remember, you must check that these are reliable sources and think about where the advice is coming from).
E-learning	Short courses and study delivered online can be a good way of further developing your knowledge around key aspects of your work practices.

Key term

Mentor refers to a person in your work setting who has more experience than you and can provide you with guidance and advice in relation to your job role and responsibilities. This person is there to offer advice more informally than your manager or employer.

If you support an individual in their own home, you can access support directly from the individual, the local authority and by attending training.

Support for your personal development can also come from people and organisations outside of the care setting where you work and can even be online. Table 14.3 lists some of these sources.

It is difficult to plan and review your development on your own. You may need support from this wide range of sources in relation to a specific area of your practice, for example when you are leading on a new work activity or completing a work task in a different way and at the same time supporting others because there has been a change in an individual's needs. You might also need their support when you want to acquire or gain new knowledge in a specialist area such as dementia care, autism or supervisions or you may want to update your knowledge of changes to legislation and standards that will impact on your working practices.

Evidence opportunity

1.5 Sources of support for planning own development

You could discuss with your assessor the different methods for planning and reviewing your development. Identify all the main sources of support available to you at work including the ones we have discussed in this section. What additional support can you access within and outside of work? You could provide a written account after your discussion with your assessor.

LO2 Be able to demonstrate commitment to own continuous development

AC 2.1 Evaluate own performance and understanding of role against: a) values, b) standards, c) skills, d) behaviours

As you will have learned in LO1 of this unit, your role as a Lead is guided by skills, behaviours and standards that are required and expected from you. These standards include codes of conduct, regulations, minimum standards and national occupational standards that set out the knowledge, understanding, skills, behaviours and competence required from you and all Lead Adult Care Workers and Lead Personal Assistants.

Your values are also important because they are what you believe to be important to you and are part of who you are and will therefore guide the decisions you make as a Lead. For example, you may believe that having family and friends is very important or you may value educational opportunities over work opportunities. You will learn more about how your values can affect your working practices in LO4, ACs 4.2 and 4.3.

It is very important therefore that you keep a close check on how well your values, skills and behaviours match these standards and regularly evaluate your performance and understanding of your job role fully to ensure that you are:

- continuing to develop in your work role
- continuing to develop others in their work roles
- ensuring the wellbeing of the individuals you provide care and support to
- maintaining safe practices
- promoting best practice.

You can evaluate your performance and understanding of your job role by:

- **reflecting:** spending time thinking about the values, skills and behaviours that are expected from you, to what extent you meet the standards expected from you, what needs to happen to ensure you meet these standards fully, and how you can make improvements to your performance and understanding of your work practices.
- **evaluating:** spending time assessing how your values, skills and behaviours impact on your work practices and working relationships in the care setting where you work. Considering whether you have been successful in ensuring that you've met the required standards and ensuring that your values, skills and behaviours do not impact on the quality of your work. Finally, considering the successful work activities you have carried out and how they have impacted on the quality of the service you've provided.

Other ways to evaluate your performance and understanding of your job role

As a Lead Adult Care Worker or Lead Personal Assistant, you should not only refer to the various standards we have discussed in LO1 to ensure that your practice is informed by these, but you should also continuously evaluate your values, skills and behaviours to ensure that they are up to date and reflect any changes in standards and practice.

Your setting and colleagues are a useful source that you can use to ensure that you are keeping your practice up to date. For example, you could ask to observe or 'shadow' a senior colleague who is experienced or is able to demonstrate good practice to see how they perform in their role and learn from their expertise. This will allow you to increase your knowledge in areas in which you may not be particularly confident. Do not be afraid to ask for these opportunities, or for advice and feedback on how you are doing. Colleagues and those senior to you want the best for their care workers, individuals and the setting, and a motivated and enthusiastic workforce that seeks such opportunities only helps the setting to maintain high standards by having people who are able and competent in their roles.

You will also need to make sure that you pay attention to what is happening around you and how health and social care issues are being reported in the media.

Training outside the setting is a good way to keep your skills up to date and to gain new ones. You can then share this knowledge with colleagues which will encourage good practice. Issues around social care are a regular topic of debate in government and there are often changes to legislation which will be documented in the news. Be on the lookout for TV documentaries focusing on issues in the health and social care sector. The news tends to cover some of the more negative issues in care homes but it is important to watch these reports as motivation to do your best to ensure good practice. You may also read care sector-related stories in newspapers and magazines. All these activities will help you become a more informed Lead Adult Care Worker or Lead Personal

Assistant with a good understanding of what is happening in the sector and what is considered current best practice.

It is your duty as a care worker to keep up to date with best practice by researching textbooks, journals and the internet to learn about new theories, data and statistics and new thinking when it comes to the care sector. Again, not only will this positively impact the care you are able to offer, but it will also mean that you are a great source of information for colleagues. As part of your research you can also approach external agencies and charities that may have a better understanding than you do, of dementia for example.

You can ask for feedback from colleagues, individuals and families in order to evaluate how you are doing and ensure you continue to develop. This can be via a formal process, such as appraisals and meetings with colleagues, or questionnaires for individuals and families, or it can be done informally in a conversation. You may find that you receive both compliments and criticism, but it is important you take both constructively and learn from both. See AC 4.6 for more information on feedback.

Whichever way you choose to research, make sure that you always question the source of the information (where it has come from) to ensure it is reliable. In an age of social media and 24-hour news channels, we are often bombarded with information that can at times be overwhelming. Some sources of information are more fact-based, others are more opinion-based. It is therefore always important to ask yourself if the source is reliable, i.e. who is offering this information and why?

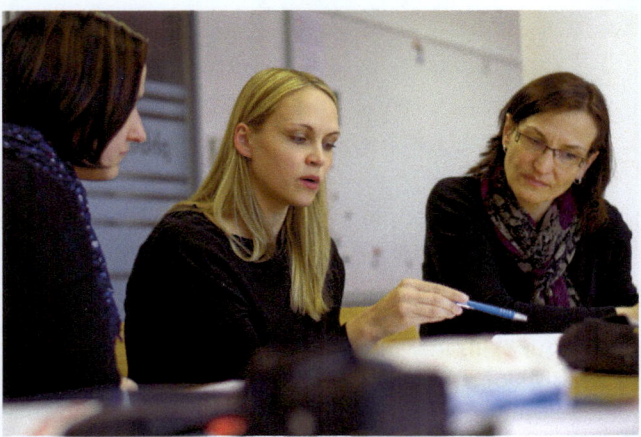

Figure 14.5 Are you keeping yourself up to date?

Research it

2.1 News reports

Find a health and social care news story you have recently heard about that interests you. How was the story reported – was it written as a news article, or reported on the news or on social media or on all three? Was the information you read or heard about this news story reported in different ways? What were the sources of the information? What were the purposes of the sources offering this information? Was the information reliable? You could discuss your thoughts with someone you work with. What were their views?

Evidence opportunity

2.1 Evaluate your performance and understanding

Discuss with your employer how you think you are meeting the values, standards, skills and behaviours that are relevant to your job role. Evaluate three aspects of your work practice that require improvement. Provide a written account.

AC 2.2 Work with others to identify and prioritise a) own learning needs, b) professional interests, c) development aspirations

As you have now identified the different sources that are available to support you in planning your development, you must now consider how others can play an important role in identifying and prioritising your development to ensure that all areas remain up to date and are still relevant to your job role and associated responsibilities. You will be observed working with others to identify and prioritise your development and you may find it helpful to review this section as well as AC 1.5 before being observed.

Learning needs

Your learning needs will change over time and therefore must be reviewed on a regular basis. For example, the learning needs you identified six weeks ago in relation to updating your knowledge around changes to data protection legislation may have already been met if you attended the course identified for you and gained the knowledge from it that you required. If, however, the course did not provide you with all the information you needed then your learning needs may still be unmet and another method to meet them must be identified. You would usually do this with your manager or employer. It could be, for example, that your manager provides you with the additional information or asks you to do some self-directed learning to find out this information yourself; you may then agree to have a discussion with your manager or employer once you have done so to confirm whether your learning needs have been met.

Self-directed learning is particularly important if you are not working in a setting with other colleagues or are self-employed. For example, if you are a private carer or a carer employed directly by the individual with care or support needs, you can obtain feedback directly from the individual and/or their family about how your care or support is being experienced and how you are perceived as a carer. In addition, you could keep your knowledge up to date by reading, watching real-life documentaries in care settings and researching lessons learned from research undertaken.

Professional interests

As well as your learning needs, you may find that your professional interests may change over time. For example, you may in your role as a Lead Adult Care Worker or Lead Personal Assistant provide leadership to a team of staff who provide services to individuals with learning disabilities, physical disabilities or mental health needs. At the time of starting in your work role it is likely that you had an interest in working alongside individuals with these needs and learning more about associated working practices.

The individuals you work with may also have specific conditions that you wish to learn more about. For example, this might be in relation to diabetes care, end of life care or use of technology in communicating with individuals with sensory loss. You will naturally wish to expand the sources you draw on to include information and support around the topics you are developing a professional interest in. It will be important for you to review and prioritise these in terms of which areas would benefit you as a practitioner working in your current Lead role.

Development aspirations

As you will learn more about in LO5, there will be many opportunities made available to you for your development. However, before you take these all on board you should think about which ones are most important for your own development, and what your aspirations are. For example, it may be that you would like to attend a conference for Lead professionals like you to further develop your leadership skills, but you have been tasked by your manager or employer to seek feedback from individuals about the quality of care and support they receive. You and your manager may decide that the latter takes priority this month as it is important that the feedback obtained from individuals is acted upon quickly and that instead, you attend the conference the following month. In this way you can access both development opportunities but at different times.

Development opportunities, as you have learned, are not only available to you through your work but may also arise naturally in your personal life. For example, a volunteering role to help at a music festival may support you in acquiring good organisational and people skills that you can then use in your current job role.

> **Research it**
>
> **2.2 Formal and informal development opportunities**
>
> Research formal and informal development opportunities that may be useful for your current role as a Lead. Explain to a colleague why these are relevant; include the skills and knowledge you plan to gain and describe how you plan to implement these in your current work role.

> **Evidence opportunity**
>
> **2.2 Work with others to identify and prioritise own learning needs, professional interests and development aspirations**
>
> Identify three people to work with to identify and prioritise your learning needs, professional interests and development aspirations. Obtain their feedback about how this worked. Reflect on your skills in working with others and the benefits of doing so effectively for your own development. For this AC, you will be observed working with others.

AC 2.3 Work with others to agree own personal and professional development plan goals

AC 2.4 Work with others to review personal and professional development plan goals

In some care settings, **personal and professional development plans (PDPs)** are also known as personal learning plans (PLPs) or personal development reviews (PDRs). What are they known as in the care setting where you work? A personal development plan is a formal record of your learning and development and identifies:

- the knowledge, skills and behaviours you have
- your strengths as well as the areas you need to improve
- your plans for the future, including how you would like to develop in your job and the goals you'd like to work towards
- the learning and support you need to improve your practice and develop in your job and career.

It is for this reason that it is vital that you have a PDP in place.

> **Key term**
>
> A **personal and professional development plan (PDP)** may have a different name but will record information such as agreed objectives for development, proposed activities to meet objectives and timescales for review.

You will agree your PDP by discussing this with your manager or supervisor during the appraisal process. This is because PDPs not only take into account your learning and development needs, but also the needs of the care setting where you work. This is to ensure that you carry out your work tasks competently, in line with your job description and your care setting's standards and agreed ways of working.

Your manager (who may also be your employer) or supervisor will ask you to plan for this discussion by reflecting on your own development, achievements and areas for development.

As part of your planning you should involve and work closely with others, including:

- **the individuals:** their comments about the care you provide can help you to reflect on your strengths and areas for improvement.
- **the carers:** their views on the support you provide to them and their relatives can help you to reflect on your abilities and behaviours.
- **advocates:** advocates speak up for individuals; they are independent of the care setting where you work so can be a useful and objective (unbiased) source of information about the quality of support you provide.
- **team members:** your colleagues who work with you on a day-to-day basis can provide you with a good insight into your strengths and the areas of your work that require further development.
- **other professionals:** as part of your role you may be required to contact other professionals who are external to the care setting where you work, such as social workers, GPs, dentists and pharmacists. You can reflect on the working relationships you have developed with them; perhaps you have received comments from them about the quality of your work, such as your communication skills or the care and support you provide.

Process for agreeing and reviewing your PDP and its goals

The process involved for agreeing and reviewing a personal development plan involves the following seven key steps:

1. Identify the skills and knowledge that are required to carry out your job role well: your job description that details your duties and responsibilities will be used as the basis of your discussion with your manager or employer.
2. Identify the skills and knowledge you have at present: you will need to gather the information you have collected from the people you have worked with in your planning.
3. Identify any gaps in your skills and knowledge (and what will be required to bridge them): you will need to discuss and agree these with your manager or employer.

4 Set goals for how to fill these gaps: you will need to discuss with your manager or employer what you would like to achieve as well as what your manager expects from you. See the section on SMART goals below. These will reflect your own goals and those of the setting in which you work.

5 Agree the ways you can bridge the gaps in your skills and knowledge: these will depend on your agreed goals. You will need to agree how you are going to do this, such as by attending a training course or working alongside a more experienced team member.

6 Agree when these gaps will be met: you and your manager will discuss and agree on what needs to be addressed urgently and what doesn't and then set realistic timescales for achieving these in the short term (six months), the medium term (one year) and the long term (two years).

7 Review your goals on a regular basis and plan your new goals for the future: you will need to discuss and agree these with your manager or employer in order to recognise what you have already achieved and what you would like to aim for next. This should document both your own and your manager's assessment of your learning and development. This is also an opportunity to update your PDP and record any training that you may have undertaken, for example. You may also need to change milestones and goals if you find they are not working. An appraisal is a good time to discuss your personal and professional development too, although you should be discussing this on an ongoing basis when meeting with your manager or employer.

Reflect on it

2.3 Your PDP

Reflect on what type of PDP you have where you work and the process you go through when working with others to agree and review it. How does the process compare to the seven steps outlined above? What are the similarities? What are the differences?

SMART PDP goals

It is important that the goals you include in your personal development plan and that you use to work with others are SMART. This means that they must be:

- **S**pecific: they must be clear and state exactly what you want to achieve. For example, an individual may be feeling low in themselves and have very little confidence as a result. Your aim may be to promote the individual's wellbeing so that they can regain their confidence, feel better in themselves and start socialising with others again.

- **M**easurable: they must have milestones or clear end-points so that you can measure how you are progressing and know when you have reached a certain goal. For example, an individual may have undergone an operation and is unable to eat by themselves or go to the toilet and dress themselves. Your goal may be to ensure that they can independently do these things in the next six months. A marker or a measurable goal may be when they are able to have their first meal on their own with very limited assistance from you in the next two months. The next marker may be when they are able to go to the toilet unassisted in the next three months.

- **A**chievable: you must be able to achieve them, in other words they must be part of your role. For example, you may decide to focus on work activities that are agreed as part of the scope of your job role and so can be achieved as part of the day-to-day support that you provide to individuals. If you see that you are on your way to achieving goals, this will serve as great motivation for achieving and progressing further. This will not only impact positively on the individuals you care for, because they experience better care as a result of your improved practice, but it will also impact positively on you and your team. Also, organising them into short, medium and long-term goals ensures that they are more achievable. For example, a short-term goal may be to help an individual with their personal care as they go through dementia. A medium-term goal may be to go on a course and train to find out more about dementia care. A long-term goal may be to support one other inexperienced colleague in this process. It may also include thinking about your long-term career plans, which might be to progress to a supervisor role.

Personal development plan

Name:　　　　　　　　　　　　　　　　　　　　Organisation:

Date PDP completed:

Part 1 – Personal analysis

What are my strengths?

What are my weaknesses and the areas that I need to further develop?

What opportunities are there available to me that can help me learn and develop?

What threats are there that may affect my plans to learn and develop?

Part 2 – Setting goals

What do I want to learn?

What do I have to do?

What skills do I want to gain?

What support will I need?

What other resources will I need?

How will I assess and evidence my achievement?

How will I show I have achieved this?

What is my target date for achieving this and reviewing my progress?

Part 3 – Personal objectives

What are my short-term goals for the next 12 months?

What are my medium-term goals for the next two to three years?

What are my longer-term goals beyond three years?

Part 4 – Review

Goal	Outcome – did I achieve this, and by agreed timescales?
1.	1.
2.	2.
3.	3.
4.	4.
5.	5.

Figure 14.6 Personal development plans vary in style and structure. This is just one example of a PDP. What does your PDP look like?

- **Realistic:** the goals you agree should be achievable in the timeframe that you are set and within the scope of your job, or you will agree on training that will enable you to achieve the goal. For example, you would not be expected to provide medical advice such as that a GP would normally give.
- **Timely or time-based:** there should be a clear timeframe for when you are expected to achieve the goal and clear milestones to aim for. That way, you and your manager can work towards these and plan any training and development needs within that schedule. Timeframes should be realistic and give you the best chance to meet them successfully (allowing you to feel encouraged to progress and meet the other goals that you are set).

You and your PDP

The most important person involved in your PDP is you. Demonstrating that you are willing to contribute to your PDP is the key to its success. You can contribute to your PDP by:

- **planning:** shows that you have prepared for a discussion with your manager or supervisor and indicates that you are keen to learn and improve your knowledge, skills and practice
- **reviewing:** being keen to review and update your personal development plan on a regular basis shows that you have a good insight into your progress regarding your learning and development
- **listening:** shows that you take seriously all comments, views and opinions received about the support you provide from all those involved in the personal development planning process. It shows that you are committed to making improvements to your practice.

As you draw up your plan make sure that it is highlighting all the things we have discussed above. In other words, ask yourself: is it outlining all my short-, medium- and long-term career goals? Will I be able to achieve these goals in these timeframes? Is the training relevant to what I want to achieve?

As well as making contributions, it is also important that you agree to your PDP and review it on a regular basis. As you have learned, planning your personal development involves meeting not only your learning and development needs but also the needs of the care setting where you work. This means that the goals that are set for you may not always be your preferred goals as they reflect the care setting's needs first and foremost. It is important not to be disappointed should this happen but instead focus on working closely and positively with your manager or employer so that you can draw up a personal development plan that meets both your needs and those of the organisation you work for.

Research it

2.3 SMART PDP goals

Setting goals for your personal development involves working closely with others. It is important that your goals are SMART: **S**pecific, **M**easurable, **A**chievable, **R**ealistic and **T**ime specific. Research the use of SMART when setting goals.

Produce an information handout about the skills needed to work with others to ensure your PDP goals are SMART.

Evidence opportunity

2.3, 2.4 Working with others to agree and review your PDP

Make arrangements to be observed working with others to agree and review your personal development plan.

You could also discuss with your assessor how you work with others to agree and review your PDP. Find out from your colleagues how they work with others to agree and review their PDPs. What skills do you share? What skills are different and why? Do you need to further develop any skills for working with others?

AC 2.5 Record progress in relation to personal and professional development in the professional development plan

You will need to demonstrate how you record your progress in relation to your personal and professional development; your practices will be observed.

Your professional development plan is a continuous record of your development at work. It is an important record because it:

- helps you to reflect on your practice
- identifies your achievements, strengths and abilities
- provides an up-to-date picture of what you have learned and how you have applied it
- provides useful information of what you aim to achieve and how you are going to do it
- reminds you to continue to develop your knowledge, skills and understanding.

PDPs can take many forms; in some care settings, they are recorded electronically, in others they are recorded on paper and held in a file. Your PDP contains personal information about you and therefore must be updated in private and stored securely when not in use. Remember the things that you have learned about completing your PDP in AC 2.3, and the various areas it must cover: for example, SMART goals with realistic timeframes and milestones, opportunities for training and development, and when and how you will review this. Remember to also record the progress you are making so that you can refer to this to evaluate how you are improving.

Reflect on it

2.5 Skills for recording progress

Reflect on the skills you need to record your progress in relation to your personal and professional development. For example, do you need to have good organisational skills and be able to write legibly?

Reflect on the qualities you need to record your progress in relation to your personal and professional development. For example, do you need to be honest and objective?

What skills and qualities do you have? Which ones do you need to improve on in relation to recording your progress for your personal and professional development?

> **Evidence opportunity**
>
> **2.5 Record progress in relation to personal development**
>
> If you have completed a PDP, review the last activity you planned. How are you progressing with it? Record your findings and share these with your employer or manager. Do they agree? Discuss this with/show this to your assessor. If discussing with your manager, this can be evidenced using a witness testimony.

LO3 Understand the value of reflective practice

AC 3.1 Define 'reflective practice' in health and social care

> **Getting started**
>
> Think about an occasion when you changed the way you practise at work because of an event that occurred. What happened? How did this impact on you, on others and on the service you provide? How did you decide what to change in terms of your practice? Did this have an impact? If so, what?

Reflective practice is another essential aspect to your work in terms of improving the quality of the service provided.

What is reflection and what does it involve?

To reflect means to think. Being able to reflect is an important skill to have as part of your work role. It involves thinking honestly about your practice, both the positives and negatives, and not being afraid to question your practice. When you reflect, you:

- take a 'step back' from your day-to-day activities and spend time thinking about a work activity you have carried out or a situation you have experienced
- examine in detail why and how you carry out your work practices
- assess your knowledge, skills and behaviours including their impact on you, the individuals you provide care and support to and others
- identify your strengths and weaknesses
- identify areas of your work practice that can be improved
- develop different ways of working that can improve your working practice
- develop new areas of learning, such as different or new approaches to situations that may arise.

> **Evidence opportunity**
>
> **3.1 What does reflective practice mean?**
>
> Develop a poster that describes what reflective practice in health and social care means.

AC 3.2 Describe models of reflection and their use in reflective practice

There are many different models of reflection that set out in a structured way the reflective process. These models are useful for helping you to understand all aspects of the reflective process. Below are examples of two models of reflection that can be used in different ways when reflecting on practice:

Driscoll's Reflective Cycle (2000) – a model of reflection that includes three stages when reflecting on your work practice.

1. **What?** This is a description of the situation, and its purpose is for you to reflect on specific aspects of that experience.
   You can reflect on:
   - What is the purpose of reflecting on the situation that happened?
   - What happened?
   - What did I see?
   - What did I do?
   - What didn't I do?
   - What did others do?
   - What was my reaction?

2. **So what?** This is the analysis of the situation you experienced, and its purpose is for you to consider the learning that arises out of the reflection process you've undertaken.
   You can reflect on:
   - So what feelings did I experience during the situation?
   - So what feelings did I experience after the situation?
   - So what, if any, were the differences between my feelings during and after the situation?
   - So what was the impact of what I did and/or didn't do?

- So what have I identified are my strengths in my practice?
- So what have I identified are my development areas in my practice?
- So what feelings did others experience during and after the situations?
- So what if any were the differences between others, and my feelings during and after the situation?

3 **Now what?** This is the proposed actions to implement following your learning, and its purpose is for you to implement the learning you've gained into your practice.

You can reflect on:
- Now what are the implications for my practice if I implement the new learning?
- Now what are the implications for my practice if I do not implement the new learning?
- Now what are the implications for others?
- Now what have I learned about my practices?
- Now what information and support do I need to carry out these proposed actions?
- Now what would I do differently if a similar situation arises again?
- Now what can I do to ensure I continue to improve my practice?

Gibbs' Reflective Cycle (1988) – a model of reflection that considers the different stages in the reflection process and the questions you should be asking yourself.

> **Evidence opportunity**
>
> **3.2 The different models of reflective practice**
>
> To help further your understanding about what reflective practice is, research the different models that can be used for reflective practice. There are many different models that can be used – for example, you may want to research: Johns, Kolb, Atkins and Murphy. Select two models that interest you and develop a leaflet for each one that explains what it is and why it is useful for understanding the different aspects involved in reflective practice.

AC 3.3 Explain the benefits and scope of reflective practice

Reflective practice does not just happen once a week or at the end of the month. It is a continuous process that you will use throughout your career and in the different roles you undertake. Reflective practice is important because it brings with it many benefits:

- **You get to know yourself:** the personal qualities you have, the areas of knowledge, understanding, skills and behaviours you have and those you need to develop. Gaining a greater understanding of who you are benefits you, as it will help you recognise how your practices influence others. This will also lead you to know more about the individuals you provide care and support to so you can ensure that you adapt your working practice to meet their unique needs and preferences.
- **You develop yourself:** by identifying opportunities to address the gaps there may be in your knowledge, skills and behaviours. For example, perhaps you have not been in a Lead job role for very long or perhaps you are experienced as a Lead but are working in a new service or with a new team. You may find that you need to access additional training from the setting where you work or guidance from another person in a similar job role to you or in a more senior position. Doing so has numerous benefits, including improving your competence and your work practice.

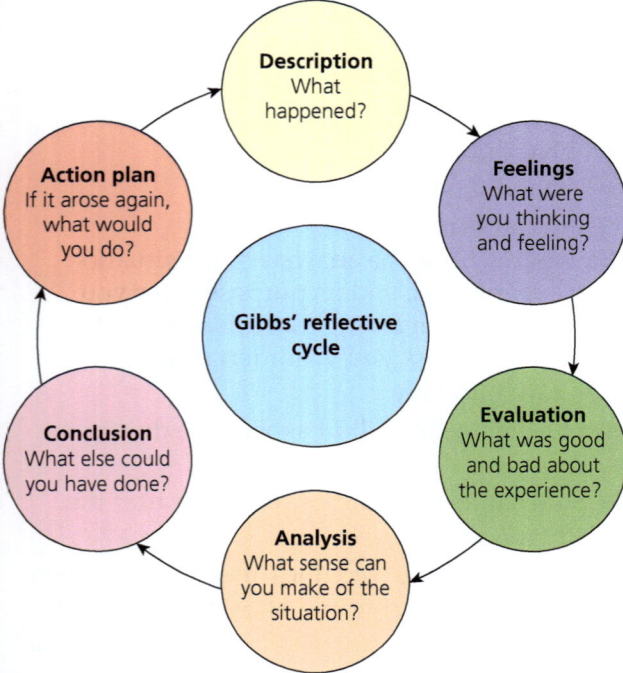

Figure 14.7 Gibbs' Reflective Cycle

- **You develop best practice:** by finding out about the working practices and approaches that are not working, you and your colleagues will be able to develop new ways of working and approaches that will have a positive influence on the care and support that you provide to individuals. Keeping a close check on these new ways of working will help you to identify best practices that you and your colleagues can apply in your day-to-day work activities. As a Lead, others you work alongside will expect you to lead by example so it is essential that your work practices as well as the information and support you provide to the team reflect current ways of working, that are in line with relevant standards as well as agreed ways of working.

Reflect on it

3.3 Reflecting on ways to improve

Using one of the reflective models you learned about in AC 3.2, reflect on the benefits of reflective practice. Discuss your findings with your manager or employer. Provide a short reflective account.

Research it

3.3, 3.4 Research and improved practice

Why is it important to stay up to date and develop your work practice, ideas, skills and knowledge? Why is it important to be aware of the different stories in the news concerning the adult care sector like the one below?

www.theguardian.com/society/2018/jun/03/data-confirms-postcode-lottery-care-for-the-old

Where else can you find out about developments in the adult care sector? For example, media reports, reviews about serious failings, conferences, internet, your **supervisor** and colleagues? Do you know about the various ways to research these? Do you know about primary and secondary research and quantitative and qualitative data? How can such research help you to improve your practice and the care you offer individuals?

Evidence opportunity

3.3 Importance of reflective practice in improving the quality of service

Produce a written account that explains why reflective practice is important. Write about the benefits and scope of reflecting on your practice and how it can help develop your knowledge and skills further.

AC 3.4 Explain how reflective practice can support continuous professional development and improvements to both own practice and the provision of quality care

You learned about reflective practice and what being a good reflector involves earlier on (see AC 3.1 and 3.2) and it would be worth recapping those sections.

Improvements to your practice

Reflecting on a situation that has taken place in the care setting where you work can lead to improved ways of working by:

- increasing your self-awareness – making you more aware of your own abilities and limitations, what situations and experiences have taught you and how you can use these to learn, improve and grow in your role
- making you more aware of the knowledge, skills and understanding you have and those you need to gain or develop or improve on
- helping you to identify suitable learning activities to meet your learning needs
- improving your work practice
- being an effective lead in improving the practice of others and leading by example.

Not only will reflecting enable you to improve your ways of working, it will also mean that you are able to inform others of what you have learned and how you have improved, which will help them to improve their ways of working too. This will in turn benefit those you care for and increase standards where you work.

Not setting time aside to reflect means that you risk your performance at work becoming poor in quality; this in turn will impact on the quality of the care you provide to individuals and the support you provide to your team members. You may also place these individuals at risk of danger, harm or abuse through poor working practices, which can have serious consequences for their lives and your career. That is not to say you should spend your time worrying about the consequences, but it is a good idea to be aware of good practice and what bad practice can mean.

> **Reflect on it**
>
> **3.4 Reflecting on a situation**
>
> Reflect on a situation you have experienced as a Lead where you work. What happened? Why? What action did you take? Why? Could you have taken different action? Why? What would you do next time should this situation happen again? Why?

> **Reflect on it**
>
> **3.4 How reflective practice has led to improved ways of working**
>
> Provide a written account explaining how being a reflective practitioner has led you to improve your performance at work and provide quality care. Discuss how you have improved two aspects of your work through reflection.
>
> You might like to think of it in these terms:
>
> - As a result of reflecting and thinking about this situation, I now know more about…
> - My skills have improved as a result of…
> - I can now do…
> - I understand that I must…

Essentially, it is only by reflecting that you can continuously improve the quality of service provided because reflective practice involves you looking at a situation and deciding if you need to change your approach or actions, either during the situation, or the next time you are faced with a similar one.

Reflection is good practice and it shows that you **care**. Just by doing this, you are showing that you are a professional and competent Lead Adult Care Worker or Lead Personal Assistant who is striving to increase in knowledge, develop their skills and provide best practice by continually finding ways to improve their practice. Reflecting will allow you to learn from what went well as well as what did not go so well. Not taking the time to reflect on your practice will mean that you and others may continue to work in the same ways, making the same mistakes and not being able to identify opportunities for learning and development.

As human beings, we often tend to focus on our mistakes, weaknesses and the things that we did not do well, or the things that we could improve. However, it is important that you also think about the things that you did well. Focusing on your strengths will mean you can tell colleagues about what went well which will encourage good practice across the team. It is also a good way to remain positive and confident with the knowledge that, while things might not go perfectly all the time, other situations have gone well. It is also a reminder that you are a competent worker able to provide high quality care and support, and support others who you work with to do the same.

In ACs 3.1, 3.2 and 3.3, we discussed what is involved in reflective practice and why it is important. You may wish to recap the learning in these ACs so you understand how to show that you can reflect meaningfully on your practice. Remember too that you will be observed doing so.

Showing that you can reflect on practice involves developing the following skills and qualities:

- **Self-awareness:** how your behaviours impact on individuals, others and your work practices
- **Honesty:** being honest with yourself about what has worked well (and what has not) and how to develop a more positive attitude
- **Commitment:** striving to improve the quality of your work practices.

6Cs

Care

Caring consistently and enough to make a positive difference to individuals' lives is essential to your role. Reflection is a key part of caring for individuals. For example, an individual may have taken offence at something you said even though you did not mean any harm. However, you will make sure that next time you are careful not to mention the same topic, so you do not cause any hurt.

It is because you genuinely care and are concerned for their wellbeing that you reflect and think about how you can improve your practice next time. Caring for individuals is only one aspect of your role; it also involves providing support to others such as your colleagues or individuals' families and carers.

Commitment

In a care setting, this refers to your dedication to providing the highest quality of service. It means continuously reflecting on how you can improve your work practices in order to improve the experience of the people who need care and support and lead by example. You can do this by thinking about the various things we have discussed in this section. Remember: during or following a work activity, you can think about the things that went well and the things that you can improve on. How will you improve your work practices? How can you ensure a safer environment? How will you communicate better? It is in this way that you can show that you are committed to being a reflective practitioner who is constantly striving to be the best they can be, who leads by example and encourages others who they support to also become reflective practitioners.

Courage

Courage refers to your dedication to doing the right thing at the right time so that the individuals in your care and support are kept safe. It takes courage to acknowledge that you did not do something so well, to take some criticism and know that you need to improve and learn.

There is nothing wrong with admitting that you could be better at something. After all, you have your interests and the best interests of the people you care for as well as those others you support and work alongside at heart. Improvements mean that you are progressing, that you are getting better at your job. Remember: do not just focus on all the things that did not go well. Also think positively – about all the things that you are doing well. This will help you continue to do the things you do well and become better at the things that you do not!

There are two different methods that you can use for reflecting on your work practice:

1. **Reflecting on a work activity after it has happened:** this is known as 'reflection on action'. If you use this method to reflect you will need to be committed to learning from the experience and then taking the necessary actions for making improvements.
2. **Reflecting on a work activity while it is happening:** this is known as 'reflection in action'. If you use this method to reflect you will need to be able to 'think on your feet' and take the necessary actions for making improvements while it is happening. Taking actions quickly requires **courage**.

Reflect on it

3.4 How do you reflect?

What is your preferred method for reflecting on your work practice – after it has happened or while it is happening? Why? Have you ever tried using the other method? Why? What skills and qualities do you think are needed for each method?

By reflecting on your practice, you will be setting a good example to others who you work with and support because they will be led by you and learn that reflective practice is an integral aspect of their work and an effective way of continuously improving the care and support you all provide.

You will also learn by working alongside your colleagues, attending meetings and having discussions where you exchange information with others. You can reflect on your practice by learning from your mistakes and successes, and develop new ways of working.

> **Evidence opportunity**
>
> **3.4 Reflect on practice to improve service**
>
> Discuss with your assessor how reflective practice can support continuous professional development as well as improvements to your practice and the provision of quality care.

LO4 Be able to use reflective practice to improve ways of working

AC 4.1 Reflect on how different types of learning activities have influenced own practice

Types of learning activities

As you know there are many different sources of support for your learning available to you both within and outside of the care setting where you work. Being an effective learner means being in control of your own learning. There are many different types of learning activities to choose from:

- **Training** usually takes place in the care setting where you work. It is usually carried out by more senior team members and can include your manager or even you if this is part of your job role. It is usually focused on specific work areas; for example it can help you and others to update your knowledge on safeguarding or further develop your practical manual and handling skills. This could also be external training carried out by an external agency or person. Whatever the training, you will need to ensure that this is relevant and will enable you to improve your work practice.
- **Learning programmes** can take place in the care setting where you work or outside of the care setting, such as in a college or an online virtual learning environment. A qualified person such as a teacher, tutor or assessor usually delivers the programme. Learning programmes can be useful for improving your knowledge and understanding that underpins your work practice as well as for further developing your skills, for example on diabetes care or even about the Level 3 Adult Care Diploma you are currently undertaking.
- **Mentoring programmes** take place in the care setting where you work. They are led by a more experienced member of the team and involve providing support to someone who has less experience, for example by guiding you through how to overcome a difficult situation you have experienced at work or supporting you to plan for a new work activity that you will then need to support others with.
- **Coaching programmes** also take place in the care setting where you work. They are led by a member of the team who is experienced and competent in a specific skill or work area. They can provide training, for example on carrying out a risk assessment or supporting an individual who has specific communication needs when interacting with others.
- **Reading and information sharing** can take place both within and outside of the care setting where you work. For example, your manager may provide you and your colleagues with a legislation update or you may read an article in the newspaper about what high quality care and support looks like, which you may then discuss with your colleagues.
- **Reflection** can take place both within and outside of your care setting, both during and after situations and experiences. For example, you may reflect on how you can adapt your communication with an individual who is not responding to you positively or you may reflect on your work achievements after your appraisal.
- **Visiting other settings** and speaking to lead care workers based there can increase your knowledge and understanding of how other settings function and learn about their ways of working. You will of course need to ask your manager and gain permission from them in order to do this. Your manager will then need to get the permission from the setting, and arrange a suitable time and for someone to show you around.

- **Individuals and their families.** It is important to remember that you will be constantly learning from the individuals that you care for daily. This may include simply learning something new about their lives or preferences. It might be something as simple as finding out that they do not like to have broccoli in their lunch, which will enable you to make sure that this is not in the meals they are given. By learning directly from individuals, you can ensure you tailor your practice to their needs.

Research it

4.1 Other theories

Research the four stages of Lewin/Kolb's cycle of experiential learning: concepts of concrete experience, reflective observation, abstract conceptualisation and active experimentation.

You might also find it useful to research Honey and Mumford's four-stage process of learning from experience and their theory of learning styles. Look into the different types of learners they have identified: activists, reflectors, theorists and pragmatists.

Reflect on it

4.1 Learning activities

Reflect on one learning activity you carried out to improve or further develop your practice. Why did you choose this activity? Was there another type of activity you could have undertaken? Why?

Evaluating the impact of learning activities

As previously discussed, it is important that you strive to improve your practice on a daily basis, continuously developing your knowledge, skills and understanding by ensuring that you are up to date with any recent developments in adult care. This means going to the library to access journals, researching on the internet, ensuring you are keeping up to date with any developments in the news and speaking to colleagues inside the setting. Being an informed practitioner who is constantly doing this as well as using learning activities such as training to develop their knowledge, skills and understanding will benefit your setting, improve your practice and thus the lives of the individuals you care for.

Evaluating how learning activities have affected your practice involves:

- **reflecting on them after they have taken place:** for example, what was the purpose of undertaking them? Did the learning activity change, develop or improve my practice? How? What evidence do I have of this?
- **weighing up the benefits:** for example, in relation to the purpose of the learning activity, did I gain what I aimed to? Perhaps more? Perhaps less? Did the learning activity's benefits make an impact on my work practice? If so, how? Who else did this impact on my practice benefit? Could these benefits be replicated, i.e. if others completed this learning activity would it benefit their practice too? Can I share any of this learning with others? Will this improve my practice as well as theirs?
- **further improvements:** for example, are there still any gaps in my learning? If so, how I can meet these outstanding learning needs? With the same type of learning activity or with a different type?

There is no point in undertaking learning activities if they do not have a positive impact on your practice. But to know whether they do so, you must EVALUATE:

- **E**xamine your practice and how it has been affected
- **V**erify that the learning you've undertaken has had the impact you intended
- **A**ssess how effective the learning activity is
- **L**earn from others, from what they tell you about how your practice has changed
- **U**ndertake further learning if you need to
- **A**im to review the goals you set yourself for your learning
- **T**ake into account your increased self-awareness of your own abilities and limitations
- **E**xperience the learning gained positively and use this to inform future learning and development.

> **Evidence opportunity**
>
> **4.1 How learning activities affect practice**
>
> Make arrangements to be observed evaluating how learning activities have affected your practice. Select a learning activity you (and a colleague, if they also took part) participated in. Discuss with your assessor the benefits. Discuss the impact on your work practices. Compare and contrast the learning gained.

AC 4.2 Describe how own values, beliefs and experiences may affect working practices

AC 4.3 Reflect on how own values, beliefs and experiences have developed since working within own role

What do we mean by values, beliefs and experiences and why is it important to be aware of them in your practice?

Your values, **belief systems** and experiences are unique to you and part of who you are, so they will inevitably influence your role as a Lead Adult Care Worker or Lead Personal Assistant, including what you do and how you do it. In a care setting, you will be working with a wide array of people from diverse backgrounds – some of whom will have similar values, attitudes and beliefs to you and some will have different ones. They may, for example, come from a different cultural or educational background to you, have conflicting political beliefs, and/or different attitudes towards a variety of things.

> **Key terms**
>
> **Belief systems** are personal to you and what you regard to be true. They can sometimes be shared with others who belong to a similar group or culture. Beliefs can be political, religious, cultural or moral and are formed throughout your life.

Much of your role as a Lead involves working closely with the people to whom you provide care and support as well as with others and is based, as you know, on close interactions and working relationships. Because your values, beliefs and experiences make up so much of the person you are, they will inevitably play a role in the relationships that you have both outside and inside the setting and will influence your work. For example, you may tend to speak more with those individuals and their families with whom you have things in common, and so take a greater interest in their choices and preferences. This may lead to you spending less time with the individuals who have different values to you, and mean that you are less empathetic in your support to them because you are not seeing things from their point of view. You might not realise you are doing this, but it will show in your work. For example, you may find that you are more patient towards some people than others or that you tend to avoid interacting with some people.

It is for this reason that you will need to be aware of your own values, beliefs and experiences because they will impact on your role and the people you work with. Being aware of them will ensure that you consider whether your own thoughts and beliefs influence individuals and others positively or negatively. It is important to remember that you may not necessarily agree with the people you support or with an individual's decisions, but you should respect them and empathise so that you can fulfil your responsibility of providing high quality care, support and leadership. This is also part of providing person-centred practice which you have learned about in Unit 306: Promoting and implementing person-centred practice

Being aware of your own values, beliefs and experiences also involves understanding what influences affect you, and how they are formed and developed during our lives from childhood to late adulthood.

How do your values, beliefs and experiences form and develop?

Everyone is different and therefore holds their own unique personal values, attitudes, beliefs and experiences. These are formed and developed during our lives from childhood to late adulthood and can be influenced by:

- **the people in our lives:** such as family, friends and teachers. How the people close to you behave towards you will in turn influence how you behave towards others. If your family and friends show you care and kindness then you are likely to act in this way towards others. If your teachers provided you with a positive educational experience this is likely to influence your values and beliefs about the importance and benefits of a good education.

- **religion:** such as Christianity, Hinduism, Islam, Sikhism, Buddhism or Judaism. These are some of the religions that are practised in the UK and have specific beliefs and practices associated with them. If you follow one of these religions and their associated practices then this will influence what you believe to be 'right' and 'wrong' (your moral values) as well as what you eat and drink and how you dress.
- **life events:** such as starting school, starting employment, moving out of the family home, marriage, divorce or death of a family member or friend. These events can all occur in our lives and impact significantly on the values, beliefs and attitudes we develop. How we survive these events will in turn influence whether we see them as positive or negative experiences and will be reflected in how we come across to others when we are supporting them through the same life events.
- **the media:** such as television, the internet, newspapers and music. What you see, read and hear about in your life can influence the values, beliefs and attitudes you form. For example, a television programme that explores what individuals value as they get older, which stresses the importance of contact with others and companionship, can in turn influence your relationships with older people by making you more aware of what is important to them. Information and stories that you read on the internet and in newspapers about best practice in the adult care sector can influence the practices you follow in the care setting where you work. Listening to music can enable you to experience its many benefits, for example relaxation and expression of how you think and feel. This may in turn lead you to supporting individuals to follow their music interests or providing music as a therapeutic activity.

Reflect on it

4.2, 4.3 Similarities and differences

Reflect on the similarities and differences between your values, beliefs and experiences and those of others you work with. What influences do you think there are on how these are formed and developed? How have your values, beliefs and experiences developed since working within your job role?

How can you ensure that your personal values, attitudes and beliefs do not negatively affect your working practice?

As you have learned, we are all different and have unique backgrounds, experiences and influences in our lives that will in turn influence what we think and feel and how we behave towards others. You may know individuals and colleagues in the care setting where you work who share your values, attitudes and beliefs but there may also be individuals and colleagues you work with who do not. It is very important that differences (that may arise between individuals or colleagues) do not impact negatively on the quality of your work and working practice.

You can do this by:

- being aware of how your personal values, attitudes and beliefs can affect the way you think, feel, interact and behave towards others. For example, you believe that families should care at home for their relatives as they get older. An older individual who has recently been admitted at the setting where you work has not yet been visited by any family members, all of whom live close by. It is important that you do not make judgements about this individual's family. Everyone is different and there may be many reasons why this individual is living in a care setting and why their family have not visited yet.
- being aware of the personal values, attitudes and beliefs that individuals and others you work with hold. For example, you are aware that one of your colleagues practises Judaism and believes that there is only one god, whereas another of your colleagues practises Hinduism and believes in multiple gods and goddesses (i.e. polytheism). You may practise a different religion and have different beliefs to both of them or you may not have a faith. Although your beliefs may be different, it is important that you respect others' beliefs and take the time to try and understand them so that you can take them into account when interacting with your colleagues. Not doing so may mean that you will not be able to develop effective team work and positive relationships with your colleagues, which in turn may impact negatively on the quality of the service provided.

- being respectful of the differences between your own, individuals and others' values, attitudes and beliefs and having a person-centred approach. This means that when working with individuals you do not let your own beliefs influence their choices and preferences, either directly through your words or indirectly through your body language. For example, you may believe that healthy eating and exercise is a good lifestyle choice, but an individual you support chooses to not eat healthily or exercise, but smokes and drinks alcohol. If the individual understands the consequences of their lifestyle choices then it is their choice to live like this, so it is important that you do not influence them with your beliefs by insisting that they eat healthily, exercise and stop smoking and drinking. If you work alongside others who are from different backgrounds and cultures, it is important that all of you work to the values of the organisation, respect and take into account each other's differences and recognise the valuable contributions each of you makes to the care and support services that are provided to individuals and their families. Not doing so may mean that you do not work well together and therefore are unable to provide high quality care and support.

Evidence opportunity

4.2, 4.3 Values, beliefs, experiences and working practice

Identify for yourself two values, two beliefs and two experiences. For each of these write down how they affect your working practice. How do you ensure that they do not have a negative impact on your working practice? Now seek feedback from someone at work who knows you well, or from your employer if appropriate. Show them what you have written down – do they agree? Reflect on their feedback. Do you need to make any improvements to your working practice? Provide a written account documenting the points mentioned here or describe in writing how an adult care worker's own values, belief systems and experiences may affect their working practice, and how your values, beliefs and experiences have developed since working in your job role.

AC 4.4 Reflect on own ability to use initiative, make decisions and take responsibility for own actions

AC 4.5 Reflect on own ability to understand the limits and accountability of your work role and when to seek advice

Using your initiative in making decisions and taking responsibility for your actions are the essential skills of an effective leader and are very much sought after by employers because they involve having the ability to:

- take action without being told to do so and before others do so
- work independently and manage your own work
- think on your feet
- believe in yourself and your abilities
- take responsibility for the decisions you make, even when others may disagree
- be courageous when difficulties arise
- be determined to overcome any difficulties that arise

Reflect on it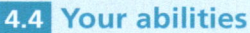

4.4 Your abilities

Reflect on an occasion when you used your initiative. How did this situation arise? What decisions did you make and why?

Understanding the limits and accountability of your work role and knowing when to seek advice are other essential skills to have because they ensure that you are carrying out your job role competently and in line with the level of expertise, knowledge and skills you have. Not having an understanding of these aspects of your job role means that you could be putting yourself, individuals and others at risk of unsafe practices.

You will find it helpful to refer to Unit 300, Responsibilities and ways of working in adult care settings/services where we explore why it's important to work within the scope of your job role including its limitations and your responsibilities.

Reflection is a useful tool that you can use for further developing and improving your skills in these areas as well as recognising which of these skills you already have so that you can continue to be a good role model to others and make a positive difference to the lives of the individuals you support. You will learn more about leadership behaviours in LO5 of this unit.

> **Evidence opportunity**
>
> **4.4, 4.5 Reflecting on your ability**
>
> Using one of the models of reflection you learned about earlier on in this unit in LO3, reflect on your ability to use your initiative, make decisions and take responsibility for your actions and understanding the limits and accountability of your work role. Think about how your reflections could improve your ways of working and why this is important. Discuss your reflections with your manager. Make sure your assessor observes you reflecting or your manager could provide a Witness Testimony.

AC 4.6 Use reflections and feedback from others to evaluate own performance and inform development

Use reflections

To be an effective reflective practitioner and provide high quality care and support it is very important that you know how to use reflections and feedback from others to evaluate your practice and inform your knowledge and development. The ability to evaluate should not be underestimated; it is a valuable skill to have and involves being able to do the following. You will need to show that you are able to do this when being observed for this AC. This will include:

- **gathering information:** for example, you may have to reflect on the areas of your practice that need improving or discuss with the individuals you provide a service to their views on the aspects of the service that are working well and those that are not, so that you can then use these reflections.
- **analysing information collated:** you could then examine in detail the improvements to your practice suggested by your colleagues, or reflect on the details of the discussions you had with the individuals you provide a service to. This will involve you carefully analysing the information you asked for as well as the information you received.
- **drawing conclusions and making judgements from your analysis:** you can use the analysis and your reflections as the basis of what to conclude from your evaluation of your work practice such as your strengths and weaknesses, or how to further develop and improve through reflection.
- **presenting information:** this may involve producing a written document that describes how you evaluated your work practice. It will involve you describing the methods you used to evaluate your practice and the reasons why. Your evaluation will also include your findings, the conclusions you reached and the recommendations from your evaluation for making improvements to your work practice.

> **Reflect on it**
>
> **4.6 Skills of evaluation**
>
> Reflect on your ability to evaluate. What skills do you have already? What skills do you need to develop? How are you going to do this? What support do you need?

Use feedback from others

To evaluate your performance at work effectively, so that it leads to you making improvements to the service you provide to individuals and to the support you provide to your team, you must be ready to receive feedback from others. At first, receiving feedback from others may seem like a daunting experience – you may be unsure about what others will say about you or how to respond to the feedback you receive. You can overcome this hurdle by focusing on the benefits of using feedback to help make you a more effective practitioner and role model to others. You will then begin to appreciate how important a role feedback plays in your continuous professional development and recognise how it can help you ensure that your strengths are reinforced and your weaknesses are converted into real improvements.

What is feedback in relation to your work performance?

Feedback, put simply, is the views of those you work alongside in relation to your work performance, such as your employer, manager, team members, colleagues, the individuals you support and their families, friends and advocates. There are many different methods of collecting feedback; some use quantitative approaches and others use qualitative approaches. Do you know the difference between the two?

- **Quantitative approaches** produce numerical data or information and are useful when obtaining feedback from a large group of people. Questionnaires, group interviews and discussion groups are all examples of quantitative approaches; the questions asked and/or the topics discussed are usually agreed with the participants to ensure the questions and topics being asked are appropriate.
- **Qualitative approaches** produce opinion-based information and are useful when obtaining feedback about people's experiences. One-to-one interviews, observations of work practice and planned events that bring people together are all examples of qualitative approaches; these methods all provide opportunities for those involved to share their views and experiences.

Using feedback

Feedback from others is only useful if you know how to respond to it. There is no point in obtaining feedback from others if you do not use it or ignore it because you disagree or find it overly critical. Remember, feedback is most helpful when it is constructive but even when it isn't, this does not necessarily mean that it is not useful or valid. If someone does give you feedback in an unhelpful way – angrily or sarcastically, for example – then you should clarify with the person what they meant. You can tell them that you can see that they're angry and want to try to understand why, so if they can tell you what they meant you will be able to understand their feedback and act upon it. It is only by doing this that you can make effective use of all types of feedback, both positive and negative.

> **Reflect on it**
>
> **4.6 Dealing with feedback**
>
> Think about an occasion when someone gave you feedback that wasn't constructive. How did you feel? Why? What do you think made this person give you their feedback in this way? How did you respond at the time? Could you have responded differently?

To help you use feedback effectively you need to do some thinking before and after you obtain it:

Before, think about…

- the reasons why you are seeking feedback. For example, is it to improve an area of your practice or did something go wrong at work? This will help you focus on the importance of using all feedback you receive.
- who you want to obtain feedback from and the reasons why. For example, is it from your manager or employer because it is in relation to an aspect of your senior/Lead role? Or is it from an individual because it is relevant to the quality of the care they received? Or is it from a team member because it is about finding out whether the team has sufficient support in place? This will help you focus on why you have chosen to obtain feedback from specific people and what you feel they have to offer you in terms of informing your development.

After, think about …

- who will be affected if you use the feedback you have obtained. Perhaps it may improve the care provided to individuals or the quality of the support you provide to those others you work with. You may also want to think about the consequences of not using the feedback on, for example, the people who provided you with feedback (they may feel that you've not taken their views seriously); the service provided (the quality of the service may worsen); and you yourself (your performance will not improve and your development may stop). This will help you focus on the impact of using feedback you receive.
- the changes that have happened since you used the feedback. Have you seen an improvement? Perhaps others have told you that they've seen an improvement. You will also need to think about what you are going to do with this information. How and with whom will you

share the improvements made? Your employer, at your next meeting; the individuals you care for, at an informal gathering such as a coffee morning; or perhaps you will inform the team members you support at the next team meeting you hold with them.

All feedback whether it is positive, negative, crucial, helpful, or unhelpful is useful and must be acted upon. This will improve your performance at work and help you to develop your skills, knowledge and understanding as well your ability to be a reflective practitioner. The reflective exemplar provides you with an opportunity to explore in more detail how you can use feedback to evaluate your work practices and inform your continuous development as a professional.

> **Evidence opportunity**
>
> **4.6 Using reflections and feedback from others to evaluate own performance and inform development**
>
> Identify an aspect of your work practice that requires improvement. Get feedback from three others and use their feedback to evaluate your performance and inform your development. You may like to do this with your employer or manager. For example, this may be in relation to how you lead the team or how you communicate with others. You will be observed using feedback you have received from others to evaluate your performance and inform your development. This could be your assessor or manager.

Reflective exemplar	
Introduction	I work as a Senior Carer in a residential care home and my role involves supervising the delivery of care to all individuals who use the service. I also lead on the implementation of all individuals' care and support documentation and provide leadership to all the care staff in all aspects of care through supervision and mentoring.
What happened	Yesterday, I held a team meeting and discussed with those present what they thought about the new location of the staff's office. Overall, the response was not positive and took me a little by surprise. Although everyone acknowledged that there was now more space in the office and that they liked the new furniture, its new location was too noisy as it was next door to the laundry room and sometimes the office was the only way to access the two residents' rooms at the end of the corridor.
	In addition, two team members added that the two residents who live at the end of the corridor are coming into the staff office more often than usual – they think this is because of the office's location because they are seeing staff enter and leave the office on a regular basis.
	We agreed to review the location of the staff office and for me to seek the whole team's opinion over the next week. I also agreed to raise this at the residents' meeting due to be held next week and speak directly to the two residents who live close to the office.
What worked well	I was pleased that the team felt able to express what they thought about the new location of the staff's office and were able to constructively tell me how this was having an impact on them, the residents and other visitors.
What did not go as well	I think I should have sought everyone's opinion much sooner and even before going ahead with the relocation of the office; this way I would have minimised the negative impact it may have had.
	I also should have made it clear to everyone what I was going to do with their feedback, how I was planning to use it, when they could expect me to reach a decision and how I would be communicating this to them.
What I could do to improve	I think I am going to speak with my manager as perhaps I need some more support to decide the best methods to use when communicating to different people what I am going to do with the feedback received. I may also see if I can find any courses that may be useful for my own development in terms of using feedback.
Links to unit's assessment criteria	ACs: 4.6

LO5 Be able to develop leadership behaviours

AC 5.1 Describe leadership behaviours in adult social care

In your work setting the ways in which you act as a Lead, including towards others, are referred to as your Leadership behaviours.

> **Reflect on it**
>
> **5.1 Leadership and you**
>
> What does leadership mean to you? What skills and behaviours do you have? Why are these useful in your job role?

The Leadership Qualities Framework published by Skills for Care in 2016 sets out a framework for good leadership behaviours that consists of seven qualities or 'dimensions' that are deemed necessary in adult social care. The first five dimensions are based on the leadership framework developed by the NHS and apply to all leaders in adult social care, and a further two dimensions apply specifically to senior staff.

The following table provides some more details of the five dimensions included within the Leadership Qualities Framework that apply to all leaders in adult social care.

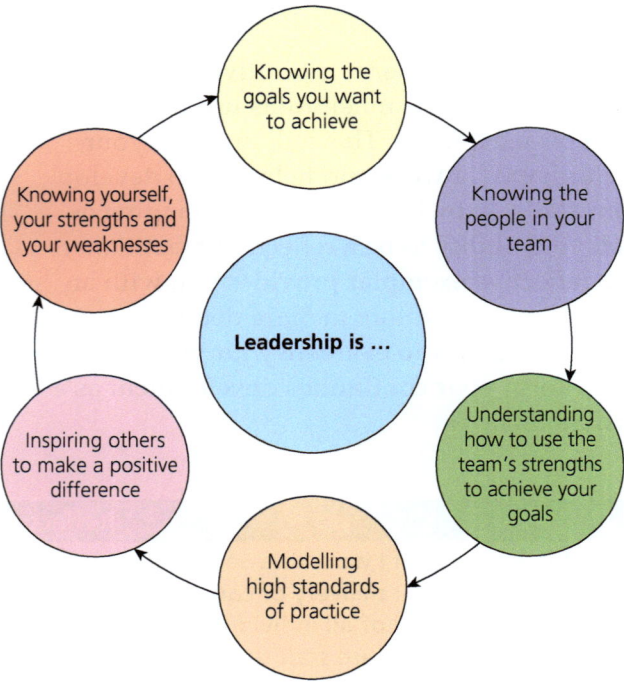

Figure 14.8 What does leadership look like?

Table 14.4 The first five dimensions or qualities included within the Leadership Qualities Framework

Leadership qualities or dimensions	Examples of behaviours
1 Demonstrating personal qualities – your personal qualities as a leader	• Developing self-awareness – being aware of how your behaviours impact on others • Managing yourself – challenging yourself to improve by trying new things as a leader • Continuing professional development – using reflection to improve your practice and supporting the professional development of others • Acting with integrity – demonstrating good values in your practice by being honest, reliable, trustworthy, warm, genuine, consistent and caring.
2 Working with others – your qualities when working effectively with colleagues within and outside of your work setting	• Developing networks – being able to influence and advocate on behalf of the organisation and sector you work in and being able to promote the sharing of information and ideas. • Building and maintaining relationships – being able to develop good working relationships that are primarily focused on the needs of individuals. • Encouraging contribution – being able to motivate others with your passion for encouraging contributions and by modelling good practice. • Acting with integrity – being able to promote a positive working environment by motivating and inspiring others to work together as one team.

Table 14.4 The five dimensions included within the Leadership Qualities Framework *continued*

Leadership qualities or dimensions	Examples of behaviours
3 Managing services – your qualities to manage services well	• Planning – being able to plan a service that encourages a culture where everything is shaped around individuals' needs, views and desires. • Managing resources – being able to ensure the necessary resources are in place for the service that has been planned. • Managing people – being able to lead from the front by modelling exemplary behaviour that gets the best out of others. • Managing performance – being able to supervise, guide and manage others to ensure best practices are encouraged and opportunities for improvement are made.
4 Improving services – your qualities to support and inspire services to be the very best they can be	• Ensuring the safety of people you support – being able to actively promote and encourage safety and whistleblowing. • Critically evaluating – being able to monitor and evaluate services by building a culture of continuous review, quality and service improvement. • Encouraging improvement and innovation – being able to empower staff to share their ideas and valuing contributions made • Facilitating transformation – being able to communicate to colleagues the benefits of making changes and encourage them to embrace these.
5 Setting direction – your qualities to make changes	• Identifying the context of change – being able to understand the challenges that the organisation faces and the impact these may have as well as the changes that need to be made. • Applying knowledge and evidence – being able to analyse available evidence of good practice before implementing changes. • Making decisions – being able to make sound judgements and decisions in all aspects of your behaviour while reflecting your values and the values of the organisation. • Evaluating impact – being able to assess what has worked well and what hasn't and the reasons why when changes have been made; being able to communicate the impact of changes to others.

Research it

5.1 Leadership in adult social care

Research the Skills for Care's Leadership Qualities Framework to find out how the guidance is used with leaders in the adult social care sector. You can find the link to the guidance here:

https://www.skillsforcare.org.uk/resources/documents/Support-for-leaders-and-managers/Developing-leaders-and-managers/Leadership-Qualities-Framework/Leadership-Qualities-Framework-Guide-for-those-in-governance.pdf

Discuss your findings with your manager.

> **Evidence opportunity**
>
> **5.1 Expected leadership behaviours**
> Develop an information handout with the leadership behaviours that are expected from all leaders in adult social care.

AC 5.2 Model high standards of practice within own work role to encourage others to make a positive difference to the lives of individuals

AC 5.3 Model high standards of practice within own work role to encourage others to make a positive difference to the work environment

In addition to the standards and expectations that are in place for Lead Adult Care Workers and Lead Personal Assistants you will also be expected to know how to model high standards of practice so that you can make a positive difference to the lives of individuals and your work environment. Modelling high standards of practice involves working effectively with others such as team members, other colleagues and those who use or commission their own health or social care services, i.e. the individuals you care for, and families, carers and advocates. As you will have learned, being a Lead involves working closely with others and doing so effectively means that you will be able to achieve the outcomes you and others want. For example, you and a colleague may want to improve the timeliness of the support provided to an individual with care needs and so it is essential that you both agree on what needs to be put in place to make this improvement. Of course, you will only be able to do this if you know what the individual's needs are and it is only by working effectively with the individual that you can get to know them and find out the information that you need to inform you and your colleague's plan of action. Modelling high standards of practice as a Lead involves setting a good example to others so that they aspire to be like you, and it also means having many different skills. Some of these are listed below.

Communicate well

The way you communicate both verbally and non-verbally will influence how effective you are as a leader. For example, if you observe a team member using unsafe work practices when handling medication and you tell them that they have done so in a loud voice and while angrily waving your hands, this may make the team member feel intimidated and be less likely to want to work with you to improve their practices. If, however, you ask to speak to the team member in private and use a polite, assertive tone to explain the reasons why their practices are unsafe they will be more likely to listen to you and work with you to reflect on their work performance so that they can ensure that they practise in safe ways. This may also involve the team member accessing further development opportunities such as training in the safe handling of medicines, or even shadowing you at work so that you can show the high standards of practice you follow and encourage them to ensure individuals are not placed at risk of harm while providing a safe working environment for all.

The way you communicate in writing and when using special methods and adaptations is also important as these can also have an impact on you working effectively with others. For example, if you are a Lead Personal Assistant and are updating the care records for an individual who commissions their own health or social care services then it is important that you use accurate and complete information only and that your records are free from jargon and discriminatory language. Not doing so can mean that the individual no longer wants you to work with them as they may feel devalued and/or disrespected by you. In this way, others who you work with can follow your lead and ensure that they complete records in a manner that is respectful to individuals and ensures an accurate audit trail that others can refer to and understand should they need to.

6Cs

Communication

When working as a Lead in an adult care setting, you will need to ensure that you develop good communication skills, and model these to others, as this is essential for developing working relationships, providing support to your colleagues and leading a team. In your lead role, you will need to ensure that you can communicate well with the individuals that you care for, their families or carers, your colleagues and others that you provide support to or guidance to. Your role and responsibilities will require you to communicate in various ways, both verbally and non-verbally. For example, one of your duties may be to assist an individual to lead their care review. A task such as this will require you to communicate well with the individual, to find out what their preferences are in relation to their care and support, what aspects they think are working well, what are not and what improvements need to be made. You will also need to be able to communicate effectively with the individual's family and other professionals that may also attend the individual's care review. This will require you to take into account their views and preferences while also maintaining the focus on the individual. (See Unit 304 Effective communication in adult care settings/services for more information.)

Foster mutual trust and respect

Developing mutual trust and respect is essential for working effectively with others because doing so will mean that others such as other team members and your colleagues will be more likely to approach you for your advice and/or guidance. This could be over, for example, safe and effective working practices or in relation to how they can further develop their knowledge and/or skills in relation to preventing infections, disposing of waste safely or moving an individual in line with their plan of care. Modelling these high standards of practice will mean that the quality of care provided to individuals will improve, and that the work environment will be a place where individuals and others can feel safe, and sure that their health and wellbeing are being promoted.

Having mutual trust and respect in your relationships with others means that as a Lead you will be promoting the value of learning from each other's experiences, knowledge and skills. In addition, working relationships based on these values promote equality and diversity because all those involved are considered equal partners and their views and contributions are therefore equally as important.

Be honest

Modelling high standards of practice also involves being honest. Honesty is integral for working effectively with others. Without honesty it is difficult to develop good working relationships as there will be no trust between all those involved. This means that misunderstandings may arise and effective communication will not be possible as people will not be willing to share anything about themselves with others. For example, imagine how you would feel if you found out that someone close to you such as a good friend or a family member was not being honest with you over something. Perhaps you would feel angry. Or let down. Or that your relationship was a lie. Honesty is therefore essential for building mutual trust and respect.

Research it

5.2, 5.3 What does being an effective leader mean?

Carry out some research where you work. Find out from the following people what being an effective leader means to them: a team member, a colleague, an individual, an individual's representative such as their family, carer or advocate. Once you have collated their feedback, did any of their responses surprise you? Were there any similarities? Were there any differences? How did their responses compare to your views and ideas about what being an effective leader means?

Case study

5.2, 5.3 Modelling high standards of practice

Matt is a Lead Personal Assistant and works within a small team delivering care and support to Justina who has **muscular dystrophy**. Matt decides on his first day at work that he wants to introduce himself to the whole team but rather than meet with them, he decides that he will send them a brief email as he feels this is a more effective way of working. Matt also emails Justina's family and explains in his email that he has not yet had time to meet Justina as he is very busy but would do so very soon.

At the end of Matt's first day, one of the Personal Assistants in the team requests to meet with him to share her concerns over Justina's mobility, which she feels has deteriorated significantly over the last few weeks. Matt explains to the Personal Assistant that, although he accepts that she knows Justina and her needs, she is not a doctor and therefore not qualified to say that Justina's mobility has deteriorated. The Personal Assistant tries again to share her concerns with Matt as she feels he has misunderstood what these are but before she can finish what she is saying Matt tells her that he has to rush off to a meeting and to not worry about this anymore. On his way out, Matt asks the Personal Assistant whether she could do him a favour and tell Justina that he will find time to meet with her but he's not really sure when that will be.

Discuss:
1 Why do you think it is important for Matt to develop his skills and behaviours?
2 How would you model high standards of practice to Matt?
3 Put together a brief presentation that you can use when supporting others in your team to model high standards of practice.

Key term

Muscular dystrophy refers to a group of conditions that affect the muscles and results in the body's muscles weakening and breaking down over time.

Be supportive

Being supportive is another skill that you will be expected to demonstrate as a Lead, and is essential for modelling high standards of practice. Without support, modelling high standards of practice would be very difficult because unless everyone feels supported in their job roles they may not feel able to carry out their day-to-day work activities effectively. You can be supportive or show your support for others in many different ways. For example, you can provide another team member with reassurance if they are finding a work task difficult, such as supporting an individual to mobilise, or listen attentively to a colleague who is finding it difficult to balance their work and family commitments.

Modelling high standards of practice involves working alongside others, respecting their differences, developing positive relationships, learning from one another and sharing knowledge, skills and experiences.

Evidence opportunity

5.2, 5.3 Modelling high standards of practice

Your assessor will observe you for these ACs. You will need to show your assessor how you model high standards of practice within your work role and how you encourage others to make a positive difference to individuals and your work setting. Remember, others may include team members, other colleagues, families, carers, advocates and those who use or commission their own health or social care services.

AC 5.4 Share ideas to improve services with others

Sharing ideas with others to improve services is another important aspect of your Lead role and integral to:

- confirming the knowledge you have to others
- developing the knowledge you have with others
- being open to learning new knowledge from others
- enabling others to respect you in your Lead role
- working in partnership with others.

This is because sharing ideas not only benefits you but also the individuals you support, their families and carers, your colleagues and the team you work within by creating an environment where everyone can learn from each other and improve. Sharing ideas is also essential for best practice and can keep you and others you work with feeling motivated and enthusiastic about new and improved ways of working. Sharing ideas in an environment where everyone feels comfortable means that you and others you work with will get to know each other and learn to work together effectively to improve services and provide quality care.

> **Reflect on it**
>
> **5.4 Share ideas**
>
> Reflect on an occasion you shared your ideas for improving an aspect of a service. Who did you share your ideas with? Why? How did you do it? What impact did your ideas have on the service and on others?

> **Evidence opportunity**
>
> **5.4 Improving services with others**
>
> You will be observed for this AC. You could ask your assessor to observe you leading a meeting or having a discussion with another colleague that involves you sharing ideas to improve an aspect of the service. You could also ask your manager to provide you with a Witness Testimony.

AC 5.5 Promote partnership approaches to supporting individuals

In Unit 300, Responsibilities and ways of working in adult care settings/services, you learned about why it is important to work in partnership with others and the skills and approaches used.

> **Reflect on it**
>
> **5.5 Partnership working**
>
> Reflect on your previous learning in Unit 300 and think about the importance of partnership approaches to supporting individuals including the consequences of not doing so.

Promoting partnership approaches to supporting individuals involves more than just working alongside individuals and supporting others to do the same. It involves working as one team, together. You can promote partnership approaches to supporting individuals by, for example:

- **encouraging contributions from individuals** – involving individuals in decision making, asking individuals for their views and sharing your ideas with individuals encourages individuals to put forward their views and ideas and makes them feel valued and included.
- **communicating effectively with individuals** – making time to listen to what individuals are saying, showing a genuine interest in individuals, being honest with them in your communications and sharing information with individuals openly and in a way they understand can ensure your working relationships with individuals are open and honest.
- **working together with individuals as one team** – creating a culture where you support individuals to achieve their goals and where you place individuals in the centre of all support and care provided encourages you and individuals to share the same goals and vision for the future and encourages collaborative working.
- **modelling good behaviours** – by being professional and using positive behaviours towards individuals such as being respectful, promoting individuals' rights, being kind and polite and being supportive will make individuals feel valued, promote their wellbeing and encourage individuals to want to work with you.

> **Reflect on it**
>
> **5.5 Promoting partnership approaches**
>
> Find out from colleagues and professionals you work with how they promote partnership approaches when supporting individuals. Reflect on the similarities and differences between the partnership approaches they use and the ones you use.

> **Evidence opportunity**
>
> **5.5 Demonstrating the promotion of partnership approaches**
>
> You will be observed for this assessment criterion by your assessor. You could demonstrate how you promote partnership approaches to supporting individuals in your day-to-day tasks over several of your work shifts. Your manager could also provide you with a Witness Testimony.

Legislation	
Act/Regulation	Key points
Health and Social Care Act 2008 (Regulated Activities) Regulations 2014, Regulation 9: Person-centred care	Providers of care must work with the individual and support them to understand and make informed choices and decisions about their care and support. You should also research the key points of the other regulations in this Act.
The Control of Substances Hazardous to Health Regulations 2002	Lead workers must ensure the safety of their own and others' work practices in relation to handling substances such as cleaning substances that may be dangerous to their health.
The Management of Health and Safety at Work Regulations 1999	Lead workers must lead by example and ensure, for example, that they take reasonable care of their own health and safety and those of others such as individuals and visitors and report any health and safety concerns they have.

Also see AC 1.3 for more information on relevant standards.

314 Understanding personal wellbeing

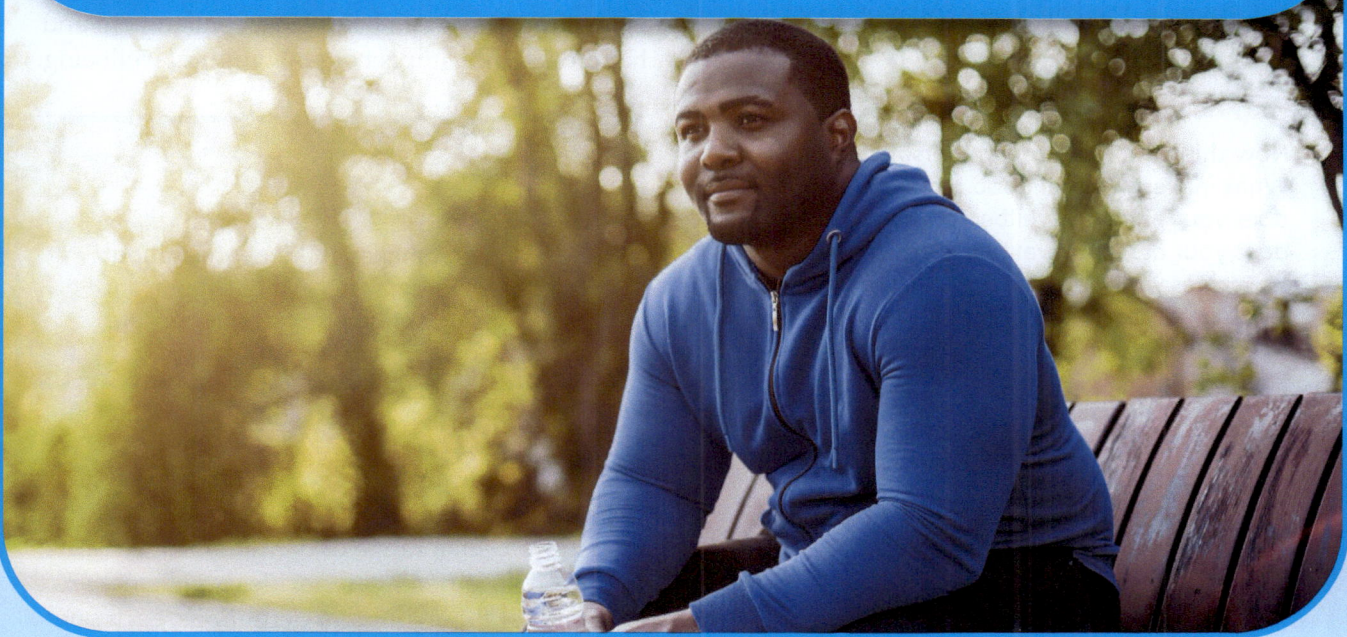

About this unit

Credit value: 3
Guided learning hours: 20

To be able to effectively support individuals with their health and wellbeing it is essential that you understand the importance of your personal wellbeing as this will directly impact on your working practices and the support you provide to individuals and others.

In this unit you will learn about the importance of your personal wellbeing, including the factors that can positively and negatively influence it and the indicators of a deterioration in your personal sense of wellbeing.

You will find out why it's important to maintain and improve your wellbeing and how it can impact on others, your role and your behaviour at work. This unit will also provide you with the opportunity to explore the strategies you use to maintain and improve your wellbeing and the sources of support that are available to you both within the care setting/service where you work and externally.

Finally, you will consider what is meant by stress and anxiety, how you can recognise indicators and triggers of both in yourself and the strategies you use for managing stress and anxiety and building resilience.

Learning outcomes

By the end of this unit you will:

LO1: Understand own wellbeing

LO2: Understand the importance of maintaining and improving own wellbeing

LO3: Know how to maintain and improve own wellbeing

LO4: Know how to manage own stress and anxiety

LO1 Understand own wellbeing

> **Getting started**
>
> Think about an occasion when you felt unwell. For example, this could be in relation to your physical wellbeing or your mental wellbeing. Why did you feel unwell? How did this affect you? How did this impact on others around you?
>
> Now think about your own personal wellbeing. What makes you feel good in yourself? How does your personal wellbeing affect you? How does your personal wellbeing affect others? How does your personal wellbeing affect your work practices?

AC 1.1 Explain what is meant by: a) own wellbeing, b) self-care, c) resilience

AC 1.2 Explain relevance of the following to own life experience: a) own wellbeing, b) self-care, c) resilience

Your wellbeing

Your wellbeing refers to your quality of life and includes your health, happiness and comfort. Your sense of wellbeing is personal to you and will therefore mean different things to different people. The acrostic below can help you to remember the many different aspects of wellbeing; you may think of others that are personal to you. You will also find it useful to reflect on your previous learning around the concept of wellbeing in Unit 308 Supporting individuals with their health and wellbeing.

Wellbeing is personal to you; a unique state of your health, happiness and comfort.

Emotional wellbeing includes having a positive outlook on life and feeling good about it.

Living a healthy lifestyle that is free from pain and distress supports your physical wellbeing.

Living a healthy lifestyle that includes feeling positive towards yourself and others supports your mental wellbeing.

Being social and having positive relationships with others supports your social wellbeing.

Economic wellbeing includes being content with your financial and housing situation.

Intellectual wellbeing includes being rational and having clear and logical thought processes.

Not being afraid to reflect on what you like about yourself as well as your purpose and reason to live forms the basis of your spiritual wellbeing.

Generating a sense of belonging, contentment and happiness is the impact of your cultural wellbeing.

> **Reflect on it**
>
> **1.1** Your personal wellbeing
>
> Reflect on what makes you feel good about yourself. Reflect on the five most important aspects to your wellbeing and why they are important to you.

Self-care

The term 'self-care' refers to the actions you take to protect and improve your wellbeing. Over time there have been a range of definitions of self-care produced by different authorities and below are examples of three different definitions, each one emphasising three different aspects of self-care:

'Self-care is about keeping fit and healthy, understanding when you can look after yourself, when a pharmacist can help, and when to get advice from your GP or another health professional. If you have a long-term condition, self-care is about understanding that condition and how to live with it.'

Source: Warner, B. (2017) Blog 'What does self-care mean and how can it help?' NHS England, 2017

'We define self-care as caring for yourself in your personal and professional roles with compassionate action and mentality … Self-care involves both your personal and professional life. Your self-care impacts the people you care about and the quality of your work, which makes self-care both a professional and personal responsibility.'

Source: The Self-care Institute, 2020

'Self-care is the ability of individuals, families and communities to promote health, prevent disease, maintain health, and cope with illness and disability with or without the support of a health worker.'

Source: World Health Organization (WHO), 2022

> **Research it**
>
> **1.1 The seven pillars of self-care**
>
> Using the weblink below, research the seven 'pillars' or 'domains' of self-care as defined by the International Self-care Foundation (ISF), a UK-registered charity.
>
> https://isfglobal.org/practise-self-care/the-seven-pillars-of-self-care/

Resilience

Your ability to manage and recover from setbacks or difficulties you experience is more commonly referred to as your resilience. Resilience involves being adaptable to unexpected events or circumstances, such as the death of a close relative or losing your job. There are different types of resilience:

- Physical resilience – this form of resilience refers to how your body deals with changes and recovers from illnesses, injuries and physical stress.
- Mental resilience – this form of resilience refers to your capacity or ability to adapt to change and unpredictability.
- Emotional resilience – this form of resilience refers to your ability to manage or regulate your emotional reactions to negative or stressful experiences.
- Social resilience – this form of resilience refers to your ability to work together with others as part of a group or community and to recover from difficult situations that can occur, such as natural disasters.

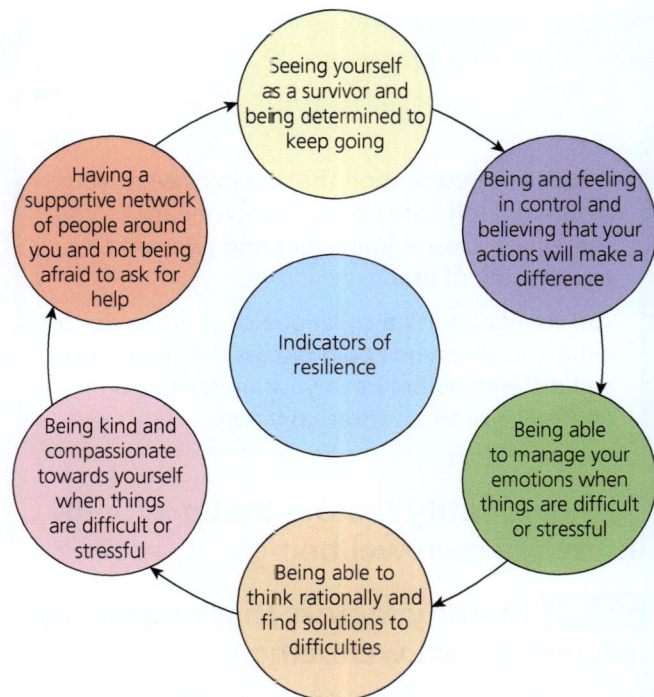

Figure 15.1 Examples of signs of resilience

Figure 15.1 provides you with some more information about the indicators of resilience. How many of these do you recognise in yourself?

Your wellbeing, your ability to self-care and your resilience are very important for your life experience and the quality of your life:

- **Why is your wellbeing important?** As you will have learned there are different aspects that make up your wellbeing. Your wellbeing is important because it affects how satisfied or happy you are with your life; the more content you are with your life the more likely you are to think positively and experience day-to-day life in a positive way even when negative or stressful things happen. Being satisfied and content with your life will also mean that your positivity will influence others around you, thus improving their wellbeing too!
- **Why is your ability to self-care important?** Taking care of yourself is important for your overall health and wellbeing, both physically and mentally. Your ability to self-care affects how you carry out your day-to-day life activities; the more time you take to look after yourself the more relaxed and confident you will feel to try new activities, for example, or deal with life's challenges, thus improving your life experience.
- **Why is building resilience important?** Taking the time to build resilience in yourself will directly impact on the quality of your life because you will learn how to stay positive in your thoughts, even in the face of adversity, and at the same time develop a degree of self-confidence or belief in yourself and your abilities, which is essential for high self-esteem; one of the key ingredients for wellbeing.

It is important to also remember that these three concepts do not work in isolation from each other. They are all intrinsically linked and together are relevant to the quality of life you develop for yourself.

> **Evidence opportunity**
>
> **1.1, 1.2** Your wellbeing, self-care and resilience
>
> Produce a presentation that explains what your wellbeing, self-care and resilience means to you, and why these are important and relevant to your quality of life.
>
> You could also ask a colleague of yours to do the same and then you could discuss the similarities and differences between your understanding and theirs of these three concepts.

> **Reflect on it**
>
> **1.3, 1.4** Factors that influence your wellbeing
>
> Reflect on three factors that positively influence your wellbeing and the reasons why and then three factors that negatively influence your wellbeing and the reasons why.

AC 1.3 Identify factors that positively influence own wellbeing

AC 1.4 Identify factors that negatively influence own wellbeing

Your wellbeing is personal to you and how you experience it will also be unique, therefore the factors that positively and negatively influence it will vary from one person to another. Table 15.1 provides you with some examples of both positive and negative factors that can contribute to your wellbeing.

> **6Cs**
>
> **Courage**
>
> It takes courage to be honest with yourself and identify the factors that negatively influence your wellbeing. Understanding what these are takes a lot of courage but it also means that you can then focus more on the positive factors that contribute to your wellbeing. Being honest with yourself means that you can then empathise with others when supporting them with their wellbeing.

The case study below will help you to further explore the factors that can influence wellbeing.

Table 15.1 Factors that positively and negatively influence wellbeing

Factors that positively influence wellbeing	Factors that negatively influence wellbeing
• Being in good physical health • Having good mental health • Regular exercise • Sufficient sleep • Participating in activities you enjoy • Doing a job that you like and that you get job satisfaction from • Being resilient and staying positive when things go wrong • Feeling confident in yourself and your abilities • Celebrating your achievements, however small • Developing a sense of purpose and meaning in your life • Spending time with people who make you feel good about yourself • Surrounding yourself with people who support you • Having healthy relationships	• Illness, i.e. physical, mental • Lack of rest/sleep • Following an unhealthy lifestyle, i.e. eating unhealthily, drinking too much alcohol, smoking, not exercising your body or mind • Stress (see LO4, AC4.1 in this unit for the meaning of this term) • Anxiety (see LO4, AC4.1 in this unit for the meaning of this term) • Financial pressures, which can lead to stress and anxiety • Not spending quality time with others that are important in your life, such as your family and friends • Spending time with others who may be negative or unhappy, which can make you feel unhappy and anxious • Unexpected life events that you do not have time to prepare for, such as the death of a relative, the break-up of a relationship or life changing injuries from an accident

Case study

1.1, 1.2, 1.3, 1.4 Understanding wellbeing

Emma lives with her partner Joel and together they have two children. Emma works long shifts in the local hospital while Joel looks after their two children aged 10 months and 22 months, who have been feeling unwell over the last few days.

Last night both children developed high temperatures and after a visit to A&E were both diagnosed with tonsilitis and prescribed antibiotics. Joel slept in the children's bedroom when they returned home in the early hours so that they did not disturb Emma who was due into work again the following day for another long shift.

In the morning, Emma tells Joel about her long shift at work and how tired she was feeling as it was so busy that she hadn't even had time for a proper break. Joel makes Emma some breakfast and then gets the children up for their breakfast. As the children seem a bit happier this morning, Emma tells Joel she is going to pop out to see a friend of hers before work. When Emma leaves, Joel spends some time playing with the children and then puts them to bed mid-morning when they begin to look tired.

Joel comes downstairs and after briefly sitting down in the kitchen falls asleep. Half an hour later Emma returns, wakes Joel up and shouts, 'Joel, the kitchen looks a mess! What have you been doing?'. Joel becomes tearful and tells Emma he feels exhausted and that he doesn't think he is very good at looking after the children as he doesn't even have time to make himself anything to eat and doesn't know if he can manage any longer.

Discuss

- What factors are impacting negatively on Joel's wellbeing?
- What factors could positively influence Joel's wellbeing?
- How could Emma support Joel?

Evidence opportunity

1.3, 1.4 Positive and negative influences

Draw a mind map of the factors that positively and negatively influence your wellbeing.

AC 1.5 Outline indicators of own sense of wellbeing
AC 1.6 Outline indicators of a deterioration in own sense of wellbeing

Recognising the signs of your own sense of wellbeing, including signs of its deterioration, will help you to maintain and improve your wellbeing by preventing it from worsening and by reducing the negative impact of deterioration on you, your self-confidence, your resilience and on others around you. You will have an opportunity to further explore how to maintain and improve your wellbeing in LO3 of this unit.

The indicators of your sense of wellbeing and its deterioration will be specific and unique to you and can include physical, emotional, psychological and social indicators. Knowing what the indicators are for you, and recognising the signs of deterioration early, will help you to stay focused and in control of your wellbeing.

Physical indicators of your sense of wellbeing can include: experiencing good physical health with absence of illness, pain and distress, participating in and enjoying physical activity, feelings of physical comfort.

Physical indicators of a deterioration in your sense of wellbeing can include: loss of appetite, eating a lot more than you usually do, dramatic weight gain, dramatic weight loss, not taking care of your personal hygiene, not washing and changing your clothes regularly, not carrying out day-to-day tasks like washing up, cleaning, doing the laundry or going food shopping, sleeping a lot more or less, poor concentration.

Emotional indicators of your sense of wellbeing can include: experiencing positive moods, experiencing positive emotions, feeling mild/even tempered, feeling relaxed, being optimistic about the future.

Emotional indicators of a deterioration in your sense of wellbeing can include: experiencing negative moods, experiencing negative emotions, increased feelings of agitation, increased feelings of irritation, feeling alone and distant from those around you, feelings of hopelessness, feeling helpless all the time, feeling overwhelmed all the time, feeling worthless, worrying more.

Psychological indicators of your sense of wellbeing can include: feeling in control, feeling secure in yourself, feeling that you're able and competent, feeling that others view you as able and competent, feeling energetic, feeling purposeful, feeling motivated, being keen and committed to improving and developing yourself, connecting with others through shared beliefs and/or outlook.

Psychological indicators of a deterioration in your sense of wellbeing can include: finding it difficult to make decisions, finding it difficult to focus on one idea or topic when talking and/or thinking, being easily distracted.

Social indicators of your sense of wellbeing can include: feelings of being confident, feelings of being accepted, feelings of belonging and being part of something, feeling safe through your social relationships with others, feeling supported through your social relationships with others, supporting others through your social relationships with them.

Social indicators of a deterioration in your sense of wellbeing can include: withdrawal from social activities you once enjoyed, not socialising with others and preferring to be on your own instead.

Evidence opportunity

1.5, 1.6 You and your wellbeing

Think about an occasion or a time in your life when you had a good sense of wellbeing and another occasion or time in your life when your sense of wellbeing deteriorated. Write a reflective account of both. For each one, briefly describe the indicators that you recognise of your own sense of wellbeing and the indicators that you recognise of a deterioration in your sense of wellbeing.

LO2 Understand the importance of maintaining and improving own wellbeing

Getting started

Reflect on an occasion when you were feeling unwell but had to go into work. How did this make you feel? How did being unwell affect your work practices and your actions at work? How did being unwell impact on others at work? Why?

AC 2.1 Explain how own wellbeing may impact on role and behaviour at work

AC 2.2 Explain how own wellbeing may impact on others

Maintaining your wellbeing and being able to recognise the early indicators of a deterioration in it is important. Not doing so can have a negative impact on your job and behaviour at work, as well as on others both in the care setting/service where you work, such as individuals, colleagues, team members, families, carers, advocates or visiting tradespeople, and others with whom you have personal relationships outside of work, such as family, partner and friends.

Impact of your wellbeing at work

Your wellbeing impacts on your work in different ways. This can be explored in terms of the aspects that make up your sense of wellbeing: social, emotional, cultural, spiritual, intellectual, economic, physical and mental.

Social wellbeing means being able to develop good working relationships not only with individuals but also with individuals' families, carers, advocates, other colleagues, team members including your supervisor/manager and tradespeople who visit. By doing so you will be demonstrating positive ways of working which welcome ideas and suggestions from others. If your social wellbeing is poor then you may prefer to work on your own, not as part of a team, and may as a result become isolated from others, thus making your role as a Lead who provides support and encouragement to others difficult to fulfil.

Emotional wellbeing means feeling positive about yourself, your job role and others around you. This will in turn encourage individuals and others you work with to approach you for advice or guidance when things go wrong. If your emotional wellbeing is poor then you may feel overwhelmed by the demands of your job role and may as a result become stressed at work, anxious about your day-to-day responsibilities or find ways of trying to avoid others so that they do not approach you.

Cultural wellbeing means you enjoy going to work and being part of a team; you will look forward to carrying out your day-to-day responsibilities and you will be more likely to take the time to get to know the individuals and others you work with so that you can learn about them too. If your cultural wellbeing is poor then you may feel that you do not belong in the care setting/service where you work, you may doubt your own abilities and may even feel excluded from the team that you lead.

Spiritual wellbeing means feeling that your life has purpose and viewing your role at work as an important one that brings out the best in you. If your spiritual wellbeing is poor then you may feel unsure about what your purpose in life is and, as a result, you may find it difficult to work with others, carry out your role and behave in a way that others expect of a Lead. It will be difficult for you to support others and set a good example as a Lead because you will not have the inner strength or belief in yourself to do so.

Intellectual wellbeing means you will have built resilience when working together with others who may have different views and ideas to yours and you will be clear in your thought processes about how to act at work when supporting individuals and when working with others. Others you work with will also feel confident in your abilities to problem solve and think through situations logically and rationally. If your intellectual wellbeing is poor, you may become disillusioned with your role at work and with the situations you have to manage as a Lead. You may also lose your sense of fulfilment and purpose at work. These negative feelings and thoughts could result in you being despondent and unmotivated when carrying out your day-to-day responsibilities.

Economic wellbeing means being content in your role and satisfied with your income. These positive feelings will translate into how you carry out your role in supporting individuals and others at work. If your economic wellbeing is poor, you may feel frustrated or fed up with your current situation and may find it difficult to be patient and understanding towards individuals and others.

Physical wellbeing means feeling healthy and being able to carry out your role effectively, even when work is busy and presents challenges. You will also be more likely to encourage individuals and others to look after and improve their physical wellbeing and be a good role model to them. If your physical wellbeing is poor, you may find it difficult to carry out some aspects of your job role, particularly if they involve supporting individuals to mobilise or take part in activities. You may also get tired more quickly and find it difficult to participate in activities with others.

Mental wellbeing means feeling confident in your own abilities at work and having positive feelings of self-worth that will enable you to work with others and lead your team through times of stress. If your mental wellbeing is poor, you will lack self-belief and confidence in yourself, which will make it very difficult for individuals and others to trust in your decisions and respect you.

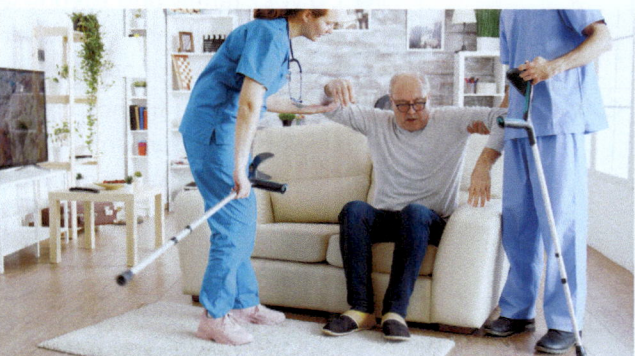

Figure 15.2 How does your wellbeing affect your job role?

Impact of your wellbeing at home

Your wellbeing doesn't just affect your job role and your working relationships, it also impacts on your life away from work, at home and in your personal relationships. You may have heard the saying, 'leave your work at work and don't bring it home' but how realistic is this? Does your wellbeing affect your personal relationships with those that are closest to you, such as your family, your partner or your friends? The answer is, yes of course it does!

Just as you considered how the different aspects of your wellbeing can impact on your job role and working relationships you must also be aware of when your wellbeing is impacting on your personal relationships and the consequences of this. To do this, you need to be aware of your sense of wellbeing and when it is deteriorating so that you can do something about it. This topic was explored in LO1 of this unit which you may find useful to review.

Below is a useful checklist with questions that you can ask yourself that will help you to assess the impact that your wellbeing is having on your personal relationships; 'Yes' replies indicate positive impacts and 'No' replies indicate negative impacts. Answer the questions as honestly as you can!

Table 15.2 Assessing the impact of your wellbeing

Wellbeing aspect	Impact on personal relationships	Yes or No
Social	<ul><li>Do you look forward to meeting your friends outside of work?</li><li>Do you enjoy being at home?</li><li>Do your family and friends enjoy being around you?</li><li>Do you try and meet up with family and friends whenever you can?</li></ul>	
Emotional	<ul><li>Do you have a positive outlook on life?</li><li>Do your family and friends say you're positive?</li><li>Do your family and friends confide in you when they are having difficulties?</li><li>Do you seek support from your family and friends when you need it?</li></ul>	
Cultural	<ul><li>Do you have a friendship group?</li><li>Do you and your family share similar/the same values?</li><li>Do you have a sense of belonging when you are around your family/friends?</li><li>Do you find it interesting to know about your family/friends' beliefs and preferences?</li></ul>	
Spiritual	<ul><li>Do you like spending time with your family/friends?</li><li>Do your family/friends like spending time with you?</li><li>Do your family/friends make you feel good about yourself?</li><li>Do your family/friends motivate you to do well?</li></ul>	
Intellectual	<ul><li>Do you think independently from your family/friends?</li><li>Do you enjoy doing things independently from your family/friends?</li><li>Do you have opportunities to be mentally stimulated by your family/friends?</li><li>Do your family/friends think of you as rational and logical in your thinking?</li></ul>	
Economic	<ul><li>Do you describe yourself as financially content?</li><li>Do your family/friends describe you as financially content?</li><li>Do you discuss finances with your family/friends?</li><li>Do you think about how you can improve your financial situation?</li></ul>	
Physical	<ul><li>Does your physical wellbeing prevent you from doing things with your family/friends?</li><li>Do you maintain your physical wellbeing?</li><li>Do your family/friends think that you maintain your physical wellbeing?</li><li>Do you feel able to discuss your physical wellbeing with your family/friends?</li></ul>	
Mental	<ul><li>Do you describe yourself as a positive person?</li><li>Do you behave positively towards your family/friends?</li><li>Do you feel worthy of the family/friends you have?</li><li>Do you feel able to discuss your mental wellbeing with your family/friends?</li></ul>	

Reflect on it

2.2 Impacts on your personal relationships

Reflect on the aspects of your wellbeing that are impacting positively on your personal relationships. How does this make you feel? Now think about the aspects that are impacting negatively on your personal relationships. How can you improve these aspects of your wellbeing?

Evidence opportunity

2.1, 2.2 Your wellbeing at work and at home

Discuss with a colleague who knows you well how your wellbeing may impact on your job role and behaviour at work and on others, both at work and at home. Remember to provide examples of how your wellbeing can have an impact and the importance of it doing so positively.

LO3 Know how to maintain and improve own wellbeing

> **Getting started**
>
> Reflect on someone you know well who was unwell. Why were they unwell? How did this impact on them? How did this impact on you? How did this impact on others who knew them? Why was it important for them to improve their wellbeing? How did they do this?

AC 3.1 Explain own strategies to maintain and improve wellbeing

Knowing how to maintain and improve your personal wellbeing is very important as not doing so, as you've already learned in LO2, can impact on your role and behaviour at work in negative ways as well as on your working and personal relationships with others both at work and at home. Table 15.3 provides some examples of strategies that you can use to maintain your wellbeing and to respond to any changes in your wellbeing when you recognise indicators of deterioration of your body and mind. Remember that certain strategies may work well for others but not you and some strategies may work well if you recognise deterioration in one aspect of your wellbeing but not necessarily for another aspect, so you must bear this in mind when putting any new strategy in place; as we have said before you're unique and so the strategy you choose to use will be specific to you and your situation.

Table 15.3 Strategies to maintain and improve wellbeing

Strategy to maintain and improve wellbeing	How to implement it
Eating a balanced diet – healthy eating	If you are feeling tired or have difficulty with the physical demands of your job role, eating a balanced diet can help to improve your physical wellbeing by providing you with the energy that your body needs to be active and keep going. Eating a healthy balanced diet also means that your body can maintain its strength and health and help prevent illness and diseases such as Type 2 diabetes (by eating a diet that is low in saturated fat and high in fibre) and heart disease (by eating fruits, vegetables, wholegrains and low-fat dairy).
Having a healthy lifestyle	If you want to improve your physical wellbeing because you recognise that you are having more frequent pain when you move around then having a healthy lifestyle can help to reduce the risk of the pain worsening or developing into illness or diseases. You can do this not only by having a healthy diet but also by avoiding alcohol and smoking, as well as introducing physical exercise as part of your daily routine such as by walking the dog or doing some gardening or going to the gym.
Exercise – getting some exercise	If you are finding it difficult to complete an activity or task that you have been asked to undertake, then taking a walk can distract you from how you are feeling at that moment in time because it involves a change of scenery for your body and mind. You can come back feeling energised again and therefore more likely to be able to problem solve with a clear mind and find creative ways of achieving what you have been asked to do. If you are finding it difficult to concentrate because you are feeling worried about understanding how to carry out a new activity at work, then participating in a quiz outside of work with a friend is a good exercise for your brain as it provides intellectual stimulation and can be a good way to reconnect with your thought processes and think logically and rationally again. It can help you to get things back into perspective.
Having proper sleep and rest	If you are feeling overwhelmed and unable to manage day-to-day activities, for example due to feeling anxious about a relative you are caring for at home, then you can improve your mental, emotional and physical wellbeing by developing a daily sleep and rest routine by ensuring that you get up and go to bed at roughly the same times every day. Having restful periods during the day, even if it's just five minutes where you can be in a quiet environment so that you feel you've taken a break, can make you feel less anxious.

Table 15.3 Strategies to maintain and improve wellbeing *continued*

Strategy to maintain and improve wellbeing	How to implement it
Meditation – relaxing your body and clearing your mind	If an unexpected situation arises at work, such as an individual becoming verbally abusive towards you, and you recognise a deterioration of your emotional health because you are frightened, then you can use meditation by taking some slow deep breaths. This can calm your body and mind very quickly, while repeating a mantra in your head such as 'I will stay calm, I will be alright' can significantly reduce your stress and anxiety levels; topics you'll learn about more in LO4.
Visualisation – imagining yourself somewhere else	If you recognise indicators that there is a deterioration of your mental wellbeing, for example because you are worried about passing an exam, then use visualisation to calm your mind from those negative thoughts. Replace those thoughts with positive ones where you feel happy with yourself because you know you've worked hard for your exam and are going to do your very best. Once your mind is calm, your body will be too as it will feel more relaxed and less in panic mode, i.e. dry mouth, sweaty hands, fast beating heart.
Having support around you – having supportive people around you	If you have moved to a new area to live in and are finding it difficult to fit in or are becoming isolated then participating in a local community group can help you to meet others who share the same or similar values and beliefs and develop new friendships. Having supportive people in your life will mean that you will have positive and healthy relationships with people that you can ask for help if you need it and talk things through, which can avoid you feeling excluded and as if you have to deal with things on your own.
Affection – getting a hug	If you have suffered the loss of someone close to you and recognise that your emotional health has deteriorated because you are frightened you will not be able to manage without them then having a loved one give you a hug can be very comforting. When you hug someone, oxytocin is released and this causes a reduction in blood pressure thus reducing stress levels and replacing these with happiness and relaxation. Being close to someone physically can provide much needed comfort at such a difficult time.
Making time for yourself – doing what you enjoy	If you are feeling unsure or doubting your purpose in life, for example due to not having job satisfaction, then you need to ensure that you take care of yourself. You can do this by taking up a favourite hobby again, treating yourself to a nice bath or watching a film or reading a book you've wanted to for a while. Making time for yourself doesn't have to take up much time; even if you do it just for ten minutes a day, or at the end of a long shift, or on your day off from work, it will provide you with something to look forward to and make you feel good in yourself.
Being kind to yourself – treating yourself with care and compassion	If you are feeling despondent about your current financial situation and you notice a deterioration in your overall wellbeing, you can treat yourself kindly by talking to yourself about your financial situation in a positive light when things are not what you'd hoped for. By being realistic with yourself about what you can and can't do, you will help yourself remain in control of your emotions and be in a better position to take action to improve your financial situation.
Being kind towards others – treating others with care and compassion	If you are leading a team and recognise that you need to improve your social wellbeing, you can focus on developing more positive working relationships with others by being kind to someone else such as taking the time to listen to what is worrying a new member of staff. This will not only help you feel that you've helped someone else and have improved their wellbeing, but you will also improve your wellbeing by making you feel good about yourself and by getting to know another member of the team.

> **Research it**
>
> **3.1 Improving mental wellbeing**
>
> Read the top tips suggested by the 'Better Health – Every Mind Matters' campaign that has been endorsed by the NHS for improving mental wellbeing by using the weblink below.
>
> www.nhs.uk/every-mind-matters/mental-wellbeing-tips/top-tips-to-improve-your-mental-wellbeing/
>
> Discuss your findings with someone who knows you well. Have you or they ever used any of these strategies for improving mental wellbeing?

> **Evidence opportunity**
>
> **3.1 Maintaining your wellbeing**
>
> Write a reflective account about the strategies that you use to enable you to maintain your wellbeing and the strategies you use when you recognise that your wellbeing has deteriorated. Perhaps you could think about an occasion or a period in your life when you used them and the reasons why.

AC 3.2 Identify sources of support available for maintaining own wellbeing

AC 3.3 Explain how to access sources of support to maintain own wellbeing

If you have tried different strategies to maintain and improve your wellbeing and they have not worked or you find that your wellbeing is still impacting negatively on your role and behaviour at work and on others, you could benefit from further support that is available from both within and outside of the care setting/service where you work. Below are some examples of the many internal and external sources of support that are available for maintaining your wellbeing; you will find it useful to know about these and how to access them even if you do not see these as relevant to you now, because they may be in the future, if not for you then for someone else such as another member of your team.

Internal sources of support and how to access them

- **Supervision** with your manager or employer is where you meet regularly and formally to discuss any issues that are affecting you at work including your wellbeing. For example, you may be finding it difficult to concentrate at work because you may be worried about an older relative you are caring for at home. Your manager or employer could discuss with you how they can support you with your current situation; for example, they may suggest you having access to a private room/office where you can phone your relative during your morning break or lunch hour to check that they are alright. They may suggest that you speak to the named welfare person in the care setting/service where you work or to an external organisation such as Age UK or a local support group for carers of older relatives and provide you with a telephone number you can ring, a website you can log onto or an information leaflet that includes additional information about these services.

- **Employee assistance schemes or programmes** are led by the employer and are designed to help employees deal with personal issues that they may be experiencing either at work or at home that are impacting negatively on their health, wellbeing and/or performance at work. For example, you may be experiencing stress and anxiety, grief and loss, concern over your own or someone else's addiction having difficulties managing your finances, managing work-related stress and/or conflict, relationship issues such as domestic abuse, divorce, childcare and parenting issues or caring for a relative.

The employee assistance scheme is confidential and therefore an employee does not need to let their employer know that they've accessed it. The scheme offers specialist support from professionals who have expertise in, for example, psychology, social work or finance. You can access the scheme by contacting them directly and accessing their support available through video, web chat, tele support, online groups or you can also refer yourself for a face-to-face, in person counselling session.

- **Mentor or buddying schemes** also provide support to employees to maintain their wellbeing. **A mentoring scheme** offers formal, structured support through a mentor, someone who works within your care setting/service and is either working at a higher level or has previous experience and training of being a mentor. The mentee (that's you) and the mentor will draw up a formal agreement at the beginning of your mentoring support to establish what support can and can't be provided and to agree on what outcomes you would like from the support so that you can both work on these together as a working partnership. The length of the mentoring agreement will depend on the outcomes to be achieved. The mentor will also offer the mentee opportunities for personal and professional development and discussions between them will be confidential.
- **A buddying scheme** offers informal support through a buddy, one of your peers or colleagues who may be working at the same level as you or in a similar role to yours in the care setting/service where you work. Unlike a mentor, a buddy does not require specialised training. A buddy provides advice and support with issues that you may be experiencing and that are impacting negatively on your wellbeing. For example, they may be able to offer advice with carrying out a work task that you are finding stressful by giving you the opportunity to shadow them so you can observe and ask them questions. A buddy will usually provide support over a short period of time.

> **Reflect on it**
>
> **3.2, 3.3 Accessing support**
>
> Reflect on the benefits for your wellbeing and your role at work of accessing support through supervision, an employee assistance scheme, a mentor or buddying scheme.

External sources of support and how to access them

- **Self-help tools** are a useful way for you to use and check your wellbeing and can come in many different forms. Some examples are included below; can you think of any others?

Online self-help tools:
- The 'How Are You?' free to use self-assessment tool endorsed by the NHS and part of the Better Health programme – a quiz that asks questions about your lifestyle and wellbeing behaviours, such as your level of physical activity, your diet and whether you smoke, to let you know how you are doing with your health and wellbeing; note that it's not a medical assessment.
- The 'How Resilient Are You?' free to use self-help tool from Mind Tools – a quiz that helps you to understand how resilient you are and that provides advice and guidance on how you can become even more resilient. In the quiz, you'll be asked to answer 16 statements and to click on the column that best describes you; when you finish you'll be asked to click on the 'Calculate My Total' button and then consider the advice that follows.

> **Research it**
>
> **3.2, 3.3 How resilient are you?**
>
> Research the Mind Tools' 'How Resilient Are You?' self-help tool using the weblink below and complete the online questionnaire. Reflect on your score, the advice provided and how you plan to use it to improve your wellbeing.
>
> www.mindtools.com/ajk5lwl/how-resilient-are-you

- **Keeping a journal** – for example, if you are in an abusive relationship then keeping a journal is a self-help tool that can help you make sense of your thoughts and feelings and can help you decide what actions you can take to improve your wellbeing and the situation you're in. You don't need to be good at writing to keep a journal; you could make voice recordings if you prefer.
- **Being creative** – if you have experienced trauma then doing a creative activity such as writing poetry or painting can help you to express your thoughts and feelings, make sense of what has happened and can at the same time improve your confidence and self-esteem. Again, you don't need to access poetry or painting activities formally through a group, you can complete these activities in private by yourself.
- **Apps and websites** also provide support to maintain your wellbeing; some examples of

both are included below (note that the apps are available to download for free on iPhone (App Store) and Android (Google Play), but they may have in-app purchases):

- Stay Alive is an online mobile phone app designed to support you or someone else you have concerns over that has suicidal and/or self-harming thoughts; it includes resources and techniques that can be used to maintain your wellbeing.
- Headspace is an online mobile phone app that provides resources on mindfulness and meditation to help maintain your wellbeing by specifically focusing on stress, anxiety and sleep.
- Mood Tools is an online mobile phone app which provides you with strategies to manage low mood and depression.
- The NHS' website can be accessed for free and contains many useful resources including guides, tools and activities to maintain your wellbeing such as exercise guidance to improve your fitness and wellbeing, information and advice about eating a healthy, balanced diet, and tips for improving your mental wellbeing.
- Mind's website can be accessed for free and contains resources, information and support on mental health and wellbeing such as how to access support and services available including professional help (a topic you'll be exploring in AC3.4 of this unit), telephone helplines that provide information about where to get help and an online community called 'Side by Side' that helps you talk about your mental wellbeing with others who have also experienced difficulties with their mental wellbeing.
- Anxiety UK's website can be accessed for free and is a national registered charity that provides many services to help maintain wellbeing including therapy services such as counselling. Counselling, online courses (for example on anxiety management) and support groups (for example via Zoom) are available to members at discounted rates via their website and have to be booked and paid for online. They also have their own magazine, 'Anxious Times' that can be ordered and downloaded from their website.

- **Local groups and networks** offer local and specialised support to maintain wellbeing; all can be accessed in person, over the telephone and online.
  - Mental Health UK offer support groups across communities to reduce the isolation that people with mental illness can experience by providing them with opportunities to meet others. The focus of the support groups varies depending on the needs of the local community, but they all provide opportunities to meet with others to enhance wellbeing, for example by engaging in sport and leisure, cooking, gardening, and meeting with others to help with understanding how to access mental illness services.
  - Network for Wellbeing is a registered charity that inspires communities to connect and take action for creating and building wellbeing by for example running a venue for retreats (Eden Rise), webinars on wellbeing, community projects and events focused on physical activity such as walking and cycling.
  - Wellbeing Networks across the UK provide information and resources on wellbeing as well as opportunities for people to meet others and get involved in their local community to improve their mental and physical wellbeing.

> **Evidence opportunity**
>
> **3.2, 3.3 Sources of support**
>
> Produce a presentation for new team members that includes the following:
>
> 1. three sources of support available in your care setting/service for maintaining wellbeing
> 2. three sources of support available outside of your care setting/service for maintaining wellbeing
> 3. an explanation of how to access each source of support for maintaining wellbeing.

AC 3.4 Explain how to access professional help if needed to support own wellbeing

Professional help to support wellbeing is also available if you feel that you would benefit from speaking to and/or meeting with a qualified professional such as a counsellor, **psychiatrist** or

psychotherapist (i.e. in relation to your thoughts and feelings) or with a dietician, physiotherapist or **occupational therapist** (i.e. in relation to your physical health and wellbeing). Depending on what type of professional help you require to support your wellbeing you can access this by:

- referring yourself to the services that accept self-referrals
- a professional referring you to the service when they have concerns over your wellbeing
- a non-professional such as a family member or friend referring you to the service when they have concerns over your wellbeing or because you have asked them to do so on your behalf as you feel unable to.

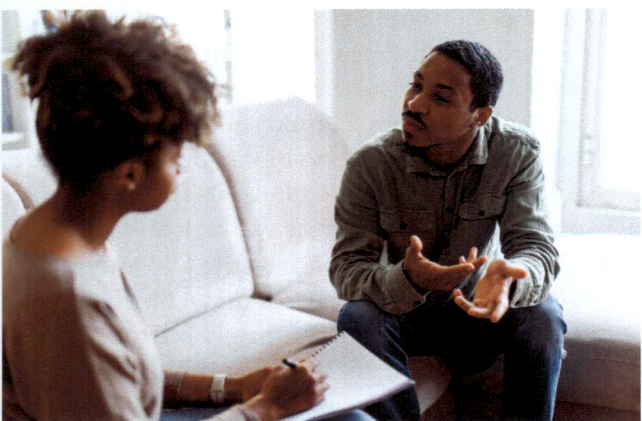

Figure 15.3 What does professional help mean to you?

There are many different types of professionals that work across a range of organisations, industries and sectors to support your wellbeing. For your mental, emotional and psychological wellbeing you may want to access a counsellor with whom you can talk through your feelings and emotions without being judged and to help you find solutions to your problems. Counsellors can work across many different organisations including in the NHS, education and workplace.

If you require help to support your mental wellbeing then you can access a psychiatrist. Psychiatrists are medically qualified doctors who specialise in the treatment and prevention of mental health conditions and can treat conditions such as anxiety and panic attacks, eating disorders and sleep disorders. Psychiatrists work in GP surgeries, outpatient clinics and hospital wards. Psychotherapists diagnose and treat emotional, social or mental health issues such as managing stress, feelings of depression, or difficulties coming to term with loss of, for example, your job or a loved one. Psychotherapists work in hospitals, local clinics, health centres and in the community.

For your physical health and wellbeing you may want to access a dietician for guidance on how to make better lifestyle and food choices to support your wellbeing. Dieticians can work in a wide range of organisations such as in the NHS, education, the sport industry and in private practice. You may need to access professional help from a physiotherapist to promote or restore your physical, psychological and social wellbeing, for example after an accident at work. Physiotherapists can be accessed in acute, community and workplace settings. **Osteopaths** can support your physical and overall wellbeing by providing treatment to the body's skeleton, its muscles, joints and ligaments and you may need to access one following, for example, a back injury that you've sustained that is causing you pain. Osteopathy is available in NHS settings in some areas; in others it is available in private practices.

> **Key terms**
>
> **Psychiatrists** are medically qualified doctors who specialises in psychiatry and can diagnose and prescribe treatments and medication.
>
> **Psychotherapists** are trained therapists who assess and treat a range of emotional, social or mental health issues.
>
> **Osteopaths** are qualified health professionals whose role it is to increase the mobility of joints, relieve muscle tension and enhance blood supply to tissues through treatments such as stretching, massage and physical manipulation.

How to access professional help

- If you are working, your employer may run an Employee Assistance Programme that you can access without going through your manager, HR or your GP. Your employer may also have an occupational health professional that you can access for additional support; usually your manager will refer you to them.
- If you are in education, your education provider may have a counselling service that you can access without going through your tutors or GP.
- Your GP may refer to you to one of the above professional help services after speaking with you.
- You can also refer yourself to one of these services; some GPs may give you a telephone number to ring so that you can refer yourself.
- You can access specific professional help such as talking therapies for mental health problems through the Improving Access to Psychological Therapy (IAPT) service, an NHS programme available in most areas of England. For this service you can refer yourself and do not need to go through your GP.
- Charities and voluntary organisations can also offer professional help to support your wellbeing and usually specialise in a specific type of support such as Cruse Bereavement Care for bereavement advice and support.
- You can also access professional help through the private sector and for some services offered you do not need to be referred to these by your GP, you can refer yourself; it is a good idea when looking for a qualified professional to support your wellbeing that you search websites that only list registered professionals, e.g. the Counselling Directory for counsellors and therapists or the British Psychological Society (BPS) for local therapists.

Evidence opportunity

3.4 Accessing professional help

Discuss with someone who knows you well how you could access professional help to support two different aspects of your wellbeing.

LO4 Know how to manage own stress and anxiety

Getting started

Think about an occasion when you felt stressed and anxious. What made you feel stressed and anxious, and why? How did you feel physically? How did you feel emotionally? Did you notice any changes in how you were behaving on a day-to-day basis? For example, did you find yourself becoming very tearful but not knowing why or did you feel very negative about yourself? Did you become irritable towards others without meaning to, or find that you couldn't sleep or concentrate very well?

AC 4.1 Explain what is meant by stress and anxiety

Our busy day-to-day lives mean that we frequently experience varying types of pressures, not just at work but also in our personal lives. It is when these pressures begin to build that they can result in us feeling unable to manage with our day-to-day activities. This is often referred to as stress.

Anxiety often accompanies stress and is when we experience an overwhelming feeling of uneasiness, including being worried or fearful in certain situations.

The national charity Anxiety UK defines anxiety as a disproportionate feeling of apprehension and dread of a situation and unlike stress, anxiety can persist even after the concern or situation has passed. Like stress, if left untreated it can affect day-to-day activities.

If stress and anxiety are not managed in their early stages, they can have a significant impact not only on people's health and wellbeing but also on the workforce in adult care settings.

In 2018, the Mental Health Foundation's study 'Stress – are we Coping?' consisted of an online poll undertaken by YouGov with a sample size of 4,619 respondents. This is the largest known study of stress levels in the UK. It found that:

- 74% of people have felt so stressed in the past year that they have been overwhelmed or unable to cope.

- 51% of adults who felt stressed reported feeling depressed, and 61% reported feeling anxious.
- 37% of adults who reported feeling stressed reported feeling lonely as a result.

Of the people who said they had felt stress at some point in their lives, 16% had self-harmed, and 32% said they had had suicidal thoughts and feelings.

Source: Mental Health Foundation, Stress Statistics, 2018

In addition, research shows that:

- in 2014, there were 8.2 million cases of anxiety reported in the UK
- in England women are almost twice as likely to be diagnosed with anxiety disorders as men.

Source: Mental Health Foundation, Stress Statistics, 2018

In 2020/21, anxiety, depression and stress accounted for 50% of all work-related ill health cases.

Source: Health and Safety Executive (2022) 'Work related Stress, Depression or Anxiety Statistics in Great Britain'

Research it

4.1 'Fight or flight' response

Research what happens in your body when you are stressed, known as the body's 'fight or flight' response. You can find a useful article about it on http://verywellmind.com.

Explain the 'fight or flight' response to a colleague.

Evidence opportunity

4.1 What is stress and anxiety?

Produce an information handout that explains the meaning of 1) stress and 2) anxiety.

AC 4.2 Explain how to recognise indicators of stress and anxiety in oneself

The first step to prevent your stress and anxiety from developing into something more serious involves being aware of the common signs and indicators. Although these vary from person to person and you may not experience all of these, it is still very important that you know about them in the event of you experiencing them in the future and so that you know you are not the only one who sometimes feels this way. It is also important that you are able to recognise these signs in others so that you can offer them support if they need it.

Signs and indicators of stress

- **Physical signs and indicators:** these can include tenseness, rapid heartbeat, high blood pressure, strokes, dizziness, nausea, diarrhoea or constipation, headaches and migraines. Other physical illnesses caused by stress include colds, cold sores and menstrual issues. These physical symptoms develop because it is how our bodies respond to stress, sometimes known as the 'fight or flight' response. 'Freeze' is another common reaction to stress.
- **Emotional signs and indicators:** these can include low moods, feeling irritable, feeling anxious, an overwhelming sense of being unable to cope, feeling unhappy or angry.
- **Mental signs and indicators:** these can include difficulties with concentration and memory, having racing thoughts and being unable to think logically.
- **Behavioural signs and indicators:** these can include being unable to sleep or sleeping too much, eating more than usual or eating a lot less, and withdrawal from situations, particularly those that involve speaking with and socialising with others.

Signs and indicators of anxiety

- **Physical signs and indicators:** a churning feeling in your stomach, feeling light-headed or dizzy, feeling restless, headaches, body aches and pains, faster breathing, sweating, feeling sick.
- **Emotional signs and indicators:** low mood, depression, feeling tense, being unable to relax, an overwhelming sense of fear or that something terrible is going to happen, excessive worrying that you cant stop.
- **Mental signs and indicators:** a surreal feeling that you're looking in on yourself and can see yourself disconnected from others, worrying that you're losing touch with reality, having racing thoughts and worries about the future.

- **Behavioural signs and indicators:** sleeping a lot or being unable to sleep, finding it difficult to wake up, needing the toilet more or less often.

> ### Reflect on it
>
> #### 4.2 Effects of stress and anxiety
>
> Reflect on the impact of the effects of stress and anxiety on you at work. For example, how might this affect the way you interact with individuals or others who visit the care setting where you work?
>
> Describe the common signs and indicators of stress and anxiety in others. How do these compare with yours?
>
> Provide a reflective account.

> ### Evidence opportunity
>
> #### 4.2 Common signs and indicators of stress and anxiety
>
> Discuss with a colleague the main ways that stress and anxiety affect you both. What signs and indicators did you have in common? What differences were there between the way you both experienced stress? Provide a written account describing common signs and indicators of stress and anxiety in self and others.

AC 4.3 Identify factors that can trigger stress and anxiety in oneself

The second step in preventing your stress and anxiety from developing into something more serious is recognising that there may be specific circumstances and factors that tend to trigger stress and anxiety in yourself and others. Again, what causes stress and anxiety is different for everyone and depends on what is important to you as well as how able you are at dealing with difficult circumstances. This is often referred to as resilience.

Figure 15.4 identifies some examples of circumstances and factors that tend to trigger stress and anxiety. It is very important to know what triggers stress and anxiety in yourself and others because in this way you will be able to recognise why you or others are behaving differently. Being supportive and empathetic is a must; not being so can add more pressure, putting you and others under even more stress. In addition, understanding the reasons why you are stressed can help you rationalise why you feel the way you do so that you can go about trying to manage it.

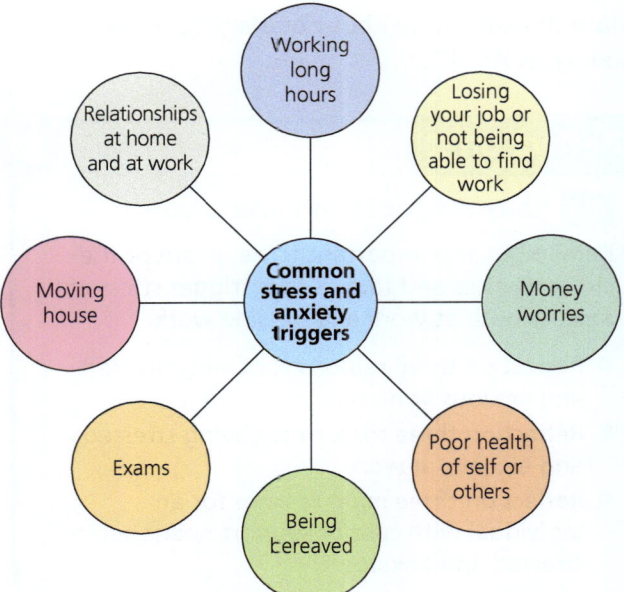

Figure 15.4 Common stress and anxiety triggers

For example, perhaps a team member you supervise at work is finding working with an individual very stressful because of their challenging needs. As result, they have become very irritable at work and have mentioned that they are not sleeping well. If you know that this is the cause of their stress and anxiety, then you can discuss with the team member what additional support they would like, for example additional training, other ideas for ways of working with the individual, or support from you when working with the individual such as working in pairs so that you can role model how to work effectively with the individual.

Another colleague may be experiencing family or relationship problems at home; consequently they are finding it difficult to concentrate at work and are getting upset frequently. You could discuss their triggers with them and suggest that they access support from someone independent to help them with the problems they are experiencing at home. You could also perhaps suggest to your employer or manager that they consider giving the person some time off work, or reduce their workload for a time limited period so they can deal with their difficulties at home. Doing so may help them to understand their stress and anxiety triggers so they are more able to take the necessary actions to manage them effectively. You will learn more about managing stress and anxiety in AC 4.5.

> **Evidence opportunity**
>
> **4.3 Circumstances and factors that trigger stress and anxiety**
>
> Identify the different factors that can trigger stress and anxiety. This can include work-related factors or those outside of work. If you work with others, you might like to compare with a colleague the differences between factors that trigger stress and anxiety. Does the impact of the triggers vary between the two of you? Assess the benefits of knowing what these triggers are and their impact. Provide a written account.

> **Reflect on it**
>
> **4.3 Reasons for stress and anxiety**
>
> Remember, it is important to be aware of the circumstances and factors that trigger stress and anxiety both at work and outside work.
>
> - Reflect on three reasons for being stressed and anxious at home.
> - Reflect on three reasons for being stressed and anxious at work.
> - Reflect on three main reasons for an individual with care or support needs being stressed and anxious.

AC 4.4 Describe how stress and anxiety may affect own reactions and behaviours towards others

As you will have learned in LO2 of this unit, your wellbeing can have a negative impact on your role and behaviour at work, as well as on others, not just in work but also at home and in your personal life. It is important therefore that you gain an understanding of how stress and anxiety can affect your reactions and behaviours towards others so that you can take action to prevent or minimise these from happening. Table 15.4 includes ten examples of how stress and anxiety can impact on the way you react and behave towards others:

Table 15.4 Examples of the ways stress and anxiety can affect your reactions and behaviours towards others

1	You may make excuses to avoid going out with family and friends because you may not want to speak with others or socialise with others due to feeling unhappy or in low mood.
2	You may try and avoid completing a work task or an activity on your own because you may feel frightened and panicky that something bad is going to happen.
3	You may try and avoid situations and/or places that make you feel stressed or anxious because you may think that others may notice that you are stressed and anxious or that you may embarrass yourself by feeling unwell or fainting.
4	You may lose your patience when supporting others at work or when things go wrong at work because you may be feeling irritable or angry.
5	You may not be able to respond to others requests for support and ideas because due to feeling stressed and anxious you may have difficulties concentrating and expressing your thoughts logically.
6	You may find it difficult to spend time with a loved one because you may be feeling as if you want to run away and escape from everyone.
7	You may feel tense and uptight most days and therefore find it difficult to relax and enjoy the day-to-day activities you participate in with others.
8	You may find it difficult to talk to others both at home and at work about day-to-day issues because you may be feeling very frustrated.

Table 15.4 Examples of the ways stress and anxiety can affect your reactions and behaviours towards others *continued*

Examples of the ways stress and anxiety can affect your reactions and behaviours towards others
9 You may find it difficult to motivate yourself and/or others at home or at work because you may be feeling very tired through lack of regular sleep because of your stress and anxiety.
10 You may feel so overwhelmed by your environment and the world around you that you may find it difficult to work alongside others on tasks and activities, as you may feel unable to cope or doubt your ability to know what to do and how to do it.

Reflect on it

4.4 Stress and anxiety

Reflect on an occasion when you felt stressed and anxious. Why were you feeling this way? How did this impact on others at work and in your personal life? What could you have done to minimise the impact of your reactions and behaviours?

The case study below provides you with an opportunity to further explore how stress and anxiety can affect reactions and behaviours towards others.

Case study

4.3, 4.4 The impact of stress and anxiety on others

Maxine is a senior carer and has just come to the end of another 12-hour shift which was unplanned as a member of staff had phoned in sick at the last minute. This was supposed to be Maxine's day off, but she felt she had to support her manager and did not want to let anyone down at the home and so agreed to work on her day off. Maxine has been feeling very tired all day and has not eaten very much because she has been so busy with the admission of a new individual to the home and with supporting two new members of staff that have recently started to work at the home.

Towards the end of her shift Maxine overhears the two new members of staff commenting on how they felt that she was a little impatient with them over completing their care records and how they didn't like the way she spoke to an individual's relative who rang up in the middle of lunchtime. This makes Maxine feel very low in herself and embarrassed over how she has let herself down in front of two new members of staff. Maxine cannot wait to leave work and get home.

When Maxine arrives home, she hears her children crying and her husband shouting out to her that he's been on his own all day looking after the children. Maxine ignores them all, runs upstairs to her room and bursts into tears.

Discuss

1. Why do you think Maxine is feeling stressed?
2. Why do you think Maxine is feeling anxious?
3. How did Maxine feeling stressed and anxious impact on others at work?
4. How did Maxine feeling stressed and anxious impact on others at home?

Evidence opportunity

4.4 The effects on your reactions and behaviours towards others

Reflect on how stress and anxiety affects your reactions and behaviours towards others and have a discussion about this with your assessor. Remember to be as honest as you can about yourself!

AC 4.5 Explain own strategies for managing stress and anxiety and building resilience

Managing my stress, my anxiety and building resilience

Once you have identified that you are displaying signs of being stressed and anxious and can identify the triggers for this then you can begin to look for a way of managing your stress and anxiety and at the same time build up your resilience for working through these difficult times. As you know everyone experiences stress and anxiety differently and therefore the ways that can be used to manage it and build resilience are varied. Remember, one size does not fit all – what works for one person may not for another.

Finding ways of managing stress and anxiety positively means that you will be more likely to avoid the ways that are not beneficial, such as by smoking heavily, 'comfort' eating, or drinking excessive amounts of alcohol; all of these are associated with serious health conditions, for example heart attacks and liver cancer.

Positive ways for managing stress and anxiety and building your resilience can include:

- **being active:** not only physically but mentally too, for example by going for a walk in the evening after a long shift at work or doing a crossword. Both activities can help with refocusing your mind and therefore reducing your body's stress and anxiety levels. You will also feel a lot calmer and able to think clearly again.
- **staying positive:** thinking about what is going well rather than dwelling on what is going wrong will help you feel more in control and able to deal with difficult situations that may arise, such as the bereavement of someone close to you; you can perhaps think about what that person would have wanted for you and how you could make them proud by showing them you are in control of your life.
- **being in contact with others:** agreeing to meet up with friends for a social occasion even when you are feeling in a low mood can prevent you from becoming isolated from others, as isolation can make you feel less confident in yourself. Meeting up with others can be a much welcomed distraction and you may find out about circumstances that your friends are experiencing that may be similar, which will help you put things in perspective.
- **helping others:** doing something for someone else can make you feel good about yourself and is a perfect way to boost your self-confidence when you are feeling anxious or withdrawn. You will at the same time meet different people and learn new skills, all examples of things that can make you feel positive about yourself and make your stress less overwhelming.
- **learning to say 'no':** this is a useful skill to have that takes some practice! It involves being in control of your stress and being aware of what your limits are.
- **making time for yourself:** it is very important to take time out to stop and think. Being calm and quiet can help you focus on what is important and put things into perspective.
- **accessing sources of support for stress:** this involves being honest and **courageous**.

6Cs

Courage

Showing courage when accessing sources of support is important so that your stress does not become worse. If it does, it could affect not only the quality of the care or support you provide to individuals but also the relationships you have with your colleagues as you may behave in ways that they are not used to, such as getting upset and becoming irritable very quickly. You can show your courage when managing stress and anxiety by not being afraid to say 'Help!'

Reflect on it

4.5 Dealing with stress and anxiety

Reflect on an occasion when you dealt with stress and anxiety negatively. Why do you think you did so? How did it make you feel? Is there anything you would do more positively if it happened again?

Evidence opportunity

4.5 Strategies for managing stress, anxiety and building resilience

Produce a presentation to your team of the strategies that you use and find helpful for managing stress and anxiety and building resilience.

AC 4.6 Describe how to access support from others when needed

How to access support from others

Formal and informal support

Meeting with your manager at work and discussing the triggers for your stress and anxiety can help with putting together a plan of action, such as providing you with additional support from a more experienced colleague when working to meet the needs of an individual whose behaviour challenges. Informal support, such as from your colleagues at work, can also be useful in terms of providing useful suggestions for managing stress, for example by socialising or talking through difficult situations that have arisen, like the bereavement of an individual with care needs who you have worked alongside for many years. Workers from outside agencies such as bereavement counsellors can also provide support and understanding at times when you need it most. You could contact a bereavement counsellor directly yourself or by being referred through your employer or GP.

Supervision

Supervision can help you have some protected time with your manager that focuses solely on how you are managing with your day-to-day responsibilities. Supervision can provide you with an opportunity to share your anxieties and discuss what can be done to manage these. This may involve accessing support from outside professionals who can provide training and information on how to develop specific skills and knowledge. Your manager can also help you to identify what circumstances you have managed well and the techniques you used to do so.

Appraisal

An appraisal provides you with time to reflect and think about what you have learned, what you have achieved and what you would like to achieve next. With the help of your manager, you will able to assess how well you have carried out your day-to-day working tasks and whether any improvements are needed. This is an opportunity to celebrate your achievements; a positive frame of mind is needed for this! It also provides you with time to think about what you would like to achieve next, for example a new skill or area of knowledge. Setting yourself targets to achieve makes you feel in control and is an excellent way to build your confidence.

Within the organisation

For more information on internal sources of support you can refer back to ACs 3.2 and 3.3 in this unit that describe how to access the employee assistance scheme, mentor or buddying systems. Your manager or employer would usually be your first source of support. There may also be a colleague or another team member that you may approach who knows you well or who has been in a similar situation to you and therefore understands how you are feeling. Your setting may provide additional support and information on dealing with stress and anxiety in the form of leaflets, or a support group.

Beyond the organisation

For more information on external sources of support you can refer back to ACs 3.2 and 3.3 in this unit that describe how to access self-help tools, apps and websites, local groups and networks. There are many different sources of support that you could access such as a confidential helpline where you can talk to someone in confidence or you could approach your trade union if you are a member. There may be a local or national group that you could approach for support. Some examples of external sources of support include:

- **SupportLine:** offers confidential emotional telephone support in the UK
- **ACAS:** provides information about managing work-related stress
- **Mind:** the mental health charity that offers information, support and guidance in relation to stress.

> **6Cs**
>
> **Care**
>
> You can only take care of and support others when you take care of yourself. If you look after your stress and anxiety and access support when you need it then you will be in a much stronger position to feel able to support others who may need support with their stress and anxiety. Improving your wellbeing will in turn improve the wellbeing of the individuals and others you care for and support.

> **Research it**
>
> **4.6 Procedures for accessing support**
>
> Research the procedures that you must follow in your work setting to access support for managing your stress and anxiety.

> **Evidence opportunity**
>
> **4.6 Managing stress and anxiety and accessing support**
>
> Compare strategies for managing stress and anxiety in yourself and others. What strategies do you find are most effective for you to manage your stress and anxiety? What strategies do others use? Assess the pros and cons of each strategy; which ones work best for managing your stress and anxiety? Why? Provide a written account.
>
> Explain to your assessor the support available in your work setting for helping you to manage your personal stress and anxiety, and how to access this. Did you find out anything you did not know about?
>
> You could also provide a written account to evidence your discussion.

Legislation	
Relevant Act	**Key points**
Data Protection Act 2018	Personal information must be recorded, used, stored and shared according to a set of principles or rules to ensure the individuals' rights are protected and the security of their personal information is maintained.
The Human Rights Act 1998	Everyone in the UK is entitled to the same rights and freedoms. This includes individuals who have care and support needs. The Act supports the promotion of individuals' rights.
The Mental Capacity Act 2005	This Act supports person-centred working by supporting individuals' rights to make their own decisions, including being provided with the necessary support to do so. It also protects the rights of individuals who lack capacity by providing guidance on who can make decisions about them and how to plan ahead for this in case it arises in the future.
The Care Act 2014	This Act supports individuals' rights to make informed decisions about their care and support and promotes a person-centred approach to care planning. It also defines the concept of wellbeing and outlines how adult care workers can promote individuals' wellbeing. Also see the Government publications: ● *Personalised Health and Care 2020*, which sets out how technology and data can be used to improve health and the way health and social care services are delivered. ● *The Adult Social Care Outcomes Framework Handbook of Definitions*, which measures how well care and support services achieve the outcomes that are the most important to people.

Glossary

Abuse occurs when someone is mistreated in a way that causes them pain and hurt. This does not just mean physical abuse but can also mean sexual or psychological or mental abuse. Neglecting someone and not caring for their needs is also a form of abuse. It is important to be aware of the different types of abuse because you will be working with vulnerable people.

ACAS is an independent organisation that provides impartial and confidential advice to employees for resolving difficulties and conflicts at work.

Active listening is a communication technique that involves understanding and interpreting what is being expressed through verbal and non-verbal communication.

Active participation means enabling individuals to be involved in their care and support and can mean that people feel in control of their day-today choices.

Advanced care plans are resources that document the care and support an individual would like to receive in the future in the event they are no longer able to speak up for themselves.

Agreed ways of working are your employer's policies and procedures that are set out to guide you in relation to your work activities, such as those in relation to safeguarding, health and safety. They may be less formally documented with smaller employers.

Alternative and augmentative technologies (AAC) refer to technologies, systems and devices that individuals can use to substitute or supplement everyday speech so that they can express themselves and communicate with others.

Alzheimer's disease is the most common cause of dementia; symptoms can include the gradual loss of memory and communication skills and a decline in the ability to think and reason clearly.

Anorexia nervosa refers to an eating disorder where people are of a low weight because they limit how much they eat and drink.

Anti-bacterials are agents that destroy and prevent the growth and spread of bacteria.

Antiseptics are agents that prevent the growth of harmful pathogens that can cause infections.

Anxiety is a feeling of fear or worry that may be mild or serious and can lead to physical symptoms such as shakiness.

Aphasia is most often caused by stroke. It is a complex language and communication disorder which affects the ability to produce or comprehend speech, and the ability to read or write. It can also be caused by disease, injury or damage to the language centres of the brain. People who suffer from aphasia experience a complete disruption to their communication; they will not understand what others say and will be unable to speak.

Approved mental health professional refers to the mental health professional responsible for co-ordinating an individual's assessment and admission to hospital when the individual is sectioned. These professionals can be nurses, adult social care workers, psychologists or occupational therapists.

Arthritis is a medical condition that affects joints by causing pain, stiffness, swelling and decreased mobility of the joints.

Assessments are resources that involve obtaining and recording information about an individual with the aim of supporting them and meeting their unique needs.

Association of Directors of Adult Social Services (ADASS) is a charity whose members are active directors of social care services and whose aim is to promote high standards of social care services.

Audit process refers to the inspection or assessment of processes for handling information. An audit process may be a more formal inspection of a company or the accounts that it holds, and a check to ensure that the information is recorded fully and accurately. This will help the setting to improve their records and how information is documented.

Audit trail refers to either the paper-based or electronic records maintained about an activity or situation.

Autism spectrum conditions (ASC) are lifelong conditions that affect how people perceive the world and interact with others. For example, they may have difficulties communicating, interacting and socialising with others.

Belief systems are personal to you and what you regard to be true. They can sometimes be shared with others who belong to a similar group or culture. Beliefs can be political, religious, cultural or moral and are formed throughout your life.

Best interests means what is right for a particular person. The Mental Capacity Act (2005) sets out a checklist of things to consider when deciding what is in a person's 'best interests'. It is not usually the role of a care worker to carry out a Best Interests Assessment.

Block alphabet is an adapted form of finger spelling taken from British Sign Language (BSL) where you use your finger to trace the outline of capital letters on the palm of the deafblind individual thus enabling communication by touch alone.

Bipolar disorder is a mental health problem that in the main affects people's mood and where they experience feeling high (referred to as manic episodes) and feeling low (referred to as depressive episodes).

Binge eating disorder refers to an eating disorder where people consume large quantities of food over a short time (referred to as binge eating) but unlike bulimia nervosa they do not try and get rid of it through.

Body fluids refers to any fluid that circulates around the body or is expelled from the body, such as blood, urine, sputum and vomit.

Boundaries are the limits that you must work within when carrying out your job role.

Braille is a method of written communication using characters that are represented by patterns of raised dots that are felt with the fingertips and is used by individuals who are blind or partially sighted.

British Sign Language (BSL) is a system used by individuals who are deaf or have a hearing impairment, to communicate and interact with others. It involves using hand signs, gestures, facial expressions and body language.

Bulimia nervosa refers to an eating disorder that involved bingeing then 'compensation' behaviours for that bingeing.

Candour refers to a way of working that involves being open and honest with individuals, your employer and others in the care setting where you work when something has gone wrong, such as incidents or near misses that may have led to harm.

Carbon footprint refers to how you measure the total greenhouse gas emissions caused by a person, organisation, service, event or product.

Care plan may be known by other names, such as a support plan, or individual plan. It is the document that sets out the agreed plan of care or support for an individual and where day-today requirements and preferences for care and support are detailed.

Care Quality Commission (CQC) is the independent regulator of health and social care services in England. They register care providers as well as monitor and inspect care services.

Care review refers to a regular meeting where individuals and others discuss whether the individual's care and support are effective and how to further meet their needs and preferences, for example.

Care settings can include adult health settings, children and young people's health settings and adult care settings. This qualification focuses on adult care settings. These include residential homes, nursing homes, domiciliary care, day centres, an individual's own home and some clinical healthcare settings.

Cerebral palsy is a neurological condition caused by damage to the brain that affects the body's movements and muscle co-ordination. Symptoms can include jerky uncontrolled movements, and stiff and floppy arms or legs.

Cleaning is the decontamination used for low infection risk items such as floors and furniture.

Clinical commissioning groups are organisations that are responsible for the provision of NHS services in England.

Clinical waste bins are bins where waste that is contaminated with body fluids (for example used dressings, bandages and disposable gloves) is disposed of as it poses a risk of infection. These are usually located in bathrooms and laundry areas.

Closed questions such as Who? Where? encourage short, less complex responses.

Codes of practice refer to the guidelines and standards that care workers are expected to follow when carrying out their roles.

Communication aids are tools that enable individuals to communicate and interact with others, for example a communication book that contains photographs and signs of people, places and objects familiar to the individual.

Community fridges are run by community groups in schools, community centres and shops and their main aim is to save fresh food from going to waste. Individuals who live and work locally can access these to meet others and eat together while learning new skills. Food includes surplus from supermarkets, local food businesses, producers, households and gardens.

Community treatment order enables you to be discharged from hospital when you have been sectioned and treated in hospital as long as you meet certain conditions such as living in a certain place or accessing medical treatment.

Complex or sensitive situations may include those that are distressing or traumatic, threatening or frightening, likely to have serious implications or consequences, of a personal nature, or involving complex communication or cognitive needs.

Confidentiality means keeping information private. Confidentiality is important in an adult care setting because it respects individuals' rights to privacy and dignity, instils trust between you and others, promotes individuals' safety and security and shows compliance with legislation such as the Data Protection Act 2018.

Consent refers to informed agreement to an action or decision; the process of establishing consent will vary according to an individual's capacity to consent.

Continence care refers to caring for an individual who unintentionally passes urine (urinary continence) or faeces (faecal incontinence) or both. This may be due to a physical health condition or to an illness such as dementia.

Continuing professional development (CPD) refers to the process of tracking and documenting the skills, knowledge and experience that you gain both formally and informally as you work, beyond any initial training. It is a record of what you experience, learn and then apply.

Counsellors are trained therapists who listens to you talk through your feelings and emotions and helps you find strategies for managing emotional issues.

Cross infection is the spread of infection from person to person, from contaminated objects, through air, food, animals and insects.

Culture refers to particular ideas, traditions and customs practised and shared by a group of people, usually from a particular country or society.

Dangerous occurrences are incidents that do not cause injury but have the potential to do so.

Data Protection Act 2018 is a set of data protection laws that protect individuals' personal information. This is the UK's implementation of the EU's General Data Protection Regulation (GDPR).

Day centres are settings that provide leisure, educational, health and wellbeing activities during the day.

Deafblind refers to an individual who has both hearing and sight loss. The combined loss of their hearing and sight means that their ability to communicate and mobilise is severely affected.

Decontamination means cleaning to a high standard, to remove or reduce harmful pathogens that cause infections.

Dementia refers to a group of symptoms that affect how a person thinks, remembers, problem-solves, uses language and communicates, and their ability to carry out tasks and activities. They occur when brain cells stop working properly and the brain is damaged by injury, or by disease such as Alzheimer's.

Depression is a medical condition causing low mood that affects your thoughts and feelings. It can range from mild to severe but usually lasts for a long time and affects your day-to-day living.

Diabetes is a health condition that occurs when the amount of glucose (sugar) in the blood is too high because the body cannot use it properly.

Dieticians are qualified health professionals whose role it is to assess, diagnose, and treat diet and nutritional issues.

Dignity in a care setting means respecting the views, choices and decision of individuals and not making assumptions about how they want to be treated.

Disclosure of abuse is when an individual tells you that abuse has happened, or is happening to them.

Disclosure and Barring Service (DBS) is a government service that makes background checks for organisations on people who want to work with children or adults with care or support needs.

Discrimination means treating people unfairly or unlawfully, because they have a disability, or are of a different race, gender or age, for example.

Disinfection is the decontamination technique used for medium infection risk items such as bedpans and bottles.

Domiciliary care is where health and social care workers provide care and support to individuals who live in their own home but require additional help such as support with household tasks or personal care.

Duty of candour refers to the standards that adult care workers and professionals must follow when mistakes are made and an individual's care goes wrong. This will include being open and honest.

Duty of care refers to the legal requirement that health and social care workers have to ensure the safety and wellbeing of individuals and others while providing care or support. This concept is covered in Unit 303 Understanding duty of care.

Dysphasia is a language disorder that is caused by damage to the brain. People with dysphasia will often have difficulty with verbal communication. It is different to aphasia because here people will experience partial loss of speech. They will still experience difficulty in comprehending and understanding language.

Empathy is the ability to understand how someone else may be feeling, or understand another person's way of thinking.

Enhanced Care Workers are care workers who have been upskilled and trained to provide, for example, increased clinical support to registered nurses in nursing homes or improve the quality of dementia care to individuals with dementia who are hospital patients.

Equality refers to ensuring equal opportunities are provided to everyone irrespective of their differences such as ages, abilities, backgrounds, religions. In an adult care setting, this also means making sure that everyone is entitled to the same rights, and opportunities.

European Convention on Human Rights protects the human rights of people that belong to the Council of Europe; it has 47 members and the UK is one of them.

European Court of Human Rights is the Council of Europe's law court and it is based in Strasbourg, France.

Female genital mutilation (FGM) refers to a practice where the female genitals are deliberately cut, injured or changed and might be done because of cultural beliefs.

Formal supervision means having regular meetings with your manager, senior or employer to discuss any issues relevant to your job role and receive feedback on what has been going well and what improvements you need to make.

The **gender pay gap** refers to the difference in the hourly earnings between men and women.

General information that is recorded and held by a public authority may include information in relation to complaints received, accidents that have taken place, and correspondence exchanged between organisations. For example, an individual may request access to find out about the number of infections there have been in a hospital or the number of accidents there have been in a residential care home so that they can decide which setting is best for their relative to access.

Hazardous materials are materials that have the potential to cause harm and illness to others, for example used dressings or PPE that has come into contact with body fluids.

Hazardous substances are substances that have the potential to cause harm and illness to others, for example cleaning detergents, medication, acids and bodily fluids such as blood and urine.

Hazards are dangers with the potential to cause harm, for example a spillage on the floor or a broken wheelchair.

Health and Safety Executive (HSE) is the independent regulator in the UK for health and safety in work settings.

Health and safety officer is a named person in an organisation who is responsible for overseeing all health and safety matters, for example reviewing health and safety procedures and investigating accidents at work.

Health and Social Care Information Centre (now called NHS Digital) is responsible for providing information and systems for handling individuals' information.

Health and wellbeing boards are health and social care organisations that work together to improve the health and wellbeing of the people living in the local area they are responsible for.

Hearing impairment refers to hearing loss that main occur in one or both ears. This can be partial or complete loss of hearing.

Hearing loop systems are specialist types of equipment that transmit sounds to individuals who use hearing aids or cochlear implants so that they can communicate with others.

Hepatitis C is a term used to describe inflammation of the liver caused by the hepatitis C virus. This is usually spread through blood-to blood contact with an infected person.

Holistic in this context refers to treating individuals as a whole person, i.e. considering all of their needs, such as physical, emotional, spiritual, etc.

Honour-based violence refers to domestic violence because the individual is perceived as having brought shame to their family or community.

ICO refers to the Information Commissioner's Office, which is the independent authority that upholds rights with regards to people's information, and promotes openness by public bodies and data privacy for individuals.

An **identifier** is a tool (for example an NHS Number) used to match people to their health records.

Identity in the context of handling information means confirmation of who a person is, for example their name, who they work for and who they are visiting.

Immune system is the body's natural defences that work together to fight disease and infections.

Inclusion means being included or involved, for example being part of a wider group, or a group of friends. In an adult care setting, this means ensuring that all individuals are able to be included or partake in everyday life regardless of any differences. This can create a sense of belonging.

Incontinence products refer to products that help people manage incontinence such as incontinence pads, waterproof sheets for beds or absorbent mats for chairs.

Independent advocates are trained independent people who are appointed to represent/speak on behalf of an individual who may be unable to speak for/represent themselves due to a disability or condition such as dementia.

Independent Mental Capacity Advocate (IMCA) refers to a person who provides support and representation for a person who lacks capacity to make specific decisions where the person has no one else to support them.

Induction is the process of introducing a worker to an organisation and work setting by showing them round and explaining the agreed ways of working, for example.

Infection refers to when germs enter the body and cause an individual to become unwell.

Information Governance Alliance includes the Department of Health, NHS England, NHS Digital and Public Health England. Its aim is to improve how people's information is handled by health and care services.

Job descriptions are documents that outline the purpose and responsibilities of your job role.

Kosher refers to foods that are permitted to be eaten under Jewish dietary laws and that can be used as ingredients in the production of additional food items.

Job descriptions are documents that outline the purpose and responsibilities of your job role.

Lack of capacity is a term used to refer to when an individual is unable to make a decision for themselves because of a learning disability, a condition such as dementia or a mental health need, or because they are unconscious.

Learning disability refers to reduced ability to think and make decisions as well as difficulty with everyday activities which affects a person for their whole life. This may, for example, include difficulties with budgeting, shopping and planning a train journey.

Legislation refers to laws that are made by the government and must be followed; these include Acts of Parliament as well as Regulations.

Lifestyle refers to the way a person lives their life; this can be related for example to their health, morals and/or finances.

Local foodbanks provide essential items free of charge to people who are struggling financially to afford these. Items can include food items as well as cleaning materials and toiletries. Items provided are usually donated by members of the public and local businesses.

Local systems may include employers' safeguarding policies and procedures as well as multi-agency protection arrangements for your local area, for example a Safeguarding Adults Board.

Makaton is a method of communication using signs and symbols that can be used by individuals who have learning disabilities.

Mental capacity refers to an individual's ability to make decisions and give consent.

Mentor refers to a person in your work setting who has more experience than you and can provide you with guidance and advice in relation to your job role and responsibilities. This person is there to offer advice more informally than your manager or employer.

Motivational interviewing techniques are positive ways of promoting an individual's strengths by, for example, using open-ended questions, i.e. those beginning with 'what' and 'how', affirmations, i.e. confirming back to the individuals their strengths and abilities, reflection and summaries.

MRSA stands for methicillin-resistant Staphylococcus aureus and is often referred to as a 'superbug' because it is difficult to treat. It is a bacterium that can cause serious infections.

Muscular dystrophy refers to a group of conditions that affect the muscles and results in the body's muscles weakening and breaking down over time.

Musculoskeletal disorders refers to injuries, damage or disorders of the joints or other tissues in the upper and lower limbs or the back.

Nanotechnology is technology that deals with the understanding and manipulation of atoms and molecules.

National Dignity Council is the lead body for the Dignity in Care campaign and supports Dignity Champions. It is made up of different organisations including health and social care organisations.

Near misses refer to incidents that have the potential to cause harm, such as a delay in administering an individual's medication or a hoist battery that runs out just before an individual is about to be moved from one position to another. It may be that the individual is not actually harmed, but they could have been, and so it is a 'near miss.'

Neglect means failing to care for someone so that their needs are not met.

Negotiation means reaching an agreement through discussion.

NEWS2 refers to the second version of the National Early Warning Score tool that was developed by the Royal College of Physicians to identify and respond to clinical deterioration in patients early. It is used across NHS services in England, including in hospitals and ambulances.

Norovirus is an infection of the stomach that causes diarrhoea and vomiting.

To be **objective** is to be fair, and not influenced by your own feelings or beliefs.

Objects of reference are used as a means of communication by individuals and can be any object which is used to represent an item, activity, place or person. For example, a fork can represent lunchtime, and a photograph of a train can represent going to visit a family member.

An **ombudsman** is a free independent service that investigates complaints against an organisation. Note that an ombudsman can only look at certain complaints from agencies. The Local Government and Social Care Ombudsman (LGO) only looks at local authority complaints, the Parliamentary and Health Service Ombudsman (PHSO) looks at NHS and government departments. There is no ombudsman for private or voluntary care services.

One-page profiles are resources that typically consist of a single page and provide an outline of what is important to the individual and how the individual would like to be supported.

Open posture means not crossing your arms or legs in front of you, which avoids you appearing defensive.

Open questions such as What? Why? How? encourage the expression of opinions and feelings.

Osteopaths are a qualified health professional whose role it is to increase the mobility of joints, relieve muscle tension and enhance blood supply to tissues through treatments such as stretching, massage and physical manipulation.

To **paraphrase** means to restate what has been said or heard in order to clarify.

PECS (Picture Exchange Communication System) is a communication system that uses visual symbols and is used with individuals who have communication difficulties and autism spectrum conditions.

Percutaneous endoscopic gastrostomy (PEG) is a small tube that is inserted through the skin into an individual's stomach when they are having difficulties swallowing so that they can receive food, fluid and medication without swallowing.

A **personal and professional development plan (PDP)** may have a different name but will record information such as agreed objectives for development, proposed activities to meet objectives and timescales for review.

Personal assistants work directly for one individual with care and support needs, usually within the individual's own home.

Personal information that is recorded and held by an organisation may include contact details as well as information about the individual's health, care needs, and family background.

Personal protective equipment (PPE) is worn by care workers to prevent infections from spreading. PPE includes disposable gloves and plastic aprons. You will be expected to know the different types of PPE and their correct and appropriate uses in your work environment. Appropriate use may, in some cases, mean that after consideration PPE is not required.

Person-centred values refer to ensuring that care provided places individuals at the heart and fits around them. Person-centred values include individuality, rights, choice, privacy, independence, dignity, respect, partnership, care, compassion, courage, communication and competence.

Physiotherapists are trained professionals who help to restore the body's movement and function when an individual is affected by injury, illness or disability through mobility exercises, for example.

Policies and procedures may include other agreed ways of working as well as formal policies and procedures, such as in relation to handling comments and complaints.

Preferences refer to an individual's wishes, likes and own personal choices, for example for food, clothes, activities and wellbeing. These may be based on an individual's beliefs, values and culture.

Prejudice refers to your bias towards something as a result of your beliefs and values and can include, for example, believing that someone with a mental health condition is at risk of being violent (which may be based on media stories or hearsay, but not on any actual experience of your own).

Professional Councils are organisations that regulate professions, such as adult social care workers who work with adults in residential care homes, in day centres and who provide care in someone's home. They can provide advice and support around working with individuals who lack capacity to make decisions.

Professional refers to carrying out your job in a skilful and knowledgeable way, showing behaviour that is moral and acceptable for the role that you are in.

Psychiatrists are a medically qualified doctor who specialises in psychiatry and can diagnose and prescribe treatments and medication.

Psychotherapists are a trained therapist who assesses and treats a range of emotional, social or mental health issues.

Race refers to the common physical characteristics associated with a group of people from the same culture and/or shared history such as skin colour, nationality, ethnic or national origins.

Radio frequency identification technology (RFID) uses radio waves to identify and track tags or labels that are attached to objects.

Recovery model is a model often used with individuals who experience mental illness. It takes a holistic view of a person's life and is lead by the person themselves and takes into account the benefits of having supportive networks and relationships for aiding mental health recovery.

Regulators are bodies that supervise a particular sector.

Rehabilitation worker refers to a person who supports individuals to live independently following an accident or illness.

Residential care homes are homes that individuals live in. Care workers will provide meals and assistance with personal care tasks such as washing, dressing, eating.

Responsible clinician refers to the mental health professional in charge of an individual's care and treatment while the individual is sectioned under the Mental Health Act.

RESTORE2 is a physical deterioration and escalation tool for care homes and nursing homes. It is based on early recognition: soft signs, NEWS2 and structured communications (SBARD).

Restraint is when an individual is held to stop them from moving.

Rights are legal entitlements to something, for example the right to have personal information held about you by an organisation kept secure.

Risk is the likelihood of hazards causing harm, for example slipping over on a spillage on the floor, an individual falling out of a broken wheelchair.

Risk assessment is a process used in work settings for identifying hazards, assessing the level of risk and putting in place processes for reducing the risk identified.

Safeguarding Adults Boards (SAB) safeguard adults with care or support needs by overseeing local adult safeguarding systems and ensuring all organisations work in partnership.

SBARD (Situation, Background, Assessment, Recommendation, Decision) is a communication tool used to escalate concerns about an individual's health deterioration quickly and fully; it can be used for both verbal and written communications.

Schizophrenia is a mental health problem where people may experience some of the following symptoms: feeling disconnected from your emotions, difficulty concentrating, hallucinations that include hearing voices and/or seeing things others don't.

SCIE is a UK charity and improvement support agency that shares knowledge of best practice across the whole social care sector, and works closely with both adults and children care services.

Seclusion is when an individual is moved to a separate room or space, away from other people.

Sectioned means that being detained in hospital under the Mental Health Act 1983.

Sector Skills Councils are organisations led by and for specific employment sectors, for example Skills for Care for the adult social care workforce and Skills for Health for the healthcare workforce.

Sensory loss refers to hearing loss, sight loss or both hearing and sight loss.

Shared Lives carer are people who open up their homes and family lives to include an adult with support needs so that they can participate and experience community and family life. The individual may stay with them for the weekend and they may even go on holiday together.

Skills for Care is the Sector Skills Council for people working in social work and social care for adults and children in the UK as well as for workers in early years, children and young people's services. It sets standards and develops qualifications for those working in the sector.

Skills for Health is the Sector Skills Council for people working in healthcare.

Social inclusion means providing opportunities for individuals to participate and be involved in their wider communities so that they feel included, have a role and are part of society. This might be through accessing public transport, socialising with friends, accessing a course at a local college or participating in a local cultural event.

Social movements refer to a group of people who come together to champion a cause and promote or prevent social, political, economic or cultural change, for example by engaging in demonstrations or picket lines.

Social workers assess, commission and coordinate care services and seek to improve outcomes for individuals, especially those who are more vulnerable. They may work in multidisciplinary teams and can specialise in areas such as mental ill-health, learning disabilities, care for older people or safeguarding.

Speech and language therapists are professionals who support individuals who have communication difficulties. They might assist those who have speech problems or difficulties using language.

Standards may include codes of conduct and practice, regulations, minimum standards, National Occupational Standards.

Standards may include codes of conduct and practice, regulations, minimum standards, National Occupational Standards.

Sterilisation is the decontamination technique used for high infection risk items, such as medical instruments used for surgery.

Stress is the body's physical and emotional reaction to being under too much pressure. It can have positive as well as negative effects, but in this unit the word is used to refer to negative stress.

Stroke refers to a life-threatening medical condition that occurs when the blood supply to part of the brain is cut off. Depending on the part of the brain it damages, it can affect how your body works, your communication and how you think and feel.

Supervisor refers to the person in your work setting that oversees your work and assesses your performance at work; this is usually your manager or, if you are a Lead Personal Assistant, your employer.

Suspicions of abuse occur when you notice indicators or are told by someone about indicators that make you think or suspect abuse is happening.

A trade union representative is a member of an organised group of workers who speaks up for the rights and interests of the employees of an organisation, for example in relation to safe working conditions.

Treaty refers to a legally binding international agreement.

UK Health Security Agency (UKHSA) is a UK government-led organisation that replaced Public Health England in 2021 and is responsible for public health including protecting the public from infections and disease.

Values are what you hold true and believe to be important to you, such as your independence, or your family. Often a person's beliefs can develop into their values.

Vetting and Barring Scheme ensures that anyone who is not fit or appropriate to work with adults and children does not do so.

Visual impairment refers to loss of vision, either severely (i.e. the individual is blind) or partially (i.e. the individual is able/unable to see to some degree).

Voice Output Communication Aids (VOCA) help individuals to communicate by speaking recorded messages and displaying words and symbols on a screen.

Whistleblowing refers to when a person exposes any kind of information or activity that is deemed illegal, unethical or not correct, for example unsafe practices, abuse, harm.

Work settings may include one specific location or a range of locations, depending on the context of a particular work role, for example a domiciliary carer who may work in individuals' own homes and in residential care homes, or an activities worker who may work in residential homes, day centres, nursing homes or in an individual's own home.

Index

6 Cs 3, 9, 11, 20, 26, 31, 431
  see also care; commitment; communication; compassion; competence; courage
abuse 33–74, 319
  of carers 57
  of children/young people 68–9
  and communication skills 140–2, 190
  and complaints procedures 72–3, 128
  definition 46–7
  disclosure 34–5, 59, 61–5, 68–9, 190–2
  discriminatory 50, 54
  domestic 49, 52–3
  and duty of care 107–8, 113–15, 128
  emotional/psychological 49, 53
  financial/material 49–50, 53, 67
  organisational 50, 54
  perpetrators 55–6, 60
  physical 49, 52
  prevention 36, 41–2, 48, 69–74, 73–4, 114
  protection from 33–46, 108
  recording 59–60, 62, 64–7, 69
  responding to 58–69, 114
  risk of 56–8, 114, 190
  sexual 49, 53, 66
  signs of 47–8, 52–9
  suspicions of 58–60, 65, 69, 75
  types of 49–54
Access to Personal Files Act 1982 197
accidents 411–12
  reporting 358, 362–4, 367–74, 383–4
accountability 20, 36, 44–5, 109, 433, 458–9
active listening 136, 139, 160–1, 180–1
active participation 69–71, 73–4, 250–3, 262–3, 269–71, 282–3
acts of omission 50–1, 54
Advance Care Plans 119, 240–2
adverse events 129–31
advice 135, 215, 268
Advisory, Conciliation and Arbitration Service (ACAS) 17, 489
Advocacy People, The 292
advocacy/advocates 7, 33, 158, 171, 182–7, 213, 280, 445
  independent 158, 182–92
agreed ways of working 4–5, 12, 18–23, 23–9
  anti-discriminatory 344
  and continuous development 440
  and data handling 219
  and health and safety 374–5, 408
  implementation 26–7
  and infection control 394
  and lone working 426
  and mental capacity 86, 89–91, 99
  and resource efficiency 27–9
  up-to-date 24–6
alcohol abuse 119, 150
allegations, untrue 21
Alzheimer's disease 149
anaphylaxis 371

anorexia nervosa 292
anti-bacterials 396, 397
antiseptics 396, 397
anxiety 88, 368, 469, 483–90
Anxiety UK 481, 483
aphasia 149, 168
apologies 112
appraisals 439, 489
approved mental health professionals 186
aprons, plastic 399, 400
arthritis 149
assertiveness 15, 30, 124, 145, 147, 172
assessments 100, 241
assessors 440
assistive technology 280, 284–6, 307
Association of Directors of Adult Social Services (ADASS) 37, 38
attitudes 97–8
audit processes 229–32
audit trails 185, 186
autism spectrum conditions (ASC) 22, 148–50, 153–4, 216–17
avoidant/restrictive food intake disorder (ARFID) 292
bacteria, pathogenic 390, 391
barriers
  to active participation 251
  to communication 152–6, 162–9
  to service access 294–5
Beat 292
belief systems 113, 146, 345–9, 456–8
bereavement 237
best interests 15, 108, 113, 115, 266–7, 319
best practice 9, 25, 251, 253, 451
biases 329–30, 339–41
binge eating disorder 292
bipolar disorder 89
bleeding 372
Blissymbols 178
block alphabet 148
body care 405
body fluids 66, 355, 356, 391, 413
body language 143, 147, 159, 173, 176, 181
boundaries 4, 5
Braille 143, 174
breathing difficulties 371, 373
British Sign Language (BSL) 143, 170, 178
buddying schemes 480
budgets, personal 351
bulimia nervosa 292
burns/scalds 372
Caldicott Principles 197
campaigns 322, 323
candour 110, 111–13, 114, 197
carbon footprint 28
cardiac arrest 368, 372
care 63, 431
  and communication 138
  continuity of 42
  definition 3

  and diversity issues 343
  and health and safety 380, 421
  and infection control 397
  and information handling 215
  and mental capacity 96
  and person-centred care 245
  and reflective practice 452
  and risk assessments 275
  and stress and anxiety 489
  and wellbeing 313
  see also duty of care
Care Act 2014 33, 49, 84, 88, 106, 126, 131, 193, 196, 201, 232, 271, 286, 315, 319, 353, 490
Care Certificates 110, 320, 436
care environment/setting 2, 16, 17, 57, 155–6
care planning 250–3
care plans 15, 119, 171, 239–42, 279
Care Quality Commission (CQC) 4, 17, 37, 39, 43–4, 111, 122, 127, 229–30, 321–2, 356, 386, 402, 433–5
care reviews 133, 134
Care and Support Advocates 184–5, 187
carers 57, 59–60, 213, 280
cerebral palsy 153, 168–9, 401
challenging situations/behaviours 41, 142–3
child-centred approaches 68
childhood abuse 68–9
Children and Families Act 2014 352
choice 71, 93, 244, 259, 266–8, 272–86
  informed 70, 79–80, 93–4, 259, 276–7, 279, 286
choking 373
Civil Contingencies Act 2004 359, 388, 427
clarification 139
cleaning 396–7
cleaning chemicals 414, 416
clinical commissioning groups (CCGs) 33, 35
clinical waste bins 394, 394–5
coaching programmes 454
Codes of Conduct 435
  Code of Conduct for Healthcare Support Workers and Adult Social Care Workers in England 108–10, 321–2, 353
codes of practice 86, 89–91, 94–6, 198–9, 204–5, 317–18, 321–2, 352–3, 432, 432–3
coercive/controlling behaviour 92
commitment 11, 29
  and complaints 125
  and continuous development 431, 441–9, 453
  and equality issues 326
  and health and safety 425
  and infection control 396
  and information handling 224, 230
  and mental capacity 96

Index

and person-centred practice 235, 245
and reflective practice 453
and safeguarding 77
and supporting choices 279
and wellbeing 298
communication 9, 132–93, 431, 433
   and advocacy services 182–92
   barriers to 152–6, 162–9
   with children/young people 68
   and choices 278, 280
   and complaints 124
   and confidentiality 187–92
   and difficult situations 140–3
   difficulties with 22, 56
   dos and don'ts 137–8
   and duty of care 123, 124
   effective 159–69
   and health and safety 410–11
   and health/wellbeing 295, 310, 313–14
   impact 160–2
   and infection control 396
   and information handling 214, 221
   and leadership 464–5
   and mental capacity 98, 99
   message of 160–2
   methods 143–8, 159–60, 172, 174–9
   needs/preferences 143–59, 169–87
   non-verbal 139, 143, 147, 174–6
   and online safety 83
   and partnership working 13, 15, 29–30, 467
   and person-centred practice 234, 245, 253–4, 262
   poor 75, 159
   and professionalism 182
   and promoting independence 282–3
   reasons for 133–6
   and relationships 135, 136–9, 162, 234
   and risk assessments 275
   and safeguarding 41–2, 68, 70, 73, 75, 83
   as service barrier 295
   styles 143–4, 145–8, 172–3
   support 144, 151–3, 156–8
   verbal 139, 143, 147, 177–8
   written 174, 464
communication aids 10
communication passports 144
communication profiles 171
communicators, alternative and augmentative 284–5
communities 246, 338–9
community fridges 293
community treatment orders 186
compassion 31, 431
   and communication 138, 167
   and duty of care 110, 117
   and equality issues 343
   and health and safety 382
   and health/wellbeing 302, 313
   and infection control 393
   and information handling 213, 215
   and mental capacity 99
   and person-centred care 245

and safeguarding 63, 70, 78
and supporting choices 279
competence 20, 70, 431
   and communication 189
   and continuous development 438
   and duty of care 108, 110
   and equality issues 336
   and health and safety 365
   and health/wellbeing 304, 313
   and infection control 394
   and information handling 196, 205, 221
   and person-centred care 245
   and restrictive practices 104
   and supporting choices 276–7
complaints 41, 72–3, 123–9, 254, 344
complex situations/behaviours 140–41, 236–9
computer viruses 208–9
concerns, responding to 123–9
conclusion-drawing 459
confidence 127, 129, 283–4
confidentiality 45, 61, 65, 156, 187–92, 197–9, 203–5, 222–5, 322, 436
   breaches 189
conflict management 1, 14–18, 31
consent 34–5, 64–5, 85, 91–102, 191, 222–3, 266–8, 278, 425
   informed 85, 100–2, 276–8
   valid 94
continence care 293
continuing professional development (CPD) 109, 322
continuous development 428–68
contrast effect 330
control, right to 319
Control of Substances Hazardous to Health (COSHH) 358–9, 387, 414–17, 427, 433, 468
counsellors 157, 483, 489
courage 26, 431
   and complaints 125
   and confidentiality breaks 189
   and equality issues 336
   and health and wellbeing 302, 313
   and infection control 393
   and information handling 230
   and person-centred care 245
   and personal wellbeing 472
   and reflective practice 453
   and restrictive practice 104
   and safeguarding 58–9, 70
   and stress 488
   and supporting choices 279
creativity 480
criminality 120, 190
cross contamination 396
cross infection 390
cultural health 257, 290
cultural wellbeing 296, 474–6
culture 92, 146–8, 154, 165, 295, 345–9
cuts 372
cyber security 197, 203, 205–11
dangerous occurrences 190, 358

data breaches 217–19
Data Protection Acts
   1998 88, 106, 200–1, 317–18, 387
   2018 24, 34, 84, 88, 127, 131, 188, 193, 196, 199, 218, 232, 271, 286, 315, 318, 352, 387, 424–5, 490
data security 197, 203, 205–11, 219–22
day centres 134
deafblind individuals 167, 171–2
decision-making 29, 44–6, 90, 98–100, 253–4, 318–19, 458–9
decontamination 396–7
delegated healthcare tasks 22–3
dementia 56, 97, 149, 153, 163, 168, 238–9, 264
dependency 56, 269
depression 88, 368
diabetes 22, 368
diet 116–18, 299, 348–9, 477, 482
dieticians 23, 482
difference 335–6, 340, 349, 458
difficult situations 140–2
digital technology 285
dignity 11–12, 37, 70, 244–5, 313
Dignity in Care 2006 37
dilemmas 115–23
direct payments 350–1
direction-setting 463
disabilities 146, 152–4
Disability Confident Employer Initiative 2014 320
disclosure of abuse 34–5, 59, 61–5, 68–9, 190–2
Disclosure and Barring Service (DBS) 34, 35, 39
discrimination 34–5, 316–17, 319–20, 326–9, 331–2, 337–45
disease
   reporting 358, 362–4, 367–74, 383–4
   see also illness
disempowerment 243, 328
disinfection 396, 397
distress 154, 164, 181, 237
diversity 316–53, 458
domiciliary care 135
Driscoll's Reflective Cycle 449–50
drowning 371
DR's ABC approach 370
duty of candour 110, 111–13, 114, 197
duty of care 11–12, 20–1, 54, 58, 107–31, 190, 225
dysphasia 149, 168
e-learning 441
eating disorders 292
economic health 116, 118, 257, 290
economic wellbeing 297, 470, 475–6
education 16, 240, 324, 395, 483
electrical equipment 359, 387, 420, 427, 480–1
electrical injury 372
Electricity at Work Regulations 1989 359, 387, 427
electronic communication devices 80, 83, 151–2, 198, 203, 308, 480–1

Index

electronic information systems 205–11
email 159, 198, 203, 209, 248
emergencies 103, 369, 370, 419–20, 426
emotional health 257, 289, 337
emotional resilience 471
emotional wellbeing 296, 470, 473–4, 476
empathy 15, 30, 111, 137, 139, 175, 216, 235
employee assistance schemes 479, 483
employers 363–4, 380, 395, 418, 479
employment 240, 338
empowerment 36, 61–2, 74, 128–9, 347, 376
enabling others 145, 147–8, 173, 236, 313
end of life care 240
energy efficiency 28
engagement 99
Enhanced Care Workers 134
environment 92, 311, 312
    see also care environment/setting
epilepsy 368, 372
equal opportunities 318, 319, 332
equality 34, 35, 316–53
Equality Act 2010 34, 84, 87, 106, 193, 319, 330–1, 353
Equality and Human Rights Commission (EHRC) 321, 336
equipment 357–9, 362–3, 366, 387, 396, 409–10, 412–13, 420, 427, 480–1
errors 111–13, 129–31, 229
European Convention on Human Rights 322, 323
European Court of Human Rights 322, 323
evacuation routes 421–2
EVALUATE approach 455
evaluations 442–3
example-setting, positive 335
eye contact 143, 147, 160, 169, 174, 181
face masks, surgical 399, 400
fact finding 10–11, 227
falls 367
families 2–3, 7, 122, 170, 213, 255, 269, 274, 280, 291, 323, 338, 441, 455–6
feedback 27, 129, 247–50, 442–3, 459–61
feelings 54, 113, 134, 484
female genital mutilation (FGM) 34, 35, 49
Female Genital Mutilation Act 2003 34
'fight or flight' response 484
filing systems 207–8, 210–11
financial matters 116, 118, 257, 290, 351
    online transactions 81–3
fire safety 359, 375, 417–22
first aid 359, 362–3, 366, 369–71, 373, 375
flexibility 145, 147–8, 161, 173, 431
flu 404
food hygiene 359, 366, 388, 406
Food Hygiene (England) Regulations 2006 359, 388
food poisoning 391
Food Safety Act 1990 359, 388
food shopping 262–3
foodbanks 293
fractures 372
Freedom of Information Act 2000 193, 197, 202, 232

friendships 3, 78–9, 122, 170, 274, 291, 323, 441, 456
fungal infections 390
gastroenteritis 404
gender equality issues 326, 330
General Data Protection Regulation (GDPR) 196
general practitioners (GPs) 8, 293, 482
gestures 143, 147, 175
Gibb's Reflective Cycle 450
gifts 6
gloves 392, 398–9
goals 13, 29, 262, 445–8
    SMART PDP 446–7, 448
Great Ormond Street Hospital 27
grievance procedures 344
guidance 135, 215, 252, 254, 279–80, 291
guidelines 24, 25
hair care 405
hand hygiene 362–4, 402–5
harassment 328
harm 47, 238
hazardous materials 358, 413–17
hazardous substances 358–9, 413–17
hazards 71–2, 280, 355, 359, 361, 363, 376–9, 383, 385
health 113, 240, 257, 287–315, 337–8, 404–5, 482
health care procedures 366
health and safety 21, 75, 354–88, 407–27
    accident/illness procedures 367–74
    in an individual's home 393, 413, 416
    fire safety 417–22
    hazardous substances 413–17
    legislation 355–60, 387–8, 408–10, 427, 433
    moving and handling 408–13
    responsibilities 355–66, 374–86
    security measures 422–7
Health and Safety at Work Act (HASAWA) 1974 356, 361–4, 377, 387, 406, 427
Health and Safety Executive (HSE) 122, 356, 360, 364, 367, 384, 386, 411–12
Health and Safety (First Aid) Regulations 1981 359, 387
health and safety officers 355, 356
health services 290–5, 299
Health and Social Care Act 2008 (Regulated Activities) Regulations 2014 111, 197, 201, 232, 271, 278, 285, 433–4
    Regulation 9 468
    Regulation 16 126–7, 131
    Regulation 20 131
Health and Social Care Act 2012 33, 84, 88, 106
Health and Social Care Information Centre (HSCIC) 198
    Code of Practice on Confidential Information 2014 198, 204
    Guide to Confidentiality 2013 198–9, 205
Health and Social Care (Safety and Quality) Act 2015 359–60
health and wellbeing boards 33, 35

health and wellbeing support groups 299–300
hearing impairment 136, 143, 148, 153, 163, 167, 175
hearing loop systems 140
hepatitis C 363, 364
homes, individuals' 230, 393, 413, 416
honesty 16, 30, 111–13, 142–3, 204, 234, 411, 454, 464
honour-based violence 49
hot and cold conditions 371
hours of work 19
Human Rights Act 1998 34, 84, 87, 106, 131, 193, 197, 202, 232, 271, 286, 315, 317, 331, 352, 490
ideas, sharing 466–7
identifiers 360
identity 288, 289, 311–12
    checks 423–5
    theft 210
illness 154, 163, 165
    see also disease
immune system 355, 356, 391, 392
Improving Access to Psychological Therapy (IAPT) 483
incidents 129–31
inclusion 109, 316–53
inclusive practice 82–3, 332–3, 350–1
incontinence products 293
independence 70, 99, 241, 244, 272–86, 313
Independent Mental Capacity Advocates (IMCAs) 158, 184, 186–7
Independent Mental Health Advocates (IMHAs) 184
individuality 70, 241, 244
induction 110
infection 27–8, 389–406
    chain of 391, 401–2
information 194–232
    access requests 424–5
    analysis 459
    back-ups 209
    gathering 459
    general 197, 198
    personal 4, 5, 6, 16, 195–7, 199–211, 213, 215, 217–25, 229–30, 232, 317–18, 424–5
    presentation 459
    provision 279, 334, 395
    sharing 5, 6, 16, 45–6, 61, 64–5, 134, 191, 222–3, 231, 454
    sources 252, 291, 300, 385–6
Information Commissioner's Office (ICO) 46, 202, 217, 218
Information Governance Alliance 198
injuries 358, 362–4, 367–74, 383–4
Innovate UK… 320
intellectual health 257, 290
intellectual wellbeing 297, 470, 475–6
internet 80–1, 83, 198, 203
interpreters 157
job descriptions 18–20, 76
job roles 130, 258–9, 456–8

Index

and accountability 458–9
agreed scope 18–21
and audit processes 229–32
clarity regarding 29
and communication skills 133
competence in 429–41
and continuous development 429–43
and duty of care 108–10
and equality issues 334–7
expectations of 432–6
and infection control 393–6
information handling 195
limits 458–9
and mental capacity 94–6, 100
and performance evaluations 441–3
and person-centred care 247–50, 258–9
personal assistants 189
and promoting choice 274–5, 279
and respect 279
and risk assessments 274–5
and safeguarding 43–5, 47–8, 52
job satisfaction 4
journalling 480
judgements 347, 459
kindness 478
knowledge 79, 365, 370, 437, 445–6
lack of 154, 165, 340
self-knowledge 450–1, 452
up-to-date 251, 336–7, 365, 370, 436, 443
kosher 348, 349
labelling others 328, 340
language 150–1, 154–7, 164–5
Lasting Power of Attorney (LPA) 119
leadership behaviours 462–8
Leadership Qualities Framework 462–3
leading by example 335
learning 79, 112–13, 130, 443–4
learning activities 454–6
learning disabilities 40–2, 41, 58, 90, 97, 137, 150–1, 153–4, 163, 168, 178, 381
legislation 286, 433–4, 490
and active participation 271
and agreed ways of working 24, 25
changes to 25
and communication 193
and complaints 126–7
and confidentiality 222
and consent 266–7
and continuous development 468
and duty of care 130
and equality issues 317–19, 352–3
and health and safety 355–60, 387–8, 408–10, 427, 433
and health and wellbeing 315
and infection control 406
and information handling 45, 196–7, 199–202, 205, 222, 225, 232
and mental capacity 86–91, 94–6
and safeguarding 33–8, 45, 84
LGBTQ+ people 325
Liberty Protection Safeguards 2019 86, 106
life events 456
life-saving treatments 103

lifestyle 50–1, 266–8, 345–9, 470, 477, 482
Lifting Operations and Lifting Equipment Regulations (LOLER) 1998 358, 387, 409, 427
lighting 155, 166
limits 22, 458–9
listening skills 124, 136, 139, 160–1, 180–1, 447
living arrangements 240
local authorities 43–4, 350–1
local systems 33–8
lone working 422–3, 426
macular degeneration 167
Makaton 136, 150, 163, 178
Management of Health and Safety at Work Regulations (MHSWR) 1999 271, 286, 356–7, 387, 406, 433, 468
managers 8, 43, 45, 60, 363–4, 385, 439, 479
Manual Handling Operations Regulations 1992 (as amended 2002) 357, 387, 408, 427
Maslow, Abraham 2
media, the 324, 456
medication 366
meditation 478, 481
mental capacity 34–5, 64, 85–106, 118–19
assessment 100
factors influencing 91–3
lack of 34, 35, 90, 91, 98, 267, 278
and legislation 86–91, 94–6
and safeguarding 42, 93–4
Mental Capacity Acts 34, 84, 87, 89, 95–7, 100, 103, 106, 118–19, 131, 193, 266, 271, 286, 315, 318–19, 353, 490
Mental Capacity Code of Practice 2005 322, 353
mental health 56, 97, 149, 257, 289, 291, 300–1, 471, 482
Mental Health Act 1983 34, 87, 89, 106, 193
Mental Health UK 481
mental wellbeing 297, 475, 476, 479, 482
mentoring 439, 441, 454, 480
methicillin-resistant Staphylococcus aureus (MRSA) 390
Mind 292, 481, 489
Mindful Employer Initiative 2004 321
mistakes 111–13, 129–31, 229
mobile phones 80, 151, 198, 203, 308, 480–1
modelling 350–1, 464–7
Modern Slavery Act 2015 33, 84
monitoring 11–12, 298–302, 303–8, 334
motivational interviewing 246–7
motor neurone disease 168–9
moving and handling 75, 357, 365, 367, 374–5, 408–13
muscular dystrophy 464
musculoskeletal disorders 355, 356, 368, 411
nanotechnology 414
National Dignity Council 322, 323
National Health Service (NHS) 218, 291, 402–3, 480, 481, 484
Health Check 299

National Institute of Health and Care Excellence (NICE) 321
National Occupational Standards (NOS) 435–6
near misses 110, 129–31
'need to know' 188
needs 25
changing 25, 263–6
health and wellbeing 313
holistic 250–3
learning 443–4
Maslow's hierarchy of 2
and person-centred practice 250–3, 259–66
neglect 33, 35, 48, 50–1, 54, 69–74, 190
negotiation 15, 16, 31
NEWS2 302, 306
'no', learning to say 488
noise levels 92, 155, 166
norovirus 390, 395
objectivity 347
objects of reference 143–5, 171–2
observations 301–2, 309–11, 431
occupational therapists 482
Office of the Public Guardian (OCG) 39
ombudsman 126
one-page profiles 240, 241, 242
online forums 441
online safety 78–84
open posture 136, 138, 160, 169, 175
openness 111–13, 127, 129, 142–3, 234, 322
operational difficulties 75
opinions 227
oppression 328
oral care 405
organisational skills 431
osteopaths 482
paper waste 28
paraphrasing 160, 161
parasites 390
partners 255, 381
partnership working 1, 3, 13–18, 29–31, 36, 70, 72, 243, 245, 313, 322, 467–8
passwords 208, 382
pathogens 390, 391
pay 19
peer support 291
percutaneous endoscopic gastronomy (PEG) 22
performance 459–60
person-centred practice 14, 19, 96, 233–71, 273–6, 283, 312–14
person-centred values 69, 70, 71, 78, 236–45, 250–3, 258, 283, 331
personal assistants 59, 60, 189, 191–2, 216–17, 401
personal budgets 351
personal care 238
personal experience 154, 163, 324, 456–8
personal histories 258, 260, 262–3
personal hygiene 405–6
personal and professional development plans (PPDs) 445–9

Index

personal protective equipment (PPE) 358, 361, 363, 392, 395, 397–401
Personal Protective Equipment at Work Regulations (PPE) 1992 358, 387, 406, 427
personal relationships 1, 2–7, 475–6
personal strengths 239, 242, 246, 260, 262, 283
personal values 97–8, 456–8
personal wellbeing 469–90
personalisation approach 350
physical assault 367
physical exercise 477, 488
physical resilience 471
physical wellbeing 297, 473, 475, 476, 482
physiological measurements 308
physiotherapists 16, 23, 482
Picture Communication System (PCS) 178
Picture Exchange Communication System (PECS) 22, 144–5
pictures 143, 179, 385
planning 5, 29, 259
poisoning 372
police 39, 43, 120
policies 4
    and agreed ways of working 24, 25
    and complaints 125–8
    and equality issues 317, 320–1
    and health and safety 360–1, 365, 374–5, 408
    and information handling 45, 197–9, 203, 205
    and personal protective equipment 400
    and restrictive practice 105–6
    and safeguarding 36–8, 43, 45, 65–6
    and working relationships 5
positive approaches 10–13, 15, 31, 488
posture
    and moving and handling 411, 412
    open 136, 138, 160, 169, 175
power, balance of 6
preferences 11–12, 113, 243, 260, 262–6, 345–9
prejudice 97–8, 258, 328–9, 334–5, 339, 345
prints 67
privacy 70, 155, 159, 166, 206–7, 244, 258, 313, 317
private sector 21, 59–60, 291, 483
procedures 4
    and agreed ways of working 24, 25
    and complaints 125–8
    and health care 366
    and health and safety 360–1, 364–5, 367–75, 408, 412, 419–20
    and identity checking 423–5
    and information sharing 45
    and moving and handling 412
    and restrictive practice 105–6
    and safeguarding 43, 45, 65–6, 76
    and working relationships 5
Professional Councils 101
professional interests 444
Professional Registration and Standards 37
professional/professionalism 4, 6, 145, 173, 182
proportionality 36
protected characteristics 330–1
Provision and Use of Work Equipment Regulations (PUWER) 1998 357, 387, 409, 427
proximity 143, 176
psychiatrists 481–2
psychological barriers 295
psychological wellbeing 473–4
psychotherapists 482
Public Interest and Disclosure Act 1998 34, 84
qualitative approaches 460
quality assurance 10–13
quality of care 4, 10, 130, 234, 243, 332, 365, 429, 437–8, 451–4
quantitative approaches 460
questions, open/closed 161, 177
race 50
racism, institutional 329
radio frequency identification 285
reablement practice 381–2
reassurance 68, 175, 369
record keeping 195, 197, 203, 206, 213–15, 223, 225–9
    access 197, 203, 220, 222
    and continuous development 448–9, 464
    and discriminatory practice 343–5
    and health and safety 358, 362, 363, 364, 373–4, 383–4, 410
    and health and wellbeing 301–2, 309–10
    and infection control 394–5
    up-to-date 225–6
Records Management Code of Practice for Health and Social Care 2016 198, 204
recovery model 246, 247
recreational drug use 150
recycling 27, 28–9
Reduce 27–9
referrals 300, 482
reflective practice 17–18, 79, 121–2, 160, 191–2, 216–17, 281, 348–9, 401, 436, 438, 442, 449–61, 461
reframing 160
regulations 433–4
regulators 39, 77, 356, 433
Regulatory Reform Order (Fire Safety) 2005 359, 387, 427
rehabilitation workers 134
relationships 135–9, 162, 190–1, 234–6, 240, 251–9, 266–8, 282, 295–8, 333
    family 2–3
    individual's 253, 254–9
    personal 1, 2–7, 475–6
    romantic 255, 381
    working 1, 2–18, 135, 188, 269–70, 385, 462
religion 456
Reporting of Injuries, Diseases and Dangerous Occurrences Regulations (RIDDOR) 2013 358, 373–4, 383–4, 387, 406
reporting procedures 19
residential care homes 134
resilience 471–2, 480, 487–8
resources 27–9, 57, 75
respect 4, 70, 128, 136, 235, 244–5, 266–8, 277, 279–81, 313, 332, 335–6, 340, 346–7, 349, 458, 464
responsibilities 1–31, 429–30, 458–9
    and audit processes 229–32
    clarity regarding 29
    and delegated healthcare tasks 22
    and health and safety 355–66, 374–86, 419
    and infection control 393–7
    and information handling 225
    and mental capacity 94–6
    and person-centred care 247–50
    and safeguarding 43–5, 47–8, 52, 68
responsible clinicians 186
rest 477
RESTORE2 302, 307
restraint 40, 102–3
restrictive practices 85, 102–106
Reuse 27–9
rights 11–12, 34, 38–43, 70–1, 79–80, 90, 94–6, 102, 113–23, 195, 199, 215, 241, 243–4, 250, 313, 316–53, 362, 380–1
    conflicts regarding 115–23
ringworm 390
risk assessments 10, 116, 273–6, 280, 356, 359, 362–3, 374–5, 377–83, 394, 397–8, 418
risk enablement 73–4
risk management 73–4, 280–2
risk-taking, managed 74, 79–80, 116, 273–6, 280–1, 381
risks 56–8, 71–2, 114, 190
    health and safety 355, 363, 376–85, 418
    of infection 391
    minimisation 376–8
    monitoring potential 383–5
    online 79–82
    reporting/recording 384–5
role modelling 29, 96, 99, 279, 376, 438
    see also modelling
room temperature 155, 166, 312
safe practice 71–2, 93–4, 108–15
Safeguarding Adult Boards (SABs) 33, 35, 38, 39, 43
Safeguarding Adult Reviews 40–2, 44
Safeguarding Adults: A National Framework… 2011 37
Safeguarding Strategy 2019 - 2025… 37
Safeguarding Vulnerable Groups Act 2006 34, 84
safeguarding/protection 32–84, 319
    agencies 38–40
    and complaints procedures 128
    and duty of care 107, 108, 113–15
    failure 40–3
    national and local context 33–46
    online 78–84
SBARD 302, 306–7, 309–10

Index

schizophrenia 88, 90
SCIE 45, 46
seclusion 40, 102
second opinions 254
sectioning 87, 89
Sector Skills Councils 386
security measures 422–7
segregation 103
self-advocacy 184, 186
self-care 54–5, 283–4, 470–1, 471–2
self-development 450
self-directed support 350
self-esteem 153, 163, 288–9, 311–12
self-fulfilling prophecy 338, 339
self-harm 47, 238
self-help 299–300, 480
self-image 288, 289, 311–12
self-kindness 478
self-knowledge/awareness 450–1, 452–3
self-neglect 51, 54
self-referrals 293, 482, 483
sensitive situations/behaviours 140–3, 236–9
sensory loss 148, 150
   see also hearing impairment; visual impairment
'shadowing' 442
Shared Lives carers 265
shock 373
sign language 146, 163, 170, 178
signs 361–3, 421–2
silence 178
skills 430–2, 437, 441–3, 445–6
Skills for Care 37, 38, 108–9, 122, 321, 433, 435, 462
Skills for Health 108–9, 321, 433, 435
skin care 405
slavery, modern 50, 53
sleep 477
sleeping tablets 382
smoke detectors 418
smoke free areas 420
social environment 311, 312
social health 257, 290, 337–8
social interaction 135, 258, 345–8, 488
social isolation 338
social media 324
social movements 322, 323
social networking sites 80–1, 83
social resilience 471
social services 291
social stories 285
social wellbeing 296, 474, 476
social workers 4
society 338–9
'soft signs' 300, 301, 302, 307
SOLER theory 160, 169
Special Educational Needs and Disability (SEND) Act 2001 318, 352
Special Educational Needs and Disability (SEND) Code of Practice 2014 318, 352
specialist organisations 122, 157
speech impairments 153

speech and language therapists 23, 157, 171
spiritual health 257, 290
spiritual wellbeing 296–7, 475, 476
staff shortages 75
standards 37–8, 243, 322, 432–6, 440–3, 464–6
statutory sector services 291
stereotypes 327, 329, 339–40
sterilisation 396–7
Stop and Watch approach 305
strength-based approaches 239–43, 246–7, 250–3, 283
stress 56, 154, 164–5, 368, 469, 483–90
stroke 56, 93, 149, 168, 171, 368, 372
summarising 160
supervision 435, 439, 479, 489
supervisors 19
support 41–2, 56, 67–8, 111, 120–3, 252, 318, 385–6, 438–41, 478–83, 488–90
   professional 481–3, 488–9
support groups 299–300, 481
support networks 239, 242, 246, 253, 290–1
support plans 171, 279
supporting others 9, 68, 111, 124, 254
   and advocacy access 185–7
   and conflict management 16–17
   and decision-making 98–100, 259, 279–80
   and health and safety 376–7
   and health and wellbeing 311–12, 314
   and infection control 395
   and information handling 211–17
   as leadership skill 466
   and partnership working 16–17, 29
   and person-centred practice 234
   and relationships 258–9
   and self-care 283–4
   skills/qualities for 216
SupportLine 489
symbols 143, 178
taking action 11, 41–2, 58–64, 76–8, 114, 328–9, 376, 383, 458–9
Talking Mats 144
tasks 18, 108
team working 8, 29–30, 333, 467
technology 280, 284–6, 307, 307–8
telehealth equipment 285
Think Personal: Act Local 37
third sector services 292
thrush 390
TILE(O) acronym 408–9
time issues 154, 165, 235, 478, 488
tiredness 154, 165
tolerance 346
touch 143, 147, 175
trade unions 122, 386, 489
trainers 441
training 43, 45, 75, 154, 165, 324, 336, 356–9, 362–3, 365–6, 370, 394, 412, 422–3, 426, 436, 440, 442–4, 454
transitions 41
translators 156–7
trauma 237

treaties 322, 323
treatment refusal 93–4
tribunals 344
trips 367
trust 4, 128, 136, 206–7, 464
UK Health Security Agency (UKHSA) 393–4
unconsciousness 93, 371, 373
uniforms 405
unsafe practice 74–8
untidiness 155–6, 166
values 11–13, 345–9, 441–3
   person-centred 69–71, 78, 236–45, 250–3, 258, 283, 331
   personal 97–8, 456–8
   shared 262
valuing others 314
Vetting and Barring Scheme 34, 35
victimisation 328
violent situations 49, 103
viruses 390
Vision for Adult Social Care… 2010 37
visitors 256
visits 454–5
visual impairment 143, 148, 163, 167–8, 175, 355
visualisation 478
vocabulary 177
voice 143, 145–6, 177, 464
Voice Output Communication Aids (VOCA) 151–2
voluntary services 8, 39, 483
waste 27–9, 392, 416–17, 420
water conservation 28
ways of working 1–31
wearable technology 307
wellbeing 240, 254–6, 257–8, 287–315, 319, 433
   care-worker 469–90
   changes in 302–11, 473–4
   and discrimination 337
   engaging individuals with 299–300, 303
   maintenance/improvement 310–11, 477–83
   monitoring 299–300, 303–8
   promotion 113, 311–15
   services/resources for 290–5, 293, 299
   types of 296–7
   and unsafe practice 75–6
whereabouts 422–3
whistleblowing 34, 35, 44, 62, 121
whole person approach 252
wishes, individual's 113, 260, 262–3
witness testimonies 66
words 143, 147, 177
work activities 18–19
working in partnership *see* partnership working
working relationships 1, 2–18, 135, 188, 269–70, 385, 462
Workplace (Health, Safety and Welfare) Regulations 1992 357, 387, 427